ICD-10 ESSENTIALS

2019

Operation PCS

Complete guide to ICD-10-PCS
coding conventions and guidelines

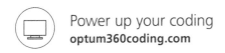

Power up your coding
optum360coding.com

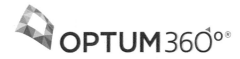

OPTUM360°®

Notice

Our Commitment to Accuracy

Copyright

Acknowledgments

Marianne Randall, CPC, *Product Manager*
Karen Schmidt, BSN, *Technical Director*
Anne Kenney, BA, MBA, CCA, CCS, *Clinical Technical Editor*
Anita Schmidt, BS, RHIT, CCS, AHIMA-approved ICD-10-CM/PCS Trainer, *Clinical Technical Editor*
Mary Walter, RHIT, CCS, *Clinical Technical Editor*
Peggy Willard, CCS, AHIMA-approved ICD-10-CM/PCS Trainer, *Clinical Technical Editor*
Stacy Perry, *Manager, Desktop Publishing*
Tracy Betzler, *Senior Desktop Publishing Specialist*
Hope M. Dunn, *Senior Desktop Publishing Specialist*
Katie Russell, *Desktop Publishing Specialist*
Kimberli Turner, *Editor*

Peggy Willard, CCS, AHIMA-approved ICD-10-CM/PCS Trainer

Ms. Willard's expertise is ICD-10-CM and PCS including in-depth analysis of medical record documentation, ICD-10-CM/PCS code and DRG assignment. In recent years she has been responsible for the creation and development of several print products and e-books designed to assist with appropriate application of ICD-10-CM and PCS coding system. Ms. Willard has several years of prior experience in Level I Adult and Pediatric Trauma hospital coding, specializing in ICD-9-CM, DRG, and CPT coding with emphasis in conducting coding audits, and conducting coding training for coding staff and clinical documentation specialists. Ms. Willard is an active member of the American Health Information Management Association (AHIMA) and the Minnesota Health Information Management Association (MHIMA).

Anita Schmidt, BS, RHIT, AHIMA-approved ICD-10-CM/PCS Trainer

Ms. Schmidt has expertise in Level I Adult and Pediatric Trauma hospital coding, specializing in ICD-9-CM, ICD-10-CM/PCS, DRG, and CPT coding. Her experience includes analysis of medical record documentation, assignment of ICD-10-CM and PCS codes, DRG validation, as well as CPT code assignments for same-day surgery cases. She has conducted coding training and auditing, including DRG validation, conducted electronic health record training, and worked with clinical documentation specialists to identify documentation needs and potential areas for physician education. Most recently she has been developing content for resource and educational products related to ICD-10-CM and ICD-10-PCS. Ms. Schmidt is an AHIMA-approved ICD-10-CM/PCS trainer, and is an active member of the American Health Information Management Association (AHIMA) and the Minnesota Health Information Management Association (MHIMA).

Contents

Case Studies

Case Studies (Alphabetical Listing)

Figures

Tables

Introduction

ICD-10 Essentials: Operation PCS is a coding reference for ICD-10-PCS focusing on application of the coding guidelines. This book provides a comprehensive look at each ICD-10-PCS guideline along with supporting examples, case studies, and in-depth coding rationale designed to ensure accurate application of the guideline in real-life coding situations. New and veteran coding professionals will find this book to be a valuable resource that explains and clarifies key coding concepts related to ICD-10-PCS.

The coding guidance found in *ICD-10 Essentials: Operation PCS* is based on the official version of the ICD-10 Procedure Coding System (ICD-10-PCS), effective October 1, 2018.

Changes reflecting the dynamic world of coding are ongoing, and Optum encourages input for inclusion in future editions of the book.

How to Use *ICD-10 Essentials: Operation PCS*

The organization of *ICD-10 Essentials: Operation PCS* follows the format of *ICD-10-PCS Official Guidelines for Coding and Reporting*. There is a chapter devoted to each of the topics covered in the guidelines as follows:

- PCS Conventions
- Medical and Surgical Body System Guidelines
- Medical and Surgical Root Operation Guidelines
- Medical and Surgical Body Part Guidelines
- Medical and Surgical Approach Guidelines
- Medical and Surgical Device Guidelines
- Obstetrics Section Guidelines
- New Technology Section Guidelines

Shaded boxes in different colors allow the user to quickly differentiate the various components of each chapter. Blue boxes enclose the focus guideline in each section. Supporting guidelines included to assist in explaining case studies are shown in orange boxes. Spotlights in yellow boxes alert the user to key facts, important information, and coding advice, while pink boxes highlight definitions.

Valuable information has been provided in case studies, tables, and figures that include illustrations and decision trees, all of which are listed in the front of the book and are easily searchable. Located in the back of the book are appendixes to supplement the material contained in the chapters, as well as an alphabetical index to search pertinent information.

PCS Guideline

As each ICD-10-PCS guideline is examined, the full, official text is presented in a blue box followed by an overview of the guideline, helpful illustrations, as well as practical applications of the guideline.

Example:

> **B2.1b** **Where the general body part values "upper" and "lower" are provided as an option in the Upper Arteries, Lower Arteries, Upper Veins, Lower Veins, Muscles and Tendons body systems, "upper" or "lower "specifies body parts located above or below the diaphragm respectively.**
>
> *Example:* **Vein body parts above the diaphragm are found in the Upper Veins body system; vein body parts below the diaphragm are found in the Lower Veins body system.**

Illustrations

Illustrations are included to provide visual support to text.

Example:

The diaphragm is a sheet of fiber and muscle that rises and falls as we breathe. It neatly bisects the human body into upper and lower halves. PCS definitions indicate that body parts above the diaphragm are to be classified as "upper" and those below it are classified as "lower."

Figure 3.7. Diaphragm

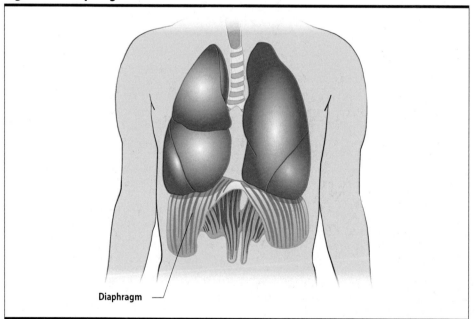

Diaphragm

AHA Coding Clinic

Official citations from AHA's *Coding Clinic* for ICD-10-PCS have been provided for conventions and guidelines, as applicable. The citations appear in red type with the year, quarter, and page of the reference, as well as the title of the question as it appears in that *AHA Coding Clinic* table of contents. *AHA Coding Clinic* citations included in this edition have been updated through second quarter 2018.

Example:

AHA Coding Clinic

2014, 3Q, 25   Revision of Transjugular Intrahepatic Portosystemic Shunt (TIPS)

Practical Application for Guidelines

Case studies in purple boxes are supplied along with full code assignment and rationale for each code with attribution of official sources used such as guidelines, official definitions, and *AHA Coding Clinic*.

Example:

Case Study 4.21. Endometrial Biopsy
The patient experienced postmenopausal uterine bleeding. A diagnostic D&C was performed through a hysteroscope to determine the cause of bleeding.

Code(s):

ØUDB8ZX   **Extraction of Endometrium, Via Natural or Artificial Opening Endoscopic, Diagnostic**

Rationale:

A dilation and curettage (D&C) is considered an extraction since the lining of the endometrium is stripped away by force. Although the initial response may be to code this biopsy using the root operation Excision, there is no body part endometrium listed in Table ØUB. Root operation Extraction (D) is the appropriate assignment.

Consulting the ICD-10-PCS index for Extraction, the entry for Endometrium lists table ØUDB. This table is found in the body system Female Reproductive System (U) with Endometrium (B) as the body part value. Endometrial biopsies are done by passing the instruments through the cervix into the uterine cavity. The hysteroscope provides the endoscopic approach Via Natural or Artificial Opening (8).

The qualifier Diagnostic (X) is used since the sample was taken to diagnose the cause of bleeding.

Root Operation Tables

To provide quick access to the root operation definitions, case studies include root operation tables that apply to the particular example.

Example:

Root Operation		
Extraction (D)	Definition:	Pulling or stripping out or off all or a portion of a body part by the use of force
	Explanation:	The qualifier DIAGNOSTIC is used to identify extraction procedures that are biopsies

PCS Guideline

Often more than one guideline must be applied in order to accurately code the entire procedure. When an additional guideline is referenced in a case study, the additional guideline may be listed in its entirety in an orange box.

Example:

PCS Guideline	
B6.1b	Materials such as sutures, ligatures, radiological markers, and temporary post-operative wound drains are considered integral to the performance of a procedure and are not coded as devices.

Spotlights

Important points are highlighted throughout the book using a yellow Spotlight box.

Example:

Spotlight
Because some surgical procedures can be performed for medical or cosmetic purposes, coding for Alteration (Ø) requires diagnostic confirmation that the surgery was in fact performed to improve appearance.

Definitions

Pink Definition boxes contain bolded terms with a definition appropriate to coding and reimbursement or coding instructions.

Example:

Definitions
allogeneic. Taken from different individuals of the same species.
syngeneic. Having to do with individuals or tissues that have identical genes, such as identical twins.
zooplastic. Tissue obtained from an animal.

Appendixes

The resources described below have been included as appendixes for *ICD-10 Essentials: Operation PCS*. These resources have been referenced throughout the text of this book and provide additional assistance to the user. Appendixes C-H are compiled from official CMS sources and updated annually.

Appendix A. ICD-10-PCS Official Guidelines for Coding and Reporting 2019

This resource lists the official conventions and guidelines in their entirety as distributed by the Centers for Medicare and Medicaid Services (CMS).

Appendix B. Components of the Medical and Surgical Approach Definitions

This resource further defines the approach characters used in the Medical and Surgical (Ø) section. Complementing the detailed definition of the approach, additional information includes whether or not instrumentation is a part of the approach, the typical access location, the method used to initiate the approach, and related procedural examples, all of which help the user determine the appropriate approach value.

Appendix C. Root Operation Definitions

This resource is a compilation of all root operations found in the Medical and Surgical-related sections (Ø-9) of the ICD-10-PCS manual. It provides a definition and in some cases a more detailed explanation of the root operation, to better reflect the purpose or objective. Examples of related procedures may also be provided.

Appendix D. Body Part Key

When an anatomical term or description is provided in the documentation but does not have a specific body part character within a table, the user can reference this resource to search for the anatomical description or site noted in the documentation to determine if there is a specific PCS body part character (character 4) to which the anatomical description or site could be coded.

Appendix E. Body Part Definitions

This resource is the reverse look-up of the Body Part Key. Each table in the Medical and Surgical section (Ø) of the ICD-10-PCS manual contains anatomical terms linked to a body part character or value. For example, in Table ØBB, Body Part (character 4) number 1 is Trachea. The body part Trachea may have anatomical structures or descriptions that may be used in procedure documentation instead of the term trachea. The Body Part Definitions list other anatomical structures or synonyms that are included in specific ICD-10-PCS body part values. According to the Body Part Definitions, in the example above, cricoid cartilage is included in the Trachea (1) body part.

Appendix F. Device Key and Aggregation Table

The Device Key relates specific devices used in the medical profession, such as stents or bovine pericardial valves, with the appropriate device character (character 6).

The Aggregation Table crosswalks specific device character value definitions for specific root operations in a specific body system to the more general device character value to be used when the root operation covers a wide range of body parts and the device character represents an entire family of devices.

Appendix G. Device Definitions

This resource is a reverse look-up to the Device Key. The user may reference this resource to see all of the specific devices that may be grouped to a particular device character (character 6).

Appendix H. Substance Key/Substance Definitions

The Substance Key lists substances by trade name or synonym and relates them to a PCS character in the Administration (3) or New Technology (X) section in the sixth-character Substance or seventh-character Qualifier column.

The Substance Definitions Table is the reverse look-up of the Substance Key, relating all substance categories, the sixth- or seventh-character values, to all trade names or synonyms that may be classified to that particular character.

Appendix I. Character Meaning Tables

This resource provides each of the character meaning tables for the Medical and Surgical related sections (Ø-9). There is a character meaning table for each body system to help identify the character members available within that section.

Index

An alphabetical index, based on key words and phrases, is supplied at the back of the book to assist users in quickly locating information specific to certain guidelines or procedures.

Example:

fractional flow reserve (FFR) **256, 257**

In this example, information regarding the fractional flow reserve procedure is found on pages 256 and 257.

Chapter 1. ICD-10-PCS Overview

History of ICD-10-PCS

The World Health Organization (WHO) has maintained the International Classification of Diseases (ICD) for recording cause of death since 1893. It has updated the ICD periodically to reflect new discoveries in epidemiology and changes in medical understanding of disease.

The International Classification of Diseases, Tenth Revision (ICD-10), published in 1992, is the latest revision of the ICD. The WHO authorized the National Center for Health Statistics (NCHS) to develop a clinical modification of ICD-10 for use in the United States. This version, called ICD-10-CM, replaced the previous U.S. clinical modification, ICD-9-CM, which had been in use since 1979. ICD-9-CM contained a procedure classification; ICD-10-CM does not.

In order to provide a procedural classification system to accompany the ICD-10-CM code set, the Centers for Medicare and Medicaid Services (CMS), the agency responsible for maintaining the inpatient procedure code set in the United States, funded a project with 3M in 1993 to develop a design for a replacement of the limited four-digit ICD-9 procedural classification. After several trials, it was determined that an entirely new system was needed and the alphanumeric, seven-digit system was developed. After requesting bids for the project, CMS contracted with 3M Health Information Systems in 1995 to design and develop the procedure classification system to replace volume 3 of ICD-9-CM. The result, ICD-10-PCS, was initially completed in 1998. The code set has been updated annually since that time. ICD-10-PCS has unique, precise codes to differentiate body parts, surgical approaches, and devices used. It can be used to identify resource consumption differences and outcomes for different procedures, and describes precisely what was done to the patient.

After legislative delays in 2013 and 2014, implementation of ICD-10-CM and ICD-10-PCS went into effect on October 1, 2015.

The development of ICD-10-PCS had as its goal the incorporation of the following major attributes:

- **Completeness:** A unique code should be available for all significantly different procedures.

- **Unique definitions:** Because ICD-10-PCS codes are constructed of individual values rather than lists of fixed codes and text descriptions, the unique, stable definition of a code in the system is retained. New values may be added to the system to represent a specific new approach, device, or qualifier, but whole codes by design cannot be given new meanings and reused.

- **Expandability:** As new procedures are developed, the structure of ICD-10-PCS should allow them to be easily incorporated as unique codes.

- **Multiaxial:** ICD-10-PCS codes should consist of independent characters, with each individual axis retaining its meaning across broad ranges of codes to the extent possible.

- **Standardized terminology:** ICD-10-PCS should include definitions of the terminology used. While the meaning of specific words varies in common usage, ICD-10-PCS should not include multiple meanings for the same term, and each term must be assigned a specific meaning.

- **Structural integrity:** ICD-10-PCS can be easily expanded without disrupting the structure of the system. ICD-10-PCS allows unique new codes to be added to the system because values for the seven characters that make up a code can be combined as needed. The system can evolve as medical technology and clinical practice evolve, without disrupting the ICD-10-PCS structure.

Several additional general characteristics were added during the development of ICD-10-PCS:

- **Diagnostic information is not included in the procedure description:** When procedures are performed for specific diseases or disorders, the disease or disorder is not contained in the procedure code. The diagnosis codes, not the procedure codes, specify the disease or disorder.

- **Explicit not otherwise specified (NOS) options are restricted:** Explicit "not otherwise specified" (NOS) options are restricted in ICD-10-PCS. A minimal level of specificity is required for each component of the procedure.

- **Limited use of not elsewhere classified (NEC) option:** There is generally no need for a "not elsewhere classified" (NEC) code option in ICD-10-PCS because all significant components of a procedure are specified. However, limited NEC options are incorporated into ICD-10-PCS where necessary. For example new devices are frequently developed, and therefore an "other device" option is necessary for use until the new device can be specifically added to the coding system.

- **Level of specificity:** All procedures currently performed can be specified in ICD-10-PCS. In the development of the system, the frequency with which a procedure is performed was not a consideration. Instead, a unique code is available for any variations of a procedure that can be performed.

Documentation Needs

Because each character in an ICD-10-PCS code represents a different detailed aspect of the procedure itself, it is necessary to have detailed clinical information about the procedure when coding.

For example, when coding the following procedure,

Laparoscopic total hysterectomy

The alphabetic index for "hysterectomy" provides the following:

Hysterectomy
Supracervical *see* Resection, Uterus ØUT9
Total *see* Resection, Uterus ØUT9

The subentries below the main term "Hysterectomy" inform the user that the most appropriate PCS table is found in the Medical and Surgical (0) section and Female Reproductive System (U) body system. Based on *AHA Coding Clinic, 2017, 4Q, 68,* the term "total" when used in relation to hysterectomy is defined as the complete removal of the uterus and the cervix; complete removal of the uterus only is considered a "supracervical" hysterectomy. Complete removal of a body part is appropriately coded with the root operation Resection rather than Excision, which implies only partial removal of a body part. If the documentation within the operative report supports the complete removal of one or both of these organs, the appropriate root operation is Resection (T).

As a "total" hysterectomy and a "supracervical" hysterectomy involve the complete removal of the uterus, the body part character provided for both index entries is Uterus (9). It is the seventh character that provides the detail as to whether a "total" or "supracervical" hysterectomy was performed. The documentation in the body of the operative report must support the complete removal of both organs regardless of whether or not the title of the operation is "total" hysterectomy. When the uterus and the cervix are completely removed, the applicable seventh character is No Qualifier (Z). If ONLY the uterus is removed, that information is communicated with seventh character Supracervical (L).

A laparoscopic approach is considered Percutaneous Endoscopic (4) in the PCS definitions. The sixth character has no specific value associated, but every PCS code must contain seven characters, so the character value of Z must be assigned. The final ICD-10-PCS code for a laparoscopic total hysterectomy is shown in the following table.

Section	Body System	Root Operation	Body Part	Approach	Device	Qualifier
Ø	U	T	9	4	Z	Z
Medical & Surgical	Female Reproductive System	Resection	Uterus	Percutaneous Endoscopic	No Device	No Qualifier

An important note about documentation is that many of the terms used in PCS code construction are well-defined in the PCS documentation and guidelines. It is the user's responsibility to apply those definitions to the physician documentation in the medical record and decide which specific character values should be assigned. This is especially crucial when determining the most appropriate root operation value. If the physician documents "total excision" and the body of the operative report indicates that the entire organ or body part was removed, the user should assign the root operation Resection rather than Excision, based on the PCS definitions. The physician is not required to document using PCS terminology and the user is not required to query a physician and request PCS terminology in the medical record documentation. This instructional information is found in the ICD-10-PCS Official Guideline A11.

PCS Organization

Overview of Structure of ICD-10-PCS

An ICD-10-PCS code is the result of a process rather than a single fixed set of digits or alphabetic characters. The process consists of combining semi-independent values from among a selection of values, according to the rules governing the construction of codes. The result of the process is a seven-character alphanumeric code. The term *procedure* in ICD-10-PCS refers to the complete specification of the seven characters.

Characters

Each character contains up to 34 possible values with each value representing a specific option for the general character definition. The alphabetic characters A–H, J–N, and P–Z, along with numbers Ø–9, are used as character values in any character position. In order to avoid confusion with numbers Ø and 1, the letters I and O are not used. The vast majority of PCS codes follow the format below, with a few exceptions related to slightly different character definitions for some of the ancillary-related types of services.

Character 1	Character 2	Character 3	Character 4	Character 5	Character 6	Character 7
Section	Body System	Root Operation	Body Part	Approach	Device	Qualifier

The second through seventh characters have the same meaning within a section but the meanings may vary between sections. For example, character 4 in the Obstetrics section does not hold the same meaning as character 4 in the Placement section. The third character in all sections captures the general type of procedure performed, while additional information is provided by the other characters.

A code is constructed by choosing a specific value for each of the seven characters. Based on details about the procedure performed, values for each character specifying the section, body system, root operation, body part, approach, device, and qualifier are assigned. Because the definition of each character is also a function of its physical position in the code, the same letter or number placed in a different position in the code has a different meaning. Codes are constructed using tables that are defined by their first three character values

Character 1: Section

Character 1	Character 2	Character 3	Character 4	Character 5	Character 6	Character 7
Section	Body System	Root Operation	Body Part	Approach	Device	Qualifier

Procedures are divided into sections that identify the general type of procedure. There are 17 sections within the PCS code book with the section being specified in the first character of the procedure code.

The sections are outlined as follows:

Medical and Surgical Section

Ø   Medical and Surgical

Medical and Surgical-related Sections

1   Obstetrics

2   Placement

3   Administration

4   Measurement and Monitoring

5   Extracorporeal or Systemic Assistance and Performance

6   Extracorporeal or Systemic Therapies

7   Osteopathic

8   Other Procedures

9   Chiropractic

Ancillary Sections

B   Imaging

C   Nuclear Medicine

D   Radiation Therapy

F   Physical Rehabilitation and Diagnostic Audiology

G   Mental Health

H   Substance Abuse Treatment

New Technology Section

X   New Technology

Section Ø is the Medical and Surgical section where the majority of PCS codes are found; sections 1–9 are designated as the Medical and Surgical-related sections; sections B–H are considered Ancillary sections; and section X is the New Technology section.

Character 2: Body System

Character 1	Character 2	Character 3	Character 4	Character 5	Character 6	Character 7
Section	Body System	Root Operation	Body Part	Approach	Device	Qualifier

The second character, Body System, provides information related to the general physiological system or anatomical region on which the procedure was performed. The categorization of procedures into these broad groupings provides quick information about the type of procedure, and makes the tables easier to navigate. All procedures with the same second character are performed on the same anatomical system or region.

The Medical and Surgical (Ø) section has 31 Body System values (as listed below) that represent a specific anatomical/physiological system such as Upper Bones (P) or a broader anatomical region such as Anatomical Regions, Upper Extremities (X).

Medical and Surgical Section (Ø) Body Systems

Ø   Central Nervous System and Cranial Nerves

1   Peripheral Nervous System

2   Heart and Great Vessels

3   Upper Arteries

4   Lower Arteries

5   Upper Veins

6   Lower Veins

7   Lymphatic and Hemic Systems

8   Eye

9   Ear, Nose, Sinus

B   Respiratory System

C   Mouth and Throat

D   Gastrointestinal System

F   Hepatobiliary System and Pancreas

G   Endocrine System

H   Skin and Breast

J   Subcutaneous Tissue and Fascia

K   Muscles

L   Tendons

M   Bursae and Ligaments

N   Head and Facial Bones

P   Upper Bones

Q   Lower Bones

R   Upper Joints

S   Lower Joints

T   Urinary System

U   Female Reproductive System

V   Male Reproductive System

W   Anatomical Regions, General

X   Anatomical Regions, Upper Extremities

Y   Anatomical Regions, Lower Extremities

Additionally, many of the Medical and Surgical-related sections (1-9) and Ancillary sections (B-H) have second-character values that represent defined PCS body systems and in some cases the second-character values are the same between sections. For example, in both the Medical and Surgical section (Ø) and the Imaging section (B) the body system (character 2) value for Upper Arteries is 3.

Medical and Surgical Section (Ø)	Imaging Section (B)
Ø Central Nervous System and Cranial Nerves	Ø Central Nervous System
1 Peripheral Nervous System	
2 Heart and Great Vessels	2 Heart
3 Upper Arteries	**3 Upper Arteries**
4 Lower Arteries	4 Lower Arteries
5 Upper Veins	5 Veins
6 Lower Veins	
7 Lymphatic and Hemic Systems	7 Lymphatic System
8 Eye	8 Eye
9 Ear, Nose, Sinus	9 Ear, Nose, Mouth and Throat
B Respiratory System	B Respiratory System
C Mouth and Throat	
D Gastrointestinal System	D Gastrointestinal System
F Hepatobiliary System and Pancreas	F Hepatobiliary System and Pancreas
G Endocrine System	G Endocrine System
H Skin and Breast	H Skin, Subcutaneous Tissue and Breast
J Subcutaneous Tissue and Fascia	
K Muscles	
L Tendons	L Connective Tissue
M Bursae and Ligaments	
N Head and Facial Bones	N Skull and Facial Bones
P Upper Bones	P Non-Axial Upper Bones
Q Lower Bones	Q Non-Axial Lower Bones
R Upper Joints	R Axial Skeleton, Except Skull and Facial Bones
S Lower Joints	
T Urinary System	T Urinary System
U Female Reproductive System	U Female Reproductive System
V Male Reproductive System	V Male Reproductive System
W Anatomical Regions, General	W Anatomical Regions
X Anatomical Regions, Upper Extremities	
Y Anatomical Regions, Lower Extremities	Y Fetus and Obstetrical

In other cases, the second-character value is unrelated to a body system and instead has a different definition that is more refined to the section in which it is found. An illustration of this is the second character for the Medical and Surgical (Ø) and Administration (3) sections. The second-character value C in the Medical and Surgical (Ø) section represents the Mouth and Throat, while the second-character value C in the Administration (3) section represents Indwelling Device.

Medical and Surgical Section (Ø)	Administration (3)
C Mouth and Throat	C Indwelling Device

Character 3: Root Operation

Character 1	Character 2	Character 3	Character 4	Character 5	Character 6	Character 7
Section	Body System	Root Operation	Body Part	Approach	Device	Qualifier

The root operation is specified in the third character and is one of the most important characters in the PCS code. The root operation identifies the objective of the procedure and is typically found in the alphabetic index. Its assignment determines which table is used for code completion. In the Medical and Surgical (Ø) section, there are 31 different root operations, each with a precise definition.

- **Alteration (Ø).** Modifying the anatomic structure of a body part without affecting the function of the body part

- **Bypass (1).** Altering the route of passage of the contents of a tubular body part

- **Change (2).** Taking out or off a device from a body part and putting back an identical or similar device in or on the same body part without cutting or puncturing the skin or a mucous membrane

- **Control (3).** Stopping, or attempting to stop, postprocedural or other acute bleeding

- **Creation (4).** Putting in or on biological or synthetic material to form a new body part that to the extent possible replicates the anatomic structure or function of an absent body part

- **Destruction (5).** Physical eradication of all or a portion of a body part by the direct use of energy, force, or a destructive agent

- **Detachment (6).** Cutting off all or a portion of the upper or lower extremities

- **Dilation (7).** Expanding an orifice or the lumen of a tubular body part

- **Division (8).** Cutting into a body part, without draining fluids and/or gases from the body part, in order to separate or transect a body part

- **Drainage (9).** Taking or letting out fluids and/or gases from a body part

- **Excision (B).** Cutting out or off, without replacement, a portion of a body part

- **Extirpation (C).** Taking or cutting out solid matter from a body part

- **Extraction (D).** Pulling or stripping out or off all or a portion of a body part by the use of force

- **Fragmentation (F).** Breaking solid matter in a body part into pieces

- **Fusion (G).** Joining together portions of an articular body part rendering the articular body part immobile

- **Insertion (H).** Putting in a nonbiological appliance that monitors, assists, performs, or prevents a physiological function but does not physically take the place of a body part

- **Inspection (J).** Visually and/or manually exploring a body part

- **Map (K).** Locating the route of passage of electrical impulses and/or locating functional areas in a body part

- **Occlusion (L).** Completely closing an orifice or the lumen of a tubular body part

- **Reattachment (M).** Putting back in or on all or a portion of a separated body part to its normal location or other suitable location

- **Release (N).** Freeing a body part from an abnormal physical constraint by cutting or by the use of force

- **Removal (P).** Taking out or off a device from a body part

- **Repair (Q).** Restoring, to the extent possible, a body part to its normal anatomic structure and function

- **Replacement (R).** Putting in or on biological or synthetic material that physically takes the place and/or function of all or a portion of a body part

- **Reposition (S).** Moving to its normal location, or other suitable location, all or a portion of a body part

- **Resection (T).** Cutting out or off, without replacement, all of a body part

- **Restriction (V).** Partially closing an orifice or the lumen of a tubular body part

- **Revision (W).** Correcting, to the extent possible, a portion of a malfunctioning device or the position of a displaced device

- **Supplement (U).** Putting in or on biological or synthetic material that physically reinforces and/or augments the function of a portion of a body part

- **Transfer (X).** Moving, without taking out, all or a portion of a body part to another location to take over the function of all or a portion of a body part

- **Transplantation (Y).** Putting in or on all or a portion of a living body part taken from another individual or animal to physically take the place and/or function of all or a portion of a similar body part

There is a clear distinction between each of the root operations listed above. The root operation *Repair* in the Medical and Surgical (Ø) section functions as a "not elsewhere classified" option; it is to be used when the procedure performed does not meet the definition of any other root operation.

Appendix C Root Operation Definitions provides additional explanation and examples of the Medical and Surgical root operations.

Character 4: Body Part

Character 1	Character 2	Character 3	Character 4	Character 5	Character 6	Character 7
Section	Body System	Root Operation	Body Part	Approach	Device	Qualifier

The body part value identifies the specific anatomical site on which the procedure was performed. Along with the value for the body system (character 2), the body part value precisely defines the procedure site. The number of body parts in the human anatomy exceeds the available character values; therefore, knowledge of general body part categories is needed. For example, a procedure performed on a sweat gland would, for PCS coding purposes, be coded to body part "Skin." Similarly, a procedure performed on the mastoid process would be coded to body part "Temporal Bone." A thorough understanding of anatomy and physiology is essential for accurate coding in PCS. To assist in locating the most appropriate body part character value, an official Body Part Key is provided that translates specific anatomical locations to the corresponding PCS value that can be found in the tables. Refer to appendix D to review the most recently released Body Part Key. Another resource, located in appendix E and referred to as Body Part Definitions, classifies alphabetically the PCS body part value with its inclusive specific anatomical body parts.

Character 5: Approach

Character 1	Character 2	Character 3	Character 4	Character 5	Character 6	Character 7
Section	Body System	Root Operation	Body Part	Approach	Device	Qualifier

Character 5 indicates the approach, or the method or technique, used to reach the procedure site. In the Medical and Surgical (Ø) section there are seven different approaches:

- **Open (Ø).** Cutting through the skin or mucous membrane and any other body layers necessary to expose the site of the procedure

- **Percutaneous (3).** Entry, by puncture or minor incision, of instrumentation through the skin or mucous membrane and any other body layers necessary to reach the site of the procedure

- **Percutaneous Endoscopic (4).** Entry, by puncture or minor incision, of instrumentation through the skin or mucous membrane and any other body layers necessary to reach and visualize the site of the procedure

- **Via Natural or Artificial Opening (7).** Entry of instrumentation through a natural or artificial external opening to reach the site of the procedure

- **Via Natural or Artificial Opening Endoscopic (8).** Entry of instrumentation through a natural or artificial external opening to reach and visualize the site of the procedure

- **Via Natural or Artificial Opening with Percutaneous Endoscopic Assistance (F).** Entry of instrumentation through a natural or artificial external opening and entry, by puncture or minor incision, of instrumentation through the skin or mucous membrane and any other body layers necessary to aid in the performance of the procedure

- **External (X).** Procedures performed directly on the skin or mucous membrane and procedures performed indirectly by the application of external force through the skin or mucous membrane

The approach value is comprised of the access location, method, and type of instrumentation.

Access location: For procedures performed on an internal body part, the access location specifies the external site through which the procedure site is reached. There are two general types of access locations: skin or mucous membranes and external orifices. Every approach value except external includes one of these two access locations. The skin or mucous membrane can be cut or punctured to reach the procedure site. All open and percutaneous approach values use this access location. The procedure site can also be reached through an external opening. External openings can be natural (e.g., mouth) or artificial (e.g., colostomy stoma).

Method: For procedures performed on an internal body part, the method specifies how the external access location is entered. An open method specifies cutting through the skin or mucous membrane and any other intervening body layers necessary to expose the procedure site. An instrumentation method specifies the entry of instrumentation through the access location to the internal procedure site. Instrumentation can be introduced by puncture or minor incision, or through an external opening. The puncture or minor incision does not constitute an open approach because it does not expose the site of the procedure. An approach can define multiple methods. For example, *Via Natural or Artificial Opening with Percutaneous Endoscopic Assistance* includes the initial entry of instrumentation to reach the procedure site and the placement of additional percutaneous instrumentation into the body part to visualize and assist in the performance of the procedure.

Type of instrumentation: For procedures performed on an internal body part, instrumentation means that specialized equipment is used to perform the procedure. Instrumentation is used in all internal approaches other than the basic open approach. Instrumentation may or may not include the capacity to visualize the procedure site. For example, the instrumentation used to perform a sigmoidoscopy permits the internal site of the procedure to be visualized, while the instrumentation used to perform a needle biopsy of the liver does not.

The term "endoscopic" as used in approach values refers to instrumentation that permits a site to be visualized.

External approach is used for procedures performed directly on the skin or mucous membrane (e.g., skin excision), as well as for those procedures performed indirectly by the application of external force (e.g., closed reduction of fracture).

Coding guidelines, as discussed in this book, help define which approach value is selected when a combination of approaches is utilized.

Appendix B compares the components (access location, method, and type of instrumentation) of each approach along with an example.

Character 6: Device

Character 1	Character 2	Character 3	Character 4	Character 5	Character 6	Character 7
Section	Body System	Root Operation	Body Part	Approach	Device	Qualifier

The device is specified in the sixth character and is assigned when the device remains in the patient's body at the conclusion of the procedure. The four general types of devices, discussed in detail in chapter 7, include:

- Biological or synthetic material that takes the place of all or a portion of a body part (e.g., skin graft, joint prosthesis).

- Biological or synthetic material that assists or prevents a physiological function (e.g., IUD).

- Therapeutic material that is not absorbed by, eliminated by, or incorporated into a body part (e.g., radioactive implant).

- Mechanical or electronic appliances used to assist, monitor, take the place of, or prevent a physiological function (e.g., cardiac pacemaker, orthopedic pin).

Materials that are incidental to a procedure, such as sutures, clips, ligatures, and temporary postoperative wound drains, are not specified in the device character. New technologies often involve a new device, therefore, it is important to check section X New Technology before assigning Other Device (Y) in the sixth-character position. In the absence of a more suitable code in section X, character 6 Other Device (Y) may be assigned until a more specific value is developed and released.

To assist in appropriate Device character value assignment, an official Device Key has been released that provides the specific manufacturer name for each device, along with its corresponding PCS Device character definition. Refer to appendix F to review the most recently released Device Key.

Many root operations have device value options, but there are six root operations whose objectives are to specifically manage a device: Change, Insertion, Removal, Replacement, Revision, and Supplement. The following table includes examples of sections and root operations in which devices are used, along with a device value with its potential procedure:

Table 1.1. Device Distribution Examples in PCS

PCS Section	Root Operation	Device Value Example	Procedure Example
Medical and Surgical	Alteration	Autologous Tissue Substitute	Nasal tip elevation using fat autograft
Medical and Surgical	Bypass	Synthetic Substitute	Femoral-popliteal bypass using synthetic graft
Medical and Surgical	Change	Drainage Device	Foley catheter exchange
Medical and Surgical	Creation	Nonautologous Tissue Substitute	Sex change operation using tissue bank graft material
Medical and Surgical	Dilation	Intraluminal Device	Percutaneous coronary angioplasty using a bare metal stent
Medical and Surgical	Drainage	Drainage Device	Drainage of pleural effusion using chest tube
Medical and Surgical	Fusion	Interbody Fusion Device	Spinal fusion using interbody fusion device such as a metal cage
Medical and Surgical	Insertion	Infusion Device, Pump	Insertion of infusion pump for pain control
Medical and Surgical	Occlusion	Extraluminal Device	Fallopian tube ligation using clips
Medical and Surgical	Removal	Spacer	Removal of joint spacer
Medical and Surgical	Replacement	Autologous Tissue Substitute	Skin graft using patient's own skin
Medical and Surgical	Reposition	Internal Fixation Device	Fracture reduction with plate and screw fixation
Medical and Surgical	Restriction	Extraluminal Device	Laparoscopic gastric banding, adjustable band
Medical and Surgical	Revision	Neurostimulator Lead	Reposition of spinal neurostimulator lead
Medical and Surgical	Supplement	Zooplastic Tissue	Pulmonary artery patch graft using bovine pericardial tissue
Obstetrics	Insertion, Removal	Monitoring Electrode	Insertion or removal of fetal monitoring electrode
Placement	Change	Cast	Forearm cast change
Placement	Compression	Pressure Dressing	Application of pressure dressing to lower leg
Placement	Dressing	Bandage	Application of bandage to chest wall
Placement	Immobilization	Splint	Splint placement to wrist
Placement	Packing	Packing Material	Nasal packing
Placement	Removal	Brace	Removal of back brace
Placement	Traction	Traction Apparatus	Traction of lower leg using traction device

Character 7: Qualifier

Character 1	Character 2	Character 3	Character 4	Character 5	Character 6	Character 7
Section	Body System	Root Operation	Body Part	Approach	Device	Qualifier

The seventh character in a PCS code represents a qualifier, which provides additional information about the procedure. It may indicate the destination of a bypass procedure or very specific information, such as whether a joint replacement device was cemented or uncemented. When the qualifier value is Diagnostic for root operations Drainage, Excision, or Extraction, it indicates that a biopsy procedure was performed. At this time, there are no official guidelines for the qualifier value (character seven) and this publication does not include a specific chapter addressing it, although many aspects of the qualifier values are discussed throughout this book.

Tables

A procedure or seven-character PCS code cannot be derived without the use of the tables. The tables make up the largest section of the PCS system. The structure of a table is always the same: the information related to the first three character values of a section is found at the top of the table. The remainder of the table contains four columns that represent the remaining four character values for valid codes. When constructing codes, the values must be selected across a row. If a character value does not appear on the same row in the table, it may not be combined to form a valid code. For example, review table ØFB below.

Ø	Medical and Surgical
F	**Hepatobiliary System and Pancreas**
B	**Excision** Definition: Cutting out or off, without replacement, a portion of a body part

Body Part Character 4	Approach Character 5	Device Character 6	Qualifier Character 7
Ø Liver 1 Liver, Right Lobe 2 Liver, Left Lobe	Ø Open 3 Percutaneous 4 Percutaneous Endoscopic	Z No Device	X Diagnostic Z No Qualifier
4 Gallbladder G Pancreas	Ø Open 3 Percutaneous 4 Percutaneous Endoscopic 8 Via Natural or Artificial Opening Endoscopic	Z No Device	X Diagnostic Z No Qualifier
5 Hepatic Duct, Right 6 Hepatic Duct, Left 7 Hepatic Duct, Common 8 Cystic Duct 9 Common Bile Duct C Ampulla of Vater D Pancreatic Duct F Pancreatic Duct, Accessory	Ø Open 3 Percutaneous 4 Percutaneous Endoscopic 7 Via Natural or Artificial Opening 8 Via Natural or Artificial Opening Endoscopic	Z No Device	X Diagnostic Z No Qualifier

Note that the first three character values are listed at the top of the table (ØFB), along with the definition of the root operation (Excision). There are three rows in this particular table, but valid codes may only be constructed moving across one row. For example, ØFB04ZX is a valid code from only the first row of this table and represents a laparoscopic excisional liver biopsy.

Section	Body System	Root Operation	Body Part	Approach	Device	Qualifier
Ø	F	B	Ø	4	Z	X
Medical & Surgical	Hepatobiliary System and Pancreas	Excision	Liver	Percutaneous Endoscopic	No Device	Diagnostic

Referring back to table ØFB, code ØFBØ7ZX is not valid because the approach Via Natural or Artificial Opening (7) is not included in the same row with body part Liver (Ø), meaning that it is an invalid combination of values. Typically, it's not anatomically possible to access the liver through a natural or artificial opening in the body. Careful table review is required to ensure that the values selected are all contained within the same row. Additionally, some of the PCS tables are very lengthy; if using an ICD-10-PCS book, rows may span more than one page in the book.

It cannot be emphasized enough that valid codes can only be selected from ONE row in any given PCS table. Many of the rows in a table can appear to be very similar or nearly identical. The user has the responsibility to determine the differences when assigning characters to construct a PCS code. The table below contains rows that are very similar.

Ø	**Medical and Surgical**				
B	**Respiratory System**				
9	**Drainage**	Definition: Taking or letting out fluids and/or gases from a body part			

Body Part Character 4	Approach Character 5	Device Character 6	Qualifier Character 7
1 Trachea 2 Carina 3 Main Bronchus, Right 4 Upper Lobe Bronchus, Right 5 Middle Lobe Bronchus, Right 6 Lower Lobe Bronchus, Right 7 Main Bronchus, Left 8 Upper Lobe Bronchus, Left 9 Lingula Bronchus B Lower Lobe Bronchus, Left C Upper Lung Lobe, Right D Middle Lung Lobe, Right F Lower Lung Lobe, Right G Upper Lung Lobe, Left H Lung Lingula J Lower Lung Lobe, Left K Lung, Right L Lung, Left M Lungs, Bilateral	Ø Open 3 Percutaneous 4 Percutaneous Endoscopic 7 Via Natural or Artificial Opening 8 Via Natural or Artificial Opening Endoscopic	Ø Drainage Device	Z No Qualifier
1 Trachea 2 Carina 3 Main Bronchus, Right 4 Upper Lobe Bronchus, Right 5 Middle Lobe Bronchus, Right 6 Lower Lobe Bronchus, Right 7 Main Bronchus, Left 8 Upper Lobe Bronchus, Left 9 Lingula Bronchus B Lower Lobe Bronchus, Left C Upper Lung Lobe, Right D Middle Lung Lobe, Right F Lower Lung Lobe, Right G Upper Lung Lobe, Left H Lung Lingula J Lower Lung Lobe, Left K Lung, Right L Lung, Left M Lungs, Bilateral	Ø Open 3 Percutaneous 4 Percutaneous Endoscopic 7 Via Natural or Artificial Opening 8 Via Natural or Artificial Opening Endoscopic	Z No Device	X Diagnostic Z No Qualifier

The first two rows of table ØB9 appear very similar. The character values for body part (character 4) and approach (character 5) are identical, but note that the values in characters 6 and 7 differ. Qualifier (character 7) value No Qualifier (Z) appears in both rows but in the second row, qualifier value Diagnostic (X), also appears. In the row with the Diagnostic value (X), only one value appears in the Device column (character 6), which is No Device (Z). This means that if a diagnostic biopsy procedure is performed, it cannot be coded together with a procedure reflecting a drainage device. The use of these character value combinations in the rows allows the system to restrict valid code construction only to those procedures that are clinically legitimate.

The tables are organized in a series, beginning with section numbers Ø–9 in numerical order, followed by the letters B–D, F–H, and X. The order of values for the second character is the same: first the numbers Ø–9 and then the letters B–D, F–H, progressing alphabetically to body system Y, making it easy to locate any given table.

Index

The ICD-10-PCS-Official Code Set includes an alphabetic index to assist the user in finding the most appropriate table from which to build PCS codes. The main term entries for procedural services are indexed in two ways:

- By root operation (e.g., Excision, Transplantation, Dilation)

- By common procedural terms

Using the previous example, for a laparoscopic excisional liver biopsy, the main term "Excision" in the index lists the following:

Excision

> Liver ØFBØ
>> Left Lobe ØFB2
>> Right Lobe ØFB1

The index provides the first three or four character values so that the user can turn to the correct table and complete the code construction. In the example above, regardless of which lobe of the liver is excised, table ØFB should be reviewed.

There are many terms that are cross-referenced in the PCS index. Many of these entries represent common procedural terms that are not designated as root operations in PCS. For example, if the term "Biopsy" is located in the index, the following appears:

Biopsy

> *see* Drainage with qualifier Diagnostic
> *see* Excision with qualifier Diagnostic
> *see* Extraction with qualifier Diagnostic

In the example for a laparoscopic excisional liver biopsy, the root operation character value B for "Excision" is selected and the "Diagnostic" portion of the procedure is reflected in the seventh-character value Diagnostic (X).

If the appropriate root operation is known, that term should be searched in the index in order to locate the corresponding PCS table most easily. Until the user becomes familiar with the root operation terms found in PCS, it may be necessary to follow the instructional notes in the index for other commonly performed procedures such as "Appendectomy," "Colostomy," or "PTCA." In many cases, the indexed entry provides the first three- or four-character values, routing the user to the appropriate table.

The index can also be used to locate specific body parts. There are many anatomical main terms listed that provide instruction for the appropriate PCS body part. For example:

Foramen magnum

> *use* Occipital Bone

Use of the alphabetic index is optional since all codes must be constructed using the tables. If the first several character values are known, codes may be constructed directly from the tables. There is no additional information in the PCS index that is not found in the tables.

List of Codes

The ICD-10-PCS List of Codes is a resource that provides each and every valid PCS code, along with its full-text description. The codes are presented in alphanumeric order and use rules that result in complete, standardized code descriptions. The official file can be found at http://www.cms.gov/Medicare/Coding/ICD10/2019-ICD-10-PCS.html.

To access the List of Codes, open the zipped file "2019 ICD-10-PCS Order File (Long and Abbreviated Titles)" and select the file "icd10pcs_order_2019.txt."

Hierarchy of Coding Advice

CMS' *ICD-10-PCS Official Guidelines for Coding and Reporting 2019* provides direction on the hierarchy to be used when coding procedures. The coding rationales provided in this product follow the advice established by CMS, as well as guidance from *AHA Coding Clinic* as appropriate. Note that conventions take precedence over guidelines. Occasionally there may be inconsistencies in advice between *AHA Coding Clinic* and guidelines or even between the guidelines and the index, tables, or definitions. It is good to always keep the following hierarchy in mind if any discrepancies between these sources are encountered.

Figure 1.1. Coding Advice Hierarchy

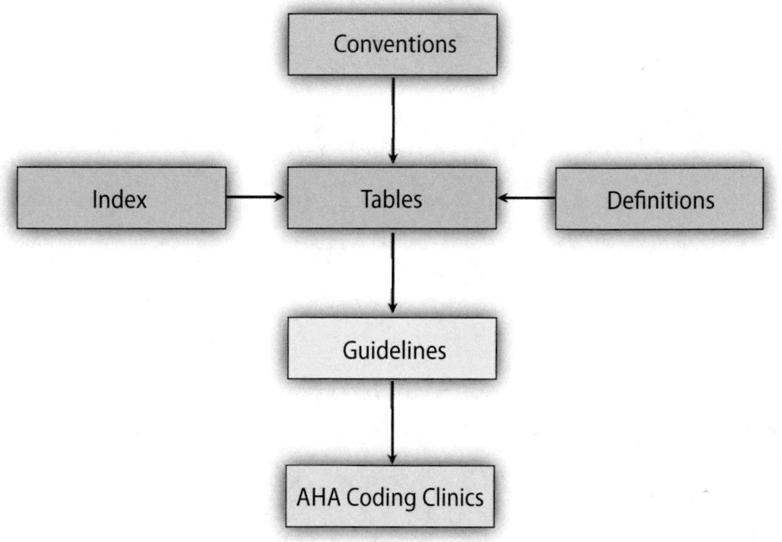

Chapter 2. PCS Conventions

General ICD-10-PCS Coding Conventions

This chapter provides the fundamentals behind the construction of ICD-10-PCS codes. Each official convention and any corresponding example, contained in the *ICD-10-PCS Official Guidelines for Coding and Reporting 2019* is provided, followed by additional and supplementary information to further interpret the convention. It should be noted that the instructions and conventions of the classification take precedence over guidelines.

The following illustration is provided to assist in learning each of the axes of classification in the Medical and Surgical section, where most of the invasive PCS procedure codes reside.

Character 1	Character 2	Character 3	Character 4	Character 5	Character 6	Character 7
Section	Body System	Root Operation	Body Part	Approach	Device	Qualifier

Convention A1

A1	**ICD-10-PCS codes are composed of seven characters. Each character is an axis of classification that specifies information about the procedure performed. Within a defined code range, a character specifies the same type of information in that axis of classification.** *Example:* **The fifth axis of classification specifies the approach in sections Ø through 4 and 7 through 9 of the system.**

As shown in the following table (Ø97), although there are multiple values listed, character 4 always represents Body Part, character 5 Approach, and character 6 Device.

Ø	**Medical and Surgical**			
9	**Ear, Nose, Sinus**			
7	**Dilation**	Definition: Expanding an orifice or the lumen of a tubular body part		

Body Part Character 4	Approach Character 5	Device Character 6	Qualifier Character 7
F Eustachian Tube, Right G Eustachian Tube, Left	Ø Open 7 Via Natural or Artificial Opening 8 Via Natural or Artificial Opening Endoscopic	D Intraluminal Device Z No Device	Z No Qualifier
F Eustachian Tube, Right G Eustachian Tube, Left	3 Percutaneous 4 Percutaneous Endoscopic	Z No Device	Z No Qualifier

Regardless of whether the specific character values represent clinical concepts or function as placeholders (e.g., No Device (Z) or No Qualifier (Z)), all seven characters must be assigned for each PCS code.

Convention A2

| A2 | One of 34 possible values can be assigned to each axis of classification in the seven-character code: they are the numbers Ø through 9 and the alphabet (except I and O because they are easily confused with the numbers 1 and Ø). The number of unique values used in an axis of classification differs as needed.

Example: Where the fifth axis of classification specifies the approach, seven different approach values are currently used to specify the approach. |

Twenty-four letters of the alphabet (letters I and O are not used) and numbers Ø through 9 allow for a total of 34 possible values for each character. For example, the character meaning table below for the Peripheral Nervous System in the Medical and Surgical section has 16 possible values in the Root Operation column because only those root operations are considered possible to perform on the peripheral nervous system. If additional root operations are added in the future, it will be determined whether the new type of procedure could be performed on the peripheral nervous system before the character is added to the table. In this way, a table does not contain combinations of characters representing invalid or impossible procedures. Please note that the following is not a PCS table from which actual codes may be constructed. This is a character meaning table from appendix I that includes all potential values for each character column in the Peripheral Nervous System. The values have not been constructed in the rows that are necessary for PCS code assignment.

Peripheral Nervous System (1)

Operation–Character 3	Body Part–Character 4	Approach–Character 5	Device–Character 6	Qualifier–Character 7
2 Change	Ø Cervical Plexus	Ø Open	Ø Drainage Device	1 Cervical Nerve
5 Destruction	1 Cervical Nerve	3 Percutaneous	2 Monitoring Device	2 Phrenic Nerve
8 Division	2 Phrenic Nerve	4 Percutaneous Endoscopic	7 Autologous Tissue Substitute	4 Ulnar Nerve
9 Drainage	3 Brachial Plexus	X External	M Neurostimulator Lead	5 Median Nerve
B Excision	4 Ulnar Nerve		Y Other Device	6 Radial Nerve
C Extirpation	5 Median Nerve		Z No Device	8 Thoracic Nerve
D Extraction	6 Radial Nerve			B Lumbar Nerve
H Insertion	8 Thoracic Nerve			C Perineal Nerve
J Inspection	9 Lumbar Plexus			D Femoral Nerve
N Release	A Lumbosacral Plexus			F Sciatic Nerve
P Removal	B Lumbar Nerve			G Tibial Nerve
Q Repair	C Pudendal Nerve			H Peroneal Nerve
R Replacement	D Femoral Nerve			X Diagnostic
S Reposition	F Sciatic Nerve			Z No Qualifier
U Supplement	G Tibial Nerve			
W Revision	H Peroneal Nerve			
X Transfer	K Head & Neck Sympathetic Nerve			
	L Thoracic Sympathetic Nerve			
	M Abdominal Sympathetic Nerve			
	N Lumbar Sympathetic Nerve			
	P Sacral Sympathetic Nerve			
	Q Sacral Plexus			
	R Sacral Nerve			
	Y Peripheral Nerve			

Convention A3

A3	The valid values for an axis of classification can be added to as needed.
	Example: If a significantly distinct type of device is used in a new procedure, a new device value can be added to the system.

ICD-10-PCS is updated annually with some characters added and some deleted to reflect current procedures.

The addition of one character value can potentially translate to a significant number of new codes since the number of different combinations of character values can be quite high.

Convention A4

A4	As with words in their context, the meaning of any single value is a combination of its axis of classification and any preceding values on which it may be dependent.
	Example: The meaning of a body part value in the Medical and Surgical section is always dependent on the body system value. The body part value Ø in the Central Nervous body system specifies Brain and the body part value Ø in the Peripheral Nervous body system specifies Cervical Plexus.

The following tables are samples of the first two pages of appendix I Character Meanings. In the first table, for the Central Nervous System and Cranial Nerves, the body part (character 4) column indicates that the value of Ø = Brain, 1 = Cerebral Meninges, 2 = Dura Mater, etc. The same column (character 4) in the next table reveals that the same values are completely different for the Peripheral Nervous System, where Ø = Cervical Plexus, 1 = Cervical Nerve, 2 = Phrenic Nerve, etc. The body part character value is inextricably related to the corresponding body system character value, which is one of the reasons that the specific rows are constructed as they are. There are many interconnected relationships between the character values moving across the row. Some devices may only be inserted using a specific type of approach; some qualifiers only apply to specific body parts. This clinical logic is used to construct the rows in the PCS tables that translate to valid character value combinations and resulting codes.

Central Nervous System and Cranial Nerves (Ø)

Operation–Character 3		Body Part–Character 4		Approach–Character 5		Device–Character 6		Qualifier–Character 7	
1	Bypass	Ø	Brain	Ø	Open	Ø	Drainage Device	Ø	Nasopharynx
2	Change	1	Cerebral Meninges	3	Percutaneous	2	Monitoring Device	1	Mastoid Sinus
5	Destruction	2	Dura Mater	4	Percutaneous Endoscopic	3	Infusion Device	2	Atrium
7	Dilation	3	Epidural Space, Intracranial	X	External	4	Radioactive Element, Cesium-131 Collagen Implant	3	Blood Vessel
8	Division	4	Subdural Space, Intracranial			7	Autologous Tissue Substitute	4	Pleural Cavity
9	Drainage	5	Subarachnoid Space, Intracranial			J	Synthetic Substitute	5	Intestine
B	Excision	6	Cerebral Ventricle			K	Nonautologous Tissue Substitute	6	Peritoneal Cavity
C	Extirpation	7	Cerebral Hemisphere			M	Neurostimulator Lead	7	Urinary Tract

Peripheral Nervous System (1)

	Operation–Character 3		Body Part–Character 4		Approach–Character 5		Device–Character 6		Qualifier–Character 7
2	Change	Ø	Cervical Plexus	Ø	Open	Ø	Drainage Device	1	Cervical Nerve
5	Destruction	1	Cervical Nerve	3	Percutaneous	2	Monitoring Device	2	Phrenic Nerve
8	Division	2	Phrenic Nerve	4	Percutaneous Endoscopic	7	Autologous Tissue Substitute	4	Ulnar Nerve
9	Drainage	3	Brachial Plexus	X	External	M	Neurostimulator Lead	5	Median Nerve
B	Excision	4	Ulnar Nerve			Y	Other Device	6	Radial Nerve
C	Extirpation	5	Median Nerve			Z	No Device	8	Thoracic Nerve
D	Extraction	6	Radial Nerve					B	Lumbar Nerve

Convention A5

A5	As the system is expanded to become increasingly detailed, over time more values will depend on preceding values for their meaning.
	Example: In the Lower Joints body system, the device value 3 in the root operation Insertion specifies Infusion Device and the device value 3 in the root operation Replacement specifies Ceramic Synthetic Substitute.

To illustrate the example in Convention A5, the following two tables from the Lower Joints body system demonstrate how the meaning of the character value can change in different root operation tables within the same body system.

Ø **Medical and Surgical** S **Lower Joints** H **Insertion**			Definition: Putting in a nonbiological appliance that monitors, assists, performs, or prevents a physiological function but does not physically take the place of a body part		
Body Part Character 4		**Approach Character 5**	**Device Character 6**		**Qualifier Character 7**
Ø Lumbar Vertebral Joint 3 Lumbosacral Joint		Ø Open 3 Percutaneous 4 Percutaneous Endoscopic	3 Infusion Device 4 Internal Fixation Device 8 Spacer B Spinal Stabilization Device, Interspinous Process C Spinal Stabilization Device, Pedicle-Based D Spinal Stabilization Device, Facet Replacement		Z No Qualifier

Ø	Medical and Surgical
S	Lower Joints
R	Replacement	Definition: Putting in or on biological or synthetic material that physically takes the place and/or function of all or a portion of a body part

Body Part Character 4	Approach Character 5	Device Character 6	Qualifier Character 7
Ø Lumbar Vertebral Joint 2 Lumbar Vertebral Disc 3 Lumbosacral Joint 4 Lumbosacral Disc 5 Sacrococcygeal Joint 6 Coccygeal Joint 7 Sacroiliac Joint, Right 8 Sacroiliac Joint, Left H Tarsal Joint, Right J Tarsal Joint, Left K Tarsometatarsal Joint, Right L Tarsometatarsal Joint, Left M Metatarsal-Phalangeal Joint, Right N Metatarsal-Phalangeal Joint, Left P Toe Phalangeal Joint, Right Q Toe Phalangeal Joint, Left	Ø Open	7 Autologous Tissue Substitute J Synthetic Substitute K Nonautologous Tissue Substitute	Z No Qualifier
9 Hip Joint, Right B Hip Joint, Left	Ø Open	1 Synthetic Substitute, Metal 2 Synthetic Substitute, Metal on Polyethylene 3 Synthetic Substitute, Ceramic 4 Synthetic Substitute, Ceramic on Polyethylene 6 Synthetic Substitute, Oxidized Zirconium on Polyethylene J Synthetic Substitute	9 Cemented A Uncemented Z No Qualifier

Because there are only 34 potential character values available for use in any character field within a section, it is necessary to duplicate values. The user is required to carefully review preceding character values and know which character values clinically match up. Valid codes will still be constructed across rows, but in some cases there may be duplicated values within one section. Currently, the majority of the duplicated values involve devices, when assigned with root operation Insertion (H) or Replacement (R). Device values need to be reviewed carefully, especially when constructing PCS codes for these two root operations.

Convention A6

A6	The purpose of the alphabetic index is to locate the appropriate table that contains all information necessary to construct a procedure code. The PCS Tables should always be consulted to find the most appropriate valid code.

Valid ICD-10-PCS codes *must* be constructed from the tables, so one of the most important steps in the code assignment process is locating the most appropriate table. The alphabetic index can assist in this location process since it is organized alphabetically by root operation or by common procedural term. It is important to note that the ICD-10-PCS alphabetic index does not contain additional information that is not in the PCS tables.

The ICD-10-PCS index can be used to access the tables. The index is a frame of reference only and the full intent of a procedure must be understood in order to assign the appropriate root operation. Common terms such as fasciotomy, osteotomy, and laminectomy may be assigned to additional root operations other than those identified in the index. The root operation assigned should be based on the procedure performed as described in the complete documentation contained in the operative report and not simply on a single descriptive term in the operative report.

Convention A7

A7	It is not required to consult the index first before proceeding to the tables to complete the code. A valid code may be chosen directly from the tables.

AHA Coding Clinic

2017, 2Q, 12   Compartment Syndrome and Fasciotomy of Foot

2017, 2Q, 13   Compartment Syndrome and Fasciotomy of Leg

2014, 2Q, 10   Transverse Abdominomyocutaneous (TRAM) Breast Reconstruction

As stated above, there is no information in the alphabetic index that is not in the PCS tables. Valid ICD-10-PCS codes *must* be constructed from the tables; however, the coding process does not need to begin with the alphabetic index. A valid code may be constructed by going directly to a table without reviewing any entries in the index. For example, after working on multiple cases involving coronary artery bypass grafting (CABG) procedures, the user may automatically know that the most appropriate table is Ø21, with the following meaning:

- Ø Medical and Surgical (Section)
- 2 Heart and Great Vessels (Body System)
- 1 Bypass (Root Operation)

Convention A8

A8	All seven characters must be specified to be a valid code. If the documentation is incomplete for coding purposes, the physician should be queried for the necessary information.

Each and every field in the seven-character ICD-10-PCS code must be completed in order for the code to be considered valid. While there are some limited not otherwise specified (NOS) and not elsewhere classified (NEC) options in PCS, they are not extensively used. If the information required to complete a character field is not found in the medical record documentation, the physician must be queried to provide the necessary information. For example, using the following table to complete a valid code for the insertion of a pacemaker generator into the subcutaneous tissue and fascia of the chest wall, the type of pacemaker must be determined. There is no option in the character six device values for an unspecified type of pacemaker generator.

Ø	Medical and Surgical
J	Subcutaneous Tissue and Fascia
H	Insertion — Definition: Putting in a nonbiological appliance that monitors, assists, performs, or prevents a physiological function but does not physically take the place of a body part

Body Part Character 4	Approach Character 5	Device Character 6	Qualifier Character 7
6 Subcutaneous Tissue and Fascia, Chest 8 Subcutaneous Tissue and Fascia, Abdomen	Ø Open 3 Percutaneous	Ø Monitoring Device, Hemodynamic 2 Monitoring Device 4 Pacemaker, Single Chamber 5 Pacemaker, Single Chamber Rate Responsive 6 Pacemaker, Dual Chamber 7 Cardiac Resynchronization Pacemaker Pulse Generator 8 Defibrillator Generator 9 Cardiac Resynchronization Defibrillator Pulse Generator A Contractility Modulation Device B Stimulator Generator, Single Array C Stimulator Generator, Single Array Rechargeable D Stimulator Generator, Multiple Array E Stimulator Generator, Multiple Array Rechargeable H Contraceptive Device M Stimulator Generator N Tissue Expander P Cardiac Rhythm Related Device V Infusion Device, Pump W Vascular Access Device, Totally Implantable X Vascular Access Device, Tunneled	Z No Qualifier

Convention A9

A9	Within a PCS table, valid codes include all combinations of choices in characters 4 through 7 contained in the same row of the table. In the example below, ØJHT3VZ is a valid code, and ØJHW3VZ is *not* a valid code.

Section: Ø Medical and Surgical

Body System: J Subcutaneous Tissue and Fascia

Operation: H Insertion: Putting in a nonbiological appliance that monitors, assists, performs, or prevents a physiological function but does not physically take the place of a body part

Body Part	Approach	Device	Qualifier
S Subcutaneous Tissue and Fascia, Head and Neck **V** Subcutaneous Tissue and Fascia, Upper Extremity **W** Subcutaneous Tissue and Fascia, Lower Extremity	**Ø** Open **3** Percutaneous	**1** Radioactive Element **3** Infusion Device	**Z** No Qualifier
T Subcutaneous Tissue and Fascia, Trunk	**Ø** Open **3** Percutaneous	**1** Radioactive Element **3** Infusion Device **V** Infusion Pump	**Z** No Qualifier

Valid PCS codes must be constructed moving across *one* row. If, for instance, an approach value appears in the character five field, but the body part value is not in the same row, the two characters may not be assigned together. Refer to another row where the two character values may appear together. In some PCS tables there are many rows, each with a different combination of values. Be sure to review the tables in their entirety, being aware that a table may encompass more than one page in the ICD-10-PCS book. The validity of a specific seven-character code can be cross-referenced with the official ICD-10-PCS Code List (https://www.cms.gov/Medicare/Coding/ICD10/2019-ICD-10-PCS.html), which contains all valid combination of character values and is all-inclusive.

Convention A10

A10	"And," when used in a code description, means "and/or," except when used to describe a combination of multiple body parts for which separate values exist for each body part (e.g., Skin and Subcutaneous Tissue used as a qualifier, where there are separate body part values for "Skin" and "Subcutaneous Tissue"). *Example:* Lower Arm and Wrist Muscle means lower arm and/or wrist muscle.

AHA Coding Clinic

2015, 2Q, 26   Pharyngeal Flap to Soft Palate

There are many instances in PCS where body parts that are adjacent or have a related function are grouped together in one character value. Examples include the following:

- Head and neck sympathetic nerve
- Mouth and throat
- Lower arm and wrist muscle

- Head and neck tendon
- Lower arm and wrist tendon
- Head and neck bursa and ligament
- Uterus and cervix
- Vagina and cul-de-sac
- Prostate and seminal vesicles
- Scrotum and tunica vaginalis
- Epididymis and spermatic cord
- Oral cavity and throat

Any procedure performed on one of the two sites listed (linked by the word "and") can be classified to that character value. The procedure does not need to be performed on both sites in order to assign that character value. It should also be noted that in the same section, a table may list the body part combination value listed above, but in other PCS tables in the same section, the specific body parts may appear as separate values. For example, as shown by the following tables, in the Female Reproductive System Table ØUP (Root Operation Removal), the body part value for Uterus and Cervix (D) appears, but in Table ØUQ (Root Operation Repair), there are separate character values, one for Uterus (9) and one for Cervix (C). Separate codes should be used when separate values exist for each body part.

Ø   Medical and Surgical
U   Female Reproductive System
P   Removal   Definition: Taking out or off a device from a body part

Body Part Character 4	Approach Character 5	Device Character 6	Qualifier Character 7
3 Ovary	**Ø** Open **3** Percutaneous **4** Percutaneous Endoscopic	**Ø** Drainage Device **3** Infusion Device **Y** Other Device	**Z** No Qualifier
3 Ovary	**7** Via Natural or Artificial Opening **8** Via Natural or Artificial Opening Endoscopic	**Y** Other Device	**Z** No Qualifier
3 Ovary	**X** External	**Ø** Drainage Device **3** Infusion Device	**Z** No Qualifier
8 Fallopian Tube	**Ø** Open **3** Percutaneous **4** Percutaneous Endoscopic **7** Via Natural or Artificial Opening **8** Via Natural or Artificial Opening Endoscopic	**Ø** Drainage Device **3** Infusion Device **7** Autologous Tissue Substitute **C** Extraluminal Device **D** Intraluminal Device **J** Synthetic Substitute **K** Nonautologous Tissue Substitute **Y** Other Device	**Z** No Qualifier
8 Fallopian Tube	**X** External	**Ø** Drainage Device **3** Infusion Device **D** Intraluminal Device	**Z** No Qualifier
D Uterus and Cervix	**Ø** Open **3** Percutaneous **4** Percutaneous Endoscopic **7** Via Natural or Artificial Opening **8** Via Natural or Artificial Opening Endoscopic	**Ø** Drainage Device **1** Radioactive Element **3** Infusion Device **7** Autologous Tissue Substitute **C** Extraluminal Device **D** Intraluminal Device **H** Contraceptive Device **J** Synthetic Substitute **K** Nonautologous Tissue Substitute **Y** Other Device	**Z** No Qualifier

Ø	Medical and Surgical	
U	Female Reproductive System	
Q	Repair	Definition: Restoring, to the extent possible, a body part to its normal anatomic structure and function

Body Part Character 4	Approach Character 5	Device Character 6	Qualifier Character 7
Ø Ovary, Right 1 Ovary, Left 2 Ovaries, Bilateral 4 Uterine Supporting Structure	Ø Open 3 Percutaneous 4 Percutaneous Endoscopic 8 Via Natural or Artificial Opening Endoscopic	Z No Device	Z No Qualifier
5 Fallopian Tube, Right 6 Fallopian Tube, Left 7 Fallopian Tubes, Bilateral 9 Uterus C Cervix F Cul-de-sac	Ø Open 3 Percutaneous 4 Percutaneous Endoscopic 7 Via Natural or Artificial Opening 8 Via Natural or Artificial Opening Endoscopic	Z No Device	Z No Qualifier

Convention A11

A11	Many of the terms used to construct PCS codes are defined within the system. It is the coder's responsibility to determine what the documentation in the medical record equates to in the PCS definitions. The physician is not expected to use the terms used in PCS code descriptions, nor is the coder required to query the physician when the correlation between the documentation and the defined PCS terms is clear. *Example:* When the physician documents "partial resection" the coder can independently correlate "partial resection" to the root operation Excision without querying the physician for clarification.

AHA Coding Clinic

2018, 2Q, 25	Third and Fourth Degree Obstetric Lacerations
2016, 3Q, 35	Use of Cemented Versus Uncemented Qualifier for Joint Replacement
2016, 3Q, 43	Peri-Pulmonary Catheter Ablation
2016, 3Q, 44	Maze Procedure
2016, 1Q, 6	Obstetric Perineal Laceration Repair
2015, 3Q, 6	Excisional and Nonexcisional Debridement
2015, 2Q, 28	Release and Replacement of Celiac Artery

Medical coders must become adept at translating the terminology found in the medical record documentation to the nomenclature used in ICD-10-PCS, particularly for root operation determination. But in doing so, users should not assume that the documentation must exactly "match" PCS terms or that the physicians must add clarification when the words do not match. If the documentation is clear and the procedure matches a PCS root operation (or approach, etc.), the user may assign the character value. In the example provided with Convention A11 (listed above), partial resection meets the full definition of Excision, since only a portion of the body part is excised.

Chapter 3. Body System Guidelines

Body System Overview

Body System: Character 2

Character 1	Character 2	Character 3	Character 4	Character 5	Character 6	Character 7
Section	Body System	Root Operation	Body Part	Approach	Device	Qualifier

The second character in each PCS code from the Medical and Surgical (Ø) section is the body system. This character designates the general body system, such as Central Nervous System and Cranial Nerves, Respiratory System, or Subcutaneous Tissue and Fascia. The body part value (character 4) is dependent upon the assignment of the body system value; therefore, the most appropriate body system value should be assigned.

It is important to understand that PCS is not separated into the same body systems as its counterpart ICD-10-CM. In ICD-10-CM, the body classification system is based on disease processes. ICD-10-PCS uses the anatomy of the human body, dividing it into specific body systems. For example, in ICD-10-CM only one chapter focuses on the diseases of the circulatory system, while ICD-10-PCS breaks the circulatory system into five separate chapters.

ICD-10-CM	ICD-10-PCS
Diseases of the Circulatory System	Heart and Great Vessels
	Upper Arteries
	Lower Arteries
	Upper Veins
	Lower Veins

The Medical and Surgical section has 31 values that represent defined PCS body systems. These body system values represent a specific anatomical/physiological system, such as Upper Bones, or a broader anatomical region, such as Anatomical Regions, Upper Extremities. For a full list of the 31 different body system values, see chapter 1 of this book.

Spotlight
The body part that is the focus of the procedure is important to note when selecting the correct body system. If the focus is the shoulder bursae or ligament, code to the body system Bursae and Ligaments. If the focus is a shoulder tendon, use body system Tendons. Cartilage does not have a body system or body part designated; it is considered part of the joint structure and is coded to the nearest joint body system.

General Guidelines

There are two guidelines associated with character 2 Body System. The first guideline discusses the appropriate use of the Anatomical Regions body systems (General, Upper Extremities, and Lower Extremities) and why specific root operations can only be found in these sections. The other guideline clarifies how PCS defines the upper and lower body system anatomy.

Guideline B2.1a

> **B2.1a**   **The procedure codes in the general anatomical regions body systems can be used when the procedure is performed on an anatomical region rather than a specific body part (e.g., root operations Control and Detachment, Drainage of a body cavity) or on the rare occasion when no information is available to support assignment of a code to a specific body part.**
>
> *Examples:* **Control of postoperative hemorrhage is coded to the root operation Control found in the general anatomical regions body systems.**
>
> **Chest tube drainage of the pleural cavity is coded to the root operation Drainage found in the general anatomical regions body systems. Suture repair of the abdominal wall is coded to the root operation Repair in the general anatomical regions body system.**

AHA Coding Clinic

2017, 2Q, 3	Qualifiers for the Root Operation Detachment
2017, 2Q, 18	Removal of Polydactyl Digits
2017, 1Q, 22	Chopart Amputation of Foot
2017, 1Q, 52	Further Distal Phalangeal Amputation
2016, 4Q, 99	Root Operation Control
2016, 4Q, 134	Changes to the ICD-10-PCS Official Guidelines for Coding and Reporting
2016, 3Q, 33	Traumatic Amputation of Fingers with Further Revision Amputation
2016, 1Q, 21	Excision of Urachal Mass
2015, 3Q, 23	Incision and Drainage of Multiple Abscess Cavities Using Vessel Loop
2015, 2Q, 25	Partial Amputation of Hallux at Interphalangeal Joint
2015, 1Q, 28	Mid-Foot Amputation
2015, 1Q, 35	Evacuation of Hematoma for Control of Postprocedural Bleeding
2013, 4Q, 119	Excision of Inclusion Cyst of Perineum

Of the 31 body systems in the Medical and Surgical section, there are three body systems designated as Anatomical Regions: General, Upper Extremities, and Lower Extremities. These body systems are only assigned in certain circumstances. A table from any of these three body systems should not be used if the procedure is performed on a location that can be designated to a more specific physiological body system. Although many of the root operations found in the more specific physiological body systems are also found in the Anatomical Regions body systems, there are two root operations almost exclusively found in the Anatomical Regions body systems: Control and Detachment.

Root Operation Control in the Anatomical Regions

Root Operation		
Control (3)	Definition:	Stopping, or attempting to stop, postprocedural or other acute bleeding
	Explanation:	The site of the bleeding is coded as an anatomical region and not to a specific body part

Control is a root operation primarily captured in the Anatomical Regions, General; Anatomical Regions, Upper Extremities; and Anatomical Regions, Lower Extremities body systems because, in general, control of bleeding is performed on a broader body area than a more specific body site.

Spotlight
In the Medical and Surgical section, the root operation Control is included in one body system outside of the Anatomical Regions: the Ear, Nose, Sinus (9) body system. This table is used to code control of bleeding from the nose (epistaxis) using body part value Nasal Mucosa and Soft Tissue (K), except when only packing is inserted to stop the bleeding. Packing is coded in the Placement (2) section with body part value Nasal (1).

Based on instruction from guideline B3.7, Control is used only if the procedure used to ultimately stop the bleeding was not attained by another root operation.

PCS Guideline	
Control vs. more definitive root operations	
B3.7	The root operation Control is defined as, "Stopping, or attempting to stop, postprocedural or other acute bleeding." If an attempt to stop postprocedural or other acute bleeding is unsuccessful, and to stop the bleeding requires performing a more definitive root operation such as Bypass, Detachment, Excision, Extraction, Reposition, Replacement, or Resection, then the more definitive root operation is coded instead of Control.
	Example: Resection of spleen to stop bleeding is coded to Resection instead of Control.

Root Operation		
Bypass (1)	Definition:	Altering the route of passage of the contents of a tubular body part
	Explanation:	Rerouting contents of a body part to a downstream area of the normal route, to a similar route and body part, or to an abnormal route and dissimilar body part. Includes one or more anastomoses, with or without the use of a device.
Detachment (6)	Definition:	Cutting off all or a portion of the upper or lower extremities
	Explanation:	The body part value is the site of the detachment, with a qualifier if applicable to further specify the level where the extremity was detached
Excision (B)	Definition:	Cutting out or off, without replacement, a portion of a body part
	Explanation:	The qualifier DIAGNOSTIC is used to identify excision procedures that are biopsies
Extraction (D)	Definition:	Pulling or stripping out or off all or a portion of a body part by the use of force
	Explanation:	The qualifier DIAGNOSTIC is used to identify extraction procedures that are biopsies

Root Operation (continued)		
Reposition (S)	Definition:	Moving to its normal location, or other suitable location, all or a portion of a body part
	Explanation:	The body part is moved to a new location from an abnormal location, or from a normal location where it is not functioning correctly. The body part may or may not be cut out or off to be moved to the new location.
Replacement (R)	Definition:	Putting in or on biological or synthetic material that physically takes the place and/or function of all or a portion of a body part
	Explanation:	The body part may have been taken out or replaced, or may be taken out, physically eradicated, or rendered nonfunctional during the Replacement procedure. A Removal procedure is coded for taking out the device used in a previous replacement procedure.
Resection (T)	Definition:	Cutting out or off, without replacement, all of a body part
	Explanation:	None

Practical Application for Guideline B2.1a Using Root Operation Control

Case Study 3.1. Hemorrhage, Postop Rectal

Upon review by the operating surgeon on the day following hemorrhoidal ligation, the patient was taken for examination under anaesthetic (EUA). Digital rectal examination (DRE) showed extensive bruising and blood coming from the rectum. Examination also found a boggy mass posteriorly with small defect at the staple line through which blood clots were coming out. Blood clots were evacuated through the defect. Staples around the defect were removed, and obvious leaking vessels were cauterized. The wound was carefully reapproximated and stapled. Hemorrhagic leakage ceased.

Code(s):

ØW3P7ZZ   Control Bleeding in Gastrointestinal Tract, Via Natural or Artificial Opening

Rationale:

Postoperative bleeding is an example of when root operation Control (3) is appropriate. In this example, the clot was evacuated, vessels cauterized, and the wound re-stapled, all of which are captured by root operation Control (3). If root operations such as Bypass (1), Detachment (6), Excision (B), Extraction (D), Reposition (S), Replacement (R), or Resection (T) had been performed, then Control (3) would not be appropriate and one of the aforementioned root operations would be reported.

The rectum is considered part of the Gastrointestinal Tract (P) in the Anatomical Regions, General (W) body system. The repair was performed Via Natural or Artificial Opening (7) with No Device (Z) and No Qualifier (Z). According to guideline B6.1b, staples are not considered a device.

PCS Guideline
Device general guideline
B6.1b   Materials such as sutures, ligatures, radiological markers and temporary post-operative wound drains are considered integral to the performance of a procedure and are not coded as devices.

> ### Case Study 3.2. Hemorrhage, Postoperative, Urethral Anastomosis
>
> Under anesthesia, the cystoscopy showed a partial disruption of the wall of the anastomosis. There was not any obvious area of the urethra that could be fulgurated with electrocautery so the perineal incision was reopened revealing no obvious perineal hematoma. The urethra was rotated to reveal the dorsal wall; the disruption was visible and bleeding was seen from the exposed spongiosum. Through the cystocope, the remaining dorsal wall stitches in the area of the disruption were excised, revealing the underlying urethral mucosa, which looked inflamed. Several interrupted anastomotic stitches of 6-0 PDS were placed in the urethral mucosa in the area of the disruption; the outer wall of the spongiosum also had 5-0 PDS stitches placed, successfully stopping the bleeding.

Code(s):

ØW3R8ZZ **Control Bleeding in Genitourinary Tract, Via Natural or Artificial Opening Endoscopic**

Rationale:

The root operation Control (3) is used when the hemorrhage occurs postoperatively and only if none of the other root operations such as Bypass (1), Detachment (6), Excision (B), Extraction (D), Reposition (S), Replacement (R), or Resection (T) are performed. In this case, Control (3) was successfully performed with stitches through the cystoscope, which is considered Via Natural or Artificial Opening, Endoscopic (8) approach since the scope is inserted directly through the urethra. The bleeding occurred at the urethra, which is reported with Genitourinary Tract (R) in the Anatomical Regions, General (W) body system.

> ### Case Study 3.3. Hemorrhage, Postoperative, Status Post-pancreatic Tumor Removal
>
> The patient was urgently returned to the operating room after surgical removal of a tumor on the tail of the pancreas. A large hemoglobin drop was noted and internal bleeding suspected. Laparotomy was reopened with a gush of blood. The spleen was noted to be friable with laceration. Urgent complete splenectomy was performed.

Code(s):

Ø7TPØZZ **Resection of Spleen, Open Approach**

Rationale:

This is an example of when guideline B2.1a is **not** applied since the procedure that was ultimately performed was done on a specific body part and not a region as the guideline directs. In this case study, the body part Spleen (P) from the Lymphatic and Hemic (7) body system is reported. It is often necessary to apply more than one guideline to reach the appropriate code. In this case, the postoperative bleeding was controlled by the complete removal or Resection (T) of the Spleen (P). As per guideline B3.7, Resection (T) is used instead of Control (3). The reopening of the laparotomy is coded to an Open (Ø) approach. There was No Device (Z) and No Qualifier (Z).

Root Operation		
Resection (T)	Definition:	Cutting out or off, without replacement, all of a body part
	Explanation:	None

> ### Case Study 3.4. Hemorrhage, After Cesarean Delivery
>
> The patient was brought back into the operating suite for control of postoperative bleeding from an abdominal wound following cesarean section. Staples were found to be pulled taunt and disrupted. The staples were excised and the wound reapproximated in layers. The staples were replaced with sutures in layers.

Code(s):

ØW3FØZZ   Control Bleeding in Abdominal Wall, Open Approach

Rationale:

Abdominal wall when indexed under "Control bleeding in" leads to a table in one of the anatomical regions body systems. Control (3) of the cesarean incision disruption required suturing of the Abdominal Wall (F) found in the Anatomical Regions, General (W) body system. An Open (Ø) approach was reported because the repair went through layers.

Spotlight
The root operation Control is also found in Anatomical Regions, Upper Extremities and Lower Extremities. For example, if postoperative or acute bleeding occurs in the right shoulder or left knee, and is not controlled with root operations such as Bypass, Detachment, Excision, Extraction, Reposition, Replacement, or Resection, the root operation Control is used with the body part Shoulder Region, Right or Knee Region, Left respectively.

Root Operation Detachment in Anatomical Regions, Upper and Lower Extremities

Root Operation		
Detachment (6)	Definition:	Cutting off all or a portion of the upper or lower extremities
	Explanation:	The body part value is the site of the detachment, with a qualifier if applicable to further specify the level where the extremity was detached

Detachment is only found in the Anatomical Regions, Upper Extremities and Anatomical Regions, Lower Extremities. Based on the definition of detachment, only the upper and lower extremities are applicable sites for an amputation. When detaching an extremity, many overlapping body layers are encountered, including skin, subcutaneous tissue, muscle, vessels, and bone. If all of the individual body layers (i.e., body systems) were reported separately, it would take multiple codes; however, the two anatomical regions, Upper or Lower Extremities, encompass all of the many body systems involved in an amputation procedure, which allows the procedure to be efficiently captured with one code. Open (Ø) approach is the only approach value option available in the Detachment tables.

A limited number of body part values do not include specific qualifier values that further identify the explicit portion of the body part being amputated; instead a whole region is captured in the detachment code. These limited body part values are listed in the following table along with illustrations and examples of their use.

Table 3.1. Detachment: Limited Body Parts

Anatomical Regions, Upper Extremity (X)	Anatomical Regions, Lower Extremity (Y)
Forequarter, Right (Ø)	Hindquarter, Right (2)
Forequarter, Left (1)	Hindquarter, Left (3)
Shoulder Region, Right (2)	Hindquarter, Bilateral (4)
Shoulder Region, Left (3)	Femoral Region, Right (7)
Elbow Region, Right (B)	Femoral Region, Left (8)
Elbow Region, Left (C)	Knee Region, Right (F)
	Knee Region, Left (G)

Figure 3.1. Detachment Forequarter

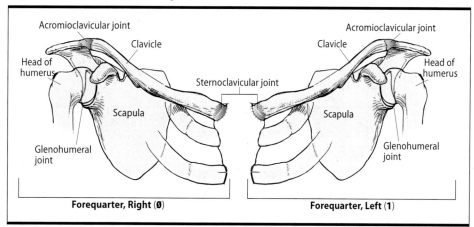

Figure 3.2. Detachment Hindquarter

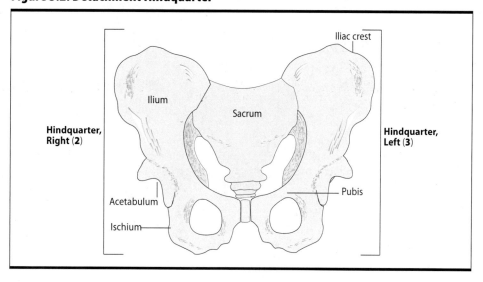

Limited Body Parts

Case Study 3.5. Amputation, Right Elbow Level

Code(s):

ØX6BØZZ   Detachment at Right Elbow Region, Open Approach

Rationale:

The Elbow Region, Right (B) has its own body part value and is not included in Upper or Lower Arm body parts.

Case Study 3.6. Amputation, Right Leg and Hip through Upper Ischium

Code(s):

ØY62ØZZ   Detachment at Right Hindquarter, Open Approach

Rationale:

The Hindquarter, Right (2) body part value includes amputation along any part of the hip bone. Hindquarter also has a bilateral body part, which would be used if applicable, rather than separate codes for left and right.

Case Study 3.7. Amputation, Right Forequarter

Code(s):

ØX6ØØZZ   Detachment at Right Forequarter, Open Approach

Rationale:

The Forequarter, Right (Ø) body part includes amputation along any part of the scapula and clavicle.

Case Study 3.8. Disarticulation, Left Knee Joint

Code(s):

ØY6GØZZ   Detachment at Left Knee Region, Open Approach

Rationale:

The Right (F) and Left (G) Knee Region have their own body part values and are not reported when below or above the knee amputation is documented. Above the knee is coded to **upper** leg body part with a qualifier of Low (3); and below the knee is coded to **lower** leg body part with a qualifier of High (1).

Specific qualifier values are used in the seventh-character position to represent the explicitly identified portion of the body part that is being amputated. The following tables, illustrations, and examples assist in determining the exact body part and qualifier value selection.

Arm and Leg

Table 3.2. Detachment Qualifier Definitions: Arms/Legs

Qualifier Definition	Upper Arm	Lower Arm	Upper Leg	Lower Leg
High: Amputation at proximal portion of the shaft of the:	Humerus	Radius/Ulna	Femur	Tibia/Fibula
Mid: Amputation at middle portion of the shaft of the:	Humerus	Radius/Ulna	Femur	Tibia/Fibula
Low: Amputation at the distal portion of the shaft of the:	Humerus	Radius/Ulna	Femur	Tibia/Fibula

Figure 3.3. Detachment of Humerus and Radius/Ulna

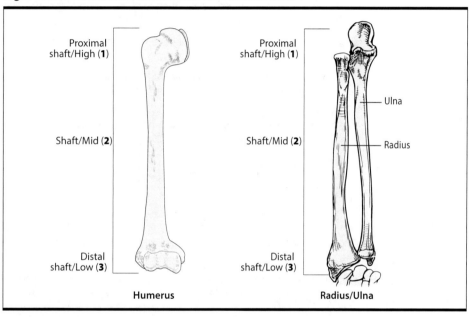

Figure 3.4. Detachment of Femur and Tibia/Fibula

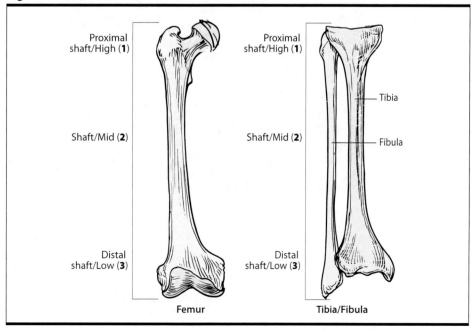

Arm and Leg

Case Study 3.9. Amputation, Right Forearm, Mid-shaft

Code(s):

0X6D0Z2   Detachment at Right Lower Arm, Mid, Open Approach

Rationale:

The right forearm includes the radius and ulna, reported with Lower Arm, Right (D) body part with a qualifier value of Mid (2). Low (3) would be the radius and ulna closest to the wrist and High (1) would be the area closest to the elbow.

Case Study 3.10. Amputation, Right Below-knee Proximal Tibia/Fibula

Code(s):

0Y6H0Z1   Detachment at Right Lower Leg, High, Open Approach

Rationale:

The qualifier High (1) refers to the portion of the tibia and fibula that is closest to the knee. Mid (2) is used for midshaft of the tibia and fibula and Low (3) is the portion closest to the ankle.

Case Study 3.11. Amputation, Midshaft Right Humerus

Code(s):

0X680Z2   Detachment at Right Upper Arm, Mid, Open Approach

Rationale:

The Upper Arm, Right (8) and Left (9) body parts only include the humerus. The qualifier Low (3) is used for amputations of the humerus just above the elbow, Mid (2) for midshaft, and High (1) for just below the shoulder. The shoulder region has its own body part value, which is used for other shoulder bones such as disarticulation at the shoulder joint.

Case Study 3.12. Amputation, Right Above-knee Distal Femur

Code(s):

0Y6C0Z3   Detachment at Right Upper Leg, Low, Open Approach

Rationale:

The Upper Leg, Right (C) and Left (D) body parts only include the femur. The qualifier Low (3) refers to the portion of the femur just above the knee, Mid (2) refers to midshaft, and High (1) just below the hip. An amputation through a hip bone is reported with a Hindquarter, Right (2), Left (3), or Bilateral (4) body part value.

Definitions
distal. In PCS when referring to a limb, the location furthest away from the point of attachment to the body.
proximal. In PCS when referring to a limb, the location closest to the point of attachment to the body.

Hand and Foot, Fingers and Toes

Table 3.3. Detachment Qualifier Definition: Hand/Foot/Fingers/Toes

Qualifier Definition	Hand	Foot
Ø Complete 1st through 5th Rays Ray: digit of hand or foot with corresponding metacarpus or metatarsus	Through carpo-metacarpal joint, wrist	Through tarso-metatarsal joint, ankle
4 Complete 1st Ray	Through carpo-metacarpal joint, thumb	Through tarso-metatarsal joint, great toe
5 Complete 2nd Ray	Through carpo-metacarpal joint, index finger	Through tarso-metatarsal joint, 2nd toe
6 Complete 3rd Ray	Through carpo-metacarpal joint, middle finger	Through tarso-metatarsal joint, 3rd toe
7 Complete 4th Ray	Through carpo-metacarpal joint, ring finger	Through tarso-metatarsal joint, 4th toe
8 Complete 5th Ray	Through carpo-metacarpal joint, little finger	Through tarso-metatarsal joint, little toe
9 Partial 1st Ray	Anywhere along shaft or head of metacarpal bone, thumb	Anywhere along shaft or head of metatarsal bone, great toe
B Partial 2nd Ray	Anywhere along shaft or head of metacarpal bone, index finger	Anywhere along shaft or head of metatarsal bone, 2nd toe
C Partial 3rd Ray	Anywhere along shaft or head of metacarpal bone, middle finger	Anywhere along shaft or head of metatarsal bone, 3rd toe
D Partial 4th Ray	Anywhere along shaft or head of metacarpal bone, ring finger	Anywhere along shaft or head of metatarsal bone, 4th toe
F Partial 5th Ray	Anywhere along shaft or head of metacarpal bone, little finger	Anywhere along shaft or head of metatarsal bone, little toe
Qualifier Definition	**Finger or Thumb**	**Toe**
Ø Complete: Amputation at the metacarpophalangeal/ metatarsal-phalangeal joint	Finger or thumb, any one 1st-5th	Toe, any one 1st-5th
1 High: Amputation anywhere along the proximal phalanx	Finger or thumb, any one 1st-5th	Toe, any one 1st-5th
2 Mid: Amputation through the proximal interphalangeal joint or anywhere along the middle phalanx	Finger or thumb, any one 1st-5th	Toe, any one 1st-5th
3 Low: Amputation through the distal interphalangeal joint or anywhere along the distal phalanx	Finger or thumb, any one 1st-5th	Toe, any one 1st-5th

Spotlight
Excision of a polydactyly digit is considered Detachment. The appropriate body part value is the one that is documented in the medical record as duplicative. The approach is Open. An example is discussed in *AHA Coding Clinic,* 2017, 2Q, 18.

Figure 3.5. Detachment Hand, Fingers, and Thumb

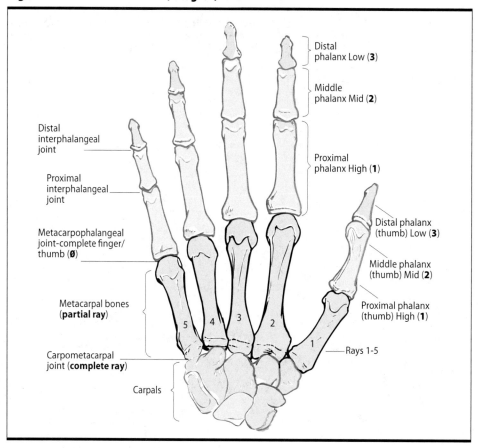

Hand and Foot

Case Study 3.13. Amputation, Second Ray Carpometacarpal Joint Left Hand

Code(s):

ØX6KØZ5   Detachment at Left Hand, Complete 2nd Ray, Open Approach

Rationale:
A Complete 2nd Ray (5) amputation is Detachment (6) of the entire index finger referred to as the 2nd ray, through the carpometacarpal joint of the Hand, Right (J) or Left (K).

Case Study 3.14. Disarticulation, Tarsometatarsal Joint of the Right Small Toe

Code(s):

ØY6MØZ8   Detachment at Right Foot, Complete 5th Ray, Open Approach

Rationale:
A Complete 5th Ray (8) amputation is Detachment (6) of the entire little toe, referred to as the 5th ray, through the tarsometatarsal joint of the Foot, Right (M) or Left (N).

Spotlight
Any detachment at the carpometacarpal or tarsometatarsal level is reported with a code from the Hand or Foot body part values as a Complete Ray. Any detachment at the metacarpal or metatarsal level is reported using the Hand or Foot body part values as a Partial Ray. Detachment involving any phalangeal joint is located in the Finger, Thumb, and Toes body part values.

Case Study 3.15. Amputation, Right Wrist Joint

Code(s):
ØX6JØZØ   Detachment at Right Hand, Complete, Open Approach

Rationale:
A complete amputation at the wrist joint is the Detachment (6) of all five rays and is coded as a Complete (Ø) Amputation of the Hand, Right (J) or Left (K).

Case Study 3.16. Amputation, Transmetatarsal of Foot at Left Big Toe

Code(s):
ØY6NØZ9   Detachment at Left Foot, Partial 1st Ray, Open Approach

Rationale:
Transmetatarsal is Detachment (6) performed across the shaft of the metatarsal bone of the first ray (big toe) rather than at the tarsometatarsal joint, and is reported as a Partial 1st Ray (9). Amputation across metatarsal bone rather than phalanx indicates that the Foot, Right (M) or Left (N) body part value is used rather than the 1st Toe, Right (P) or Left (Q) body part value.

Figure 3.6. Detachment Foot and Toes

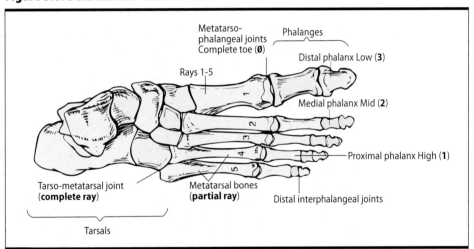

Fingers, Thumb, and Toes

Case Study 3.17. Disarticulation, DIP Joint, Right Thumb

Code(s):
ØX6LØZ3   Detachment at Right Thumb, Low, Open Approach

Rationale:
The qualifier Low (3) in this Detachment (6) means through the distal interphalangeal (DIP) joint of the Thumb, Right (L).

Case Study 3.18. Amputation, Left Fourth Toe Mid-proximal Phalanx

Code(s):
ØY6WØZ1   Detachment at Left 4th Toe, High, Open Approach

Rationale:
The qualifier High (1) in this Detachment (6) refers to any location along the proximal phalanx of the 4th Toe, Left (W).

Case Study 3.19. Disarticulation, Right Ring Finger, PIP Joint

Code(s):
ØX6SØZ2   Detachment at Right Ring Finger, Mid, Open Approach

Rationale:
The qualifier Mid (2) represents the Detachment (6) at the proximal interphalangeal (PIP) joint of the Ring Finger, Right (S).

Case Study 3.20. Amputation, Left Index Finger at Metacarpal-phalangeal Joint

Code(s):
ØX6PØZØ   Detachment at Left Index Finger, Complete, Open Approach

Rationale:
The qualifier Complete (Ø) is used for the Detachment (6) of Index Finger, Left (P) or Right (N) when the finger is amputated at the metacarpal-phalangeal joint but **not** carried down into the shaft of the metacarpal bone.

Practical Application for Guideline B2.1a using Root Operation Detachment

Case Study 3.21. Amputation, Below the Knee (BKA)

The patient was placed supine under general anesthesia. The right lower extremity was prepped and draped in the usual sterile fashion. An occlusive dressing was applied to the foot up to the level of the ankle. Anterior and posterior skin incisions were outlined with a marking pen. The anterior skin incision was made 6 cm below the tibial tuberosity and extended medially and laterally toward the edges of the gastrocnemius muscle. The skin incision was extended distally on either side parallel to the tibia for 12 cm to 15 cm, creating a posterior flap. The skin and subcutaneous tissues were incised down to the fascia. The greater and short saphenous veins were ligated and divided. The fascia and the muscles in the anterior and lateral compartment were divided, exposing the anterior tibial vessels, which were ligated and divided. The interosseous membrane was then incised. The tibial periosteum was incised circumferentially with electrocautery at the same level of the skin and muscle division. Using a periosteal elevator, the tibial periosteum was stripped proximally for 2 cm. The tibia was transected 2 cm proximal to the skin incision. The fibula was exposed, dissected circumferentially, and transected. The amputation was then completed, transecting the soleus muscle obliquely and the gastrocnemius muscle at the same level as the posterior flap. Bleeding soleal veins and posterior tibial and peroneal vessels were clamped and oversewn with 2-0 silk sutures. Sharp bony edges were filed, eliminating any bony prominences over the anterior aspect of the tibia. The fascia of the anterior and posterior muscle flaps were approximated with interrupted absorbable sutures. The skin was approximated with interrupted 3-0 nylon sutures/skin staples and dressed with 4 × 4 gauze, Kerlix, and an Ace bandage.

Code(s):
ØY6HØZ1   Detachment at Right Lower Leg, High, Open Approach

Rationale:
The tibial tuberosity is at the top of the tibia just below the patella. Detachment (6) was performed only 6 cm or approximately 2 inches below the tibial tuberosity, which is in the proximal or High (1) portion of the tibia/fibula shaft of the Lower Leg, Right (H) in the Anatomical Regions, Lower Extremities (Y) body system. This operative report describes all of the body layers that are involved in an amputation and demonstrates the efficiency of PCS with root operation Detachment (6) in the Anatomical Regions, Upper Extremities (X) and Lower Extremities (Y) body systems.

Case Study 3.22. Amputation, Transmetatarsal (Ray) Toe

The right foot was prepped and draped in a sterile fashion. An elliptical skin incision was performed at the level of the metatarsophalangeal joint at 30° to the longitudinal axis of the metatarsal bone of the second toe. A circular incision was performed at the metatarsophalangeal level and extended on the dorsal aspect of the foot along the metatarsal bone. The incision was deepened to the level of the bone, dividing all tendinous attachments. The periosteum overlying the metatarsal bone was elevated with a periosteal elevator. The bone was then transected at the midmetatarsal level, 1.5 cm to 2 cm proximal to the level of the skin incision. Hemostasis was secured and the wound was irrigated. The skin was closed with interrupted sutures of 4-0 nylon. The patient tolerated the procedure well and was taken to the postanesthesia care unit in stable condition.

Code(s):

ØY6MØZB   Detachment at Right Foot, Partial 2nd Ray, Open Approach

Rationale:
Although this Detachment (6) is referred to as a toe amputation, because it was performed midway along the metatarsal bone, it is represented by body part value Foot, Right (M). A "ray" includes the phalanx and the metatarsal bone of the toe. The cut was made along the metatarsal bone shaft of the second toe, or Partial 2nd Ray (B) rather than a Complete 2nd Ray (5), which includes the tarsometatarsal joint. Physician education may be necessary to ensure complete documentation of the toes and bones involved because an unspecified option does not exist.

Root Operation Drainage in the Anatomical Regions, General Body System

Root Operation		
Drainage (9)	Definition:	Taking or letting out fluids and/or gases from a body part
	Explanation:	The qualifier DIAGNOSTIC is used to identify drainage procedures that are biopsies

Although Drainage is found in several body systems, drainage of fluid from a body cavity is reported with a body part from the Anatomical Regions, General body system (e.g., Pericardial Cavity, Pelvic Cavity, Peritoneal Cavity, or Pleural Cavity, Right and Left).

Practical Application for Guideline B2.1a using Root Operation Drainage

Case Study 3.23. Paracentesis for Ascites

The abdomen was prepped and draped in a sterile fashion using chlorhexidine scrub. 1% lidocaine was used to numb the skin, soft tissue, and peritoneum. The paracentesis catheter was inserted and advanced with negative pressure until colored fluid was aspirated. Approximately three liters of ascitic fluid was drained. The catheter was removed and no leaking was noted. A band-aid was placed over the puncture wound. The patient tolerated the procedure well without any immediate complications.

Code(s):

ØW9G3ZZ   Drainage of Peritoneal Cavity, Percutaneous Approach

Rationale:
Ascites is a collection of fluid in the abdominal cavity, also referred to as the Peritoneal Cavity (G), which is located in the Anatomical Regions, General (W) body system. Paracentesis is a procedure in which a needle or catheter is used to drain fluid from the abdomen. The correct root operation Drainage (9) is performed via a catheter, which is a Percutaneous (3) approach. The device character

for No Device (Z) is the appropriate selection for this case as the drainage tube was removed at the end of the procedure. The paracentesis was performed for therapeutic purposes, which is No Qualifier (Z).

Spotlight
When a catheter (drainage device) is left in following a procedure, the sixth character is Drainage Device (Ø) instead of No Device (Z).

Case Study 3.24. Thoracentesis, Right Pleural Space

After obtaining written informed consent and after the appropriate infiltration level was confirmed by ultrasound, the patient's right side was prepped and draped in a sterile manner. 1% lidocaine was used to anesthetize the surrounding skin. A finder needle was used to locate fluid and clear yellow fluid was obtained. A 10-blade scalpel was used to make the incision. The thoracentesis catheter was threaded without difficulty and the right pleural space was aspirated. Initial fluid was clear. With positioning of the plastic catheter, there was some mild bleeding, which stopped by the end of the procedure. A total of 800 mL of blood-tinged fluid was removed without difficulty.

Code(s):

ØW993ZZ   Drainage of Right Pleural Cavity, Percutaneous Approach

Rationale:

Thoracentesis is removal of fluid from the space between the lungs and chest wall called the pleural "space." When referencing Drainage (9) in the index, it is important to note the distinction between the pleural space/cavity and the pleura itself in order to access the correct table in PCS. A pleural effusion is excess fluid in the pleural space (i.e. cavity). The tissue lining the lungs is the pleura. Body system value Anatomical Region, General (W) and body part Pleural Cavity, Right (9) are appropriate in this scenario. Only a small incision was made to fit the catheter, reported with Percutaneous (3) approach. This thoracentesis was performed for therapeutic purposes with the catheter withdrawn at the end of the procedure, reported with No Device (Z) and No Qualifier (Z).

Guideline B2.1b

B2.1b	Where the general body part values "upper" and "lower" are provided as an option in the Upper Arteries, Lower Arteries, Upper Veins, Lower Veins, Muscles and Tendons body systems, "upper" or "lower "specifies body parts located above or below the diaphragm respectively.
	Example: **Vein body parts above the diaphragm are found in the Upper Veins body system; vein body parts below the diaphragm are found in the Lower Veins body system.**

AHA Coding Clinic

2017, 1Q, 30   Insertion of Umbilical Artery Catheter

2017, 1Q, 31   Central Catheter Placement in Femoral Vein

2014, 3Q, 25   Revision of Transjugular Intrahepatic Portosystemic Shunt (TIPS)

The diaphragm is a sheet of fiber and muscle that rises and falls as a person breathes. As shown in the following illustration, the diaphragm neatly bisects the human body into upper and lower halves; PCS definitions indicate that body parts above the diaphragm are classified as "upper" and those below it are classified as "lower."

Figure 3.7. Diaphragm

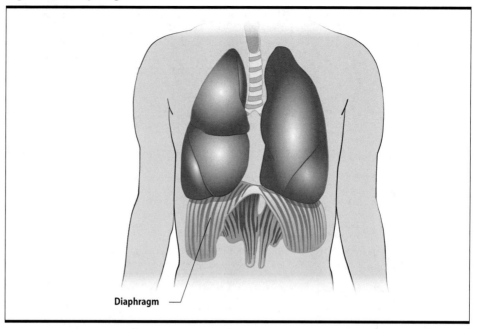

Diaphragm

Use of Character Meaning Tables

Occasionally it may be difficult to determine the correct body system in which a specific body part is found (e.g., body parts that are near the location of the diaphragm). In these circumstances, the Character Meaning Tables are a good resource and can be found in appendix I of this book or in Optum360's *ICD-10-PCS: The Complete Official Code Set* book. Each table defines the root operations, body parts, approaches, devices, and qualifiers available for use in a particular body system. These tables should not be used to build the full, seven-character code; they are simply a resource that assists the user in discerning the correct body system needed to begin building the code.

For example, attempting to locate the correct body systems for the **innominate artery**, **hemiazygos vein**, or **thoracolumbar vertebral joint** body parts may prove difficult unless detailed knowledge of the anatomy is known. The Character Meaning Tables provide a quick reference to determine the appropriate body system for these body parts. The partial tables listed in the following examples are from Optum360's Character Meaning Tables.

Definition
innominate artery. Also known as the brachiocephalic artery or the brachiocephalic trunk, the innominate artery branches directly off the arch of the aorta and supplies blood to the head and neck, as well as the right arm.

Upper Arteries (3) Body System Character Meaning Table

Operation–Character 3	Body Part–Character 4	Approach–Character 5	Device–Character 6	Qualifier–Character 7
1 Bypass	0 Internal Mammary Artery, Right	0 Open	0 Drainage Device	0 Upper Arm Artery, Right
5 Destruction	1 Internal Mammary Artery, Left	3 Percutaneous	2 Monitoring Device	1 Upper Arm Artery, Left OR Drug-Coated Balloon
7 Dilation	2 Innominate Artery	4 Percutaneous Endoscopic	3 Infusion Device	2 Upper Arm Artery, Bilateral
9 Drainage	3 Subclavian Artery, Right	X External	4 Intraluminal Device, Drug-eluting	3 Lower Arm Artery, Right
B Excision	4 Subclavian Artery, Left		5 Intraluminal Device, Drug-eluting, Two	4 Lower Arm Artery, Left
C Extirpation	5 Axillary Artery, Right		6 Intraluminal Device, Drug-eluting, Three	5 Lower Arm Artery, Bilateral

Figure 3.8. Map of Upper Arteries

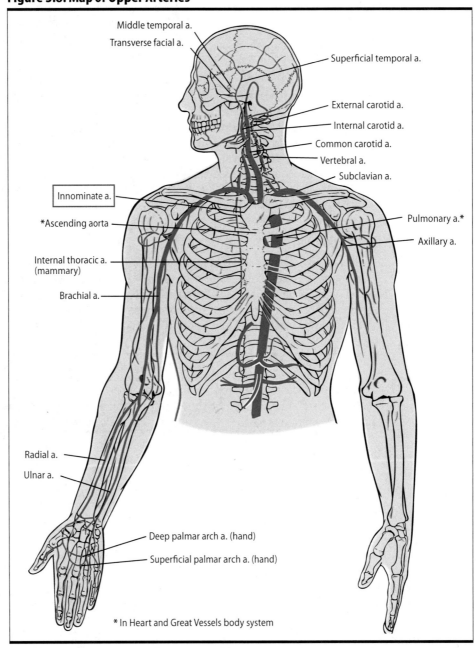

Middle temporal a.
Transverse facial a.
Superficial temporal a.
External carotid a.
Internal carotid a.
Common carotid a.
Vertebral a.
Subclavian a.
Innominate a.
*Ascending aorta
Pulmonary a.*
Axillary a.
Internal thoracic a. (mammary)
Brachial a.
Radial a.
Ulnar a.
Deep palmar arch a. (hand)
Superficial palmar arch a. (hand)

* In Heart and Great Vessels body system

Definition
hemiazygos vein. Vein that begins in the left ascending lumbar vein and receives blood from several of the intercostal veins on the left side of the body. One of the vessels that joins the hemiazygos vein is the left subcostal vein.

Upper Veins (5) Body System Character Meaning Table

Operation–Character 3		Body Part–Character 4		Approach–Character 5		Device–Character 6		Qualifier–Character 7	
1	Bypass	Ø	Azygos Vein	Ø	Open	Ø	Drainage Device	1	Drug-Coated Balloon
5	Destruction	1	Hemiazygos Vein	3	Percutaneous	2	Monitoring Device	X	Diagnostic
7	Dilation	3	Innominate Vein, Right	4	Percutaneous Endoscopic	3	Infusion Device	Y	Upper Vein
9	Drainage	4	Innominate Vein, Left	X	External	7	Autologous Tissue Substitute	Z	No Qualifier
B	Excision	5	Subclavian Vein, Right			9	Autologous Venous Tissue		

Figure 3.9. Map of Upper Veins

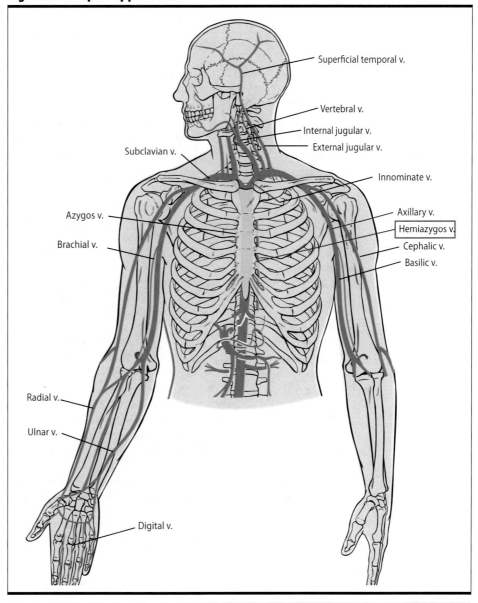

Definition
thoracolumbar vertebral joint. Joint that is included in the Upper Joints body system, along with the thoracic joints. However, the lumbar vertebral joints are contained in the Lower Joints body system.

Upper Joints (R) Body System Character Meaning Table

Operation–Character 3	Body Part–Character 4	Approach–Character 5	Device–Character 6	Qualifier–Character 7
H Insertion	6 Thoracic Vertebral Joint		A Interbody Fusion Device	Z No Qualifier
J Inspection	7 Thoracic Vertebral Joint, 2 to 7		B Spinal Stabilization Device, Interspinous Process	
N Release	8 Thoracic Vertebral Joint, 8 or more		C Spinal Stabilization Device, Pedicle-Based	
P Removal	9 Thoracic Vertebral Disc		D Spinal Stabilization Device, Facet Replacement	
Q Repair	A Thoracolumbar Vertebral Joint		J Synthetic Substitute	
R Replacement	B Thoracolumbar Vertebral Disc		K Nonautologous Tissue Substitute	

Practical Application for Guideline B2.1b

Case Study 3.25. Endarterectomy, Right Carotid Arteries
Indications: A 79-year-old with symptomatic severe right internal carotid artery stenosis, extending to the right common artery bifurcation, has opted to proceed with carotid endarterectomy. Options and complications have been discussed.
Technique: After the regional block anesthetic was administered, the patient's right neck was prepped and draped in the usual sterile manner. A longitudinal skin incision was made overlying the anterior border of the sternocleidomastoid, along with a 10-blade scalpel. The incision was deepened through the platysma with Bovie cautery and was retracted laterally. The internal jugular was identified along with the facial vein. The common internal and external carotid arteries were exposed and isolated. The vagus and hypoglossal nerves were identified and preserved. Intravenous heparin was administered and clamps were placed on the internal, external, and common carotid arteries in sequential order. Arteriotomy of the distal common was made and extended into the internal carotid artery. A highly friable plaque lesion was encountered from the bifurcation through the distal internal carotid artery. The plaque was transected proximally in the common carotid artery. In the distal internal carotid artery, the plaque was feathered off, leaving a smooth endpoint. An eversion endarterectomy of the external carotid artery was performed in continuity. All debris from the endarterectomized segment was removed. No tacking sutures were deemed necessary. A bovine patch was tailored and secured in position from the common carotid to the internal carotid using a Prolene suture. Flushing irrigation was conducted to restore flow to the external and internal carotid arteries. Hemostasis was achieved and multilayer closure was performed using Vicryl sutures. The patient tolerated the procedure and was moved to the recovery area in stable condition.

Code(s):

Ø3CKØZZ **Extirpation of Matter from Right Internal Carotid Artery, Open Approach**

Ø3UKØKZ **Supplement Right Internal Carotid Artery with Nonautologous Tissue Substitute, Open Approach**

Rationale:

The left common carotid artery originates from the aorta, just above the heart, and runs up the left side of the neck where it divides (bifurcates) into the left internal and external carotid arteries. The right common carotid originates from the subclavian artery, a branch off the aorta, and runs up through the right neck branching into the right internal and external carotid arteries. The external carotids supply blood to the face, scalp, jaws, and mouth. The internal carotids supply blood to the cerebral branches of the brain. When the internal carotids are occluded, it can cause a transient ischemic attack (TIA) or stroke (CVA).

Figure 3.10. Carotid Arteries

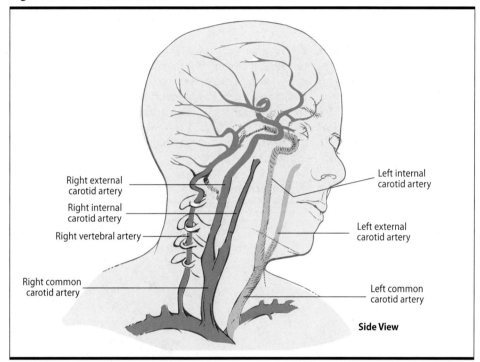

When consulting the Character Meaning Tables in appendix I, the carotid arteries, right and left, can only be found in the Medical and Surgical (Ø), Upper Arteries (3) table. With the first two characters of the code identified as Ø3, the Upper Arteries (3) body system and its associated tables can be used to build the code. In an endarterectomy, the vessel is incised and opened. The plaque is peeled away from the wall of the artery, which is reported with root operation Extirpation (C). Instructions in guideline B4.1c state that procedures performed on a continuous section of a tubular body part are coded to the furthest anatomical site from the point of entry. The Internal Carotid Artery, Right (K) is the body part reported. An Open (Ø) approach was used to access the site and perform the arteriotomy, which is an incision through the arterial wall and is inherent in the procedure as part of accessing the site.

PCS Guideline	
B4.1c	If a procedure is performed on a continuous section of a tubular body part, code the body part value corresponding to the furthest anatomical site from the point of entry.
	Example: A procedure performed on a continuous section of artery from the femoral artery to the external iliac artery with the point of entry at the femoral artery is coded to the external iliac body part.

Root Operation		
Extirpation (C)	Definition:	Taking or cutting out solid matter from a body part
	Explanation:	The solid matter may be an abnormal byproduct of a biological function or a foreign body; it may be imbedded in a body part or in the lumen of a tubular body part. The solid matter may or may not have been previously broken into pieces.
Supplement (U)	Definition:	Putting in or on biological or synthetic material that physically reinforces and/or augments the function of a portion of a body part
	Explanation:	The biological material is nonliving, or is living and from the same individual. The body part may have been previously replaced, and the SUPPLEMENT procedure is performed to physically reinforce and/or augment the function of the replaced body part.

Since ICD-10-PCS is a new coding system for capturing procedural codes, there are still many uncertainties. There will be more guidance in the years to come so it is important to stay abreast of these important updates. For instance, it may seem logical to assume that the patch graft is an inherent part of the procedure closure, but current guidance from *AHA Coding Clinic,* 2014, 4Q, 37; and 2016, 1Q, 31, instruct that a bovine patch artery repair is reported with the root operation Supplement (U) with the device value of Nonautologous Tissue Substitute (K). *AHA Coding Clinic,* 2016, 2Q, 11, discusses the separate reporting of the Dacron® patch graft using Supplement (U) with Synthetic Substitute (J).

Figure 3.11. Endarterectomy

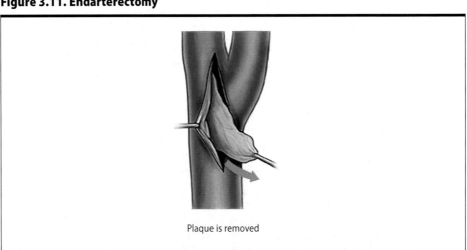

Plaque is removed

Case Study 3.26. Transjugular Intrahepatic Portosystemic Shunt (TIPS)

The patient was brought into the interventional radiology suite and sedation was administered. Skin and subcutaneous tissues were anesthetized with 1% buffered lidocaine. Under fluoroscopic guidance, the left internal jugular vein was accessed and a wire and catheter were passed down to the level of the hepatic vein. The needle was run to the identified portal vein and a balloon was inflated and a stent advanced across the liver to the portal vein. The catheter was exchanged for a 5-French pigtail catheter. With this in the portal vein, hemodynamic pressure monitoring was performed. After ensuring portal pressure decrease, the catheter was withdrawn and a bandage applied with pressure to the insertion site.

Code(s):

Ø6183J4   **Bypass Portal Vein to Hepatic Vein with Synthetic Substitute, Percutaneous Approach**

4AØ43B2   **Measurement of Venous Pressure, Portal, Percutaneous Approach**

Rationale:

For this example, it is important to understand the objective of the procedure and the anatomy involved. The normal pathway of blood through the liver begins with blood entering the liver through the portal vein. This blood is coming from the vessels of the intestines and spleen. Once filtered through the liver, the blood leaves the liver via the hepatic vein. Patients with portal hypertension have a damaged liver that cannot keep up with blood filtration causing the blood to find alternate routes or to back up into the portal vein.

The objective of the TIPS procedure is to alter the route of the blood around the liver (e.g., bypass), from the portal vein directly into the hepatic vein, to reduce the pressure on the blood vessels. The creation of an alternate route is best described by root operation Bypass (1).

Root Operation		
Bypass (1)	Definition:	Altering the route of passage of the contents of a tubular body part
	Explanation:	Rerouting contents of a body part to a downstream area of the normal route, to a similar route and body part, or to an abnormal route and dissimilar body part. Includes one or more anastomoses, with or without the use of a device.

Guideline B2.1b states that where the general body part values "upper" and "lower" are provided as an option, "upper" or "lower "specifies body parts located above or below the diaphragm respectively. Since the site of the procedure is at the liver level of the portal and hepatic vein, which is situated beneath the diaphragm, Lower Veins (6) is the appropriate body system.

This example demonstrates how the following Character Meaning Table can also be consulted to determine that the portal vein is part of the Lower Veins (6) body system. The next step is to use the index to find the correct table for this bypass procedure or go directly to the tables in the Lower Veins (6) body system.

Lower Veins (6) Body System Character Meaning Table

Operation–Character 3	Body Part–Character 4	Approach–Character 5	Device–Character 6	Qualifier–Character 7
1 Bypass	**Ø** Inferior Vena Cava	**Ø** Open	**Ø** Drainage Device	**4** Hepatic Vein
5 Destruction	**1** Splenic Vein	**3** Percutaneous	**2** Monitoring Device	**5** Superior Mesenteric Vein
7 Dilation	**2** Gastric Vein	**4** Percutaneous Endoscopic	**3** Infusion Device	**6** Inferior Mesenteric Vein
9 Drainage	**3** Esophageal Vein	**7** Via Natural or Artificial Opening	**7** Autologous Tissue Substitute	**9** Renal Vein, Right
B Excision	**4** Hepatic Vein	**8** Via Natural or Artificial Opening Endoscopic	**9** Autologous Venous Tissue	**B** Renal Vein, Left
C Extirpation	**5** Superior Mesenteric Vein	**X** External	**A** Autologous Arterial Tissue	**C** Hemorrhoidal Plexus
D Extraction	**6** Inferior Mesenteric Vein		**C** Extraluminal Device	**P** Pulmonary Trunk
H Insertion	**7** Colic Vein		**D** Intraluminal Device	**Q** Pulmonary Artery, Right
J Inspection	**8** Portal Vein		**J** Synthetic Substitute	**R** Pulmonary Artery, Left
L Occlusion	**9** Renal Vein, Right		**K** Nonautologous Tissue Substitute	**T** Via Umbilical Vein
N Release	**B** Renal Vein, Left		**Y** Other Device	**X** Diagnostic

The root operation Bypass (1) describes the objective of the procedures, which reroutes blood flow by bypassing the liver "from" the higher pressure Portal Vein (8) directly "to" the lower pressure hepatic vein. The Bypass (1) is created through a tract through the liver and is completed by placing a special mesh tube known as a stent, represented by Synthetic Substitute (J). Based on guideline B3.6a, the body part Portal Vein (8) identifies the body part bypassed "from" and the qualifier indicates the body part bypassed "to," which in this case is the Hepatic Vein (4). This procedure was performed through a catheter with external imaging represented by the Percutaneous (3) approach.

PCS Guideline
Bypass Procedures
B3.6a   Bypass procedures are coded by identifying the body part bypassed "from" and the body part bypassed "to." The fourth character body part specifies the body part bypassed from, and the qualifier specifies the body part bypassed to.   *Example:* Bypass from stomach to jejunum, stomach is the body part and jejunum is the qualifier.

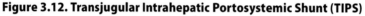

After the bypass is created, the portal hypertension or pressure is measured to ensure that it has sufficiently decreased. This is reported with the root operation Measurement (Ø) from the Measurement and Monitoring (4) section. The Venous (4) system is the body system where the Pressure (B) is being measured with the Percutaneous (3) approach. The qualifier further identifies Portal (2) as the specific venous system.

Figure 3.12. Transjugular Intrahepatic Portosystemic Shunt (TIPS)

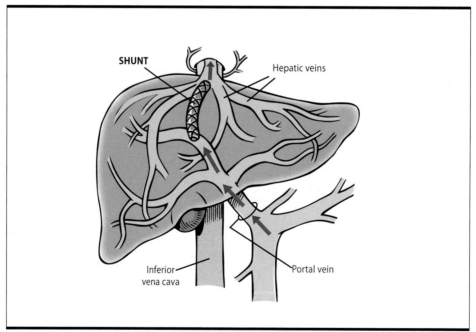

Table 3.4. Body System Table of Arteries and Veins

In addition to the Character Meaning Tables found in appendix I, the following table, which includes a complete listing of the Upper and Lower Veins, Upper and Lower Arteries, and the Heart and Great Vessels, assists in the selection of the correct body system.

Heart and Great Vessels	Upper Arteries	Lower Arteries	Upper Veins	Lower Veins
Ø Coronary Artery, 1 Artery	Ø Internal Mammary Artery, Rt	Ø Abdominal Aorta	Ø Azygos Vein	Ø Inferior Vena Cava
1 Coronary Artery, 2 Arteries	1 Internal Mammary Artery, Lt	1 Celiac Artery	1 Hemiazygos Vein	1 Splenic Vein
2 Coronary Artery, 3 Arteries	2 Innominate Artery	2 Gastric Artery	3 Innominate Vein, Rt	2 Gastric Vein
3 Coronary Artery, 4 or More Arteries	3 Subclavian Artery, Rt	3 Hepatic Artery	4 Innominate Vein, Lt	3 Esophageal Vein
4 Coronary Vein	4 Subclavian Artery, Lt	4 Splenic Artery	5 Subclavian Vein, Rt	4 Hepatic Vein
Q Pulmonary Art, Rt	5 Axillary Artery, Rt	5 Superior Mesenteric Artery	6 Subclavian Vein, Lt	5 Superior Mesenteric Vein
R Pulmonary Art, Lt	6 Axillary Artery, Lt	6 Colic Artery, Rt	7 Axillary Vein, Rt	6 Inferior Mesenteric Vein
S Pulmonary Vein, Rt	7 Brachial Artery, Rt	7 Colic Artery, Lt	8 Axillary Vein, Lt	7 Colic Vein
T Pulmonary Vein, Lt	8 Brachial Artery, Lt	8 Colic Artery, Mid	9 Brachial Vein, Rt	8 Portal Vein
V Superior Vena Cava	9 Ulnar Artery, Rt	9 Renal Artery, Rt	A Brachial Vein, Lt	9 Renal Vein, Rt
W Thoracic Aorta, Descending	A Ulnar Artery, Lt	A Renal Artery, Lt	B Basilic Vein, Rt	B Renal Vein, Lt
X Thoracic Aorta, Ascending/Arch	B Radial Artery, Rt	B Inf Mesenteric Art	C Basilic Vein, Lt	C Com Iliac Vein, Rt
Y Great Vessel	C Radial Artery, Lt	C Com Iliac Art, Rt	D Cephalic Vein, Rt	D Com Iliac Vein, Lt
	D Hand Artery, Rt	D Com Iliac Art, Lt	F Cephalic Vein, Lt	F Ext Iliac Vein, Rt
	F Hand Artery, Lt	E Int Iliac Artery, Rt	G Hand Vein, Rt	G Ext Iliac Vein, Lt
	G Intracranial Artery	F Internal Iliac Artery, Lt	H Hand Vein, Lt	H Hypogastric Vein, Rt
	H Common Carotid Artery, Rt	H External Iliac Artery, Rt	L Intracranial Vein	J Hypogastric Vein, Lt
	J Common Carotid Artery, Lt	J External Iliac Artery, Lt	M Internal Jugular Vein, Rt	M Femoral Vein, Rt
	K Internal Carotid Artery, Rt	K Femoral Artery, Rt	N Internal Jugular Vein, Lt	N Femoral Vein, Lt
	L Internal Carotid Artery, Lt	L Femoral Artery, Lt	P External Jugular Vein, Rt	P Saphenous Vein, Rt
	M External Carotid Artery, Rt	M Popliteal Artery, Rt	Q External Jugular Vein, Lt	Q Saphenous Vein, Lt
	N External Carotid Artery, Lt	N Popliteal Artery, Lt	R Vertebral Vein, Rt	T Foot Vein, Rt
	P Vertebral Artery, Rt	P Anterior Tibial Artery, Rt	S Vertebral Vein, Lt	V Foot Vein, Lt
	Q Vertebral Artery, Lt	Q Anterior Tibial Artery, Lt	T Face Vein, Rt	Y Lower Vein
	R Face Artery	R Post Tibial Art, Rt	V Face Vein, Lt	
	S Temporal Artery, Rt	S Post Tibial Art, Lt	Y Upper Vein	
	T Temporal Artery, Lt	T Peroneal Art, Rt		
	U Thyroid Artery, Rt	U Peroneal Art, Lt		
	V Thyroid Artery, Lt	V Foot Artery, Rt		
	Y Upper Artery	W Foot Artery, Lt		
		Y Lower Artery		

Chapter 4. Root Operation Guidelines

Root Operation Overview

Root Operation: Character 3

Character 1	Character 2	Character 3	Character 4	Character 5	Character 6	Character 7
Section	Body System	Root Operation	Body Part	Approach	Device	Qualifier

The root operation, specified by the third character, is the most essential building block of ICD-10-PCS codes. It defines the objective, or what was actually performed during the procedure, and is typically used as a main term in the alphabetic index. Because the terms used in the documentation by the physician may not be the same terms as the root operations, understanding the definition of each root operation and the types of procedures typically assigned to each is essential for appropriate ICD-10-PCS coding. The full Root Operation Definitions table, found in appendix C, includes the definitions, explanations, and examples of the 31 root operations found in the Medical and Surgical Section and in the following additional sections that utilize the root operation value:

- Administration

- Chiropractic

- Extracorporeal or Systemic Assistance and Performance

- Extracorporeal or Systemic Therapies

- Measurement and Monitoring

- Obstetrics

- Osteopathic

- Other Procedures

- Placement

The root operation guidelines comprise the majority of the PCS Official Guidelines and help to further expand upon the definition and explanations that are provided for each root operation. The first two guidelines are considered general guidelines and apply to all of the remaining root operation guidelines.

General Guidelines

Guidelines B3.1a and B3.1b provide instruction on the proper application of the root operation definition and explanation. The root operation, which is the third character in each PCS code, defines the objective of the procedure and determines the table from which the rest of the character values are selected to construct the seven-character code. The general guidelines are vital to the interpretation of all root operations. Guideline B3.1a explains, in basic terms, the importance of the root operation definition, while guideline B3.1b relates to the components and procedural steps that are inherent in or integral to the performance of the procedure as provided in the definition and explanation.

Guideline B3.1a

B3.1a	In order to determine the appropriate root operation, the full definition of the root operation as contained in the PCS Tables must be applied.

AHA Coding Clinic

2018, 1Q, 11	Repair of Internal Hernia at Petersen Space
2017, 4Q, 107	Total Ankle Replacement versus Revision
2017, 2Q, 12	Compartment Syndrome and Fasciotomy of Foot
2017, 2Q, 13	Compartment Syndrome and Fasciotomy of Leg

Each root operation has a precise definition that describes the objective of the surgical procedure. Most definitions are comprised of more than one concept, all which must be applied to complete the meaning. Since root operations define the procedure's objective, numerous *AHA Coding Clinics* make reference to the root operation definitions. Only the few that specifically call out Guideline B3.1a are listed here.

Root Operation Definition Examples

Root Operation		
Resection (T)	Definition:	Cutting out or off, without replacement, all of a body part

The full definition of Resection (T) consists of three concepts:

1. Cutting out or off

2. Without replacement

3. All of a body part

Root Operation		
Excision (B)	Definition:	Cutting out or off, without replacement, a portion of a body part
	Explanation:	The qualifier DIAGNOSTIC is used to identify excision procedures that are biopsies

The definition of Excision (B) consists of three concepts:

1. Cutting out or off

2. Without replacement

3. A portion of a body part

Excision (B) and Resection (T) contain two of the same concepts: each procedure involves "cutting out or off" and the procedure is done "without replacement." However, in a Resection (T), "all of a body part" is removed, while in Excision (B) a "portion of a body part" is removed. If the excised or resected body part is replaced or transplanted in the same operative episode, the root operation changes to Replacement (R) or Transplantation (Y) since the definition of Excision (B) and Resection (T) clearly state "without replacement."

Root Operation		
Replacement (R)	Definition:	Putting in or on a biological or synthetic material that physically takes the place and/or function of all or a portion of a body part
	Explanation:	The body part may have been taken out or replaced, or may be taken out, physically eradicated, or rendered nonfunctional during the REPLACEMENT procedure. A REMOVAL procedure is coded for taking out the device used in a previous replacement procedure.

The definition of Replacement (R) consists of three concepts:

1.   Putting in or on

2.   Biological or synthetic material

3.   That physically takes the place and or function of all or a portion of a body part

Root Operation		
Transplantation (Y)	Definition:	Putting in or on all or a portion of a living body part taken from another individual or animal to physically take the place and/or function of all or a portion of a similar body part
	Explanation:	The native body part may or may not be taken out, and the transplanted body part may take over all or a portion of its function

The definition of Transplantation (Y) consists of four concepts:

1.   Putting in or on

2.   All or a portion of a living body part

3.   From another individual or animal

4.   To physically take the place and/or function of all or a portion of a similar body part

Replacement (R) and Transplantation (Y) contain two of the same concepts: each procedure involves "putting in or on" and the material put in or on "physically takes the place and/or function of all or a portion of a body part." If the body part is replaced with a device consisting of "biological or synthetic material," the root operation Replacement (R) best describes the intent. If replaced by a living body part from another individual or animal, the root operation Transplantation (Y) is appropriate.

Root Operation Explanation

Most root operation definitions include not only a definition, but also an explanation that expands the definition. In addition, root operation definitions may include examples that demonstrate correct usage. The entire definition, which includes the explanation, must be taken into consideration when determining the root operation that best matches the objective of the procedure as documented in the operative report.

Spotlight
Two root operations in the Medical and Surgical section, Insertion (H) and Resection (T), have only a definition and includes/examples in the definitions table.

For the root operation Excision (B), the explanation in the preceding example expands on the definition of Excision with information regarding the use of the qualifier Diagnostic (X) to identify a biopsy. The explanations for Replacement (R) and Transplantation (Y) instruct that removal of the body part is included in these root operations. While removal of the body part is not reported separately, the Replacement (R) explanation does clarify that when a device used in a previous replacement procedure is taken out during the same operative session, Removal (P) is also coded.

The following excerpt from the CMS Official ICD-10-PCS Manual shows the definition, explanation, and includes/examples for three root operations.

ICD-10-PCS Value	Definition
Alteration	**Definition:** Modifying the anatomic structure of a body part without affecting the function of the body part **Explanation:** Principal purpose is to improve appearance **Includes/Examples:** Face lift, breast augmentation
Bypass	**Definition:** Altering the route of passage of the contents of a tubular body part **Explanation:** Rerouting contents of a body part to a downstream area of the normal route, to a similar route and body part, or to an abnormal route and dissimilar body part. Includes one or more anastomoses, with or without the use of a device. **Includes/Examples:** Coronary artery bypass, colostomy formation
Change	**Definition:** Taking out or off a device from a body part and putting back an identical or similar device in or on the same body part without cutting or puncturing the skin or a mucous membrane **Explanation:** All CHANGE procedures are coded using the approach EXTERNAL **Includes/Examples:** Urinary catheter change, gastrostomy tube change

A thorough review of the information contained in this excerpt demonstrates the level of detail contained in the definitions and explanations of root operations. For example:

- Alteration (Ø)
  - modifies the structure
  - must not affect the function of the body part
  - used only for cosmetic purposes
- Bypass (1)
  - used only for tubular body parts
  - reroutes the passage of the contents
  - reroutes contents downstream

- can reroute to a similar or abnormal route
- can reroute to a similar or dissimilar body part
- includes one or more anastomoses (surgical connections)
- can be accomplished with or without a device
- Change (2)
    - only involves removal and replacing a device, not a body part
    - device that is changed may be identical or similar
    - device changed must be removed from and replaced in or on the same body part
    - procedures can only be coded to the approach External

Practical Application for Guideline B3.1a

This section provides a number of case studies that require determining the objective of the procedure as documented in the operative report and applying the full root operation definition to determine the correct root operation.

Case Study 4.1. Mastectomy with Reconstruction

Procedure: Bilateral mastectomy with bilateral free TRAM flap reconstruction.

Starting with the right breast, the plain incision was marked along the skin. Tissues and flaps were injected with Marcaine with epinephrine solution and a transverse elliptical incision was made in the breast of the skin to include the nipple areolar complex, as well as the recent biopsy site. Breast tissue along with the pectoralis major fascia was dissected off the pectoralis major muscle. The dissection was started medially and extended laterally toward the left axilla. The breast was removed. The same procedure was done on the left side. The abdomen was marked and rectus flaps dissected on the right and left side. Each flap was transferred to the chest area and venous and arterial anastomosis was performed with good blood flow. Drains were placed in the patient's abdomen and the abdomen was closed in three layers. The patient tolerated the procedure well and was transferred in stable condition.

Code(s):

ØHRVØ76	Replacement of Bilateral Breast using Transverse Rectus Abdominis Myocutaneous Flap, Open Approach
ØKBKØZZ	Excision of Right Abdomen Muscle, Open Approach
ØKBLØZZ	Excision of Left Abdomen Muscle, Open Approach

Rationale:
Although the entire right and left breasts are resected during this operative session, meeting the objective of "all of a body part being cut out or off," this procedure also involves replacement of the breasts with autologous tissue in the same operative episode. Because the definition of Resection (T) stipulates that replacement is not performed, Resection (T) cannot be coded. The root operation Replacement (R) is defined as "putting in or on biological or synthetic material that physically takes the place and/or function of all or a portion of a body part." The explanation of Replacement (R) further identifies that the body part may have been taken out before or is taken out during the current replacement procedure. For this scenario, the breasts are removed AND replaced in one operative session, capturing the full definition of Replacement (R).

Spotlight

Multiple procedures guideline B3.2c does not apply to the mastectomy with breast reconstruction during the same surgical episode as the resection and reconstruction procedures are not two distinct and independent objectives being performed on the breasts. Instead, one root operation, Replacement (R), encompasses the removal and reconstruction of the breasts in one singular objective.

Only one code is needed for the replacement of the right and left breast, based on the bilateral body part guideline B4.3. If the identical procedure is performed on both sides of a body part and a bilateral body part value exists, only a single procedure code is used. In this case, the correct body part is Breast, Bilateral (V). See the following Bilateral body part guideline.

PCS Guideline
Bilateral body part values
B4.3   Bilateral body part values are available for a limited number of body parts. If the identical procedure is performed on contralateral body parts, and a bilateral body part value exists for that body part, a single procedure is coded using the bilateral body part value. If no bilateral body part value exists, each procedure is coded separately using the appropriate body part value. *Example:* The identical procedure performed on both fallopian tubes is coded once using the body part value Fallopian Tube, Bilateral. The identical procedure performed on both knee joints is coded twice using the body part values Knee Joint, Right and Knee Joint, Left.

An Open (Ø) approach was used to remove and replace the breasts.

The muscle grafts are captured by the device value Autologous Tissue (7) since the graft material was taken from the patient's own body.

The qualifier value in this code provides additional information about the type of autologous tissue graft used to replace the breast. In this case study, the breasts are replaced using a Transverse Rectus Abdominis Myocutaneous Flap (6), more commonly called a TRAM flap. A TRAM flap consists of abdominal skin, subcutaneous fat, and the rectus abdominis muscle, as well as the blood vessels.

Based on guideline B3.9, Excision for graft, an autograft obtained from a different body part in order to complete the objective of the procedure is coded separately. The rectus abdominis muscles are two large muscles on the right and left side of the anterior aspect of the abdomen extending from the xiphoid process to the symphysis pubis. In order to reconstruct both breasts, the right and the left rectus abdominis muscles, along with the overlying tissue and blood supply, are excised. In table ØKB there is not a specific body part value for rectus abdominis muscle. According to the Body Part Definitions (appendix E), the rectus abdominis muscle is included in the Right (K) and Left (L) Abdominal Muscle body part values. Replacing both breasts with a free TRAM flap requires excision of the right and left rectus abdominis muscles. Two codes are needed for the excision of the right and left abdominal muscle because no bilateral body part value is offered in table ØKB.

PCS Guideline
Excision for graft
B3.9   If an autograft is obtained from a different procedure site in order to complete the objective of the procedure, a separate procedure is coded. *Example:* Coronary bypass with excision of saphenous vein graft, excision of saphenous vein is coded separately.

Spotlight
If the flaps are moved into place with the vascular and nervous supply intact rather than dissected and anastomosed, the appropriate root operation is Transfer (X). The definition of Transfer (X) does not include the removal of the body part, necessitating a second code for the Resection (T) of the breasts. No codes are reported for Excision (B) of the grafts.

Case Study 4.2. Revision, Left Knee

A patient presents to surgery for revision of left total knee replacement. The previous components were removed and new femoral, tibial, and patellar components were inserted. Cement was used to secure the new components.

Code(s):

ØSRDØJ9	**Replacement of Left Knee Joint with Synthetic Substitute, Cemented, Open Approach**
ØSPDØJZ	**Removal of Synthetic Substitute from Left Knee Joint, Open Approach**

Rationale:

Although the surgeon documented revision, the correct root operation according to ICD-10-PCS definitions is Replacement (R). Revision is used when the objective of the procedure is to correct the position or function of a previously placed device, without removing the entire device.

Root Operation		
Replacement (R)	Definition:	Putting in or on a biological or synthetic material that physically takes the place and/or function of all or a portion of a body part
	Explanation:	The body part may have been taken out or replaced, or may be taken out, physically eradicated, or rendered nonfunctional during the REPLACEMENT procedure. A REMOVAL procedure is coded for taking out the device used in a previous replacement procedure.
Revision (W)	Definition:	Correcting, to the extent possible, a portion of a malfunctioning device or the position of a displaced device
	Explanation:	Revision can include correcting a malfunctioning or displaced device by taking out or putting in components of the device such as a screw or pin

The procedure is taking place on the body part Knee Joint, Left (D), which can be found in the Lower Joints (S) body system. Synthetic Substitute (J) is used for the device and the qualifier is Cemented (9). The only approach listed in Table ØSR is Open (Ø).

Guideline B3.1a directs the coder to review the entire definition for proper code assignment. The explanation for Replacement specifies that removal of the device should also be coded. Using root operation Removal (P), the correct code assignment is body system Lower Joints (S), body part Knee Joint, Left (D), and device Synthetic Substitute (J).

Guideline B3.1b

Guideline B3.1b explains how the root operation definition and explanation, when used together and in their entirety, help identify the parts of a procedure that are inherent to the operation.

B3.1b	**Components of a procedure specified in the root operation definition and explanation are not coded separately. Procedural steps necessary to reach the operative site and close the operative site, including anastomosis of a tubular body part, are also not coded separately.** ***Examples:*** **Resection of a joint as part of a joint replacement procedure is included in the root operation definition of Replacement and is not coded separately.** **Laparotomy performed to reach the site of an open liver biopsy is not coded separately. In a resection of sigmoid colon with anastomosis of descending colon to rectum, the anastomosis is not coded separately.**

AHA Coding Clinic

2018, 1Q, 13	Bilateral Cuboid Osteotomy for Repair of Congenital Talipes Equinovarus
2018, 1Q, 15	Pubic Symphysis Fusion
2017, 3Q, 8	Removal of Silo and Closure of Gastroschisis
2017, 3Q, 10	Repair of Chiari Malformation
2017, 3Q, 17	Posterior Sagittal Anorectoplasty
2017, 3Q, 17	Resection of Schwannoma and Placement of Duragen and Lorenz Cranial Plating System
2017, 1Q, 29	Newborn Resuscitation using Positive Pressure Ventilation
2017, 1Q, 38	Mitral Valve Repair and Chordae Tendineae Transfer
2016, 4Q, 134	Changes to the ICD-10-PCS Official Guidelines for Coding and Reporting
2016, 3Q, 3	Stoma Creation & Takedown Procedures
2016, 3Q, 26	Insertion of Gastrostomy Tube
2016, 3Q, 27	Endoscopic Retrograde Cholangiopancreatography with Sphincterotomy and Insertion of Pancreatic Stent
2016, 3Q, 31	Femoral to Peroneal Artery Bypass with In-Situ Saphenous Vein Graft and Lysis of Valves
2016, 3Q, 32	Rotator Cuff Repair, Tenodesis, Decompression, Acromioplasty and Coracoplasty
2016, 3Q, 33	Traumatic Amputation of Fingers with Further Revision Amputation
2016, 3Q, 39	Infrarenal Abdominal Aortic Aneurysm Repair with Iliac Graft Extension
2016, 2Q, 22	Esophageal Lengthening Collis Gastroplasty with Nissen Fundoplication and Hiatal Hernia
2016, 2Q, 23	Thoracic Outlet Syndrome and Release of Brachial Plexus
2016, 2Q, 29	Decompressive Craniectomy with Cryopreservation and Storage of Bone Flap
2016, 1Q, 16	Pulmonary Valvotomy and Dilation of Annulus
2015, 3Q, 14	Endoprosthetic Replacement of Humerus and Tendon Reattachment
2015, 3Q, 15	Vascular Ring Surgery with Release of Esophagus and Trachea
2015, 3Q, 29	Placement of Adhesion Barrier
2015, 2Q, 7	Urinary Calculi Fragmentation and Evacuation
2014, 4Q, 42	Right Colectomy with Side-to-Side Functional End-to-End Anastomosis
2014, 3Q, 13	Orthotopic Liver Transplant with End to Side Cavoplasty
2014, 3Q, 28	Ileostomy Takedown and Parastomal Hernia Repair
2014, 3Q, 30	Spinal Fusion & Fixation Instrumentation
2014, 3Q, 31	Corneal Amniotic Membrane Transplantation
2014, 1Q, 3-4	Lysis of Adhesions
2013, 2Q, 37	Coronary Artery Release Performed During Coronary Artery Bypass Graft

This guideline addresses components of procedures that are not reported separately. Some of these procedural components are specifically identified in the root operation and explanation. Other components may not be specifically identified, but because these components are integral to the procedure they are not reported separately.

Spotlight
Most root operations have a definition and an explanation. The explanation contains supplementary information related to the root operation, such as what is or is not included. It is essential that both the definition and the explanation be reviewed when choosing a root operation.

To illustrate a case where the definition and explanation specifically identify integral components, consider the root operations Fragmentation (F) and Extirpation (C). Both involve breaking solid matter into pieces. The explanation for Fragmentation (F) specifies that the solid matter is broken into pieces but **is not removed;** when Extirpation (C) is performed, these solid matter pieces **are removed.** The breaking into pieces of the solid matter, Fragmentation (F), is considered a component of Extirpation (C) and therefore should not be coded separately (*AHA Coding Clinic,* 2015, 2Q, 7).

Root Operation		
Extirpation (C)	Definition:	Taking or cutting out solid matter from a body part
	Explanation:	The solid matter may be an abnormal byproduct of a biological function or a foreign body; it may be imbedded in a body part or in the lumen of a tubular body part. The solid matter may or may not have been previously broken into pieces.
Fragmentation (F)	Definition:	Breaking solid matter in a body part into pieces
	Explanation:	Physical force (e.g., manual, ultrasonic) applied directly or indirectly is used to break the solid matter into pieces. The solid matter may be an abnormal byproduct of a biological function or a foreign body. The pieces of solid matter are not taken out.

Since not all integral components are specifically identified in the root operation definition or explanation, it is important to understand which components are integral to a procedure and which are separately reportable. In some instances, the inherent components are easily identified, such as the procedural steps required to access or close the operative site. One common example of an inherent procedure is anastomosis following excision or resection of a segment of the colon. Once all or a portion of the colon segment is removed, the remaining sections of the colon must be rejoined, or anastomosed, for the colon to be functional again and to not spill fecal matter into the abdominal cavity. Therefore, the anastomosis is a procedural step and is an integral component of the procedure and is not reported separately. Further education and physician queries may be required to determine whether one step of a procedure is routinely included in another.

Spotlight
Much has been published in *AHA Coding Clinics* pertaining to integral components of procedures. An extensive list of dates and titles is provided after Guideline B3.1b in this resource to assist in locating the specific advice for accurate reporting of many specific procedures.

Practical Application for Guideline B3.1b

> ### Case Study 4.3. Takedown, Hartmann Ostomy
>
> The patient was brought to the operating room, placed in the lithotomy position, and prepped and draped in sterile fashion. The rectum was cleaned and irrigated prior to the sterile preparation. The ostomy site was closed with a running silk suture. A midline incision was made and the abdomen opened. A short segment of the descending colon was mobilized, visually inspected, and the colostomy portion of the bowel was trimmed. A 2.0 prolene suture was used as a purse-string and the anvil of a (25 mm to 34 mm range) circular EEA stapler was placed and the purse-string was tied. The descending colon was reduced inside the abdominal cavity. The fascia was approximated with a 0 Vicryl purse-string suture and the splenic flexure mobilized to ensure a tension-free anastomosis. The omentum was removed from the pelvis and rectum identified. This was further mobilized. There was enough length after mobilization had taken place to perform a side-to-side colorectal anastomosis. A GIA 60 laparoscopic green load was performed followed by a TA60 to close the enterotomies. The fascia of the ostomy site was closed with number 1 PDS suture in a figure-of-eight fashion and approximated the abdominal wall with running number 1 looped PDS suture. Skin incision was approximated with skin staples, and the ostomy site was approximated with skin staples.

Code(s):

ØDSMØZZ   Reposition Descending Colon, Open Approach

Rationale:

Hartmann procedures are often performed when a diseased portion of the colon needs to be emergently excised followed by the creation of a temporary stoma. The distal, nonfunctioning end is sealed and left in the abdominal cavity. When the colon has had time to heal, the procedure is taken down or reversed and intestinal continuity restored. To perform the reversal, the stoma and distal ends of the bowel are reanastomosed and the bowel is placed back into its proper anatomical abdominal location. According to *AHA Coding Clinic*, 2016, 3Q, 3, the root operation Reposition (S) best describes the objective of the procedure. According to guideline B3.1b, the anastomosis of the colon and rectum are considered components of the procedure and are not coded separately. Often the ends of the bowel are slightly excised or trimmed to ensure a neat anastomosis. This trimming is also considered integral to the procedure. The operative report indicates that the Descending Colon (M) was the body part "reduced" or moved back into its normal anatomical location via an Open (Ø) approach.

Root Operation		
Reposition (S)	Definition:	Moving to its normal location, or other suitable location, all or a portion of a body part
	Explanation:	The body part is moved to a new location from an abnormal location, or from a normal location where it is not functioning correctly. The body part may or may not be cut out or off to be moved to the new location.

Case Study 4.4. Removal, Hardware from Left Humerus

The left elbow was prepared and draped in the usual sterile fashion. A small stab wound was made directly over the prominent screws going into the humerus medially and laterally. Dissection was carried down bluntly in the screw head with hemostat, and the screw head was delivered through the incision. Both screws were removed without difficulty. Great care was taken to avoid the ulnar nerve, which was located lateral to the incision and was palpable throughout the procedure. The incision was closed with 5-0 nylon interrupted sutures, and the dressing consisted of Owens gauze, 4x4; sterile Webril; and a posterior mold.

Code(s):

ØPPGØ4Z   **Removal of Internal Fixation Device from Left Humeral Shaft, Open Approach**

Rationale:

Removal of internal hardware cannot be performed without first incising the skin and/or other body layers to reach the internal hardware. Since the stab wound and dissection are procedural steps necessary to reach the operative site, they are part of the approach and are not coded separately. This is captured with fifth character Open (Ø) for the approach method. The sutures and dressing are also necessary and expected procedural steps required to properly close the operative site and keep the operative site free from infection and are not reported separately.

Root Operation		
Removal (P)	Definition:	Taking out or off a device from a body part
	Explanation:	If a device is taken out and a similar device put in without cutting or puncturing the skin or mucous membrane, the procedure is coded to the root operation CHANGE. Otherwise, the procedure for taking out a device is coded to the root operation REMOVAL.

Root operation Removal (P) is used strictly for the removal of a device, not a body part. Screws that were previously inserted into the left humerus for the purpose of fixating a prior fracture are removed and are captured with the sixth-character device value Internal Fixation Device (4). The body system Upper Bones (P) contains the correct body part Humeral Shaft, Left (G). The Body Part Definitions table in appendix E verifies that the Humeral Shaft body part value includes the distal end of the humerus, which is located in the vicinity of the elbow as indicated in the operative report.

Body Part Definitions Table	
ICD-10-PCS Value	**Definition**
Humeral Head, Left **Humeral Head, Right**	Includes: Greater tuberosity Lesser tuberosity Neck of humerus (anatomical)(surgical)
Humeral Shaft, Left **Humeral Shaft, Right**	Includes: Distal humerus Humerus, distal Lateral epicondyle of humerus Medial epicondyle of humerus

Multiple Procedures

Coding multiple procedures is required under a number of circumstances. The guidelines in this section are general multiple procedure guidelines that address four instances in which reporting more than one code is necessary to completely describe the procedure. The general multiple procedure guidelines address the following circumstances:

- Same root operation on distinct body parts defined by different body part value. When a procedure represented by the same root operation is performed on different body parts each defined by its own individual PCS body part value, multiple codes are assigned for each body part represented by a separate body part value.

- Same root operation on distinct body parts represented by the same body part value. When the same root operation is repeated on anatomically different body parts that are all classified into the same body part value, the same code is repeated for each separate and distinct anatomical body part.

- Distinct root operations. When multiple root operations with different objectives are performed on the same body part as defined by the same body part value, a code for each distinct root operation is assigned.

- Initial approach converted to another approach. When a procedure is attempted using one approach but must be converted to another approach to complete the procedure, a code is assigned for each approach.

In addition to the general multiple procedure guidelines covered here, there are multiple procedure guidelines specific to certain body systems, root operations, and body parts that are addressed throughout this book.

A final consideration when coding multiple procedures is the selection of the principal procedure. CMS outlines specific instructions to follow in that determination, which can be found in the *ICD-10-PCS Official Coding Guidelines for Coding and Reporting* in appendix A of this book.

Guideline B3.2a

B3.2	**During the same operative episode, multiple procedures are coded if:**
	a. The same root operation is performed on different body parts as defined by distinct values of the body part character.
	Examples: **Diagnostic excision of liver and pancreas are coded separately.**
	Excision of lesion in the ascending colon and excision of lesion in the transverse colon are coded separately.

AHA Coding Clinic

2018, 1Q, 15	Pubic Symphysis Fusion
2017, 3Q, 7	Senning Procedure (Atrial Switch)
2017, 3Q, 9	Ileocolic Intussusception Reduction via Air Enema
2017, 2Q, 21	Arthroscopic Anterior Cruciate Ligament Revision using Autograft with Anterolateral Ligament Reconstruction
2017, 1Q, 20	Preparatory Nasal Adhesion Repair Before Definitive Cleft Palate Repair
2017, 1Q, 52	Further Distal Phalangeal Amputation
2016, 4Q, 89	Branched and Fenestrated Endograft Repair of Aneurysms
2016, 4Q, 134	Changes to the ICD-10-PCS Official Guidelines for Coding and Reporting
2016, 2Q, 12	Resection of Malignant Neoplasm of Infratemporal Fossa
2016, 2Q, 17	Photodynamic Therapy for Treatment of Malignant Mesothelioma
2015, 2Q, 8	Urinary Calculi Fragmentation and Evacuation

2014, 4Q, 32   Open Reduction Internal Fixation of Fracture with Debridement
2014, 4Q, 33   Radical Prostatectomy
2014, 4Q, 40   Dilation of Gastrojejunostomy Anastomosis Stricture
2013, 3Q, 28   Total Hysterectomy

This guideline addresses procedures that are performed on separate and distinct body parts. The body part is represented by the fourth character in the PCS structure. When the root operation (character 3) is the same but there are multiple body parts, a code for each body part value is needed. Multiple procedures covered by this guideline have the same root operation, but different body part values. In some cases, procedures with multiple body part values are in the same body system and coded from the same table; however, in other cases, the same root operation may be performed on body parts in different body systems requiring that codes be assigned from a root operation table found in another body system.

Case Study 4.5. Lysis, Adhesions, Ileum and Jejunum

Code(s):

ØDNB4ZZ   **Release Ileum, Percutaneous Endoscopic Approach**

ØDNA4ZZ   **Release Jejunum, Percutaneous Endoscopic Approach**

Rationale:
In this example, the same root operation Release (N) is coded for multiple body parts, Ileum (B) and Jejunum (A), within the same Gastrointestinal (D) body system. Both codes can be found in table ØDN.

Case Study 4.6. Repair, Skin of Left Ear and Repair of Subcutaneous Tissue of Face

Code(s):

ØHQ3XZZ   **Repair Left Ear Skin, External Approach**

ØJQ1ØZZ   **Repair Face Subcutaneous Tissue and Fascia, Open Approach**

Rationale:
In this example, Repair (Q) is done on the Left Ear (3) and Face (1); however, these body parts are in different body system tables. Repair of the skin of the ear is part of the Skin and Breast (H) body system, while repair of the subcutaneous tissue of the face is part of the Subcutaneous Tissue and Fascia (J) body system. The two codes in this example are not found in the same table.

Spotlight
In order to code from the correct body system, it is important to note the tissue layer (e.g., skin or subcutaneous) and the specific body part (ear or face) where the procedure was performed. In the preceding example, a body part value for face is included in the Skin and Breast (H) body system, but it would be the incorrect body system as this procedure was performed on the subcutaneous tissue of the face.

Practical Application for Guideline B3.2a

Case Study 4.7. Upper Endoscopy with Biopsy

After adequate sedation, the Olympus video endoscope was inserted into the mouth and advanced toward the duodenum. Mucosa appeared normal. The duodenum appeared normal. The scope was brought back toward the stomach. The antrum and angularis appeared slightly erythematous, so biopsies were taken from the **pyloric antrum**. The scope was retroflexed to visualize the mucosa of rugal folds, the body, and fundus of the **stomach**. At the body, there were shallow ulcerations with no stigmata of bleeding, but biopsies were taken to rule out erosive gastritis. At the **cardia**, there was a large fungating ulcerated mass appreciated, which was oozing blood. Biopsies were taken of this mass, which was very firm and likely representing a carcinoma. The scope was then anteflexed and brought back to the distal esophagus. All of the esophageal mucosa appeared normal. The squamocolumnar junction appeared normal as well. The scope was removed and the procedure terminated. The patient tolerated the procedure well. There were no immediate complications.

Code(s):

ØDB48ZX   **Excision of Esophagogastric Junction, Via Natural or Artificial Opening Endoscopic, Diagnostic**

ØDB68ZX   **Excision of Stomach, Via Natural or Artificial Opening Endoscopic, Diagnostic**

ØDB78ZX   **Excision of Stomach, Pylorus, Via Natural or Artificial Opening Endoscopic, Diagnostic**

Rationale:

Consulting the alphabetic index under Biopsy provides three root operations to which a biopsy procedure may be coded: Drainage, Excision, or Extraction. The appropriate root operation for this procedure is Excision (B) because small portions of tissue were cut out, without replacement, of the body part. Excision was performed on body parts within the Gastrointestinal System (D) body system so all procedures are coded from the same root operation table ØDB.

Root Operation		
Excision (B)	Definition:	Cutting out or off, without replacement, a portion of a body part
	Explanation:	The qualifier DIAGNOSTIC is used to identify excision procedures that are biopsies

Even though all three biopsies were taken from the stomach area, three codes are required. In PCS, the stomach is divided into three body parts with distinct values. Biopsies were obtained from each of these separate and distinct body parts, including the Esophagogastric Junction (4), Stomach (6), and Stomach, Pylorus (7).

Upon initial review of the case study, it might appear that the cardia should be coded with body part value Stomach (6); however, according to the Body Part Key, the cardia is coded to the Esophagogastric Junction (4). The esophagogastric junction is located between the esophagus and the stomach and is also called the cardia, cardioesophageal junction, or gastroesophageal (GE) junction. It is a valve that opens to allow passage of contents from the esophagus to the stomach and closes to prevent stomach contents from refluxing from the stomach back into the esophagus.

The body part Stomach (6) includes the fundus and the body. The fundus is the upper portion of the stomach lying directly below the esophagogastric junction and the body is the lower portion lying just above the pylorus.

The body part Stomach, Pylorus (7) includes three structures: the pyloric antrum, pyloric canal, and pyloric sphincter. The pyloric antrum connects to the body of the stomach and leads to the pyloric canal followed by the pyloric sphincter, which is connected to the duodenum.

The approach was performed with an endoscope, which is a flexible tube with a light and camera for visualization and a channel through which instruments are passed. The approach was performed through the esophagus. This approach meets the definition Via Natural or Artificial Opening Endoscopic (8).

The acronym for a procedure performed with an endoscope introduced through the esophagus and advanced into the stomach and duodenum is EGD (esophagogastroduodenoscopy). EGD describes the approach and body parts visualized; however, it does not describe the surgical procedures performed. An EGD can be performed for diagnostic or therapeutic purposes. In this case, multiple biopsies were performed. Biopsies are typically obtained using a biopsy forceps used to excise tissue samples.

There is no device (Z) and the correct qualifier is Diagnostic (X) since these are clearly stated as biopsies. See guidelines B3.4a and B3.4b for additional information on coding biopsies.

Case Study 4.8. Tonsilloadenoidectomy

The patient was taken to the operative suite and prepped for surgery. A Crowe-Davis mouth gag was inserted and suspended from the Mayo stand. A Blair drape was placed. A red rubber catheter was inserted through the nasal cavity and used to elevate the soft palate. The nasopharynx was examined. The adenoid pad was removed using a suction cautery technique. This area was packed with gauze sponges. Attention was turned to the right tonsil, which was grasped with an Allis clamp and dissected from the underlying constrictor muscle of the pharynx using a coagulating Bovie current. The left tonsil was similarly grasped and removed using the same coagulating Bovie current.

Bleeding in both tonsil areas was controlled with suction Bovie. Packing was removed from the nasopharynx and bleeding was controlled in this area using a suction Bovie cauterizing the entire adenoid bed. The entire pharynx was then copiously irrigated with sterile saline. With no significant bleeding, the Crowe-Davis mouth gag was removed and the patient was extubated.

Code(s):

ØCTPXZZ   **Resection of Tonsils, External Approach**

ØCTQXZZ   **Resection of Adenoids, External Approach**

Rationale:

In a tonsilloadenoidectomy, the tonsils and the adenoids are removed in their entirety. According to root operation definitions, complete removal of a body part is reported with Resection (T) rather than Excision (B). Therefore, the root operation for coding this procedure is Resection (T). The tonsils and adenoids are part of the body system Mouth and Throat (C).

Root Operation		
Resection (T)	Definition:	Cutting out or off, without replacement, all of a body part
	Explanation:	None

Two codes are needed to describe a procedure when the same root operation is performed on two distinct body parts as indicated by the body part values. Tonsils (P) and Adenoids (Q) are represented by distinct body part values so two codes are required to code a tonsilloadenoidectomy.

Tonsils and adenoids are bilateral structures with tonsil and adenoid tissue present on the right and left side. Some body parts have separate right and left body part characters for bilateral structures. When this is the case and the procedure is performed bilaterally, a code is required for each side. However, this is not the case for the tonsils and adenoids because PCS does not include separate body parts for the right and left tonsils and adenoids. Procedures performed on the tonsils or adenoids, whether the procedure is performed on one side or both, are reported by the body part character for Tonsils (P) or Adenoids (Q), respectively.

Figure 4.1. Tonsils and Adenoids

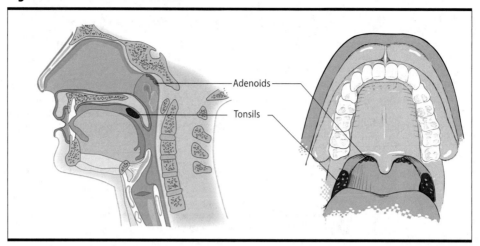

Adenoids

Tonsils

The next character to consider is the approach and two approach values are available: Open (Ø) and External (X). Tonsillectomy and adenoidectomy procedures are performed on body parts within the mouth and throat and the tonsils and adenoids are visible without the use of instrumentation so the correct approach is External (X). This follows the direction of Guideline B5.3a.

PCS Guideline
External approach
B5.3a   Procedures performed within an orifice on structures that are visible without the aid of any instrumentation are coded to the approach External. *Example:* Resection of tonsils is coded to the approach External.

Case Study 4.9. Stripping, Greater Saphenous Veins, Right and Left Leg

After adequate anesthesia was obtained, the left lower extremity was prepped and a diagonal incision was made. A self-retaining retractor was placed and the incision was carried down through the subcutaneous tissues until the greater saphenous vein was identified. The vein was isolated with a right angle. The vein was followed proximally until multiple tributary branches were identified. These were ligated with #3-0 silk suture. The dissection was carried to the femorosaphenous vein junction. This was identified and #0 silk suture was placed proximally and distally and ligated inbetween. The proximal suture was tied down. Distal suture was retracted and a vein stripping device was placed within the greater saphenous vein. An incision was created at the level of the knee. The distal segment of the greater saphenous vein was identified and the left foot was encircled with #0 silk suture and tied proximally and ligated. The distal end of the vein stripping device was passed through at its most proximal location. The device was attached to the vein stripping section and the greater saphenous vein was stripped free from its canal within the left lower extremity. This procedure was repeated on the right leg.

Code(s):

Ø6DP3ZZ   **Extraction of Right Saphenous Vein, Percutaneous Approach**

Ø6DQ3ZZ   **Extraction of Left Saphenous Vein, Percutaneous Approach**

Rationale:

Vein stripping is used to treat varicose veins by removing or tying off a large vein in the leg called the superficial saphenous vein. The saphenous veins are found in the Lower Veins (6) body system in PCS.

Extraction (D) is the appropriate root operation as force is needed to remove the vein. The ICD-10 PCS root operation definition listed in appendix C for Extraction (D) uses vein stripping as an example.

Since there are different body part values for Saphenous Vein, Right (P) and Left (Q), the stripping (Extraction) procedures are coded separately. The vein stripping device is inserted through small incisions meeting the definition of Percutaneous (3) approach.

Root Operation		
Extraction (D)	Definition:	Pulling or stripping out or off all or a portion of a body part by the use of force
	Explanation:	The qualifier DIAGNOSTIC is used to identify extraction procedures that are biopsies

Case Study 4.10. Transplant, Pancreas and Kidney

Procedure: Pancreas/left kidney transplant using organ bank pancreas and kidney.

A patient with kidney failure due to Type 1 diabetes presented for a kidney-pancreas transplant. A midline incision was made in the abdomen. The organ bank kidney was placed in the left side of the lower abdomen and the pancreas was placed on the right side of the lower abdomen. Both transplanted organs came from one deceased donor.

Code(s):

ØFYGØZØ   **Transplantation of Pancreas, Allogeneic, Open Approach**

ØTY1ØZØ   **Transplantation of Left Kidney, Allogeneic, Open Approach**

Rationale:

Organ transplants are coded using the root operation Transplantation (Y).

Root Operation		
Transplantation (Y)	Definition:	Putting in or on all or a portion of a living body part taken from another individual or animal to physically take the place and/or function of all or a portion of a similar body part
	Explanation:	The native body part may or may not be taken out, and the transplanted body part may take over all or a portion of its function

According to guideline B3.2a, each transplant must be coded separately in ICD-10-PCS since two body parts, Pancreas (G) and Kidney, Left (1), received transplants. These body parts are also listed in different body systems. The Pancreas (G) is in the Hepatobiliary System and Pancreas (F) body system while the Kidney, Left (1) is in the Urinary System (T) body system.

An incision was used to reach and visualize the operative site meeting the approach definition of Open (Ø). There are no device choices listed in the transplantation tables so No Device (Z) is the appropriate device value.

In selecting the qualifier (character 7), a complete understanding of transplant types is necessary. Allogeneic (Ø)—taken from different individuals of the same species—is the appropriate choice in this case.

Definitions
allogeneic. Taken from different individuals of the same species.
syngeneic. Having to do with individuals or tissues that have identical genes, such as identical twins.
zooplastic. Tissue obtained from an animal.

Case Study 4.11. Bronchoscopy with Pulmonary Toilet

A patient with severe pneumonia with opacification of the left hemithorax with poor secretion clearance presented for surgery. The tracheostomy tube was changed to a size 6 Bivona. A standard pediatric bronchoscope was advanced through the trach. There was copious purulent secretion emanating from the posterior segment of the **right lower lobe of the bronchus;** secretions were suctioned. The upper and middle bronchial lobes were grossly normal except for mild erythema and occasional mucous. The scope was advanced into the left mainstem bronchi. It was met with copious purulent secretions in the **left main**. This was suctioned and the scope advanced further. The **left upper lobe bronchi, lingula, and lower lobe** with all the segments on the left were full of purulent secretions. This was suctioned out. Given the amount of secretions, chest percussion with a vest was instituted. The bronchoscope was again advanced down the left for more aggressive suctioning. The patient tolerated the procedure well.

Code(s):

ØB968ZZ   **Drainage of Right Lower Lobe Bronchus, Via Natural or Artificial Opening Endoscopic**

ØB9B8ZZ   **Drainage of Left Lower Lobe Bronchus, Via Natural or Artificial Opening Endoscopic**

Rationale:

Bronchoscopy is a procedure in which a hollow, flexible tube called a bronchoscope is inserted into the airways to provide a view of the tracheobronchial tree. Therapeutic use includes the suctioning of retained secretions as is indicated in this example. Drainage (9) is the appropriate root operation since secretions (fluid) in the bronchi were suctioned out.

Root Operation		
Drainage (9)	Definition:	Taking or letting out fluids and/or gases from a body part
	Explanation:	The qualifier DIAGNOSTIC is used to identify drainage procedures that are biopsies

The specific bronchial lobes can be found in the Respiratory (B) body system. Although each bronchial lobe is listed as a separate body part, only the body part drained that is furthest from the point of entry is coded. This is in accordance with PCS guidelines that apply to coding of tubular body parts and supported by advice given in *AHA Coding Clinic,* 2017, 1Q, 51. In this case study, two codes are needed to capture the removal of fluid from the Lower Lobe Bronchus, Right (6), and the Lower Lobe Bronchus, Left (B). Only the body part character differs in these codes. The following illustration depicts the location of the body parts of the tracheobronchial tree.

In this case, the bronchoscope was inserted through the tracheostomy, which is an artificial opening, and the bronchoscope was used to visualize the bronchi, meeting the approach definition of Via Natural or Artificial Opening Endoscopic (8). No tubes or devices were left in the chest at the completion of the procedure, so the device value for No Device (Z) was used. Since this procedure was done for therapeutic rather than diagnostic purposes, the qualifier is No Qualifier (Z).

Figure 4.2. Tracheobronchial Tree

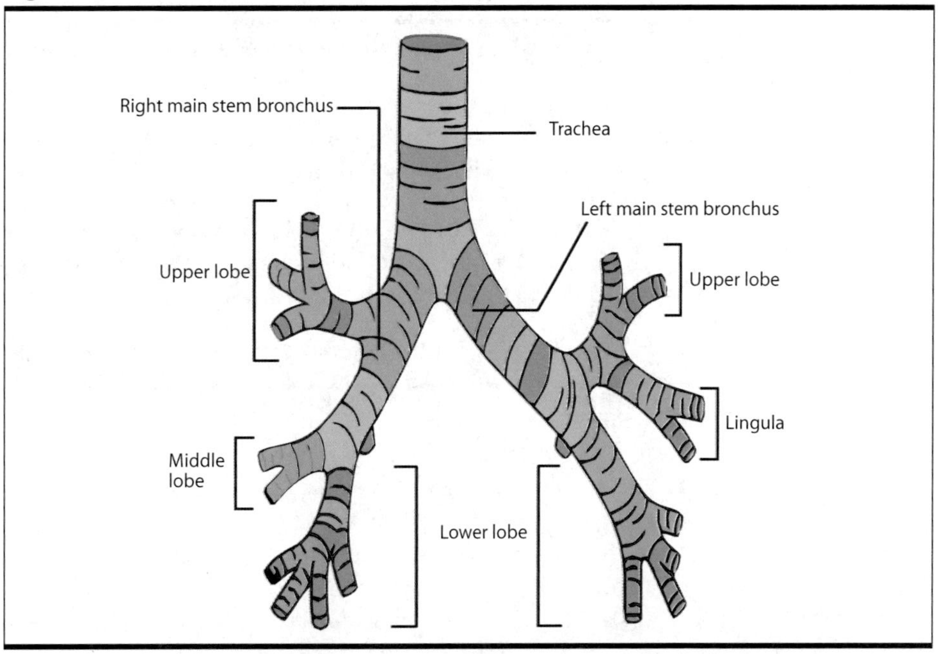

Spotlight
When bronchoalveolar lavage (BAL) is documented, the appropriate body part is lung since the alveolar is lung tissue and the correct qualifier is Diagnostic (X) as noted in *AHA Coding Clinic,* 2017, 1Q, 51.

Guideline B3.2b

> **B3.2**   **During the same operative episode, multiple procedures are coded if:**
>
> **b. The same root operation is repeated in multiple body parts, and those body parts are separate and distinct body parts classified to a single ICD-10-PCS body part value.**
>
> *Examples:* **Excision of the sartorius muscle and excision of the gracilis muscle are both included in the upper leg muscle body part value, and multiple procedures are coded.**
>
> **Extraction of multiple toenails are coded separately.**

AHA Coding Clinic

2017, 2Q, 12	Compartment Syndrome and Fasciotomy of Foot
2017, 2Q, 13	Compartment Syndrome and Fasciotomy of Leg
2016, 4Q, 134	Changes to the ICD-10-PCS Official Guidelines for Coding and Reporting
2015, 2Q, 19	Multiple Decompressive Cervical Laminectomies
2014, 4Q, 16	Excision of Multiple Uterine Fibroids
2014, 3Q, 26	Coil Embolization of Gastroduodenal Artery with Chemoembolization of Hepatic Artery

In PCS, some body part values include anatomical structures that are separate and distinct body parts. A good understanding of anatomy, along with use of the Body Part Definitions Table, is required to accurately apply guideline B3.2b.

A list of many separate and distinct body parts included in a particular body part value can be found in the Body Part Definitions Table in appendix E of this book. The Body Part Definitions table lists the ICD-10-PCS value for the body part in the first column and the anatomical structures that are included in the PCS body part in the second column labeled Definition. However, it should be noted that some terms in the Definition column are synonyms and not separate and distinct body parts. Only procedures performed on separate and distinct body parts are coded separately.

The upper leg muscles are used in the example provided for guideline B3.2b above. There are 14 muscles reported with the body part Upper Leg Muscle, Right and Upper Leg Muscle, Left. An excerpt from the Body Part Definitions Table for the Upper Leg Muscle is provided below.

ICD-10-PCS Value	Definition

Upper Leg Muscle, Left
Upper Leg Muscle, Right
	Includes:
	  Adductor brevis muscle
	  Adductor longus muscle
	  Adductor magnus muscle
	  Biceps femoris muscle
	  Gracilis muscle
	  Pectineus muscle
	  Quadriceps (femoris)
	  Rectus femoris muscle
	  Sartorius muscle
	  Semimembranosus muscle
	  Semitendinosus muscle
	  Vastus intermedius muscle
	  Vastus lateralis muscle
	  Vastus medialis muscle

When documentation identifies that the same root operation was performed on multiple distinct and separate muscles included in body part Upper Leg Muscle, Right or Upper Leg Muscle, Left, the same procedure code is reported for each separate and distinct muscle. This means that the same seven-character code is repeated multiple times.

Practical Application for Guideline B3.2b

Case Study 4.12. Fracture Repair, Orbital Bone

The patient was struck in the face by a baseball, resulting in a complex facial injury. Upon further evaluation, nondisplaced fractures were noted in the orbital portions of the right maxilla and right zygomatic bones. Treatment included the insertion of plates at both sites via an open approach.

Code(s):

ØNHPØ4Z	**Insertion of Internal Fixation Device into Right Orbit, Open Approach**
ØNHPØ4Z	**Insertion of Internal Fixation Device into Right Orbit, Open Approach**

Rationale:

The orbit consists of seven bones that are part of the Head and Facial Bones (N) body system, including the maxilla, lacrimal bone, ethmoid, palatine bone, sphenoid, frontal bone, and zygomatic bone, all shown in the illustration that follows. Since the orbital portions of the maxilla and zygomatic bone were treated and they are two separate and distinct anatomical body parts included in the Body Part Definitions Table for Orbit, Left and Orbit, Right, two codes are required.

Figure 4.3. Orbital Structures

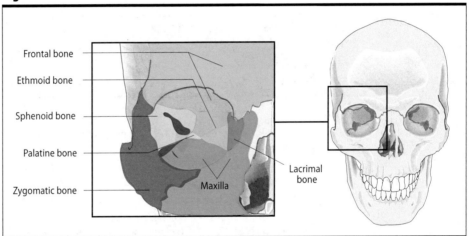

ICD-10-PCS Value	Definition
Orbit, Left **Orbit, Right**	Includes: Bony orbit Orbital portion of ethmoid bone Orbital portion of frontal bone Orbital portion of lacrimal bone Orbital portion of maxilla Orbital portion of palatine bone Orbital portion of sphenoid bone Orbital portion of zygomatic bone

Plates are fixation devices that are coded using root operation Insertion (H), which is defined as "putting in a nonbiological appliance that monitors, assists, performs, or prevents a physiological function but does not physically take the place of a body part." The following Guideline B3.15 specifies that nondisplaced fractures are coded to the procedure performed, which is Insertion (H) of plates in this example, as opposed to a displaced fracture, which is coded to root operation Reposition (S).

PCS Guideline
Reposition for fracture treatment
B3.15   Reduction of a displaced fracture is coded to the root operation Reposition and the application of a cast or splint in conjunction with the Reposition procedure is not coded separately. Treatment of a nondisplaced fracture is coded to the procedure performed. *Examples*: Casting of a nondisplaced fracture is coded to the root operation Immobilization in the Placement section. Putting a pin in a nondisplaced fracture is coded to the root operation Insertion.

Although the code description identifies the body part as Orbit, Right (P), it is appropriate to list the code twice since the procedure was performed on two separate and distinct bones comprising the orbit—the orbital portion of maxilla and the orbital portion of zygomatic bone—which are classified as a single body part character.

The approach is listed as Open (Ø) and the plates are represented by Internal Fixation Device (4).

Case Study 4.13. Angioplasty, Pulmonary Vein

Non-drug eluting stents were placed percutaneously in the left inferior and superior pulmonary veins to treat severe pulmonary vein stenosis (PVS) that resulted after catheter ablation of atrial fibrillation (AF).

Code(s):

Ø27T3DZ   **Dilation of Left Pulmonary Vein with Intraluminal Device, Percutaneous Approach**

Ø27T3DZ   **Dilation of Left Pulmonary Vein with Intraluminal Device, Percutaneous Approach**

Rationale:

Stents hold the vein open after a catheter has been placed and a special balloon has been inflated to widen the passage through the vein. The stent stays in the vein while the catheter and balloon are taken out. Therefore, the correct root operation for this procedure is Dilation (7).

Root Operation		
Dilation (7)	Definition:	Expanding an orifice or the lumen of a tubular body part
	Explanation:	The orifice can be a natural orifice or an artificially created orifice. Accomplished by stretching a tubular body part using intraluminal pressure or by cutting part of the orifice or wall of the tubular body part.

The PCS index for Dilation, Vein, Pulmonary directs the user to table Ø27T for the Left Vein (T). Reviewing the Body Part Definitions table, which can be found in appendix E, the Pulmonary Vein, Left includes the left inferior and left superior pulmonary veins. Reporting the same code twice is appropriate in this procedure since both veins are separate and distinct body parts classified to a single ICD-10-PCS body part value.

ICD-10-PCS Value	Definition

Pulmonary Vein, Left	Includes:
	
	    Left inferior pulmonary vein
	    Left superior pulmonary vein

A Percutaneous approach (3) was used with the correct device value being Intraluminal Device (D) since non-drug eluting stents were placed.

Guideline B3.2c

B3.2	**During the same operative episode, multiple procedures are coded if:**
	c. Multiple root operations with distinct objectives are performed on the same body part.
	Example: **Destruction of sigmoid lesion and bypass of sigmoid colon are coded separately.**

AHA Coding Clinic

2018, 1Q, 12   Percutaneous Balloon Valvuloplasty & Cardiac Catheterization with Ventriculogram

2017, 3Q, 12   Therapeutic and Diagnostic Paracentesis

2017, 3Q, 21   Augmentation Cystoplasty with Indiana Pouch and Continent Urinary Diversion

2017, 3Q, 22   Laparoscopic Esophagomyotomy (Heller Type) and Toupet Fundoplication

2017, 2Q, 17   Billroth II (Distal Gastrectomy with Gastrojejunostomy)

2017, 2Q, 19   Thoracic Outlet Decompression with Sympathectomy

2015, 2Q, 21   Annuloplasty Ring

Root operations specify the intent or objective of a procedure. One operative session may involve many procedural objectives all performed on the same body part, necessitating reporting multiple procedure codes. Each root operation (character 3) documented in the operative report should be coded even when the body part (character 4) remains the same. The only exception to this is when one root operation is considered inherent or integral to another root operation as identified in the definition and/or explanation. Refer to guideline B3.1b for more information on the components of procedures that are not reported separately.

Practical Application for Guideline B3.2c

> **Case Study 4.14. Annuloplasty**
>
> A 60-year-old female with mitral valve incompetence was admitted for a mitral valve reconstruction. Posterior leaflet repair and Carpentier-Edwards ring annuloplasty were performed using an open approach. Redundant leaflet tissue was excised. Defects in the valve leaflets were closed with sutures. The chordae tendineae were shortened with sutures. Valve closure was assessed after the repair and determined to be adequate.

Code(s):

Ø2UGØJZ	**Supplement Mitral Valve with Synthetic Substitute, Open Approach**
Ø2BGØZZ	**Excision of Mitral Valve, Open Approach**

Rationale:

In this example, two different root operations were performed on the same body part Mitral Valve (G), which is listed in the body system Heart and Great Vessels (2) table. The procedure was completed using an Open (Ø) approach.

The annuloplasty ring does not replace the valve but instead is a device used to improve and reinforce the shape and size of the valve. Since its function is to reinforce and restore the mitral value to its proper size, Supplement (U) is the correct root operation. The Carpentier-Edwards ring is a synthetic product; therefore, the device character is Synthetic Substitute (J).

Root Operation		
Supplement (U)	Definition:	Putting in or on biological or synthetic material that physically reinforces and/or augments the function of a portion of a body part
	Explanation:	The biological material is non-living, or is living and from the same individual. The body part may have been previously replaced, and the SUPPLEMENT procedure is performed to physically reinforce and/or augment the function of the replaced body part.

The second part of this procedure includes the removal of extra tissue. Not all of the tissue is removed, so Excision (B) is the root operation used. No Device (Z) is used.

Root Operation		
Excision (B)	Definition:	Cutting out or off, without replacement, a portion of a body part
	Explanation:	The qualifier DIAGNOSTIC is used to identify excision procedures that are biopsies

---

Case Study 4.15. Delivery with Fetal Rotation

Procedure: Routine vaginal delivery following internal (or transcervical) fetal rotation due to face-brow presentation.

With the pregnant patient in a knee-chest position, knees slightly apart, the physician inserted a hand into the patient's vagina. Grasping the head firmly and during a contraction, the baby's head was turned to an anterior position. The amniotic sac was artificially ruptured, and shortly thereafter the baby was delivered vaginally without difficulty.

Code(s):

1Ø EØ XZZ	**Delivery of Products of Conception, External Approach**
1Ø SØ 7ZZ	**Reposition Products of Conception, Via Natural or Artificial Opening**
1Ø 9Ø 7ZC	**Drainage of Amniotic Fluid, Therapeutic from Products of Conception, Via Natural or Artificial Opening**

Rationale:
Procedures performed on the body part Products of Conception (Ø) are only found in the Obstetrics (1) section. The products of conception include the fetus, amnion, umbilical cord, and placenta.

Rotating the fetus prior to delivery is classified as Reposition (S). This root operation has the same meaning in the Obstetrics section as in the Medical and Surgical section. The root operation Delivery (E) is also applicable in this example for the manually assisted delivery of the baby. It is appropriate to code the Reposition (S) and the Delivery (E) since two different root operations were performed on the same body part.

Obstetrics Section (1)

Root Operation		
Reposition (S)	Definition:	Moving to its normal location, or other suitable location, all or a portion of a body part
	Explanation:	The body part is moved to a new location from an abnormal location, or from a normal location where it is not functioning correctly. The body part may or may not be cut out or off to be moved to the new location.
Delivery (E)	Definition:	Assisting the passage of the products of conception from the genital canal
	Explanation:	None
Drainage (9)	Definition:	Taking or letting out fluids and/or gases from a body part
	Explanation:	None

In order to perform the reposition, the provider inserted his/her hand directly into the vagina, which meets the approach definition of Via Natural or Artificial Opening (7). The only approach option for a manually assisted delivery is External (X).

An additional code is reported for rupture of the amniotic sac. This code is also located in the Obstetrics section (1) and since the objective of the procedure is to drain the amniotic fluid, the correct root operation is Drainage (9). Products of Conception (Ø) is the only body part value offered in the Drainage (1Ø9) table. The amniotic fluid is further specified with the seventh-character qualifier, which offers Amniotic Fluid, Therapeutic (C) or Amniotic Fluid, Diagnostic (U), as well as other fetal fluid values. Since this rupture was performed to facilitate the delivery and not for diagnostic purposes, Amniotic Fluid, Therapeutic (C) is the appropriate qualifier. The rupture was performed using approach Via Natural or Artificial Opening (7).

Guideline B3.2d

B3.2d	**During the same operative episode, multiple procedures are coded if:**
	d. The intended root operation is attempted using one approach, but is converted to a different approach.
	Example: **Laparoscopic cholecystectomy converted to an open cholecystectomy is coded as percutaneous endoscopic Inspection and open Resection.**

AHA Coding Clinic

2015, 1Q, 33   Robotic-Assisted Laparoscopic Hysterectomy Converted to Open Procedure

Procedures are sometimes initiated using one approach and then converted to another approach when the procedure cannot be completed using the initial approach. In the event that the surgical approach needs to be changed intraoperatively, the procedure using the original approach and the actual procedure performed need to be coded. A common mistake is coding both procedures using the same approach.

Practical Application for Guideline B3.2d

Case Study 4.16. Cholecystectomy, Laparoscopic, Converted to Open
Procedure: Laparoscopic cholecystectomy converted to open procedure, suture repair of intraoperative laceration of abdominal aorta.
In the operating suite, the patient was prepped, draped, and positioned. Anesthesia was maintained with fentanyl and isoflurane in oxygen/air. Trocars were inserted through small abdominal incisions. Pneumoperitoneum was induced by insufflation of the abdomen. The patient was repositioned at 30° with a head-up tilt. Approximately 30 minutes post-trocar insertion, during the gallbladder dissection, arterial hypertension rapidly decreased (from 28 to 18 mm Hg). The patient developed bradycardia. The procedure was immediately converted to an open abdominal approach. Pneumoperitoneum was released, instruments withdrawn, and ports removed. The abdomen was opened via a subcostal incision in the right upper quadrant. The skin and fascia were dissected down to the abdominal cavity and retractors placed. Abdominal exploration identified intraperitoneal bleeding from a tiny rent in the infrarenal abdominal aorta, possibly during trocar insertion. The aorta was isolated and clamped. The approximate 1 mm rent was immediately sutured and hemostasis was achieved.
Transection of the gallbladder was resumed at the level of the cystic duct using GIA stapler. The stump was reinforced with 2-0 Vicryl suture. The gallbladder was filled with numerous 3 mm to 5 mm stones. The specimen was removed and the right upper quadrant was irrigated extensively. No stones were identified inside the peritoneal cavity. The aorta was again checked for hemostasis. No bleeding or oozing was identified. A JP drain was placed in the right upper quadrant area close to the cystic duct and stump. The abdominal wound was closed in layers. Dry sterile dressing was applied. The patient was extubated in the operating room and taken to the recovery room in stable condition.

Code(s):

ØFJ44ZZ	**Inspection of Gallbladder, Percutaneous Endoscopic Approach**
ØFT4ØZZ	**Resection of Gallbladder, Open Approach**
Ø4QØØZZ	**Repair Abdominal Aorta, Open Approach**

Rationale:

In this example, the procedure was converted from laparoscopic to open when the patient became unstable. Further investigation indicated that there was a laceration (rent) in the lower (infrarenal) abdominal aorta. The gallbladder removal was ultimately completed via an open approach after the rent was repaired.

Proper code assignment includes three codes: a code for the Inspection (J) procedure via Percutaneous Endoscopic (4) approach to represent the initial laparoscopic attempt, a code for the Repair (Q) of the Abdominal Aorta (Ø) via Open (Ø) approach, and a code for the Resection (T) of the Gallbladder (4) via Open (Ø) approach. Inspection (J) and Resection (T) were completed on the body part Gallbladder (4) using different approaches.

Root Operation		
Inspection (J)	Definition:	Visually and/or manually exploring a body part
	Explanation:	Visual exploration may be performed with or without optical instrumentation. Manual exploration may be performed directly or through intervening body layers.
Repair (Q)	Definition:	Restoring, to the extent possible, a body part to its normal anatomic structure and function
	Explanation:	Used only when the method to accomplish the repair is not one of the other root operations
Resection (T)	Definition:	Cutting out or off, without replacement, all of a body part
	Explanation:	None

Case Study 4.17. Cystolithotomy, Laparoscopic, Converted to Open

The patient was brought to the operating room and given intravenous ceftriaxone sodium and general laryngeal mask anesthesia. He was prepped, draped, and placed in a modified dorsal lithotomy position. The flexible cystoscope was placed to evaluate the prostatic urethra and bladder. The bladder was filled to capacity with sterile water mixed with gentamicin. One stone could easily be seen. With a lighted flexible scope the area was marked with the marking pen. A 1.5 cm incision was made transversely in the midline on the mark. A 12 mm direct-vision laparoscopic trochar was placed through the incision and directly into the bladder. The stone was more challenging than expected. A decision was made to do an open removal. The trocar was removed and an incision was made in the lower abdomen. The bladder was opened and the stone removed.

Code(s):

ØTCBØZZ	**Extirpation of Matter from Bladder, Open Approach**
ØTJB4ZZ	**Inspection of Bladder, Percutaneous Endoscopic Approach**

Rationale:

Cystolithotomy is a minimally invasive surgical procedure used for the removal of bladder stones when the stones have been deemed too large to pass naturally. It can be performed percutaneously with endoscopy or endoscopically though a transurethral (via natural or artificial opening) approach. In this instance, the laparoscope was inserted directly into the bladder wall through a small incision in the abdomen. The laparoscope allows for visualization of the bladder, which meets the approach definition of Percutaneous Endoscopic (4). Since the stone removal using this method was unsuccessful, only the Inspection (J) of the Bladder (B) body part is coded as a Percutaneous Endoscopic (4) procedure.

A second code is needed to capture the stone removal. Changing techniques to an Open (Ø) approach, solid matter was taken out of the Bladder (B). This meets the root operation definition of Extirpation (C).

Root Operation		
Inspection (J)	Definition:	Visually and/or manually exploring a body part
	Explanation:	Visual exploration may be performed with or without optical instrumentation. Manual exploration may be performed directly or through intervening body layers.
Extirpation (C)	Definition:	Taking or cutting out solid matter from a body part
	Explanation:	The solid matter may be an abnormal byproduct of a biological function or a foreign body; it may be imbedded in a body part or in the lumen of a tubular body part. The solid matter may or may not have been previously broken into pieces.

Discontinued or Incomplete Procedures

Guideline B3.3

B3.3   **If the intended procedure is discontinued or otherwise not completed, code the procedure to the root operation performed. If a procedure is discontinued before any other root operation is performed, code the root operation Inspection of the body part or anatomical region inspected.**

Example: **A planned aortic valve replacement procedure is discontinued after the initial thoracotomy and before any incision is made in the heart muscle, when the patient becomes hemodynamically unstable. This procedure is coded as an open Inspection of the mediastinum.**

AHA Coding Clinic

2017, 1Q, 50	Dry Aspiration of Ankle Joint
2017, 1Q, 50	Failed Lumbar Puncture
2015, 3Q, 9	Aborted Endovascular Stenting of Superficial Femoral Artery
2015, 3Q, 10	Coronary Angioplasty with Unsuccessful Stent Insertion
2015, 1Q, 29	Discontinued Carotid Endarterectomy
2015, 1Q, 35	Attempted Removal of Foreign Body from Cornea

Procedures may be discontinued for many reasons, including an unstable patient, inability to cross a vessel, or a failed attempt at removing a foreign body. The code used for a discontinued procedure should capture the extent to which the procedure was performed. If no other root operation was performed, Inspection (J) should be used.

Root Operation		
Inspection (J)	Definition:	Visually and/or manually exploring a body part
	Explanation:	Visual exploration may be performed with or without optical instrumentation. Manual exploration may be performed directly through intervening body layers.

In order to apply this guideline properly, it is imperative to understand the anatomy of and the typical procedural/surgical steps taken in each procedure. In the example provided with guideline B3.3, the patient had a thoracotomy performed, which is an incision into the chest wall that exposes the heart, lungs, and other organs in the chest/thoracic cavity. The mediastinum is the septum or partition in the chest cavity that contains the heart. The procedure is coded as an inspection of the mediastinum because no incision was made into the heart itself (as would be required for an aortic valve replacement procedure). Refer to the following illustration of the mediastinum.

Figure 4.4. Mediastinum

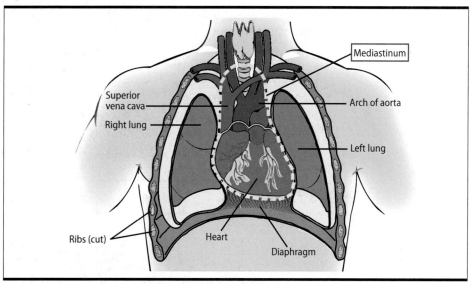

Practical Application for Guideline B3.3

Case Study 4.18. Cystoureteroscopy with Unsuccessful Removal of Calculus

After induction of general anesthesia, the patient was placed in the lithotomy position. Genitalia were prepped and draped in the usual sterile fashion. A #21-French cystoscope was inserted under camera vision. The urethra was unremarkable. Prostate was normal. The scope was passed into the bladder. The bladder mucosa was normal throughout. Under fluoroscopic control, a guidewire was placed up the right ureter and bypassed the stone. This was difficult at first, but the guidewire was eventually manipulated around the stone into the proximal collecting system. A rigid ureteroscope was negotiated up the right ureter alongside the guidewire up to the stone, which was at approximately the junction of the upper third and the middle two-thirds of the ureter. The stone was quite large and occupied the entire lumen of the ureter. After multiple unsuccessful attempts were made to remove the stone, the guidewire and ureteroscope were removed.

Code(s):

ØTJ98ZZ   **Inspection of Ureter, Via Natural or Artificial Opening Endoscopic**

Rationale:

In this procedure, a ureteroscope was used to visually inspect the bladder and the ureter, which are part of the Urinary (T) body system and are shown in the illustration that follows. Because the calculus removal was unsuccessful, the intended procedure was considered discontinued and the procedure is coded to the completed objective, which was root operation Inspection (J).

ICD-10 PCS guideline B3.11b shown following, states that the most distal body part should be used if more than one tubular body part is inspected, which is the ureter in this case. Because there is no body part value for right ureter listed under Inspection, the general body part Ureter (9) is assigned.

The approach is Via Natural or Artificial Opening Endoscopic (8) since the ureteroscope is inserted directly into the urethra.

PCS Guideline
Inspection procedures
B3.11b   If multiple tubular body parts are inspected, the most distal body part (the body part furthest from the starting point of the inspection) is coded. If multiple non-tubular body parts in a region are inspected, the body part that specifies the entire area inspected is coded. *Examples:* Cystoureteroscopy with inspection of bladder and ureters is coded to the ureter body part value. Exploratory laparotomy with general inspection of abdominal contents is coded to the peritoneal cavity body part value.

Figure 4.5. Urinary Tract

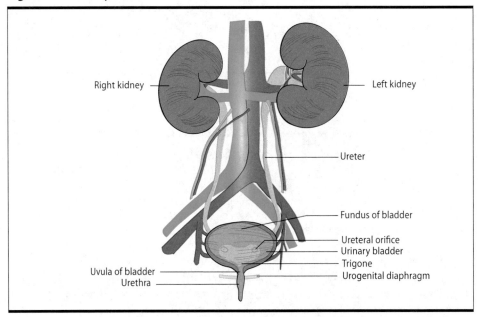

Right kidney — Left kidney — Ureter — Fundus of bladder — Ureteral orifice — Urinary bladder — Trigone — Urogenital diaphragm — Uvula of bladder — Urethra

---

Case Study 4.19. Colonoscopy, Partial

Procedure: Planned screening colonoscopy that due to poor prep, progressed only to the sigmoid colon.

After adequate sedation was achieved, the patient was placed in the left lateral decubitus position and a digital rectal exam was performed. This examination was within normal limits. A well-lubricated colonoscope was inserted into the rectum and advanced under direct visualization to the level of the sigmoid colon. The sigmoid colon was identified by visual and anatomic landmarks; however, the procedure was terminated at this level due to poor prep. The scope was completely retrieved upon exiting the anal canal. The patient was transferred to the recovery room in stable condition.

Code(s):
ØDJD8ZZ   **Inspection of Lower Intestinal Tract, Via Natural or Artificial Opening Endoscopic**

Rationale:
A screening colonoscopy is reported using root operation Inspection (J). When referencing the Inspection table in the Gastrointestinal (D) body system, note that the body part values are less detailed than they are in the other tables, distinguishing only the upper and lower gastrointestinal tracts, stomach, omentum, mesentery, and peritoneum. The correct body part, Lower Intestinal Tract (D), encompasses the entire large intestine with the sigmoid colon and, therefore, does not allow the user to indicate that the colonoscopy ended at the sigmoid colon.

The scope is inserted directly into the rectum, resulting in an approach assignment of Via Natural or Artificial Opening, Endoscopic (8). In this case, although the procedure was not completed as originally planned, the code remains the same for the limited (reduced) colonoscopy as it would for the entire colonoscopy.

Figure 4.6. Large Intestine

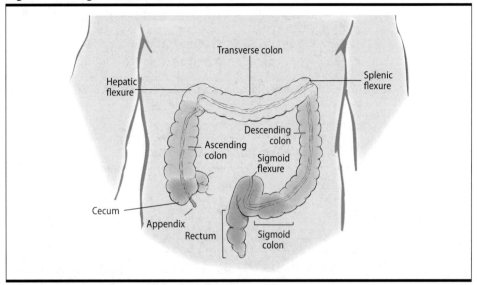

Case Study 4.20. Foreign Body, Unsuccessful Removal

A 9-year-old male was stabbed in the right thigh with a stick while playing. The area of the injury is sore and the patient's mother thinks there is still a foreign body in the wound. The mother tried to get out the sliver of wood but according to the mother it was too painful. Plan to remove foreign body from thigh.

The patient was brought to the surgery room, and his thigh was prepped and draped in the usual sterile fashion. The area was injected with a local anesthetic and irrigated with a normal saline flush. Using a small retractor, the edges of the wound were opened. After multiple attempts were made to remove the splinter, all of which were unsuccessful, the wound was irrigated again and a sterile dressing was applied.

Code(s):
ØHJPXZZ   Inspection of Skin, External Approach

Rationale:
The foreign body was not removed in this case. Therefore, the only root operation that applies is Inspection (J), with Skin and Breast (H) as the appropriate body system and Skin (P) assigned for the body part. There are no values in the Inspection (J) table that further specify the body part.

An External (X) approach was used as the entire procedure took place without the use of a scope, needle, or incision.

Biopsy Procedures

Guideline B3.4a

B3.4a **Biopsy procedures are coded using the root operations Excision, Extraction, or Drainage and the qualifier Diagnostic.** *Examples:* **Fine needle aspiration biopsy of fluid in the lung is coded to the root operation Drainage with the qualifier Diagnostic.** **Biopsy of bone marrow is coded to the root operation Extraction with the qualifier Diagnostic.** **Lymph node sampling for biopsy is coded to the root operation Excision with the qualifier Diagnostic.**

AHA Coding Clinic

2017, 4Q, 41-42	Extraction Procedures
2016, 4Q, 134	Changes to the ICD-10-PCS Official Guidelines for Coding and Reporting
2016, 1Q, 23	Endoscopic Ultrasound with Aspiration Biopsy of Common Hepatic Duct
2016, 1Q, 24	Endoscopic Brush Biopsy of Esophagus
2016, 1Q, 26	Bronchoalveolar Lavage, Endobronchial Biopsy and Transbronchial Biopsy
2016, 1Q, 27	Fiberoptic Bronchoscopy with Brushings and Bronchoalveolar Lavage
2015, 4Q, 16	Changes to the ICD-10-PCS Official Guidelines for Coding and Reporting Biopsy procedures
2014, 1Q, 8	Diagnostic Lumbar Tap
2014, 1Q, 26	Correction Notice: Transbronchial Needle Aspiration Lymph Node Biopsy
2013, 4Q, 111	Root Operation for Bone Marrow Biopsy
2013, 4Q, 111-112	Transbronchial Needle Aspiration Lymph Node Biopsy

Biopsies are performed in order to sample tissue for abnormalities. Samples sent to the laboratory may not always be for the purpose of diagnostic testing. It is critical to understand that only those specimens tested to "diagnose" a condition are considered biopsies.

When coding a biopsy, the method used to secure the sample is key to selecting the correct root operation. Guideline B3.4a states that only three root operations should be used when coding a biopsy: Excision, Extraction, or Drainage.

Root Operation		
Excision (B)	Definition:	Cutting out or off, without replacement, a portion of a body part
	Explanation:	The qualifier DIAGNOSTIC is used to identify excision procedures that are biopsies
Extraction (D)	Definition:	Pulling or stripping out or off all or a portion of a body part by the use of force
	Explanation:	The qualifier DIAGNOSTIC is used to identify extraction procedures that are biopsies
Drainage (9)	Definition:	Taking or letting out fluids and/or gases from a body part
	Explanation:	The qualifier DIAGNOSTIC is used to identify drainage procedures that are biopsies

A bone marrow biopsy is coded with root operation Extraction (D) with qualifier Diagnostic (X) since a larger caliber needle is used to collect the bone marrow core (cylindrical sample), which requires force. The body part value for Bone Marrow can be found in the Lymphatic and Hemic (7) body system with the choice of Bone Marrow Sternum (Q), Iliac (R), or Vertebral (S). Additionally, endometrial biopsies are also coded using root operation Extraction (D). Although bone marrow biopsies and endometrial biopsies may appear to be excisional in nature, they are actually performed via an extraction type of procedure.

Practical Application for Guideline B3.4a

Case Study 4.21. Biopsy, Endometrial

The patient experienced postmenopausal uterine bleeding. A diagnostic D&C was performed through a hysteroscope to determine the cause of bleeding.

Code(s):
ØUDB8ZX   **Extraction of Endometrium, Via Natural or Artificial Opening Endoscopic, Diagnostic**

Rationale:
A dilation and curettage (D&C) is considered an extraction since the lining of the endometrium is stripped away by force. Although the initial response may be to code this biopsy using the root operation Excision, there is no body part endometrium listed in Table ØUB. Root operation Extraction (D) is the appropriate assignment.

Consulting the ICD-10-PCS index for Extraction, the entry for Endometrium lists table ØUDB. This table is in the body system Female Reproductive System (U) with Endometrium (B) as the body part value. Endometrial biopsies are done by passing the instruments through the cervix into the uterine cavity, in this case via a hysteroscope, which correlates with approach value Via Natural or Artificial Opening Endoscopic (8).

The qualifier Diagnostic (X) is used since the sample was taken to diagnose the cause of bleeding.

Root Operation		
Extraction (D)	Definition:	Pulling or stripping out or off all or a portion of a body part by the use of force
	Explanation:	The qualifier DIAGNOSTIC is used to identify extraction procedures that are biopsies

Case Study 4.22. Biopsy, Shave

A shave biopsy is performed on a skin lesion on the left cheek.

Code(s):
ØHB1XZX   **Excision of Face Skin, External Approach, Diagnostic**

Rationale:
A superficial shave biopsy can be used to diagnose questionable dermatologic lesions, including possible malignancies. Biopsies of the skin are coded using body system Skin and Breast (H).

A shave biopsy samples only a part of a lesion; therefore, the root operation Excision (B) is appropriate. Consulting table ØHB, no listing for cheek is available, so body part Skin, Face (1) must be used.

A surgical knife (scalpel) is used to scrape off the skin to be biopsied. Since this is done directly on the skin, an External (X) approach is coded.

The procedure is performed with the intent to sample the lesion, which is reflected with qualifier, Diagnostic (X).

Root Operation		
Excision (B)	Definition:	Cutting out or off, without replacement, a portion of a body part
	Explanation:	The qualifier DIAGNOSTIC is used to identify excision procedures that are biopsies

Case Study 4.23. Biopsy, Needle Core of Thyroid Nodule

A 62-year-old female was admitted with a painless, palpable, solitary thyroid nodule on the right lobe discovered on routine physical examination last week. Because of this suspicious finding, compounded by a family history of thyroid cancer, needle core biopsy was performed. Biopsy results yielded a diagnosis of papillary carcinoma.

Code(s):

ØGBH3ZX   Excision of Right Thyroid Gland Lobe, Percutaneous Approach, Diagnostic

Rationale:

A needle core biopsy uses a wider needle than what is used in a fine-needle aspiration. The needle used is a hollow tube that extracts a core of tissue for testing. Excision (B) is the appropriate root operation since a portion of the body part is being removed for evaluation.

The thyroid gland is part of the Endocrine (G) body system. Review of table ØGB reveals three body part values for thyroid: Thyroid Gland Lobe, Left (G), Thyroid Gland Lobe, Right (H), and Thyroid Gland Isthmus (J). Coders should assign the most specific character value available, if possible. Therefore, Thyroid Gland Lobe, Right (H) is the appropriate body part character value.

Needle biopsies meet the definition of Percutaneous (3) approach with the qualifier being Diagnostic (X).

Root Operation		
Excision (B)	Definition:	Cutting out or off, without replacement, a portion of a body part
	Explanation:	The qualifier DIAGNOSTIC is used to identify excision procedures that are biopsies

Case Study 4.24. Biopsy, Aspiration Needle

Procedure: Aspiration needle biopsy of the right inguinal lymph node.

The right inguinal area was prepped and draped in the usual sterile fashion. An incision was made over the abscess and carried down until the lymph node was visualized. After identification of the lymph node, a needle was inserted. The lymph node tissue was removed and sent to pathology. Pressure was applied to the area and Steri-strips were used to close the area.

Code(s):

Ø7DH3ZX   Extraction of Right Inguinal Lymphatic, Percutaneous Approach, Diagnostic

Rationale:

The term Biopsy in the ICD-10-PCS index directs the user to Drainage, Excision, or Extraction. Although aspiration of a lymph node seems to imply the removal of fluid from the lymph node, it is actually tissue that is aspirated. The tissue in this case was aspirated via a needle and not actually excised making Extraction (D) the most appropriate choice. (*AHA Coding Clinic,* 2017, 4Q, 41)

Lymph nodes are part of the Lymphatic and Hemic (7) body system. Review of table Ø7D includes the body part Lymphatic Right, Inguinal (H).

The biopsy is performed using a needle, making the approach Percutaneous (3) since the lymph node is accessed by puncture. A biopsy is a diagnostic procedure, so the qualifier value is Diagnostic (X).

Root Operation		
Extraction (D)	Definition:	Pulling or stripping out or off all or a portion of a body part by the use of force
	Explanation:	The qualifier DIAGNOSTIC is used to identify extraction procedures that are biopsies

Case Study 4.25. Biopsy, Transthoracic Needle

Procedure: Right upper lobe transthoracic fine needle biopsy for the evaluation of a suspicious lung nodule.

After the skin was cleansed, fluoroscopy was used to guide the needle into the right upper lobe nodule. After multiple samples were withdrawn and sent to pathology, the needle was removed and a small bandage was placed over the area.

Code(s):
ØBDC3ZX   Extraction of Right Upper Lung Lobe, Percutaneous Approach, Diagnostic

Rationale:
When performing a transthoracic needle biopsy, a fine needle is passed through the skin and into the lung mass where a sample of the mass is removed (aspirated) and sent to the laboratory to be evaluated. Extraction (D) is the correct root operation for this procedure.

Root Operation		
Extraction (D)	Definition:	Pulling or stripping out or off all or a portion of a body part by the use of force
	Explanation:	The qualifier DIAGNOSTIC is used to identify extraction procedures that are biopsies

Figure 4.7. Fine Needle Biopsy

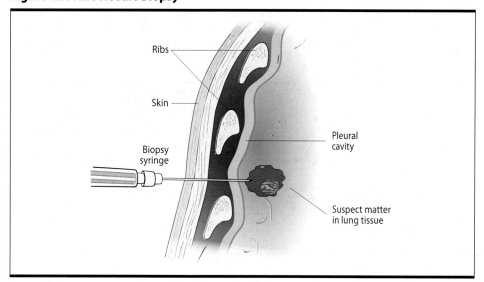

The Upper Lung Lobe, Right (C) body part is found in the Respiratory (B) body system. A needle is used to extract the sample meeting the definition for Percutaneous (3) approach. Since the sample is being sent to pathology for evaluation, Diagnostic (X) is the correct qualifier.

Case Study 4.26. Biopsy, Burr Hole, Brain

A patient was admitted to undergo stereotactic brain biopsy. The stereotactic frame was assembled, placed over the skull, and secured with pins. Under CT guidance, the calvarium (roof of the skull) was entered using a burr drill. A biopsy needle was inserted through the burr hole to obtain the specimen.

Code(s):

ØØBØ3ZX	**Excision of Brain, Percutaneous Approach, Diagnostic**
8EØ9XBG	**Computer Assisted Procedure of Head and Neck Region, With Computerized Tomography**

Rationale:

The Central Nervous System and Cranial Nerves (Ø) body system contains the body part Brain (Ø), which was biopsied in this example.

In the ICD-10-PCS index, the main term Biopsy directs the user to Drainage, Excision, or Extraction. No fluid is removed and although a needle was used to obtain the tissue, there is no choice in the Extraction table for the Brain body part. Since the purpose of this procedure was to remove tissue, the root operation Excision (B) is assigned. The qualifier Diagnostic (X) is assigned to report the excision for diagnostic purposes (e.g., biopsy).

A needle was used to remove the specimen, which meets the approach definition of Percutaneous (3).

Root Operation		
Excision (B)	Definition:	Cutting out or off, without replacement, a portion of a body part
	Explanation:	The qualifier DIAGNOSTIC is used to identify excision procedures that are biopsies

To obtain an accurate location of the biopsy target, stereotactic computer assistance was used. This can be performed with or without a frame. If required by the facility, the frame, which is placed over the skull and held securely in place with pins, can be reported with 2W3ØXYZ Immobilization of Head using Other Device (Y), from the Placement section. CT or MRI is used with the stereotactic computer assistance to confirm the precise location of the burr hole and biopsy. This computer-assisted procedure is found in the Other Procedures (8) section using the Head and Neck Region (9) as the body region. The computer-assisted imaging was performed via an External (X) approach. The procedure method, Computer Assisted (B), is captured with the sixth character and the qualifier specifies whether specific imaging such as With Computerized Tomography (G) was used.

Spotlight

Stereotactic computer assistance should not be confused with Stereotactic Radiosurgery, which includes various types of radiation therapy and is found in the Radiation Therapy (D) section.

Case Study 4.27. Amniocentesis

Procedure: Amniocentesis of pregnant patient with single fetus, at 20 weeks gestation for genetic testing.

The abdomen was prepped and draped. Using a sterile covered ultrasound transducer with guide, a pocket of fluid was located. The 20-gauge needle was inserted into the pocket of amniotic fluid and 20 cc of clear yellow amniotic fluid was withdrawn. The fluid was sent for genetic testing. The patient tolerated the procedure without difficulty.

Code(s):

10903ZU	**Drainage of Amniotic Fluid, Diagnostic from Products of Conception, Percutaneous Approach**
BY4CZZZ	**Ultrasonography of Second Trimester, Single Fetus**

Rationale:

Amniocentesis can be used to diagnose fetal defects during pregnancy. A sample of the amniotic fluid, which surrounds a fetus in the womb, is collected through a pregnant woman's abdomen using a needle and syringe.

Drainage (9) is the appropriate root operation since fluid was removed; the qualifier Diagnostic (U) is used when the fluid is removed for further study. For obstetric procedures, body system Obstetrics (1), there is only one body part character available, Products of Conception (0).

The approach is Percutaneous (3) since a needle was used to reach the amniotic fluid.

Root Operation		
Drainage (9)	Definition:	Taking or letting out fluids and/or gases from a body part
	Explanation:	None

If the facility reports the imaging, a second code is added to represent the ultrasonography. The ultrasound transducer is the hand-held probe that rubs over the body, receives the echoes from the sound waves, and sends them to the computer to create a picture called the sonogram. The Imaging (B) section is organized by body system, which includes Fetus and Obstetrical (Y), and then by imaging type, such as Ultrasonography (4). Since the patient has one fetus and is in the 20th gestational week, the appropriate body part character is Second Trimester, Single Fetus (C).

Definition
trimester. Counted from the first day of the last menstrual period and defined as follows:
• 1st trimester: less than 14 weeks, 0 days
• 2nd trimester: 14 weeks, 0 days to less than 28 weeks, 0 days
• 3rd trimester: 28 weeks, 0 days until delivery

Case Study 4.28. Biopsy, Spinal Tap

The patient was positioned for tap. Aseptic solution was applied to the skin and a local anesthetic injected at the puncture site. The biopsy needle was inserted at L3-L4. Cerebrospinal fluid was withdrawn and specimen prepared for analysis. The needle was removed and the wound dressed.

Code(s):

ØØ9U3ZX   **Drainage of Spinal Canal, Percutaneous Approach, Diagnostic**

Rationale:

Lumbar puncture (spinal tap) is performed in the lumbar region of the lower back. During lumbar puncture, a needle is inserted between two lumbar bones (vertebrae) to remove a sample of cerebrospinal fluid—fluid that surrounds the brain and spinal cord to protect them from injury. Since fluid was removed, Drainage (9) is the appropriate root operation for this biopsy.

For a lumbar spinal tap/drain or an aspiration via a lumbar drain port, the body part Spinal Canal (U) should be used rather than Spinal Cord. If the objective of the procedure is diagnostic, use Diagnostic (X) for the qualifier (*AHA Coding Clinic*, 2014, 1Q, 8). The spinal canal refers to the hollow passage through which the spinal cord runs and is filled with cerebrospinal fluid. Since fluid was removed from the canal during a spinal tap, Spinal Canal (U) is the appropriate body part. The spinal canal is part of the Central Nervous and Cranial Nerves (Ø) body system.

The biopsy was performed using a needle, making the approach Percutaneous (3).

Root Operation		
Drainage (9)	Definition:	Taking or letting out fluids and/or gases from a body part
	Explanation:	The qualifier DIAGNOSTIC is used to identify drainage procedures that are biopsies

Case Study 4.29. Biopsy, Bronchoscopy

Procedure: Bronchoscopy with brushing biopsy of left lower lobe of bronchus.

The patient was brought to the endoscopy suite and sedated using IV Versed. The fiberoptic scope was inserted into the mouth, through the trachea, and passed through to the bronchial tree. The left lower lobe was examined. Using fluoroscopic guidance to validate appropriate placement, the tip of the bronchoscope was placed into the posterior segment of the left lower lobe and brushings were taken. The sample was sent for histology. The bronchoscope was removed.

Code(s):

ØBDB8ZX   **Extraction of Left Lower Lobe Bronchus, Via Natural or Artificial Opening Endoscopic, Diagnostic**

Rationale:

Bronchoscopy is used to view the trachea and bronchial tubes as depicted in the following illustration. During a brushing, a soft, sterile brush resembling a pipe cleaner is inserted through a tube in the scope and used to gently brush (scrape) lung tissue or a lesion. When the brush is withdrawn, cells adhere to it and are taken to the laboratory for further evaluation. Extraction (D) is the appropriate root operation for the bronchial brush biopsy since tissue and cells were removed for evaluation instead of fluid, supported by *AHA Coding Clinic,* 2016, 1Q, 26.

Figure 4.8. Bronchoscopy

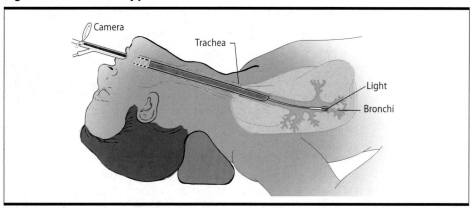

The lungs are part of the Respiratory (B) body system. Table ØBD lists a specific body part character for Lower Lobe Bronchus, Left (B). The scope was inserted directly through a natural opening, so the approach is Via Natural or Artificial Opening Endoscopic (8).

Diagnostic (X) is used for the qualifier since the samples taken will undergo further study.

Root Operation		
Extraction (D)	Definition:	Pulling or stripping out or off all or a portion of a body part by the use of force
	Explanation:	The qualifier DIAGNOSTIC is used to identify extraction procedures that are biopsies

Case Study 4.30. Biopsy, Laparoscopic Liver and Evacuation of Ascites

The patient was taken to the operating room and placed in the supine position. General anesthesia was induced. A Hasson cutdown technique was utilized in a supraumbilical location. Upon gaining entry into the peritoneal cavity, a very large amount of ascitic fluid was siphoned free prior to placing a 5 mm trocar. Once the 5 mm trocar was placed, the patient's abdomen was insufflated with carbon dioxide to create a pneumoperitoneum to approximately a total of 15 mmHg. The patient tolerated the insufflation well.

A 30-degree laparoscope was inserted. Examination of the liver showed it to be nodular in appearance with a large amount of ascitic fluid, which was not purulent. Additional trocars were placed, 11 mm in the subxiphoid region and another 5 mm in the right upper quadrant. At this time, approximately 6 liters of ascitic fluid was evacuated to gain entry to the liver parenchyma because it was submerged in all of the ascites.

FNA biopsies were taken from the liver parenchyma x2. Once this was completed, three liver biopsies were obtained with the use of laparoscopic scissors, passed off the field, and sent to pathology. Hemostasis was intact with the use of Bovie electrocautery at the liver edge. A piece of Surgicel was applied within the liver biopsy sites. The liver bed was reexamined and shown to be hemostatic. The trocars were removed under direct vision. No bleeding was noted at the trocar sites. The abdomen was allowed to collapse. The 5 mm trocar and laparoscope were removed.

The fascia from the xiphoid, along with the supraumbilical locations, was closed with 2-0 Vicryl in a figure-of-eight fashion. Skin incisions were closed with staples. The patient was awoken from anesthesia and transported back to the bone marrow transplant unit in stable condition and extubated. All sponge, needle, and instrument counts were correct at the end of the case.

Code(s):

ØW9G4ZZ	Drainage of Peritoneal Cavity, Percutaneous Endoscopic Approach
ØFDØ4ZX	Extraction of Liver, Percutaneous Endoscopic Approach, Diagnostic
ØFBØ4ZX	Excision of Liver, Percutaneous Endoscopic Approach, Diagnostic

Rationale:

Ascites refers to abnormal accumulation of fluid in the abdominal (peritoneal) cavity. Treatment may include removing fluid. The ICD-10-PCS index lists table ØW9G for Drainage, Peritoneal Cavity.

Guideline B2.1a also instructs that the general anatomical regions body systems be used when the procedure is performed on a region instead of a specific body part and lists drainage of a body cavity as an example. Review of table ØW9G confirms that body system Anatomical Regions, General (W), root operation Drainage (9), and body part Peritoneal Cavity (G) are correct.

PCS Guideline
General guidelines
B2.1a   The procedure codes in the general anatomical regions body systems can be used when the procedure is performed on an anatomical region rather than a specific body part (e.g., root operations Control and Detachment, Drainage of a body cavity) or on the rare occasion when no information is available to support assignment of a code to a specific body part.
Examples: Control of postoperative hemorrhage is coded to the root operation Control found in the general anatomical regions body systems.
Chest tube drainage of the pleural cavity is coded to the root operation Drainage found in the general anatomical regions body systems. Suture repair of the abdominal wall is coded to the root operation Repair in the general anatomical regions body system.

In this example, the evacuation of ascites is considered therapeutic and not diagnostic. No further tests were done on the ascitic fluid. Therefore, the seventh-character qualifier for the drainage of peritoneal cavity should be No Qualifier (Z).

A total of five liver biopsies were taken. Two tissue samples were aspirated via fine needle from the liver parenchyma, which is described by the root operation Extraction (D). Three more tissue samples were obtained with laparoscopy scissors, which is reported with the root operation Excision (B). Although there were five biopsies in total, all were taken from the same body part Liver (Ø), in the body system Hepatobiliary System and Pancreas (F), so only one code is needed for the Extraction (D) and one for the Excision (B).

The liver biopsies were completed via Percutaneous Endoscopic (4) approach. The qualifier is Diagnostic (X) since the samples were sent to pathology for further study.

Root Operation		
Drainage (9)	Definition:	Taking or letting out fluids and/or gases from a body part
	Explanation:	The qualifier DIAGNOSTIC is used to identify drainage procedures that are biopsies
Excision (B)	Definition:	Cutting out or off, without replacement, a portion of a body part
	Explanation:	The qualifier DIAGNOSTIC is used to identify excision procedures that are biopsies
Extraction (D)	Definition:	Pulling or stripping out or off all or a portion of a body part by the use of force
	Explanation:	The qualifier DIAGNOSTIC is used to identify extraction procedures that are biopsies

Case Study 4.31. Biopsy, Bone Marrow

The skin over the iliac crest was cleansed with antiseptic solution and a local anesthetic was injected to numb the skin. The biopsy needle was inserted into the bone. The core of the needle was removed and the needle pressed forward and rotated in both directions. An adequate sample of bone marrow was obtained within the needle. The needle was removed and pressure applied to the biopsy site. A bandage was applied.

Code(s):

Ø7DR3ZX   Extraction of Iliac Bone Marrow, Percutaneous Approach, Diagnostic

Rationale:
Bone marrow biopsies are coded using the root operation Extraction (D). Bone Marrow is found in the Lymphatic and Hemic Systems (7) body system with three body part (character 4) values available:

Q	**Bone Marrow, Sternum**
R	**Bone Marrow, Iliac**
S	**Bone Marrow, Vertebral**

This example lists the Iliac (R) crest as the body part. The biopsy was performed using a needle, making the approach Percutaneous (3). Since this was performed as a biopsy, the qualifier Diagnostic (X) is used.

Root Operation		
Extraction (D)	Definition:	Pulling or stripping out or off all or a portion of a body part by the use of force
	Explanation:	The qualifier DIAGNOSTIC is used to identify extraction procedures that are biopsies

Biopsy Followed by More Definitive Treatment

Guideline B3.4b

B3.4b	**If a diagnostic Excision, Extraction, or Drainage procedure (biopsy) is followed by a more definitive procedure, such as Destruction, Excision or Resection at the same procedure site, both the biopsy and the more definitive treatment are coded.**
	Example: **Biopsy of breast followed by partial mastectomy at the same procedure site, both the biopsy and the partial mastectomy procedure are coded.**

AHA Coding Clinic

2017, 3Q, 12   Therapeutic and Diagnostic Paracentesis

Root Operation		
Excision (B)	Definition:	Cutting out or off, without replacement, a portion of a body part
	Explanation:	The qualifier DIAGNOSTIC is used to identify excision procedures that are biopsies
Extraction (D)	Definition:	Pulling or stripping out or off all or a portion of a body part by the use of force
	Explanation:	The qualifier DIAGNOSTIC is used to identify extraction procedures that are biopsies
Drainage (9)	Definition:	Taking or letting out fluids and/or gases from a body part
	Explanation:	The qualifier DIAGNOSTIC is used to identify drainage procedures that are biopsies
Destruction (5)	Definition:	Physical eradication of all or a portion of a body part by the direct use of energy, force, or a destructive agent
	Explanation:	None of the body part is physically taken out
Resection (T)	Definition:	Cutting out or off, without replacement, all of a body part
	Explanation:	None

The diagnostic objective of the biopsy is to determine the nature of the lesion or tissue. In addition, a separate procedure may be performed on the same site during the same surgical episode in order to fulfill a therapeutic objective. The assignment of separate codes, one for the biopsy and one for the therapeutic procedure, provides a means of capturing these separate objectives. A second guideline, B3.2c, which covers multiple procedure coding guidelines, provides further support for assigning separate codes for these separate objectives.

PCS Guideline
Multiple procedures
B3.2   During the same operative episode, multiple procedures are coded if:
c. Multiple root operations with distinct objectives are performed on the same body part.
Example: Destruction of sigmoid lesion and bypass of sigmoid colon are coded separately.

Practical Application for Guideline B3.4b

Case Study 4.32. Biopsy and Brain Tumor Removal

Procedure: Left temporal craniotomy and removal of brain tumor.

The patient was placed in the supine position, shoulder rolled, and the head turned to the right side. The entire left scalp was prepped and draped in the usual fashion after being placed in a two-point, skeletal fixation. Next, an inverted-U fashion base over the asterion was made over the temporoparietal area of the skull. A free flap was elevated after the scalp was reflected using the burr hole and craniotome. The bone flap was placed aside and soaked in the bacitracin solution. The dura was opened in an inverted-U fashion. Using the Stealth, a large cystic mass was visualized just below the cortex in the white matter, anterior to the trigone of the ventricle. Heading through the vein of Labbe, taking great care to preserve it, the tumor was visualized where it almost made it to the surface. A small corticectomy was made using the Stealth for guidance. Leaving the small corticectomy, the large cavity was entered. The very abnormal tissue was **biopsied** and submitted to pathology. A frozen section diagnosis of glioblastoma multiforme was given. With the operating microscope and Greenwood bipolar forceps, the tumor was systematically debulked. The tumor was very vascular. **Removal of the tumor** was continued until all visible tumors were removed. It appeared that there were two gliotic planes circumferentially, as seen through the ventricle. After removing all visible tumor grossly, the cavity was irrigated multiple times and meticulous hemostasis was obtained. The dura was closed primarily with 4-0 Nurolon sutures with the piece of DuraGen placed over this in order to increase chances for a good watertight seal. The bone flap was replaced and sutured with the Lorenz titanium plate system. The muscle fascia galea was closed with interrupted 2-0 Vicryl sutures. Skin staples were used for skin closure.

Code(s):

ØØBØØZX	Excision of Brain, Open Approach, Diagnostic
ØØBØØZZ	Excision of Brain, Open Approach
8EØ9XBZ	Computer Assisted Procedure of Head and Neck Region

Rationale:

A biopsy was done in this procedure as a diagnostic test, which led to a diagnosis of glioblastoma multiforme. An additional procedure was performed during the same operative episode for the tumor removal. Although performed on the same body part, both procedures are coded according to guideline B3.4b.

Two codes are used to capture this procedure, with the qualifier character being the differentiating value. For both codes, the body system is Central Nervous System and Cranial Nerves (Ø) with the body part Brain (Ø); the root operation Excision (B) meets the objective of only removing portions of the brain; and the procedure was completed through an opening in the skull for an Open (Ø) approach.

The seventh character for the biopsy is coded using qualifier value Diagnostic (X); the seventh character of No Qualifier (Z) is used for the tumor removal excision code.

Root Operation		
Excision (B)	Definition:	Cutting out or off, without replacement, a portion of a body part
	Explanation:	The qualifier DIAGNOSTIC is used to identify excision procedures that are biopsies

An additional code is reported to represent the use of the Stealth System. The Stealth is a stereotactic navigational system, indicating that this is a Computer Assisted Procedure (B) found in the Other Procedures (8) section with a body part for Head and Neck Region (9). No other imaging (e.g., fluoroscopy, MRI, CT) was mentioned so No Qualifier (Z) is used.

Since the bone flap was immediately replaced, it is considered inherent to the procedure as part of the closure. DuraGen, when applied as part of the closure, is also not coded separately. (*AHA Coding Clinic*, 2017, 3Q, 17)

> ### Case Study 4.33. Thoracentesis, Diagnostic and Therapeutic
>
> **History:** Right pleural effusion. History of right hepatectomy.
>
> **Technical Report:** Informed consent was obtained and witnessed. The patient was brought to the ultrasound suite and placed in a recumbent position. A time-out and pause and confirm was performed. The right thorax was prepped and draped in a sterile fashion. Under ultrasound guidance and following cutaneous anesthesia, a 5-French one-step catheter was advanced into the right pleural fluid above a rib. A total of 750 liters of serosanguineous fluid was removed. Following aspiration, the catheter was removed and a bandage was applied. The patient was sent for a chest radiograph.
>
> **Findings:** Limited ultrasound confirms the presence of a pleural effusion.
>
> **Impression:** Successful ultrasound guided **diagnostic and therapeutic** right-sided thoracentesis with aspiration of 750 ml of serosanguineous fluid. Sample was submitted to the laboratory for further analysis per referring physician.

Code(s):

ØW993ZZ	**Drainage of Right Pleural Cavity, Percutaneous Approach**
BB4BZZZ	**Ultrasonography of Pleura**

Rationale:

A thoracentesis procedure was performed to drain fluid from the cavity between the lungs and chest wall (the pleural space). A needle was placed through the skin overlying the chest wall and advanced into the pleural space. Fluid was drawn into the needle. This procedure is coded using root operation Drainage (9) since fluid was removed, not tissue.

Root Operation		
Drainage (9)	Definition:	Taking or letting out fluids and/or gases from a body part
	Explanation:	The qualifier DIAGNOSTIC is used to identify drainage procedures that are biopsies

Figure 4.9. Pleural Fluid Sample

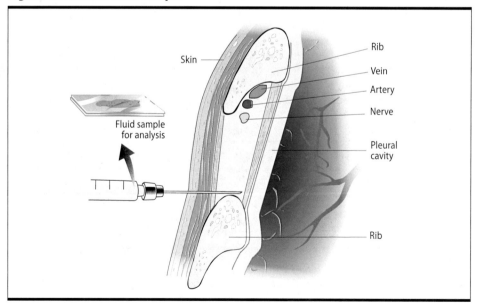

The ICD-10-PCS index directs the coder to *see* Drainage, Anatomical Regions, General ØW9 for Thoracentesis. The advice in the following Guideline B2.1a further demonstrates that the appropriate body system for drainage of a body cavity is the Anatomical Regions, General (W).

PCS Guideline
General guidelines
B2.1a   The procedure codes in the general anatomical regions body systems can be used when the procedure is performed on an anatomical region rather than a specific body part (e.g., root operations Control and Detachment, Drainage of a body cavity) or on the rare occasion when no information is available to support assignment of a code to a specific body part. *Examples:* Control of postoperative hemorrhage is coded to the root operation Control found in the general anatomical regions body systems. Chest tube drainage of the pleural cavity is coded to the root operation Drainage found in the general anatomical regions body systems. Suture repair of the abdominal wall is coded to the root operation Repair in the general anatomical regions body system.

Review of table ØW9 lists bilateral body parts for the pleural cavity with body part Pleural Cavity, Right (9) as the correct value. A Percutaneous (3) approach is used since a needle was used to puncture the skin in order to reach the pleural space.

When there is a diagnostic and therapeutic component to the same procedure, only the therapeutic is reported, using seventh character No Qualifier (Z). The X qualifier is exclusively for diagnostic procedures.

Spotlight
If a diagnostic procedure is followed by a therapeutic procedure on a different body part or using a different approach, two separate codes are needed to capture the diagnostic and therapeutic procedures. This advice is consistent with *AHA Coding Clinic,* 2017, 3Q, 12.

Depending on the facility requirements, code BB4BZZZ can capture the ultrasound guidance used to guide the needle into the pleura.

Case Study 4.34. Mohs Surgery

Pre-Op Diagnosis: Biopsy proven basal cell carcinoma nasal dorsum, skin.

Post-Op Diagnosis: Basal cell carcinoma nasal dorsum, skin.

Pre-Op Size: 1.5 x 1.9 cm

Post-Op Size: 2.2 x 2.5 cm

Indication: Patient with biopsy confirmed basal cell carcinoma of the skin of the dorsum of the nose for Mohs micrographic surgical excision due to the tumor location in an area with high incidence of recurrence and with poorly defined borders.

Procedure: Mohs micrographic surgery for basal cell carcinoma of the nose. Two-stage procedure: 1st stage = 4 tissue blocks; 2nd stage = 6 tissue blocks.

The surgical site was injected with plain Marcaine 0.5% solution for local anesthesia and prepped and draped in sterile fashion. Prior to each stage, the surgical site was tested for anesthesia and reanesthetized as needed and again prepped and draped in a sterile fashion. The clinically visible tumor was carefully defined and debulked prior to the first stage, determining the extent of the surgical excision. With the first stage, a thin layer of tumor-laden tissue was excised with a narrow margin of normal appearing skin, using the Mohs technique. The wound was dressed and the patient returned to the waiting room. A map was prepared to correspond to the area of skin that was excised. The tissue was prepared for the cryostat and sectioned into four tissue blocks. Each section was coded, cut, and stained for microscopic examination. The entire base and margins of the excised piece of tissue were examined by the surgeon. The areas noted to be positive were mapped for excision in the second stage. The patient was returned to the operating room and reanesthetized and prepped and draped in sterile fashion. The positive areas identified in the mapping from the previous stage were removed with the Mohs technique and reprocessed for analysis. During the second stage excision, six tissue blocks were prepared. No tumor was identified after the final stage of surgery. The patient tolerated the procedure well without any complication. After discussion with the patient regarding the various options, it was decided that the best closure option for the size and location of the defect was referral to plastic surgery for nasal reconstruction using a median forehead flap for optimal functional and cosmetic results.

Code(s):

ØHB1XZZ   **Excision of Face Skin, External Approach**

Rationale:

Review of the operative report indicates the objective of the procedure was to remove a skin lesion from the dorsum of the nose. Root operation Excision (B) is coded when a portion of a body part is cut off without replacement. Body system Skin and Breast (H) is coded using body part Skin, Face (1) to specify the location of the lesion removed. An External (X) approach was used since the procedure was performed directly on the skin.

Root Operation		
Excision (B)	Definition:	Cutting out or off, without replacement, a portion of a body part
	Explanation:	The qualifier DIAGNOSTIC is used to identify excision procedures that are biopsies

Since a previous biopsy had already confirmed basal cell carcinoma, the tissue being sent for pathological examination during this procedure was used only to define the margins of the tumor, and not as a diagnostic test. Therefore, only one code is reported to reflect the removal of the skin lesion and because this is therapeutic treatment and not diagnostic, a seventh character of Diagnostic (X) would not be appropriate. The correct seventh character is No Qualifier (Z).

Case Study 4.35. Biopsy and Polyp Removal via Colonoscopy

Colonoscopy was performed with biopsy and electrocautery at descending colon of oozing vasculature consistent with angiodysplasia. Four polyps were removed by snare technique from the sigmoid, ascending, and transverse colon.

Code(s):

ØDBM8ZX	Excision of Descending Colon, Via Natural or Artificial Opening Endoscopic, Diagnostic
ØD5M8ZZ	Destruction of Descending Colon, Via Natural or Artificial Opening Endoscopic
ØDBN8ZZ	Excision of Sigmoid Colon, Via Natural or Artificial Opening Endoscopic
ØDBK8ZZ	Excision of Ascending Colon, Via Natural or Artificial Opening Endoscopic
ØDBL8ZZ	Excision of Transverse Colon, Via Natural or Artificial Opening Endoscopic

Rationale:

All of the procedures in this case were performed on the colon, which is part of the Gastrointestinal (D) body system.

Two guidelines support the use of multiple procedure codes: B3.4b, which is the focus of this section, and also guideline B3.2a that is explained below. A biopsy of the descending colon was performed followed by destruction of the oozing vasculature. Guideline B3.4b supports coding the biopsy and the definitive treatment performed on the same body part.

The biopsy is coded using root operation Excision (B) with qualifier Diagnostic (X). The electrocautery of the body part Descending Colon (M) was for definitive treatment and is captured by root operation Destruction (5), with No Qualifier (Z).

Root Operation		
Excision (B)	Definition:	Cutting out or off, without replacement, a portion of a body part
	Explanation:	The qualifier DIAGNOSTIC is used to identify excision procedures that are biopsies
Destruction (5)	Definition:	Physical eradication of all or a portion of a body part by the direct use of energy, force, or a destructive agent
	Explanation:	None of the body part is physically taken out

Guideline B3.2a addresses the need to code multiple procedures when the same root operation is performed on different body parts that have a distinct body part character. The polyps removed by snare technique are all considered Excision (B) procedures. Three separate codes are required because there are separate body part characters for the Sigmoid Colon (N), Ascending Colon (K), and Transverse Colon (L). The qualifier for the removal of the polyps is No Qualifier (Z) since the removal was for a definitive purpose, not diagnostic.

PCS Guideline
Multiple procedures
B3.2   During the same operative episode, multiple procedures are coded if: a. The same root operation is performed on different body parts as defined by distinct values of the body part character.   *Examples:* Diagnostic excision of liver and pancreas are coded separately.   Excision of lesion in the ascending colon and excision of lesion in the transverse colon are coded separately.

A colonoscopy was performed using a colonoscope, a flexible tube with a camera and a source of light at its tip. The tip of the colonoscope was inserted into the anus and advanced slowly, under visual control, into the rectum and through the colon. This procedure meets the approach definition of Via Natural or Artificial Opening Endoscopic (8).

Overlapping Body Layers

Guideline B3.5

> **B3.5** **If the root operations Excision, Repair or Inspection are performed on overlapping layers of the musculoskeletal system, the body part specifying the deepest layer is coded.**
>
> *Example:* **Excisional debridement that includes skin and subcutaneous tissue and muscle is coded to the muscle body part.**

AHA Coding Clinic

2016, 3Q, 20   Excisional Debridement of Sacrum
2016, 3Q, 20   VersaJet™ Nonexcisional Debridement of Leg Muscle
2016, 3Q, 21   Nonexcisional Debridement of Infected Lumbar Wound
2016, 3Q, 21   Nonexcisional Pulsed Lavage Debridement
2016, 3Q, 22   Debridement of Bone and Tendon Using Tenex Ultrasound Device
2015, 3Q, 3-8   Excisional and Nonexcisional Debridement
2014, 3Q, 14   Application of Thera Skin® and Excisional Debridement

The integumentary and musculoskeletal systems of the body are composed of multiple layers of tissue. The outermost layers are the skin, subcutaneous tissue, and fascia. Below these tissues are the muscles, tendons, bursae, ligaments, bones, and joints. In PCS, these body layers are represented by 10 body systems as follows:

- Skin and Breast (H)
- Subcutaneous Tissue and Fascia (J)
- Muscles (K)
- Tendons (L)
- Bursae and Ligaments (M)
- Head and Facial Bones (N)
- Upper Bones (P)
- Lower Bones (Q)
- Upper Joints (R)
- Lower Joints (S)

Some root operations, specifically Excision (B), Repair (Q), and Inspection (J), may be performed on multiple body layers during the same operative session. Each of these root operations are described in the table below.

Root Operation		
Excision (B)	Definition:	Cutting out or off, without replacement, a portion of a body part
	Explanation:	The qualifier DIAGNOSTIC is used to identify excision procedures that are biopsies
Repair (Q)	Definition:	Restoring, to the extent possible, a body part to its normal anatomic structure and function
	Explanation:	Used only when the method to accomplish the repair is not one of the other root operations
Inspection (J)	Definition:	Visually and/or manually exploring a body part
	Explanation:	Visual exploration may be performed with or without optical instrumentation. Manual exploration may be performed directly or through intervening body layers.

When performing an Excision (B), Repair (Q), or Inspection (J), each individual layer may need to be excised, repaired, or inspected as the operation progresses. When one of these root operations is performed on overlapping body layers, only one code is assigned reflecting the deepest layer on which the surgical procedure was performed.

In addition to this guideline related to coding procedures performed on overlapping body layers, a number of additional guidelines apply to Excision (B), Repair (Q), and Inspection (J). In order to ensure that the correct root operation is selected, all root operation guidelines must be reviewed and applied.

Practical Application for Guideline B3.5

Case Study 4.36. Repair, Stab Wound to Thigh

The patient presented to the ED with a stab wound to the left thigh. On initial examination, it appeared as if the wound was fairly superficial with penetration barely into the subcutaneous tissue. However, the wound was bleeding extensively so the patient was sent to the OR. After being prepped, draped, and placed under local sedation, the area around the wound was injected with Marcaine. Exploration of the wound found that it was deeper than expected, lacerating the quadriceps muscle. All the tissue surrounding and down to the muscle appeared viable except for a small section of skin that was scraped back to healthy tissue. The muscle was sutured closed followed by sutures in the subcutaneous tissue and skin. The patient left the OR in stable condition.

Code(s):

ØKQRØZZ   **Repair Left Upper Leg Muscle, Open Approach**

Rationale:

The wound was restored to its normal structure with sutures, meeting the root operation definition of Repair (Q). Although every layer of the wound was sutured in order to completely close the defect, only the muscle repair is coded as it was the deepest layer repaired. Muscle repair is captured by the Muscles (K) body system. Since the thigh muscle was repaired, a review of table ØQK shows that body part Upper Leg Muscle, Left (R) is used. The wound was repaired through an open wound for an approach of Open (Ø).

Case Study 4.37. Arthroscopy, Diagnostic Shoulder

The patient was laid supine upon the operative table. The right shoulder was marked for the procedure. After receiving interscalene block general anesthetic by the anesthesia department, the patient was placed in a modified beach chair position and prepped and draped in the usual sterile manner. Small stab incisions were made in the creation of the anterior, accessory anterior, and accessory posterior arthroscopic portals. A standard arthroscope was introduced. A full and complete diagnostic arthroscopy was carried out by visualizing and probing the subacromial space, subacromial bursa, biceps tendon, coracoacromial ligament, supraspinatus, subscapularis, infraspinatus, capsule-labral complex, glenoid labrum, humeral head, and glenoid. All were within normal limits.

Code(s):

ØRJJ4ZZ   **Inspection of Right Shoulder Joint, Percutaneous Endoscopic Approach**

Rationale:

A diagnostic arthroscopy was done to look within a joint so Inspection (J) is the appropriate root operation.

In this example, muscles, tendons, bursae, ligaments, as well as the joint itself, were visualized. Guideline B3.5 instructs that when multiple overlapping layers are inspected, only the deepest layer is coded, which in this case is the Shoulder Joint, Right (J). The shoulder is part of the Upper Joints (R) body system. A scope was inserted and used to visualize the joint, which meets the approach definition of Percutaneous Endoscopic (4). No Device (Z) and No Qualifier (Z) are used.

Figure 4.10. Shoulder Anatomy

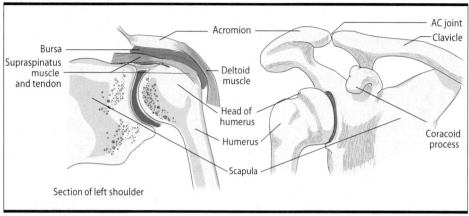

Section of left shoulder

Spotlight

Note that guideline B3.5 only refers to procedures on the overlapping layers of the musculoskeletal system. In contrast, guidelines B3.11b and B4.1c provide instruction regarding tubular and other non-musculoskeletal, non-tubular body parts. For instance, individual body parts or the deepest body parts are not reported for a diagnostic laparoscopy of multiple abdominal body parts (non-tubular); rather, a code from the Anatomical Regions, General (W), such as Peritoneal Cavity (G), is used to represent all of the body parts. An inspection on tubular body parts, such as the bladder and ureter, is coded to ureter to represent the most distal body part inspected.

Case Study 4.38. Debridement, Decubitus Ulcer

Procedure: Debridement of stage IV necrotic sacral decubitus ulcer.

The patient was properly prepped and draped under local sedation. A 0.25% Marcaine was injected circumferentially around the necrotic decubitus ulcer. A wide excision and debridement of the necrotic decubitus ulcer was taken down into the right gluteus maximus muscle adjacent to the sacrum and all necrotic tissue was electrocauterized and removed. All bleeding was cauterized with electrocautery and a Kerlix stack was placed and a pressure dressing applied. The patient was sent to recovery in satisfactory condition.

Code(s):
ØKBNØZZ   Excision of Right Hip Muscle, Open Approach

Rationale:
This example states that tissue was excised as well as electrocauterized for a root operation of Excision (B). In order to fully excise all of the damaged areas of this wound, the skin, subcutaneous, and muscle layers were removed. Even though tissue was excised from multiple body layers, representing multiple PCS body systems, only a single code for the deepest layer is assigned. In this case, the body system value for Muscle (K) is used.

Body part Hip Muscle, Right (N) is coded with an approach of Open (Ø). The gluteus maximus muscle is included in the Hip Muscle, Right (N) according to the Body Part Key (appendix D). The tissue was removed for therapeutic purposes so No Qualifier (Z) is used for the seventh character.

Beyond the Guidelines

Coding Debridement

AHA Coding Clinic

2018, 1Q, 14	Excisional Debridement of Breast Tissue and Skin
2017, 4Q, 41-42	Extraction Procedures
2016, 3Q, 20	Excisional Debridement of Sacrum
2016, 3Q, 20	VersaJet™ Nonexcisional Debridement of Leg Muscle
2016, 3Q, 21	Nonexcisional Debridement of Infected Lumbar Wound
2016, 3Q, 21	Nonexcisional Pulsed Lavage Debridement
2016, 3Q, 22	Debridement of Bone and Tendon Using Tenex Ultrasound Device
2015, 3Q, 3-8	Excisional and Nonexcisional Debridement
2015, 3Q, 13	Nonexcisional Debridement of Cranial Wound with Removal and Replacement of Hardware
2015, 1Q, 23	Non-Excisional Debridement with Lavage of Wound
2015, 1Q, 34	Arthroscopic Meniscectomy with Debridement and Abrasion Chondroplasty
2014, 4Q, 32	Open Reduction Internal Fixation of Fracture with Debridement
2014, 3Q, 14	Application of TheraSkin® and Excisional Debridement
2014, 3Q, 18	Placement of Reverse Sural Fasciocutaneous Pedicle Flap

Debridement is the removal of unhealthy tissue, whether it is devitalized, contaminated, or infected, in order to promote the healing of adjacent healthy tissue. Due to the proximity of the musculoskeletal body layers, the damaged tissue is often not isolated to just one specific layer and debridement may require the removal of tissue from all of the layers affected.

The two primary methods used to carry out a debridement procedure are nonexcisional and excisional. The root operation employed depends on the method applied: Extraction (D) for nonexcisional debridement and Excision (B) for excisional debridement. The use of a sharp surgical instrument alone does not justify the use of root operation Excision (B). It must be clear in the documentation that the definition of the root operation Excision (B) was met, meaning tissue was deliberately cut or excised away with a sharp instrument. According to *AHA Coding Clinic,* 2015, 3Q, 5, excisional debridement may be reported if the physician documents "excisional debridement."

Root Operation		
Excision (B)	Definition:	Cutting out or off, without replacement, a portion of a body part
	Explanation:	The qualifier DIAGNOSTIC is used to identify excision procedures that are biopsies
Extraction (D)	Definition:	Pulling or stripping out or off all or a portion of a body part by the use of force
	Explanation:	The qualifier DIAGNOSTIC is used to identify extraction procedures that are biopsies

It is not always easy to determine whether tissue has been deliberately excised from a wound. Certain devices and surgical terms identified in the documentation can provide clues as to whether a nonexcisional or excisional method was used. The following instruments are commonly used in debridement procedures: scalpel, wire, electrocautery tip, saw, blade, or scissors. Although use of one of these instruments may be a clue as to whether or not an excisional debridement has been performed, the use of these instruments alone does not always justify root operation Excision (B). Documentation must state that tissue was cut away, excised, or trimmed using these sharp instruments.

Nonexcisional debridement can also be carried out via the use of these same sharp instruments. However, the documentation will reflect only minor removal of tissue using terms such as brushing, washing, pulse lavage, curettage, decortication, or scraping, which does not meet the definition of

Excision (B). Instead, the code should be built using root operation Extraction (D) (*AHA Coding Clinic,* 2015, 3Q, 3).

Table 4.1. Extraction and Excision Terms/Devices

Extraction (D)		Excision (B)	
Term	**Device**	**Term**	**Device**
scraping	scalpel	excision	bone saw
curettage	curette	cutting	scalpel
irrigating	VersaJet		electrocautery tip
lavage	Pulsavac		scissors
brushing			wire
washing			

One important aspect of debridement coding is knowing how a surgical tool was used. The previous table shows that a scalpel can be used for excisional and nonexcisional debridement. How the scalpel is used dictates which root operation, Excision (B) or Extraction (D), is the most appropriate. For example, a scalpel can scrape tissue out of a wound (Extraction) or cut tissue out of a wound (Excision).

Careful review of the documentation is critical so that the appropriate root operation is chosen. If the documentation does not clearly describe an excisional or a nonexcisional debridement, the provider should be queried.

Spotlight
"ICD-10 PCS does not provide a default if the debridement is not specified as 'excisional' or 'nonexcisional'" (*AHA Coding Clinic,* 2015, 3Q, 7).

Practical Application for Coding Debridement

Case Study 4.39. Debridement, Hand
The patient presented with cellulitis of her right hand caused by an unknown source, potentially a wood sliver. The provider performed a 4 sq cm excisional debridement of the skin of the right hand using a scalpel, going only to the level of the dermis. The wound was appropriately dressed.

Code(s):
0HBFXZZ   Excision of Right Hand Skin, External Approach

Rationale:
In this example, the physician documents excisional debridement as well as the use of a scalpel; root operation Excision (B) is appropriate. An External (X) approach was used since the procedure was performed directly on the skin. The body part Skin, Right Hand (F) can be found in the Skin and Breast (H) body system.

Case Study 4.40. Debridement, Foot Ulcer with Versajet
The patient developed a nonhealing necrotic ulcer of the left foot. A VersaJet debrider was used to perform debridement of the skin, subcutaneous tissue, and fascia.

Code(s):
0JDR0ZZ   Extraction of Left Foot Subcutaneous Tissue and Fascia, Open Approach

Rationale:

VersaJet is considered a nonexcisional debridement procedure according to *AHA Coding Clinic,* 2015, 3Q, 5. Root operation Extraction (D) is assigned for nonexcisional debridement. Since skin, subcutaneous tissue, and fascia was debrided, guideline B3.5 instructs the coder to assign a code for the deepest layer. Therefore, body system Subcutaneous Tissue and Fascia (J) is coded using a body part value of Subcutaneous Tissue and Fascia, Left Foot (R). Table ØJD lists approach choices of Open (Ø) and Percutaneous (3). Open (Ø) is the most appropriate approach for a VersaJet procedure.

Case Study 4.41. Debridement, Stasis Ulcers with Pulsavac

Procedure: Debridement of stasis ulcers of the lower extremities.

Having obtained adequate general endotracheal anesthesia, the patient was prepped from the pubis to the toes. The legs were examined and Pulsavac was used on the wounds bilaterally with 3 liters of saline with Bacitracin. Each wound was inspected. The ulcer on the right lower leg had adequate hemostasis and required only minor scraping of fibrinous debris from the skin and subcutaneous tissue and muscle. In the left lower leg wound, a scalpel was used to excise necrotic tissue down to the muscle. A wound VAC was placed on the left lower leg ulcer with adequate seal. Tegaderm was applied to the right leg wound. The patient tolerated the procedure well and returned to the recovery room in satisfactory condition.

Code(s):

ØKDSØZZ   **Extraction of Right Lower Leg Muscle, Open Approach**

ØKBTØZZ   **Excision of Left Lower Leg Muscle, Open Approach**

Rationale:

This procedure involved an excisional method of debridement as well as a nonexcisional method. The ulcer on the right lower leg was healthier and only required a minimal amount of scraping to clean the wound of fibrinous debris. Root operation Extraction (D) is used when scraping, brushing, or other forms of minor tissue removal are used. Extraction (D) is the appropriate root operation for non-excisional debridement of the Lower Leg Muscle, Right (S).

The wound bed of the left lower leg ulcer was not as healthy, requiring the necrotic tissue to be excised with a scalpel. Because tissue was deliberately cut away, this method of debridement meets the definition of Excision (B). The deepest layer debrided on this side was the muscle and therefore the code was built from the Excision (B) table in the Muscles (K) body system, with a body part of Lower Leg Muscle, Left (T).

Both procedures were performed using an Open (Ø) approach with No Device (Z) and No Qualifier (Z).

Bypass Procedures

Three guidelines apply to the root operation Bypass. The first guideline (B3.6a) addresses identification of "from" and "to" sites for all bypass procedures with the exception of coronary arteries. The second and third bypass procedure guidelines (B3.6b and B3.6c) are specific to the coronary arteries.

Guideline B3.6a

B3.6a	**Bypass procedures are coded by identifying the body part bypassed "from" and the body part bypassed "to." The fourth character body part specifies the body part bypassed from, and the qualifier specifies the body part bypassed to.** ***Example:* Bypass from stomach to jejunum, stomach is the body part and jejunum is the qualifier.**

AHA Coding Clinic

2017, 4Q, 36-38	Fontan Completion Procedure
2017, 4Q, 64-65	New Qualifier Values
2017, 4Q, 78	Intraoperative Treatment of Vascular Grafts
2017, 3Q, 5	Femoral Artery to Posterior Tibial Artery Bypass Using Autologous and Synthetic Grafts
2017, 3Q, 15	Bypass of Innominate Vein to Atrial Appendage
2017, 3Q, 16	Abdominal Aortic Debranching with Bypass of External Iliac Artery to Bilateral Renal Arteries and Superior Mesenteric Artery
2017, 3Q, 21	Augmentation Cystoplasty with Indiana Pouch and Continent Urinary Diversion
2017, 2Q, 17	Billroth II (Distal Gastrectomy with Gastrojejunostomy)
2017, 2Q, 22	Carotid Artery to Subclavian Artery Transposition
2017, 1Q, 19	Norwood Sano Procedure
2017, 1Q, 31	Left to Right Common Carotid Artery Bypass
2017, 1Q, 32	Peroneal Artery to Dorsalis Pedis Artery Bypass Using Saphenous Vein Graft
2017, 1Q, 34	Lymphovenous Bypass Following Mastectomy
2017, 1Q, 37	Perineal Urethrostomy
2016, 3Q, 37	Insertion of Arteriovenous Graft Using HeRO Device
2013, 4Q, 125	Stage II Cephalic Vein Transposition (Superficialization) of Arteriovenous Fistula
2013, 4Q, 126-127	Creation of Percutaneous Cutaneoperitoneal Fistula

Bypass Procedure Objective

The primary objective of a Bypass is to avoid, go around, or "bypass" a tubular body part. Bypass may be performed to reroute the contents of a tubular body part around a blocked region as is seen in a coronary artery bypass procedure or to prevent the tubular contents from entering a portion of the tubular body part as is seen in gastric bypass procedures performed to treat obesity.

Root Operation		
Bypass (1)	Definition:	Altering the route of passage of the contents of a tubular body part
	Explanation:	Rerouting contents of a body part to a downstream area of the normal route, to a similar route and body part, or to an abnormal route and dissimilar body part. Includes one or more anastomoses, with or without the use of a device.

Bypass Coding

Factors to remember when coding a bypass include:

- Bypass only applies to tubular body parts. When consulting the PCS tables, if Bypass is not offered in a particular body system it is because that body system does not contain any tubular body parts.
- The body part being bypassed is not removed from the body. Although the route of passage for the contents of the tubular body part is altered, the removal of the body part is not part of the overall objective of Bypass. **Note:** If the body part is removed, refer to root operations Excision and Resection. Bypass may be performed when:
  - removal of the body part is more detrimental to the patient than bypassing it
  - removal of the body part is more technically challenging than bypass of the body part
  - the intent of the bypass is to allow the bypassed area to heal so that in time the original route can once again be utilized
  - other functional features of the bypassed body part are needed even though contents may no longer pass through the bypassed body part
- Bypass follows the natural and often downstream course of the tubular body parts. The contents of the tubular body part are rerouted from an upstream site to a site further downstream.
- The route of the bypass may follow:
  - a normal route and similar body part
  - an abnormal route and dissimilar body part
- Bypass requires one or more anastomoses
- Bypass may be performed with or without the use of a device

Determining the "From" and "To" Sites

One of the more challenging aspects of coding bypass procedures is identifying the fourth character (body part) "from" and seventh character (qualifier) "to" sites. In order to select the correct "from" and "to" bypass sites, the typical course of contents through the tubular body part must be understood.

Spotlight
It is the **contents** of the tubular body part that are being rerouted. The contents may be rerouted to a similar or dissimilar body part.

Tubular contents have a natural flow through the body, with a beginning, middle, and end, typically flowing in a downstream course. The "from" site, which is rarely altered, represents the site from which the normal flow of contents is rerouted. It is important to understand that the "from" site can be at any point along the natural course of the tubular body part; it does not have to be at the very beginning tubular structure. For example, the digestive tract is one long tube, beginning at the oropharynx and ending at the anus. A bypass may be performed around a portion of the duodenum following an injury to allow the injured portion of duodenum to heal. In this case, the bypass begins and ends in the duodenum.

The "to" site identifies the new destination for the tubular contents. Bypass procedures may connect the tubular body part to a similar or dissimilar site. A similar site is a more distal site in the tubular body part, while a dissimilar site is one that is not part of the tubular body part. The primary objective of the procedure can help determine whether the "to" site is a similar or dissimilar body part.

Examples:

Tubular Contents Rerouted Along Similar Route to Similar Body Part

Procedure: Right femoral popliteal bypass graft using autologous tissue graft.

Objective: The tubular content (blood) is rerouted around a blocked area in the right femoral artery using bypass graft to the right popliteal artery to maintain blood supply to lower right leg and foot.

"From" site: Right femoral artery.

"To" site: Right popliteal artery.

Explanation: If the natural course of contents goes from point A to B to C, and the procedure alters this course so that contents no longer go through point B but instead go directly into point C (and B was not removed), then a bypass has been performed, rerouting the contents to a similar body part. In this example, point A is the "from" site and point C is the "to" site.

Tubular Contents Rerouted Along Alternate Route to Dissimilar Body Part

Procedure: Colostomy creation, transverse colon to skin.

Objective: The tubular content (stool) is rerouted out of the body through an opening created in the abdominal wall and skin (non-tubular body part) instead of passing through the remaining colon, rectum, and then out the anus.

"From" site: Transverse colon.

"To" site: Cutaneous.

Explanation: If the natural course of contents goes from point A to B to C, and the procedure alters the course of contents from point A to a site extraneous to this course, such as the skin, completely bypassing points B and C, this would be an example of rerouting contents to a dissimilar body part.

Spotlight
If the "from" or "to" site is not readily apparent in the operative report, the Bypass root operation table for that body system should be referenced. If what has been identified as the "from" or "to" site in the documentation is not found in the root operation table, it could mean the documentation has been misinterpreted and Bypass is not the correct root operation.

Practical Application for Guideline B3.6a

The following case studies provide practical examples of a variety of bypass procedures, along with rationale for the character values assigned for each code.

Case Study 4.42. Roux-en-Y Gastric Bypass

Procedure: Laparoscopic robotic-assisted Roux-en-Y gastric bypass with intraoperative upper endoscopy.

The abdomen was insufflated and trocars were placed, including robotic trocars. The omentum was divided at the level of the ligament of Treitz up to the transverse colon. The bowel was divided transversely at a point 60 cm distal to the ligament of Treitz. Once this was completed, a point 125 cm to this was selected and a side-to-side jejunojejunostomy was carried out. Stay sutures were placed. Enterotomies were created using the Harmonic scalpel. The side-to-side anastomosis was created using a stapling device and no reinforcement material. The open end of the anastomosis was closed transversely using staple with Seamguard reinforcement. The horizontal transection of the stomach was carried down using a stapling device and no reinforcement. The vertical transection of the stomach was carried out using a stapling device and Seamguard reinforcement. Subsequent to this time, the proximal Roux limb was brought up to the pouch and held in place with a single suture placed with the Endo Stitch device.

At this point, the robotic portion of the operation was begun. The da Vinci robotic assistance was brought to the operating room table and docked to the operating trocars without difficulty. The operation was begun using the da Vinci assistance by placing a single row of posterior running 2-0 Ethibond suture. The gastrotomy and enterotomy were created using the da Vinci robotic scissors as well as electrosurgical cautery. The endoscope was passed through the orifice of the stomach and the orifice of the small intestine to ensure adequate size of the anastomosis. Once this was completed, the inner layer of the anastomosis was completed by placing a posterior row of running sutures. The anterior layer of the anastomosis was closed over the endoscope with sutures. The anterior portion of the anastomosis was imbricated along its length using a suture. Once this was completed, a bowel clamp was placed on the Roux limb. Insufflation with the endoscope revealed no leakage of air under a fluid level of sterile saline. The anastomosis was patent and not bleeding.

Code(s):

ØD164ZA	**Bypass Stomach to Jejunum, Percutaneous Endoscopic Approach**
8EØW4CZ	**Robotic Assisted Procedure of Trunk Region, Percutaneous Endoscopic Approach**

Rationale:

Two procedure codes are required. The bypass procedure is reported with a code from the Medical and Surgical (Ø) section. Robotic assistance is reported with a code from the Other Procedure (8) section.

The bypass procedure, code ØD164ZA, was performed on the stomach and jejunum, which are part of the body system Gastrointestinal System (D). The objective of this procedure was to bypass a portion of the stomach by creating a small stomach pouch, which also bypassed the entire duodenum. Both of these are considered tubular body parts; this objective fits the definition of root operation Bypass (1). The natural route—stomach to duodenum to jejunum—was altered so that the stomach contents bypassed the duodenum and instead moved directly into the jejunum.

The body part character represents the origin of the flow of contents through a tubular body part and is the "from" site. In this case, the "from" site is Stomach (6). Laparoscopic approach meets the definition of Percutaneous Endoscopic (4) approach. Some bypass procedures require the use of a biologic or synthetic device to reroute the tubular contents. However, a Roux-en-Y procedure involves direct anastomosis of the jejunum to the stomach so the correct device value is No Device (Z). The qualifier for most bypass procedures represents the destination of the Bypass and is the "to" site. In this case, the qualifier Jejunum (A) is the destination or "to" site.

Figure 4.11. Roux-en-Y Gastric Bypass

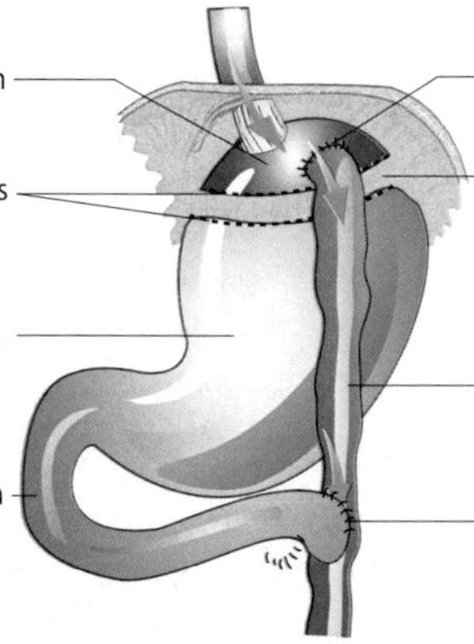

In addition to the bypass procedure code, a second code, 8E0W4CZ, is assigned for the use of robotic assistance to accomplish the procedure. Robotic assistance is sometimes used in conjunction with minimally invasive procedures, such as laparoscopy, because it allows for greater precision, flexibility, and control when complex procedures such are gastric bypass are performed.

Robotic assisted procedures are classified in the section Other Procedures (8). The Other Procedures section contains medical and surgical related procedures that do not fit well into one of the other more specific PCS sections. The body system Physiological Systems and Anatomical Regions (E) in this case identifies an anatomical region, which will be more specifically identified by the fourth character body region. Robotic assistance was used to place sutures and create the gastrotomy and enterotomy. The robotic-assistance body region for a Roux-en-Y gastric bypass is the Trunk Region (W). The root operation is Other Procedures (0), which is defined as methodologies that attempt to remediate or cure a disorder or disease. Robotic assistance was used as an adjunct to the Roux-en-Y gastric bypass performed to treat morbid obesity. The robotic-assistance was performed using the same laparoscopic approach as the Roux-en-Y gastric bypass, defined as Percutaneous Endoscopic (4) approach. The method used is captured by the value Robotic Assisted Procedure (C) in character 6. There are no qualifiers associated with robotic assistance so the value No Qualifier (Z) is assigned.

Case Study 4.43. Ileal Conduit

The patient was placed in the supine position. A left median incision was made because of the location of the ileal-conduit with stoma. The small bowel anastomosis was performed to provide 15 cm of ileal conduit. The GIA-55 stapler was used for the bowel and for the anastomosis. The TA-60 was used to secure the side of the side-to-side small bowel anastomosis. The mesenteric trap was closed. The left ureter was placed under the sigmoid mesentery after freeing both ureters and placed into the right lower quadrant.

The small bowel that was used for ileal conduit had the two staple lines removed. The left ureter was sewn to the one end of the bowel loop and the right ureter was anastomosed to the anterior mesenteric border of the mid portion of the ileal conduit. The opposite loop end was brought into the stoma in the right lower quadrant, which had been selected by the stoma nurse and secured in place with sutures to the rectus fascia and skin with pretty good eversion so as to consider the patient's obesity.

The patient's pulse was checked. Excellent hemostasis was obtained. The wound was irrigated again and the midline incision was closed with running sutures. The skin was closed with staples. Dressings were applied. Stoma and faceplate in binder. The patient tolerated the procedure well.

Code(s):

ØT18Ø7C   **Bypass Bilateral Ureters to Ileocutaneous with Autologous Tissue Substitute, Open Approach**

ØDBBØZZ   **Excision of Ileum, Open Approach**

Rationale:

Two codes are required for this case study. The first code captures the bypass procedure and the second captures excision of the ileum from which the ileal conduit was created.

Bypass procedure code ØT18Ø7C describes the bypass of both ureters using an ileal conduit. The ureters were rerouted along a different route to a dissimilar body part to bypass the bladder and urethra. The body system in which the bypass was performed is the Urinary System (T). Both ureters were rerouted and there is a bilateral body part value so rerouting of both ureters is captured by the single body part value Ureters, Bilateral (8) in the fourth-character position. The ureters are the "from" site of the bypass. An ileal conduit was used to divert urine from the ureters to a cutaneous site, rerouting the urine away from the bladder. A tubular body part was rerouted so the root operation Bypass (1) was performed. The procedure was performed through a left median incision, which is an Open (Ø) approach. The conduit was created from a segment of the patient's small intestine (autologous tissue), more specifically the ileum. The segment of ileum used to reroute the urine was captured by the device value for Autologous Tissue Substitute (7). The left and right ureters were anastomosed to the ileal conduit, which was stapled to an opening created in the abdomen. The abdomen or more specifically the skin of the abdomen was the final "to" site. Abdomen is not listed as a qualifier, but the skin represented by the qualifier Cutaneous is. However, because the ureters were first attached to the ileal conduit, which was attached to the skin to create a stoma, the qualifier Ileocutaneous (C) more specifically describes the "to" site. A bag is attached to the stoma to collect the urine that has been rerouted.

When an autograft is obtained from a separate site, an additional code is reported. The excision of the ileum is a separate site, which means it is not a component of the bypass procedure. Code ØDBBØZZ is required to capture this component of the procedure, according to guideline B3.9.

PCS Guideline
Excision for graft
B3.9   If an autograft is obtained from a different procedure site in order to complete the objective of the procedure, a separate procedure is coded. *Example:* Coronary bypass with excision of saphenous vein graft, excision of saphenous vein is coded separately.

Even though the primary procedure is being performed to reroute the ureters, this secondary procedure involves removing a portion of small intestine to create the ileal conduit. The Gastrointestinal System (D) is the value assigned for the body system for the Excision (B) procedure. The fourth-character body part value Ileum (B) captures the specific site of the excision.

Root operation Excision (B) involves cutting out or off, without replacement, a portion of a body part. In this case, a portion of the ileum was cut out to create the ileal conduit. The excision was performed through a left median incision, which correlates with an Open (Ø) approach. Even though a portion of the ileum was excised and used as an autograft, the autograft is captured in the Bypass (1) root operation. The Excision root operation does not involve a device so No Device (Z) is the correct value. The excision was not performed for diagnostic purposes so the correct qualifier is No Qualifier (Z).

Case Study 4.44. Aortobifemoral Bypass

After prepping and draping the patient, groin incisions were opened and the common femoral vein and its branches isolated and loops placed around the vessels. The abdomen was opened with some radiation changes noted in the wall and sections of the small bowel. A retractor was placed and the aorta and iliac arteries mobilized. The aorta was measured and an 11 x 6 bifurcated Microvelour graft selected. An end-to-end anastomosis was made connecting the graft to the aorta. The limbs of the graft were taken down through tunnels to the femoral arteries where end-to-side anastomosis was performed. All incisions were closed with sutures and staples and sterile dressings applied.

Code(s):

Ø41ØØJK   **Bypass Abdominal Aorta to Bilateral Femoral Arteries with Synthetic Substitute, Open Approach**

Rationale:

The objective of an aortobifemoral bypass is to improve blood flow in the lower extremities by rerouting blood around narrowed or blocked vessels. A "Y" shaped synthetic graft is positioned upside down with the single end connected or anastomosed to the abdominal aorta and each split end connected to the left and right femoral arteries distal to the diseased portion of the vessels.

The body system Lower Arteries (4) contains the aorta and femoral arteries. Open (Ø) approach was selected because both groin regions and the abdomen were incised and each area of anastomosis directly visualized. The body part Abdominal Aorta (Ø) is the "from" site. A Microvelour graft is a Synthetic Substitute (J) device. The qualifier Femoral Arteries, Bilateral (K) represents the "to" site.

Case Study 4.45. Subclavian/Carotid Artery Transposition

The patient was placed on the operating table in the supine position. A general endotracheal anesthetic was administered. The patient received preoperative antibiotics. The chest and neck were prepped with DuraPrep and draped sterilely. An incision was made a fingerbreadth above the left clavicle from near the sternal notch laterally approximately 8 cm. Dissection was carried through the dermis, subcutaneous tissue, and platysma with cautery. The clavicular head of the sternomastoid muscle was identified and divided with cautery. Medially, the internal jugular vein was identified and dissected circumferentially. The common carotid artery was identified and dissected circumferentially. Next, the anterior scalene muscle was divided and the subclavian artery identified. The subclavian artery was dissected circumferentially at this point, and the dissection was continued proximally identifying the thyrocervical trunk and internal mammary artery. Dissection was continued proximally by gently retracting the jugular vein medially. The vertebral artery was eventually identified and dissection was continued proximal to the structure. After five minutes of anticoagulation, the subclavian artery was clamped with a Satinsky clamp proximal to the vertebral artery. The subclavian artery was clipped distally with an angled DeBakey clamp. The vertebral artery was controlled with a vessel loop. The subclavian artery was transected proximal to the vertebral artery with the Metzenbaum scissors. The subclavian artery was oversewed in two layers of running 4-0 Prolene with an inner layer done as a horizontal mattress layer and the outer layers in over-and-over layer. The clamp was removed and hemostasis was excellent. The subclavian artery was examined carefully at the orifice of the vertebral artery. The artery was fairly normal at this level with the exception of some mild plaquing near the orifice of the vertebral artery. This caused no significant stenosis.

(Continued)

Case Study 4.45. (Continued)

Next, the carotid artery was controlled proximally and distally with vascular clamps, and a lateral arteriotomy was made. An end-to-side anastomosis was performed between the common carotid artery and subclavian artery with the posterior wall completed first with running 6-0 Prolene. The anastomosis was continued anteriorly. Prior to completing the anastomosis, vigorous flushing was performed and the anastomosis was irrigated copiously with heparinized saline solution. The anastomosis was brought to completion. Flow was restored first to the left arm, then the vertebral artery, and finally to the carotid artery. Hemostasis along the suture line was excellent. All structures were carefully checked, including the thoracic duct. At this point, hemostasis was excellent. The scalene fat pad was reapproximated over the repair with interrupted 2-0 Vicryl suture. A Blake drain was placed over the scalene fat pad and brought out lateral to the incision. The clavicular head of the sternocleidomastoid muscle was closed with interrupted 2-0 Vicryl suture. The platysma was closed with running 3-0 Vicryl, and the skin was closed with running 4-0 Monocryl. The epidermis was sealed with Dermabond and a dry, sterile dressing was placed. The drain was secured with a nylon suture. The patient was awakened in the room and demonstrated baseline motor and cranial nerve function. The patient was taken to recovery in stable condition.

Code(s):

Ø31JØZY   **Bypass Left Common Carotid Artery to Upper Artery, Open Approach**

Rationale:

Transposition of the subclavian artery may be performed to treat a blockage in the subclavian artery proximal to the transection site or in the aorta. This procedure may also be performed in preparation for insertion of a thoracic aorta endograft in a patient with a thoracic aneurysm. Most procedures classified to the root operation Bypass include the term bypass in the procedure description or in the operative report. However, the above case study uses only the term transposition to describe the procedural objective of altering the route of blood flow by bypassing a blockage proximal to the transected site in the subclavian artery. To assist with the visualization of this procedure, an illustration follows the rationale.

It is important to apply the full definition and explanation of the root operations as instructed by general guideline B3.1a. A thorough review of the documentation, or using an anatomical illustration, can establish the objective without the statement of the specific terminology (e.g., Bypass) in the root operation title. The inclusion or absence of a root operation in a particular body system, or body part in a certain root operation table, also assists in determining the correct code. Additionally, the index listing for Transposition includes Bypass.

The body system Upper Arteries (3) includes arteries in the head, neck, and chest region, which include the carotid and subclavian arteries. The objective of this arterial transposition procedure was to alter the route of blood flow, meeting the definition of root operation Bypass (1). Although it is the left subclavian artery that was cut and moved, the "from" site (body part) is **not** the subclavian artery. The "from" site (body part value) and the "to" site (qualifier value) relate to how the blood will flow through the vessels once the subclavian artery has been transposed. When the left subclavian artery is transposed, instead of getting its blood supply from the aorta, it will get its blood supply from the left common carotid artery. For this reason, the correct body part is Common Carotid Artery, Left (J) as it represents the "from" site. The procedure was performed under direct vision through a chest incision so the approach value is Open (Ø). This transposition procedure does not use any type of tissue or synthetic graft. The left common carotid and left subclavian arteries were anastomosed to each other, so the device value No Device (Z) is assigned. The subclavian artery is the "to" site. However, there is not a value for subclavian artery in the qualifier column for the body part Left Common Carotid Artery. The qualifier Upper Artery (Y) is the best choice as the subclavian artery is not considered an intracranial or extracranial artery.

Figure 4.12. Subclavian/Carotid Artery Transposition

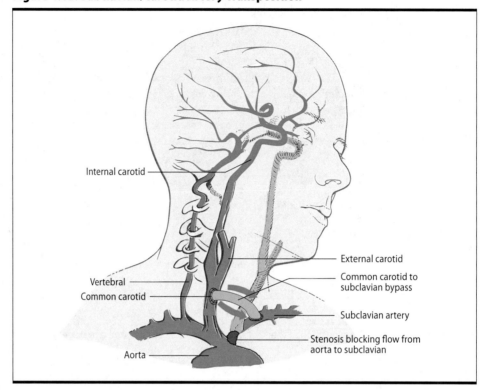

Internal carotid

External carotid

Common carotid to subclavian bypass

Vertebral

Common carotid

Subclavian artery

Stenosis blocking flow from aorta to subclavian

Aorta

Guidelines B3.6b and B3.6c

B3.6b   **Coronary artery bypass procedures are coded differently than other bypass procedures as described in the previous guideline. Rather than identifying the body part bypassed from, the body part identifies the number of coronary arteries bypassed to, and the qualifier specifies the vessel bypassed from.**

Example: **Aortocoronary artery bypass of the left anterior descending coronary artery and the obtuse marginal coronary artery is classified in the body part axis of classification as two coronary arteries, and the qualifier specifies the aorta as the body part bypassed from.**

AHA Coding Clinic

2017, 4Q, 78   Intraoperative Treatment of Vascular Grafts

2016, 4Q, 134   Changes to the ICD-10-PCS Official Guidelines for Coding and Reporting

2015, 2Q, 3-5   Coronary Artery Intervention Site

> **B3.6c**   **If multiple coronary arteries are bypassed, a separate procedure is coded for each coronary artery that uses a different device and/or qualifier.**
>
> *Example:* **Aortocoronary artery bypass and internal mammary coronary artery bypass are coded separately.**

AHA Coding Clinic

2016, 4Q, 134   Changes to the ICD-10-PCS Official Guidelines for Coding and Reporting
2016, 1Q, 27   Aortocoronary Bypass Graft Utilizing Y-Graft

In the root operation table for coronary artery bypass procedures (Ø21), the fourth- and seventh-character meanings are the opposite of what they are in bypass tables for other body systems. The fourth character (body part) represents the "to" site for coronary artery bypass procedures while the seventh character (qualifier) represents the "from" site. It is important to note that the "from" site represents the source of the blood supply **post** bypass.

The body part values for coronary artery bypass graft (CABG) procedures representing the "to" site do not designate the specific coronary arteries bypassed. Instead, they designate the number of coronary arteries bypassed. There are four body part values available:

> Ø   Coronary Artery, One Artery
> 1   Coronary Artery, Two Arteries
> 2   Coronary Artery, Three Arteries
> 3   Coronary Artery, Four or More Arteries

The seventh-character value represents the vessel that feeds the bypassed areas. The Aorta (W) and the Internal Mammary Artery, Left (LIMA) (9) are the two most frequently used "from" sites in CABG procedures, rerouting the blood from the aorta or LIMA around a blocked area in the coronary artery to a section of that artery that is patent and able to support blood flow. In addition to values for the aorta and LIMA, the seventh-character qualifier includes values for Coronary Artery (3), Internal Mammary Artery, Right (8), Thoracic Artery (C), and Abdominal Artery (F), which are other "from" sites that are sometimes used in CABG procedures.

Carefully reading the operative report and noting the bypass "from" sites is key to correct application of guideline B3.6c. This guideline is essentially a multiple procedure coding guideline. It defines situations when more than one code is necessary in order to capture the full operative objective. There are two variables that affect how many codes are required: how many "from" sites are used and how many different types of devices are used. To summarize:

- If multiple bypass "to" arteries are connected to the same "from" qualifier site using the same device or no device, one code is assigned for the bypass procedure.
- If multiple bypass "to" arteries are connected to different "from" qualifier sites or multiple devices are used, multiple codes must be assigned for the bypass procedure.

The following CABG decision tree may help determine the number of codes required.

Figure 4.13. CABG Decision Tree

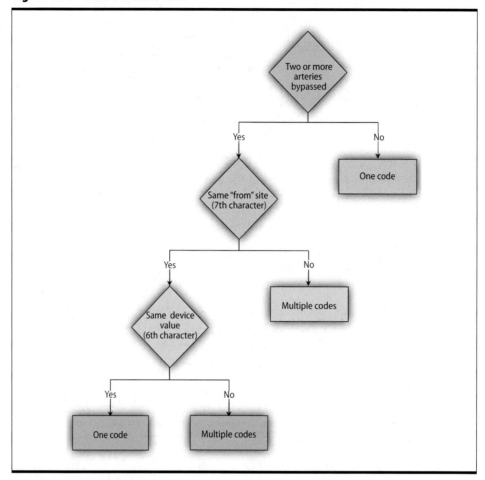

Practical Application for Guidelines B3.6b and B3.6c

The following case studies provide examples of coding CABG procedures. While one or more codes may be required for the CABG procedure, CABG procedures often require additional codes to capture other aspects of the procedure, such as harvesting of autografts and cardiopulmonary bypass. The following guideline is applied frequently for the harvesting of the autografts.

PCS Guideline
Excision for Graft
B3.9 If an autograft is obtained from a different procedure site in order to complete the objective of the procedure, a separate procedure is coded.
Example: Coronary bypass with excision of saphenous vein graft, excision of saphenous vein is coded separately.

Case Study 4.46. CABG

Procedure: CABG x 3.

Open saphenous vein graft harvest from the left thigh followed by bypass from the aorta to the right coronary artery, left circumflex, and left descending artery.

Code(s):

021209W   **Bypass Coronary Artery, Three Arteries from Aorta with Autologous Venous Tissue, Open Approach**

06BQ0ZZ   **Excision of Left Saphenous Vein, Open Approach**

Figure 4.14. Coronary Artery Bypass

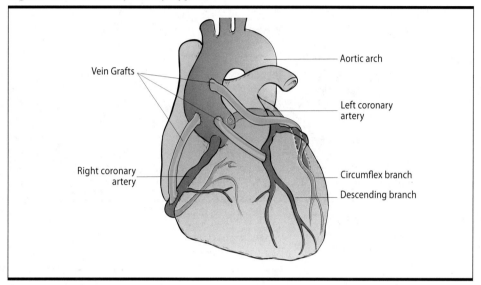

Rationale:

Only code 021209W is necessary to report the bypass procedure described in this case study. Even though three separate coronary arteries have been bypassed, all three sites were bypassed from the aorta using saphenous vein grafts as the device.

Procedures on the coronary arteries are classified to the body system Heart and Great Vessels (2). CABG is performed to reroute the flow of blood around a blockage in the coronary, which meets the definition of the root operation Bypass (1). Bypass procedures on the coronary arteries are specific to the number of coronary artery sites bypassed. In this case study, the right coronary artery, left circumflex artery, and left descending artery were bypassed, so the body part Coronary Artery, Three Arteries (2) is used. The approach value is Open (0) because it utilized direct access and visualization of the heart. Some CABG procedures require the use of a graft to reroute blood around the blocked coronary artery. Graft material is considered a device in PCS. Grafts may be autologous, meaning that the graft material is harvested from the patient's body, and autologous grafts may be venous or arterial. Synthetic grafts and nonautologous cadaver grafts are also used. In this case, all graft material was harvested from the patient's left saphenous vein, so the device is Autologous Venous Tissue (9). The "from" site of the graft is captured by qualifier Aorta (W).

A second code, 06BQ0ZZ, is required for excision of the left saphenous vein based on guideline B3.9, which stipulates that a separate procedure code can be applied when the autograft is obtained from a different body part.

The graft was harvested from the left saphenous vein, which is anatomically located in the thigh and is classified in the body system Lower Veins (6). Only a portion of the body part Saphenous Vein, Left (Q) was excised for use as graft material in the CABG procedure, meeting the root operation Excision (B) definition. Excision of a venous graft can be performed using a variety of approaches, but in this case, the approach is specified as Open (Ø). For the sixth-character device, the value is No Device (Z). The excision of the left saphenous vein was performed for therapeutic as opposed to diagnostic purposes so the qualifier is No Qualifier (Z).

Case Study 4.47. CABG x 5

The patient was placed in supine position and prepared and draped as usual. The chest was opened through a median sternotomy incision and the heart exposed. The left greater saphenous vein was harvested from the lower extremity. The right radial artery was harvested and the left mammary was taken down and prepared. The patient was placed on cardiopulmonary bypass.

The first anastomosis was the saphenous vein to the posterior descending right coronary artery performed in an end-to-side fashion.

The second anastomosis was between the saphenous vein and the distal right coronary artery in a side-to-side fashion just distal to the acute margin.

An end-to-side anastomosis was performed between the radial artery and the marginal branch of the circumflex, as well as a side-to-side anastomosis between the radial artery and the diagonal branch of the left anterior descending coronary artery.

Finally, the left internal mammary and the left anterior descending coronary artery were anastomosed in an end-to-side fashion. The saphenous vein was anastomosed to the ascending aorta and the radial artery was anastomosed to the left internal mammary artery.

Prior to coming off cardiopulmonary bypass, the left atrial appendage, measuring 5 cm x 4 cm x 3 cm, was excised and stapled at the base for hemostasis. The sternum was approximated with peristernal wires, the subcutaneous tissue in layers, and the skin with sutures. Leg wounds and arm wounds were closed. Dressings were placed on all of the wounds. The patient was transferred to the intensive care unit in fair condition.

Code(s):

Ø21109W	**Bypass Coronary Artery, Two Arteries from Aorta with Autologous Venous Tissue, Open Approach**
02110A9	**Bypass Coronary Artery, Two Arteries from Left Internal Mammary with Autologous Arterial Tissue, Open Approach**
02100Z9	**Bypass Coronary Artery, One Artery from Left Internal Mammary, Open Approach**
03BBØZZ	**Excision of Right Radial Artery, Open Approach**
06BQØZZ	**Excision of Left Saphenous Vein, Open Approach**
02B70ZK	**Excision of Left Atrial Appendage, Open Approach**
5A1221Z	**Performance of Cardiac Output, Continuous**

Rationale:
In the above scenario, three codes are required to capture the five bypasses performed. The decision tree questions and answers as they apply to this case study are as follows:

Was there more than one artery bypassed?   **Yes. Five arteries were bypassed:**

Right posterior descending artery

Distal right coronary artery

Circumflex artery

Diagonal branch of the left anterior descending artery (LAD)

Left anterior descending artery (LAD)

Was there more than one "from" site?   **Yes. Two from sites were documented:**

Aorta

Left internal mammary artery

Was there more than one type of device used?   **Yes. Two devices were documented:**

Saphenous vein graft

Radial artery graft

In addition to the codes for the coronary artery bypass procedures, two different types of autografts were harvested so two excision procedures must be reported. The left atrial appendage was excised, which is also reported. The final code assigned is for the cardiopulmonary bypass procedure. Rationale for each code assigned is provided below.

A single code, Ø21109W, captures the bypass of the posterior descending right coronary artery and the distal right coronary artery. Both bypasses are "from" the aorta and use a saphenous vein graft, so the same qualifier and device apply.

Since two vessels were bypassed, body part Coronary Artery, Two Arteries (1) is used. A sternotomy incision exposing the heart indicates an Open (Ø) approach. The saphenous vein graft was harvested from the patient and is captured by the device value for Autologous Venous Tissue (9). The "from" site is captured by qualifier value Aorta (W).

Another single code, Ø2110A9, captures the bypass of the marginal branch of the circumflex artery and the diagonal branch of the LAD. The radial artery was used as graft material for both of these arteries and both coronary arteries were bypassed from the left internal mammary artery. This graft was connected to each of these arteries in a sequential fashion, meaning one radial artery section was used but connected to two separate coronary arteries. The radial artery graft was then anastomosed to the left internal mammary artery.

The body system is Heart and Great Vessels (2). The root operation is Bypass (1). The marginal branch of the circumflex artery and the diagonal branch of the LAD are captured by the body part Coronary Artery, Two Arteries (1). A segment of the radial artery was harvested from the patient and used as the graft material at these two arteries. This is captured by the device Autologous Arterial Tissue (A). The "from" site in coronary artery bypass procedures is captured by the qualifier. Both coronary arteries were bypassed from the Internal Mammary, Left (9).

The final bypass code, Ø2100Z9, illustrates the use of the left internal mammary artery not as a graft or device material but as the "from" site from which blood travels into the coronary artery. In this case, the left internal mammary and the left anterior descending coronary artery were anastomosed in an end-to-side fashion to each other eliminating the need for a tissue or synthetic graft.

The internal mammary artery was attached to only one coronary artery so the body part Coronary Artery, One Artery (Ø) is used. When a bypass is performed by direct anastomosis of the "from" and "to" sites, no graft is used so the device value No Device (Z) applies. The "from" site is captured by the qualifier value Internal Mammary, Left (9).

Spotlight
When an artery, such as the left internal mammary artery, is transected at one end only, mobilized, and the cut end attached to a coronary artery, the artery is not considered a device and the value No Device (Z) is assigned. Only when an artery is excised as a free graft (i.e., completely detached from its previous blood supply), is it considered a device.

Excision of the radial artery, Ø3BBØZZ, which was used as a free graft, is reported as a separate procedure based on guideline B3.9. The graft was harvested from the right radial artery, which is classified in the body system Upper Arteries (3). Only a portion of the right radial artery was harvested, meeting the definition of the root operation Excision (B). A portion of the body part Radial Artery, Right (B) was excised for use as graft material in the CABG procedure. Excision of an arterial graft can be performed using a variety of approaches, but in this case the approach was specified as Open (Ø). Harvesting of the radial artery graft does not require a device so No Device (Z) is used. Excision of the right radial artery was performed for a therapeutic as opposed to a diagnostic purpose so the qualifier is No Qualifier (Z).

Excision of the left greater saphenous vein, which was used as a free graft, is reported as a separate procedure based on guideline B3.9 using 06BQ0ZZ. The graft was harvested from the left greater saphenous vein, which is classified in the body system Lower Veins (6). A portion of the body part Saphenous Vein, Left (Q) was excised for use as graft material in the CABG procedure, meeting the root operation Excision (B) definition. Excision of a venous graft can be performed using a variety of approaches, but in this case the approach was specified as Open (0). The correct device value is No Device (Z). The excision of the left saphenous vein was performed for a therapeutic as opposed to a diagnostic purpose so the qualifier is No Qualifier (Z).

The left atrial appendage is a small pouch extending off the main body of the left atrium and excision of the left atrial appendage is a separate procedure reported with 02B70ZK. For the purposes of PCS coding, the left atrial appendage is considered a part of the left atrium although it has different pathophysiological, anatomical, and embryological characteristics independent from the main body. These distinct characteristics could be why the left atrial appendage is provided as an additional qualifier (seventh character) for the left atrium row in the Excision table (02B). The left atrial appendage is part of the heart so the body system Heart and Great Vessels (2) applies. Only part of the left atrium, specifically the atrial appendage, was excised so the correct root operation is Excision (B). Since there is not a specific body part value for left atrial appendage, Atrium, Left (7) is used. The correct device value is No Device (Z). Atrial Appendage, Left (K) is available as a qualifier to more specifically identify the part of the left atrium that was excised.

Cardiopulmonary bypass (CPB) is classified in the Extracorporeal or Systemic Assistance and Performance (5) section and reported with 5A1221Z. A code from this section of medical and surgical related procedures is used when equipment outside of the body is used to assist or perform a physiological function. Finding the correct code for CPB by going directly to the root operation tables in this section is difficult because it requires an understanding of the value definitions for each character. For this reason, the best way to find the correct code for CPB is to use the index. The terms Bypass, cardiopulmonary provide the complete code 5A1221Z.

The section character value is Extracorporeal or Systemic Assistance and Performance (5), and the second character is Physiological Systems (A). Since there is only one value for the second character, all codes in this section contain the value Physiological Systems (A). CPB is used during some procedures performed on the heart and involves the use of a machine (CPB pump) that takes over heart and lung functions. This is captured by the root operation Performance (1), which is defined as completely taking over a physiological function by extracorporeal means. Cardiac (2) is the body system value. The fifth character is for the duration of the extracorporeal performance. CPB is used continuously during the surgical procedure so the duration value Continuous (2) applies. The sixth-character function offers two choices within the body system Cardiac (2): output and pacing. Output (1) best describes the function performed. The only qualifier available in this row is No Qualifier (Z).

Control Versus More Definitive Root Operations

Guideline B3.7

> **B3.7**   **The root operation Control is defined as, "Stopping, or attempting to stop, postprocedural or other acute bleeding." If an attempt to stop postprocedural or other acute bleeding is unsuccessful, and to stop the bleeding requires performing a more definitive root operation such as Bypass, Detachment, Excision, Extraction, Reposition, Replacement, or Resection, then the more definitive root operation is coded instead of Control.**
>
> *Example:* **Resection of spleen to stop bleeding is coded to Resection instead of Control.**

AHA Coding Clinic

2018, 1Q, 19   Argon Plasma Coagulation of Duodenal Arteriovenous Malformation

2018, 1Q, 19   Control of Epistaxis via Silver Nitrate Cauterization

2017, 4Q, 105   Control of Gastrointestinal Bleeding

2017, 4Q, 106   Control of Bleeding of External Naris Using Suture

2017, 4Q, 106   Nasal Packing for Epistaxis

2016, 4Q, 99   Root Operation Control

2016, 4Q, 134   Changes to the ICD-10-PCS Official Guidelines for Coding and Reporting

2015, 1Q, 35   Evacuation of Hematoma for Control of Postprocedural Bleeding

2014, 4Q, 44   Bakri Balloon for Control of Postpartum Hemorrhage

2013, 3Q, 22   Control of Intraoperative Bleeding

2013, 2Q, 38   Evacuation of Clot Post-Partum

The root operation Control (3) is used when the sole objective of a procedure is to stop bleeding, regardless of whether the bleeding is postoperative or an acute hemorrhage unrelated to a procedure. Active bleeding from the body site or area in question does not need to be present in order to use the root operation Control. Control methods may be required in order to prevent future or recurrent bleeding.

Control, as a root operation, is primarily captured in the Anatomical Regions, General; Anatomical Regions, Upper Extremities; and Anatomical Regions, Lower Extremities body systems. This correlates with the explanation of Control because, in general, control of bleeding is performed on a broader body area than a more specific body site. However, the root operation Control is included in one other body system: Ear, Nose, Sinus (9) when used on body part value Nasal Mucosa and Soft Tissue (K).

Root Operation		
Control (3)	Definition:	Stopping, or attempting to stop, postprocedural or other acute bleeding
	Explanation:	The site of the bleeding is coded as an anatomical region and not to a specific body part

Only certain methods used to attain control of postoperative or acute bleeding can be captured with the root operation Control (3). These methods include, but are not limited to, pressure balloon, cautery, suture, clipping, or drainage of the operative site. If any of the above methods are unsuccessful at stopping the acute or postoperative bleeding and a more definitive procedure such as Bypass, Detachment, Excision, Extraction, Reposition, Replacement, or Resection is required, the more specific root operation should be reported instead of the root operation Control (3). Packing is coded using Table 2Y4 of the Placement (2) section rather than the root operation Control.

Spotlight
Almost all of the root operations in the Medical and Surgical (Ø) section are considered a more definitive procedure when used to control bleeding, except for the root operation Repair (Q). Repair should only be used when no other root operation is applicable, based on its definition, explanation, and includes/examples. When the objective of a procedure is to control bleeding, the root operation Control (3) is considered the more definitive procedure than root operation Repair (Q). (*AHA Coding Clinic*, 2017, 4Q, 106)

Some postoperative bleeding is normal or expected after a surgical procedure; control of normal postoperative bleeding should not be reported separately. If excessive postoperative bleeding occurs, requiring a return to the operating room or a control method atypical to achieving adequate hemostasis, the root operation Control (3) should be considered. Irrigation and evacuation of blood clots may be necessary to clear the operative field and effectively stop the bleeding and is an inherent component of the root operation Control. If irrigation or evacuation of blood clots is performed at a different body site, it becomes a separately reportable procedure.

Practical Application for Guideline B3.7

Case Study 4.48. Hemorrhage, Epistaxis

A patient taking nonsteroidal anti-inflammatory drugs (NSAID) while on anticoagulants was admitted for severe, ongoing epistaxis. Tears were observed after evacuation of the clot and irrigation of the right naris. The bleeding mucosa was treated with epinephrine injection followed by sutures and silver nitrate. The patient was advised to discontinue NSAID use.

Code(s):

Ø93K7ZZ **Control Bleeding in Nasal Mucosa and Soft Tissue, Via Natural or Artificial Opening**

Rationale:
The root operation Control (3) includes the evacuation of the clot and irrigation of the procedure site. Sutures and administration of epinephrine and silver nitrate are inherent in the Control (3) procedure. The Ear, Nose and Sinus (9) body system is the only body system outside the General Anatomical body systems that includes a table for the root operation Control. The only body part in that table is Nasal Mucosa and Soft Tissue (K).

The approach was through the nasal passage with no mention of endoscopy correlating to Via Natural or Artificial Opening (7) for the approach value. No Device (Z) and No Qualifier (Z) values complete the code.

Case Study 4.49. Cauterization for Postoperative Hemorrhage

A patient was returned to the operative suite for cauterization control of persistent postoperative hemorrhage status post-outpatient cervical conization. Through a transvaginal approach, the origin of the hemorrhage was directly visualized and isolated. The cervix was irrigated and the vessel cauterized, achieving hemostasis.

Code(s):

ØW3R7ZZ **Control Bleeding in Genitourinary Tract, Via Natural or Artificial Opening**

Rationale:
The objective of this procedure was to control the postoperative bleeding. Root operation Control (3) includes any irrigation or evacuation necessary to clear the affected body site.

This Control procedure is coded to the Anatomical Regions, General (W) body system. The appropriate body part character for cervix is Genitourinary Tract (R).

Transvaginal is defined as across or through the vagina and was visualized without the assistance of a scope, which meets the definition of Via Natural or Artificial Opening (7) approach.

Case Study 4.50. Hemorrhage, Postpartum

Indications: Postpartum bleeding.

The patient continued to experience postpartum bleeding and was taken to the operating room following vaginal delivery. A D&C (dilation and curettage) was performed and a Bakri balloon was inserted and inflated. No significant vaginal bleeding was found after the Bakri was removed.

Code(s):

10D17ZZ   **Extraction of Products of Conception, Retained, Via Natural or Artificial Opening**

Rationale:

If only the Bakri balloon had been used, the correct root operation would be Control (3) (*AHA Coding Clinic*, 2014, 4Q, 44). In this case, however, a D&C was performed, indicating that material (products of conception) was removed from inside the uterus. The "dilation" refers to dilation of the cervix and "curettage" refers to the scraping or removal of tissue lining the uterine cavity with a curette. Products of conception include all components of the pregnancy, such as the fetus, umbilical cord, amnion, placenta, and embryo.

Guideline C2, which follows, specifies that procedures performed following a delivery for the evacuation of retained products of conception are coded in the Obstetrics (1) section, using root operation Extraction (D) and the body part Products of Conception, Retained (1).

Dilation involves widening the opening of the lower part of the uterus (the cervix) to allow insertion of an instrument through the vaginal opening; the approach is Via Natural or Artificial Opening (7).

PCS Guideline
Procedures following delivery or abortion
C2   Procedures performed following a delivery or abortion for curettage of the endometrium or evacuation of retained products of conception are all coded in the Obstetrics section, to the root operation Extraction and the body part Products of Conception, Retained. Diagnostic or therapeutic dilation and curettage performed during times other than the postpartum or post-abortion period are all coded in the Medical and Surgical section, to the root operation Extraction and the body part Endometrium.

Root Operation		
Extraction (D)	Definition:	Pulling or stripping out or off all or a portion of a body part by the use of force
	Explanation:	None

> ### Case Study 4.51. Hemorrhage, Postadenoidectomy
>
> Earlier in the day the patient had an adenoidectomy; the patient returned later the same day with postoperative adenoidectomy bleeding. After satisfactory anesthesia was established, a mouth gag was inserted. The clots were removed from the nasopharynx, the nose and nasopharynx were irrigated, and diffuse low-grade bleeding from the adenoid bed was identified and controlled with cautery. The area was carefully observed for a period of about 10 minutes, and no further bleeding occurred. Silver nitrate was applied to the adenoid bed.

Code(s):

ØW33XZZ   Control Bleeding in Oral Cavity and Throat, External Approach

Rationale:

Cautery is a common method used in the control of postoperative bleeding. When consulting the PCS index under Control bleeding in, body part adenoid is not found. In general, control of bleeding is coded to the general anatomical regions body systems per guideline B2.1a. In this case, the Anatomical Regions, General (W) body system should be used. Oral Cavity and Throat (3) is the appropriate body part character.

PCS Guideline
General guidelines
B2.1a   The procedure codes in the general anatomical regions body systems can be used when the procedure is performed on an anatomical region rather than a specific body part (e.g., root operations Control and Detachment, Drainage of a body cavity) or on the rare occasion when no information is available to support assignment of a code to a specific body part.
Examples: Control of postoperative hemorrhage is coded to the root operation Control found in the general anatomical regions body systems.
Chest tube drainage of the pleural cavity is coded to the root operation Drainage found in the general anatomical regions body systems. Suture repair of the abdominal wall is coded to the root operation Repair in the general anatomical regions body system.

The approach is External (X) in this case since no additional instrumentation was used to visualize the adenoids. This follows the direction given in guideline B5.3a.

PCS Guideline
External approach
B5.3a   Procedures performed within an orifice on structures that are visible without the aid of any instrumentation are coded to the approach External.
Example: Resection of tonsils is coded to the approach External.

Case Study 4.52. Hemopericardium Evacuation

Indication: Postoperative bleeding following emergency CABG x4.

The patient had diffuse oozing from all the raw surface areas. There was a small arterial bleeder from the lower aspect of the right side of the sternum. There was some oozing at the distal anastomosis to the right coronary artery.

The patient was taken from the intensive care unit to the operating room and placed on the operating room table in the supine position. General anesthesia was given via an endotracheal tube previously placed. After this was performed, the chest, abdomen, and lower extremities were prepped and draped in the usual sterile fashion. Sutures from the previous procedure were removed, as well as the sternal wires.

A sternal retractor was placed. Evacuation of the hemopericardium was performed. All of the clots in the pericardium and chest cavity were removed. The chest cavity was irrigated with antibiotic solution. Careful examination of all the suture lines was performed. Some oozing was noticed at the distal anastomosis of the right coronary artery and this was secured with a 7-0 Prolene suture.

The other suture lines were checked and neither one showed any bleeders. After the sternal retractor was removed, an arterial bleeder from the sternum was noticed. It was controlled with a Bovie cautery.

After adequate hemostasis was obtained, the chest tubes were placed back to their original position. The sternum was approximated with #6 stainless steel wires. The chest wall was closed in layers. The patient tolerated the procedure and was transferred to the cardiovascular recovery unit in stable condition.

Code(s):

| ØW3DØZZ | **Control Bleeding in Pericardial Cavity, Open Approach** |
| ØW38ØZZ | **Control Bleeding in Chest Wall, Open Approach** |

Rationale:

Two codes are required to capture the control of hemorrhage at the two separate sites. The evacuation of clots in the pericardium and suture of the right coronary artery are captured using body part Pericardial Cavity (D); body part Chest Wall (3) reflects the cautery done in the sternum. This follows multiple procedure guideline B3.2a.

PCS Guideline
Multiple procedures
B3.2   During the same operative episode, multiple procedures are coded if: a. The same root operation is performed on different body parts as defined by distinct values of the body part character. *Examples:* Diagnostic excision of liver and pancreas are coded separately. Excision of lesion in the ascending colon and excision of lesion in the transverse colon are coded separately.

In order to control the postoperative bleeding, the original incision was reopened, which is coded using an Open (Ø) approach.

Excision Versus Resection

The distinction between Excision (B) and Resection (T) relates to whether the **entire body part is removed**, in which case Resection (T) applies, or whether only a **portion of the body part is removed**, in which case Excision (B) applies. Determining when to code Excision (B) versus when to code Resection (T) requires a good understanding of the concept of body part in ICD-10-PCS.

Root Operation		
Excision (B)	Definition:	Cutting out or off, without replacement, a portion of a body part
	Explanation:	The qualifier DIAGNOSTIC is used to identify excision procedures that are biopsies
Resection (T)	Definition:	Cutting out or off, without replacement, all of a body part
	Explanation:	None

Guideline B3.8

> **B3.8** **PCS contains body parts for anatomical subdivisions of a body part, such as lobes of the lungs or liver and regions of the intestine. Resection of the specific body part is coded whenever all of the body part is cut out or off, rather than coding Excision of a less specific body part.**
>
> *Example:* **Left upper lung lobectomy is coded to Resection of Upper Lung Lobe, Left rather than Excision of Lung, Left.**

AHA Coding Clinic

2018, 1Q, 22	Resection of Lymph Node Chains
2016, 2Q, 12	Resection of Malignant Neoplasm of Infratemporal Fossa
2016, 1Q, 30	Axillary Lymph Node Resection with Modified Radical Mastectomy
2015, 3Q, 26	Femoral Head Resection
2014, 4Q, 34	Skin-Sparing Mastectomy
2014, 4Q, 35	Vitrectomy with Air/Fluid Exchange
2014, 3Q, 6	Ileocecectomy Including Cecum, Terminal Ileum and Appendix
2014, 3Q, 6	Right Colectomy
2014, 3Q, 9	Radical Resection of Level I Lymph Nodes
2014, 3Q, 10	Selective Excision of Paratracheal Lymph Nodes
2013, 3Q, 28	Total Hysterectomy
2013, 1Q, 24	Excision versus Resection of Remaining Ovarian Remnant Following Previous Excision

Any anatomical site listed in the PCS tables with a unique character 4 body part value is considered a body part in PCS. The body part may be an anatomical site, such as the neck muscles; a whole organ, such as the spleen; or a subdivided organ where each subdivision has a unique body part value. For example, in the Gastrointestinal (D) body system the root operation tables ØDT for Resection (T) and ØDB for Excision (B) contain five different body part values for the esophagus. These include:

- Esophagus, Upper (1)
- Esophagus, Middle (2)
- Esophagus, Lower (3)
- Esophagogastric Junction (4)
- Esophagus (5)

By assigning values to the subdivisions of the esophagus, the anatomical site requiring surgical attention can be more specifically identified. Because five body part values are available for the esophagus, it is possible to identify whether the surgical procedure involved the entire esophagus or just a portion of the esophagus (i.e., the upper, middle, or lower esophagus or the esophagogastric junction).

Spotlight
When a subdivided organ is resected in its entirety, only one code with a body part value representing the whole organ is needed. Appending multiple codes to identify each subdivision resected is not appropriate. For example, open resection of the upper, middle, and lower right lobes of the lung codes to ØBTKØZZ Resection of Right Lung, Open Approach and **not** to the following:
ØBTCØZZ   Resection of Right Upper Lung Lobe, Open Approach ØBTDØZZ   Resection of Right Middle Lung Lobe, Open Approach ØBTFØZZ   Resection of Right Lower Lung Lobe, Open Approach

Listed in the following table are examples of organs with specific body part subdivisions in ICD-10-PCS. In some cases there is a body part value for the entire anatomical site or organ as well as body part values for subdivided parts.

Table 4.2. Body Part Subdivision Examples

Body System	Major Organ	Body Part Values
Respiratory System (B)	Bronchus	Main Bronchus, Right (3) Upper Lobe Bronchus, Right (4) Middle Lobe Bronchus, Right (5) Lower Lobe Bronchus, Right (6) Main Bronchus, Left (7) Upper Lobe Bronchus, Left (8) Lingula Bronchus (9) Lower Lobe Bronchus, Left (B)
	Lung	Upper Lung Lobe, Right (C) Middle Lung Lobe, Right (D) Lower Lung Lobe, Right (F) Upper Lung Lobe, Left (G) Lung Lingula (H) Lower Lung Lobe, Left (J) Lung, Right (K) Lung, Left (L) Lungs, Bilateral (M)
Gastrointestinal System (D)	Esophagus	Esophagus, Upper (1) Esophagus, Middle (2) Esophagus, Lower (3) Esophagogastric Junction (4) Esophagus (5)
	Small Intestine	Small Intestine (8) Duodenum (9) Jejunum (A) Ileum (B) Ileocecal Valve (C)

Body System	Major Organ	Body Part Values
Gastrointestinal System (D) (continue)	Large Intestine	Large Intestine (E)
		Large Intestine, Right (F)
		Large Intestine, Left (G)
		Cecum (H)
		Ascending Colon (K)
		Transverse Colon (L)
		Descending Colon (M)
		Sigmoid Colon (N)
		Rectum (P)
		Anus (Q)
		Anal Sphincter (R)
	Stomach	Stomach (6)
		Stomach, Pylorus (7)
Hepatobiliary System and Pancreas (F)	Liver	Liver (Ø)
		Liver, Right Lobe (1)
		Liver, Left Lobe (2)
Endocrine System (G)	Thyroid Gland	Thyroid Gland Lobe, Left (G)
		Thyroid Gland Lobe, Right (H)
		Thyroid Gland Isthmus (J)
		Thyroid Gland (K)
Urinary System (T)	Bladder	Bladder (B)
		Bladder Neck (C)
	Kidney	Kidney, Right (Ø)
		Kidney, Left (1)
		Kidney, Bilateral (2)
		Kidney Pelvis, Right (3)
		Kidney Pelvis, Left (4)
		Kidney (5)

The subdivided body part is not always a specific organ. Some PCS body systems have more generalized body parts that are subdivided based on the anatomical area. In the Muscles (K) body system, for example, muscles of the arm are split into Upper Arm Muscles and Lower Arm Muscles with further classification based on laterality.

Spotlight
Many bilateral body parts are given unique body part values to distinguish the left side from the right. Although a subdivided body part may also carry the distinction of laterality, this is a separate characteristic to further define that subdivided body part.

Practical Application for Guideline B3.8

Case Study 4.53. Excision, Tumor Mid Esophagus

A transthoracic esophagectomy was performed to remove a tumor located in the middle esophagus. The upper esophagus was anastomosed to the lower esophagus.

Code(s):

ØDT2ØZZ   Resection of Middle Esophagus, Open Approach

Rationale:

The brief operative description specifies that the upper and lower esophagus were reconnected (anastomosed) indicating that the entire middle esophagus was removed. The Esophagus, Middle (2) is an anatomical subdivision of the esophagus found in the Gastrointestinal (D) body system. Because it has its own body part value and was removed in its entirety, it is appropriate to code the removal to the root operation Resection (T).

A transthoracic esophagectomy involves making an incision through the chest, which meets the definition of an Open (Ø) approach.

Case Study 4.54. Lobectomy, Video-assisted Thoracoscopic (VATS)

The patient was intubated and positioned, the hemithorax cleaned with antiseptics, and drapes placed. An incision was made at the seventh intercostal rib space and the thoracoscope with camera inserted. Two additional ports were placed: one at the fifth intercostal level and another at the ausculatory triangle port. Using the scope, the entire right lung was inspected. The middle lobe had a large mass in the lower apex of the lobe. The upper and lower lobes appeared normal but a biopsy of both lobes was taken for pathological examination. With sharp dissection, the middle lobe was excised and an endostapler used for vessel and bronchial ligation. The lung lobe was placed in an endobag and removed from one of the port sites. The right lung was again inspected and no bleeding was evident. All instrumentation was removed, the ports removed, and the incisions closed.

Code(s):

ØBTD4ZZ   Resection of Right Middle Lung Lobe, Percutaneous Endoscopic Approach

ØBBC4ZX   Excision of Right Upper Lung Lobe, Percutaneous Endoscopic Approach, Diagnostic

ØBBF4ZX   Excision of Right Lower Lung Lobe, Percutaneous Endoscopic Approach, Diagnostic

Rationale:

The right lung has three lobes: upper, middle, and lower. Each of these lobes or subdivisions has been given their own PCS body part value. Because each lobe has its own body part value, root operation Resection (T) can be utilized without the entire right lung being removed. Each lobe can be resected or excised independent of the other lobes. In this case study, multiple procedure codes are required because two distinct procedural objectives were accomplished (resection and excision) and the same root operation (excision) was performed on multiple distinct body parts (right upper lobe and right lower lobe).

Root Operation		
Excision (B)	Definition:	Cutting out or off, without replacement, a portion of a body part
	Explanation:	The qualifier DIAGNOSTIC is used to identify excision procedures that are biopsies
Resection (T)	Definition:	Cutting out or off, without replacement, all of a body part
	Explanation:	None

Figure 4.15. Lung Lobes

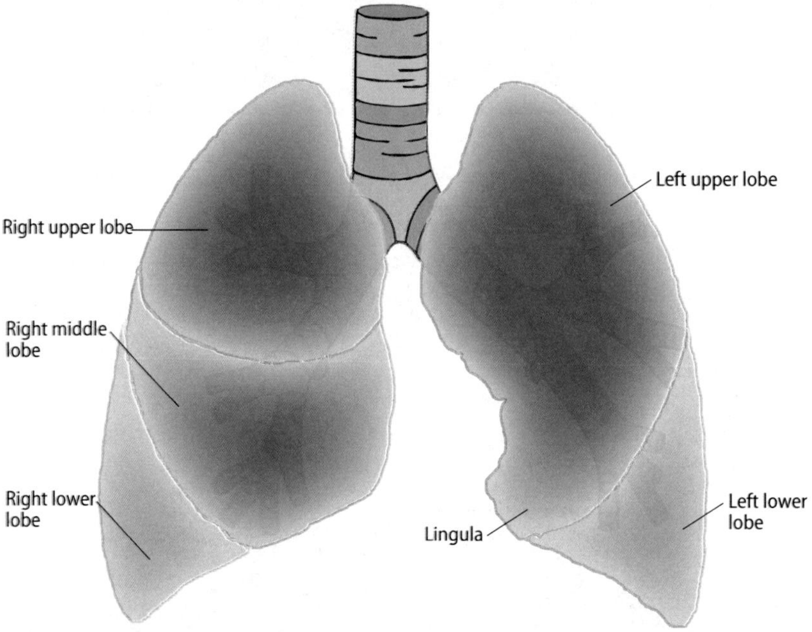

The first objective of this procedure was to remove the entire middle lobe. The body system is the Respiratory System (B), the root operation is Resection (T), and the body part is the Middle Lung Lobe, Right (D). The procedure was performed through port sites using a tiny camera that transmits images to a video monitor called a thoracoscope to visualize the resection site, making the approach Percutaneous Endoscopic (4).

In addition to the right middle lobe lobectomy, two biopsies were taken: one of the Upper Lung Lobe, Right (C) and one of the Lower Lung Lobe, Right (F). Based on the following multiple procedure guideline B3.2a, two Excision (B) codes are appropriate because an excision was performed on different body parts as defined by distinct values of the body part character. Biopsy procedures are inherently diagnostic and a qualifier value of Diagnostic (X) is appended to both excision codes.

PCS Guideline
Multiple procedures
B3.2 During the same operative episode, multiple procedures are coded if:
a. The same root operation is performed on different body parts as defined by distinct values of the body part character.
Examples: Diagnostic excision of liver and pancreas are coded separately.
Excision of lesion in the ascending colon and excision of lesion in the transverse colon are coded separately.

Case Study 4.55. Lymphadenectomy

The physician performed a regional abdominal lymphadenectomy via a midline abdominal incision. The abdominal contents were exposed, allowing location of the lymph nodes. A celiac lymph node grouping was dissected away from the surrounding tissue, nerves, and blood vessels, and removed. A biopsy of a lumbar lymph node on the left side, as well as one superior mesenteric lymph node, was also performed, and tissue sent to pathology. The incision was closed with sutures or staples.

Code(s):

Ø7TDØZZ	**Resection of Aortic Lymphatic, Open Approach**
Ø7BDØZX	**Excision of Aortic Lymphatic, Open Approach, Diagnostic**
Ø7BBØZX	**Excision of Mesenteric Lymphatic, Open Approach, Diagnostic**

Rationale:

Lymph nodes are separated into stations or chains, identifying a cluster of nodes, with nomenclature based on their anatomical location. Instead of giving each lymph node station a specific body part value, the stations are grouped to a more general lymphatic body part. For example, the Body Part Key classifies the inferior mesenteric lymph node, pararectal lymph node, and superior mesenteric lymph node stations to body part value Lymphatic, Mesenteric (B). Due to the anatomical dispersal of these mesenteric lymph nodes, one lymph node station can be operated on without affecting the other lymph node stations.

In this procedure, the entire celiac lymph node grouping, also referred to as a chain, was removed. When all or most lymph nodes in a chain are removed, it is classified as a Resection (T). The Body Part Key (appendix D) classifies the celiac lymph node to the body part value Lymphatic, Aortic (D). An Open (Ø) approach was used, with no device or qualifier.

In addition to the removal of the celiac lymph node chain, sampling of nearby lymph nodes in the lumbar and mesenteric areas was also performed. Using the Body Part Key as a reference, it is determined that the lumbar lymph nodes are classified to the same body part value as the celiac lymph nodes, Lymphatic, Aortic (D). It may seem counter intuitive that a PCS body part can be partially removed and completely removed at the same time, but due to the unique anatomical structure and division of the lymphatic system it is possible for Resection (T) and Excision (B) to apply. The sampling of the lumbar lymph node is represented by root operation Excision (B) and body part Lymphatic, Aortic (D).

According to the following excerpt from the Body Part Key, the superior mesenteric lymph node is classified to the body part Lymphatic, Mesenteric (B). Because only one node was sampled from this lymph node group, Excision (B) is used as the root operation.

Sampling of the lymph nodes was performed via an Open (Ø) approach and is considered diagnostic, which is represented in both excision codes with the seventh-character Diagnostic (X).

Term	ICD-10-PCS Value
Celiac lymph node	Lymphatic, Aortic
Lumbar lymph node	Lymphatic, Aortic
Superior mesenteric lymph node	Lymphatic, Mesenteric

Spotlight

A lymph node level is synonymous to a lymph node chain. When the intent is to remove most of a level or chain of lymph nodes, regardless of whether the entire chain was removed, the appropriate root operation is Resection (T). Resection is used when the majority of a chain is removed to reflect a distinction between procedures removing chains of lymph nodes (Resection) as opposed to a single node (Excision). See *AHA Coding Clinics*, 2018, 1Q, 22; 2016, 1Q, 30.

Case Study 4.56. Hemicolectomy, Right

The abdomen was prepped and draped in the usual sterile fashion. A midline laparotomy incision was made with a #10 blade scalpel and subcutaneous tissues were separated with electrocautery down to the anterior abdominal fascia. Once divided, the intraabdominal cavity was accessed and bowel was protected as the rest of the abdominal wall was opened in the midline. The entire ileocecal region up to the transverse colon was mobilized into the field. Next, a window was made 5 inches from the ileocecal valve and a GIA-75 was fired across the ileum. A second GIA device was fired across the proximal transverse colon, just sparing the middle colic artery. The dissection was carried down along the mesentery, down to the root of the mesentery. The mesentery vessels were hemostated and tied with #0-Vicryl suture sequentially, ligated in between. Once this specimen was submitted to pathology, the wound was inspected. There was no evidence of bleeding from any of the suture sites. Next, a side-by-side anastomosis was performed between the transverse colon and the terminal ileum. A third GIA-75 was fired side-by-side and GIA-55 was used to close the anastomosis. A patent anastomosis was palpated. The anastomosis was then protected with a #2-0 Vicryl #0-muscular suture. The mesenteric root was closed with a running #0-Vicryl suture to prevent any chance of internal hernia. The suture sites were inspected and there was no evidence of leakage. Next, the intraabdominal cavity was thoroughly irrigated with sterile saline and the anastomosis was carried into the right lower gutter. Omentum was used to cover the intestines, which appeared dilated and indurated from the near obstruction. The abdominal wall was reapproximated and the fascial layer closed using two running loop PDS sutures meeting in the middle with good approximation of both the abdominal fascia. Additional sterile saline was used to irrigate the subcutaneous fat and the skin was closed with sequential sterile staples.

Code(s):
ØDTFØZZ   Resection of Right Large Intestine, Open Approach

Rationale:
The gastrointestinal system is composed of a series of anatomical structures, beginning at the mouth and ending at the anus. The colon or large intestine is the final structure in the series, running from its connection to the small intestine to the rectum. The large intestine is represented in several different ways within the PCS tables. One body part character represents the large intestine as a whole unit. Two body part characters divide the large intestine into Large Intestine, Right (F) and Large Intestine, Left (G) halves. Finally, each segment of the large intestine has a distinct body part character. These include the following:

- Cecum (H)
- Appendix (J)
- Ascending Colon (K)
- Transverse Colon (L)
- Descending Colon (M)
- Sigmoid Colon (N)

A right hemicolectomy typically involves the removal of the cecum, appendix, ascending colon, and all or a portion of the transverse colon.

Figure 4.16. Large Intestine

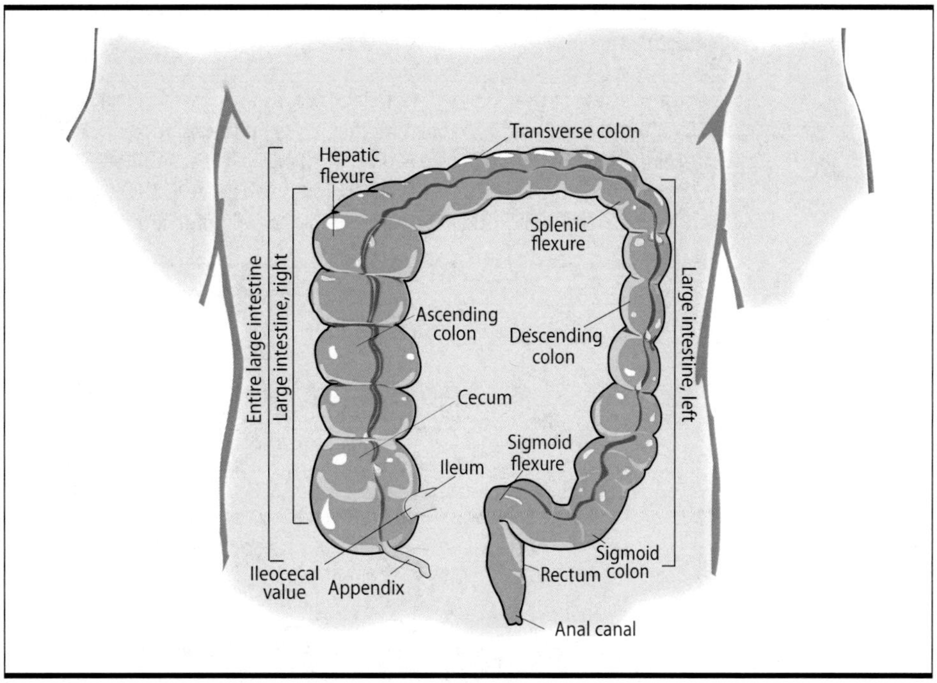

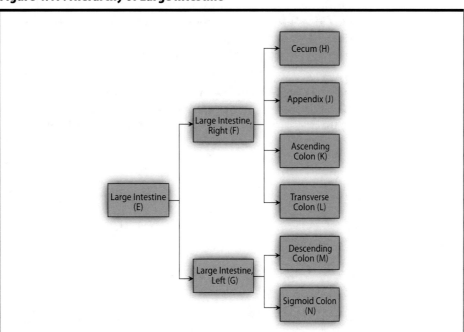

Following multiple procedure guideline B3.2a, it might be assumed that a code should be assigned for each body part that has a distinct value within the PCS table. However some body parts, such as the large intestine, are broke out into hierarchical body part characters. The cecum, appendix, ascending colon, transverse colon, descending colon, and sigmoid colon collectively make up the entire large intestine. When all of these sections are removed, the body part value Large Intestine (E) is coded because this one body part encompasses all of the individual segments. When all of the intestinal segments that collectively make up the right large intestine are removed (i.e., cecum, appendix, ascending colon, and transverse colon), only the body part value Large Intestine, Right (F) is coded (*AHA Coding Clinic,* 2014, 3Q, 6).

Figure 4.17. Hierarchy of Large Intestine

In this example, the entire Large Intestine, Right (F) was removed, which is coded as Resection (T). A large incision was made through the abdominal wall to gain access into the abdominal cavity, meeting the approach definition of Open (Ø).

Careful review of the operative note is critical as the extent of the disease may require resection beyond those segments of intestine that make up the right colon. Additional codes may be necessary to identify partial excision of the ileum or descending colon. The anastomosis between the terminal ileum and the transverse colon is considered inherent to the procedure and is not coded separately. This guidance is found in general guideline B3.1b.

PCS Guideline
General guidelines
B3.1b   Components of a procedure specified in the root operation definition and explanation are not coded separately. Procedural steps necessary to reach the operative site and close the operative site, including anastomosis of a tubular body part, are also not coded separately.
Examples: Resection of a joint as part of a joint replacement procedure is included in the root operation definition of Replacement and is not coded separately.
Laparotomy performed to reach the site of an open liver biopsy is not coded separately. In a resection of sigmoid colon with anastomosis of descending colon to rectum, the anastomosis is not coded separately.

Case Study 4.57. Excision, Foot Aneurysm

Procedure: Excision of right dorsal foot superficial venous aneurysm.

The patient was brought into the surgical suite and placed in the supine position on the operating table. Cardiopulmonary monitoring was initiated and sedation performed. The area of the aneurysm was prepped and draped. The skin overlying the abscess was anesthetized with 1% lidocaine mixed with 0.5% Marcaine. The skin was opened with a #15 blade overlying the abnormal vasculature. All abnormal venous structures and branches were ligated with 2-0 and 3-0 silk and excised. Hemostasis was completed. The skin was closed with 5-0 Monocryl and the wound was dressed with Dermabond, gauze, and Kerlix. The patient tolerated the procedure well.

Code(s):
Ø6BTØZZ   Excision of Right Foot Vein, Open Approach

Rationale:
Only a part of the foot vein was removed, specifically the portion with the abnormal vasculature, so Excision (B) is the correct root operation. There is no Resection (T) table for the Lower Veins (6) body system, which further supports the decision to use Excision (B). An incision was made that indicates an Open (Ø) approach and the procedure was therapeutic, so seventh-character No Qualifier (Z) applies.

Beyond the Guidelines

While all body parts can have a portion removed (excised), not every body part can be completely removed (resected) because of its anatomical configuration. One way to determine whether a body part can be resected is to consult the PCS Index. For example, the term Nerve in the PCS Index is not a subheading under the main term Resection (T). However, it is a subheading under main term Excision (B). Review of the tables in the Peripheral Nervous System (1) section show that an Excision (B) table is represented but a Resection (T) table is not. Based on the lack of entries in the index and the absence of a table for Resection (T) in the Peripheral Nervous System (1) section, it can be ascertained that a peripheral nerve cannot be completely resected. Other examples of body systems that do not contain the Resection table include:

- Upper Arteries (3)
- Lower Arteries (4)
- Upper Veins (5)
- Lower Veins (6)
- Subcutaneous Tissue and Facia (J)
- Anatomical Regions, General (W)
- Anatomical Regions, Upper Extremities (X)
- Anatomical Regions, Lower Extremities (Y)

Whether a body part is represented in the Resection (T) table also depends on its functional role in that body system. In many cases, body parts can only be removed in their entirety with immediate replacement and thus is found in the root operation Replacement (R) table rather than the Resection (T) table. The definition of root operation Replacement (R) includes the removal of the body part being replaced. For example, the Aortic Valve (F) is an anatomic structure in the heart that must be present in order for the heart to function properly. Without it, the patient cannot survive. Therefore, the Aortic Valve value (F) is not a body part value offered in the Resection (T) table but instead is found in the Replacement (R) table.

Root Operation		
Replacement (R)	Definition:	Putting in or on a biological or synthetic material that physically takes the place and/or function of all or a portion of a body part
	Explanation:	The body part may have been taken out or replaced, or may be taken out, physically eradicated, or rendered nonfunctional during the REPLACEMENT procedure. A REMOVAL procedure is coded for taking out the device used in a previous replacement procedure.

For body systems that do have an Excision (B) table and a Resection (T) table, it is helpful to review the differences and similarities in the body part values provided in each of these tables, not only to identify organs that have subdivisions but to recognize those body parts that can or cannot be coded as resected. In the following table, the body part values from the Excision (B) table and Resection (T) table in the Heart and Great Vessels (2) body system are delineated. The choices for body part values in the Resection (T) table are minimal compared to the choices in the Excision (B) table. All of the body parts that are missing from the Resection (T) table with the exception of Coronary Vein (4) can only be reported as Replacement (R) if they are completely removed. For examples of the use of the root operation Replacement (R), see Chapter 7. Device Guidelines.

Table 4.3. Excision/Resection

Body Part—Character 4 from Heart and Great Vessels (2) Body System	
Excision (B) Table	**Resection (T) Table**
Coronary Vein (4)	
Atrial Septum (5)	Atrial Septum (5)
Atrium, Right (6)	*See Replacement (R)*
Atrium, Left (7)	*See Replacement (R)*
Conduction Mechanism (8)	Conduction Mechanism (8)
Chordae Tendineae (9)	Chordae Tendineae (9)
Papillary Muscle (D)	Papillary Muscle (D)
Aortic Valve (F)	*See Replacement (R)*
Mitral Valve (G)	*See Replacement (R)*
Pulmonary Valve (H)	Pulmonary Valve (H)
Tricuspid Valve (J)	*See Replacement (R)*
Ventricle, Right (K)	*See Replacement (R)*
Ventricle, Left (L)	*See Replacement (R)*
Ventricular Septum (M)	Ventricular Septum (M)
Pericardium (N)	Pericardium (N)
Pulmonary Trunk (P)	*See Replacement (R)*
Pulmonary Artery, Right (Q)	*See Replacement (R)*
Pulmonary Artery, Left (R)	*See Replacement (R)*
Pulmonary Vein, Right (S)	*See Replacement (R)*
Pulmonary Vein, Left (T)	*See Replacement (R)*
Superior Vena Cava (V)	*See Replacement (R)*
Thoracic Aorta, Descending (W)	*See Replacement (R)*
Thoracic Aorta, Ascending/Arch (X)	*See Replacement (R)*

Spotlight
An important element to note in definitions Excision and Resection is that neither would be coded separately if immediate Replacement is performed.

Excision for Graft

Guideline B3.9

> **B3.9**   **If an autograft is obtained from a different procedure site in order to complete the objective of the procedure, a separate procedure is coded.**
>
> *Example:* **Coronary bypass with excision of saphenous vein graft, excision of saphenous vein is coded separately.**

AHA Coding Clinic

2018, 1Q, 7	Placement of Fat Graft following Lumbar Decompression Surgery
2017, 3Q, 5	Femoral Artery to Posterior Tibial Artery Bypass Using Autologous and Synthetic Grafts
2017, 3Q, 7	Senning Procedure (Atrial Switch)
2017, 1Q, 23	Reconstruction of Mandible Using Titanium and Bone
2017, 1Q, 31	Left to Right Common Carotid Artery Bypass
2017, 1Q, 32	Peroneal Artery to Dorsalis Pedis Artery BypassUsing Saphenous Vein Graft
2016, 4Q, 134	Changes to the ICD-10-PCS Official Guidelines for Coding and Reporting
2016, 3Q, 29	Closure of Bilateral Alveolar Clefts
2016, 2Q, 23	Repair of Tetralogy of Fallot with Autologous Pericardial Patch Graft
2016, 1Q, 27	Aortocoronary Bypass Graft Utilizing Y-Graft
2015, 2Q, 12	Transfer of Free Flap to Reconstruct Orbital Defect
2015, 1Q, 30	Total Hip Replacement Surgery Using Stem Cell Autograft
2014, 3Q, 8	Coronary Artery Bypass Graft Utilizing Internal Mammary as Pedicle Graft
2014, 3Q, 22	Transsphenoidal Removal of Pituitary Tumor and Fat Graft Placement
2014, 2Q, 6	Posterior Lumbar Fusion with Discectomy
2014 1Q, 10	Repair of Thoracic Aortic Aneurysm & Coronary Artery Bypass Graft
2013, 2Q, 39	Ankle Fusion, Osteotomy, and Removal of Hardware

Many procedures require the use of a graft to accomplish the procedural objective. Grafts may be obtained from the patient, classified as autografts (autologous), or from a tissue bank, classified as allografts (nonautologous). In addition, autografts may be obtained from the surgical site or from a separate site. Reporting an additional code for excision or harvesting of an autograft applies only when a separate incision is required and the graft is obtained from a different body part. This guideline is applicable to free grafts only, meaning the body part must be completely excised from and not connected in any way to its normal anatomical location.

Free Graft Versus Other Graft

Some procedural objectives can be accomplished by multiple surgical techniques with some techniques requiring a free graft and other techniques making use of other types of grafts. A good example is a transverse rectus abdominis myocutaneous flap (TRAM), which includes skin, subcutaneous tissue, and muscle and is used for breast reconstruction postmastectomy. The TRAM flap can be a free flap, which is completely dissected and moved to the chest wall to replace a breast requiring a code for the excision of the graft, or it can be a pedicled graft in which the graft is transferred with its vascular and nervous structures intact. The pedicled graft does not require an additional code for harvesting.

Saphenous Vein, Radial Artery, and Internal Mammary Grafts

The greater and lesser saphenous veins, as shown in the following illustration, are commonly used conduits for coronary artery bypass grafts. ICD-10-PCS does not differentiate between greater or lesser saphenous veins, but rather by laterality resulting in body part values Saphenous Vein, Right (P) and Saphenous Vein, Left (Q).

Figure 4.18. Greater and Lesser Saphenous Veins

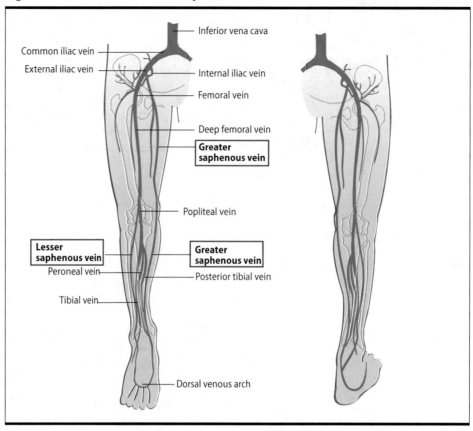

The radial artery, located in the arm, is often used as a conduit for the CABG procedure. The harvesting of the saphenous vein and radial artery require an additional code for the excision of the grafts. The internal mammary artery as shown on the following illustration is still attached to its origin, referred to as a pedicled graft. Although it is also used as a conduit, since it is a pedicled graft, an additional code is not required for the harvesting or excision.

Figure 4.19. LIMA Pedicle Graft, Radial Arterial Graft, and Saphenous Vein Graft

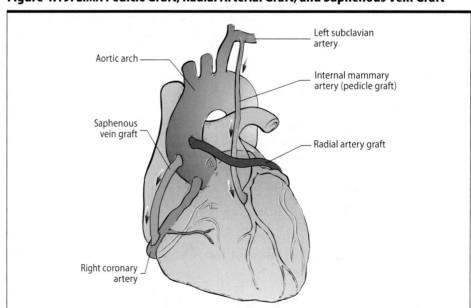

Spotlight
Although more commonly used as pedicle grafts, internal mammary arteries may also be harvested or excised as free grafts, for use in CABG procedures. When the internal mammary artery is completely excised for use as a conduit, the excision of the internal mammary artery can be reported separately. The qualifier values Internal Mammary, Right (8) and Internal Mammary, Left (9) are no longer applicable in the Bypass (1) procedure code when the right or left internal mammary artery is utilized as a free graft.

Local Versus Remote Autografts

Another important element of guideline B3.9 is that the body part being used as graft material must come from a different body part than where the graft material will be placed. Locally harvested graft material is not coded separately. For example, bone autografts may be harvested from a remote site or may be obtained from bone excised at the surgical site. In a spinal fusion procedure, if the bone is harvested from a remote site such as the iliac crest, the graft excision is reported separately; however, if bone chips from the surgical approach are used in the spinal fusion procedure, these local bone chips are considered to be integral to the fusion procedure and are not reported separately.

Practical Application for Guideline B3.9

Case Study 4.58. CABG, Coronary Artery Bypass Graft

Procedure: Saphenous vein graft from aorta to the RCA, LIMA to LAD.

The patient was brought to the operating suite, where she was placed under general anesthesia. Once adequate sedation was achieved, the patient was prepped and draped in the usual sterile fashion.

The left greater saphenous vein was removed. Hemostasis was achieved at the site with the use of silk clips and ligatures. The area was irrigated with saline and antibiotics and closed using 5-0 Prolene sutures. Attention was turned to the chest, where a sternotomy was performed using the sternal saw and the left internal mammary artery was located. Using a self-retraining retractor, the left internal mammary artery was mobilized and harvested as a pedicle from the anterior chest wall using electrocautery and hemoclips. Distal pedicle was divided and the left internal mammary artery was prepared for grafting. The patient was placed on cardiopulmonary bypass for the remainder of the procedure. The right coronary artery was identified and grasped. An arteriotomy was performed in order to attach the saphenous vein graft using 7-0 Prolene. Attention was turned to the left anterior descending artery. The left internal mammary was placed with an end-LIMA-to-side LAD anastomosis. The blood flow was resumed to all grafts and the patient was removed from cardiopulmonary bypass without any complications. The heart began a normal rhythm spontaneously.

The sternum was repaired using sternal wires. The rest of the wound was closed in layers in the usual fashion, and sterile dressings were applied. The patient tolerated the procedure well and was escorted to the recovery room in stable condition.

Code(s):

021009W	**Bypass Coronary Artery, One Artery from Aorta with Autologous Venous Tissue, Open Approach**
02100Z9	**Bypass Coronary Artery, One Artery from Left Internal Mammary, Open Approach**
06BQ0ZZ	**Excision of Left Saphenous Vein, Open Approach**
5A1221Z	**Performance of Cardiac Output, Continuous**

Rationale:

ICD-10-PCS includes guidelines that address how to report coronary artery bypass grafts. Guideline B3.6b specifies that the fourth-character body part identifies the body part bypassed "to" (coronary artery), including the number of arteries involved, and the seventh-character qualifier identifies the body part bypassed "from." This is the reverse of other bypass reporting.

Root Operation		
Bypass (1)	Definition:	Altering the route of passage of the contents of a tubular body part
	Explanation:	Rerouting contents of a body part to a downstream area of the normal route, to a similar route and body part, or to an abnormal route and dissimilar body part. Includes one or more anastomoses, with or without the use of a device.

PCS Guideline
Bypass procedures
B3.6b Coronary artery bypass procedures are coded differently than other bypass procedures as described in the previous guideline. Rather than identifying the body part bypassed from, the body part identifies the number of coronary arteries bypassed to, and the qualifier specifies the vessel bypassed from.
Example: Aortocoronary artery bypass of the left anterior descending coronary artery and the obtuse marginal coronary artery is classified in the body part axis of classification as two coronary arteries, and the qualifier specifies the aorta as the body part bypassed from.

Additionally, guideline B3.6c provides direction about the use of multiple codes when different devices and/or qualifiers are used.

PCS Guideline
Bypass procedures
B3.6c If multiple coronary arteries are bypassed, a separate procedure is coded for each coronary artery that uses a different device and/or qualifier.
Example: Aortocoronary artery bypass and internal mammary coronary artery bypass are coded separately.

In this example, two bypass codes are needed. One code is reported for the Bypass (1) from the Aorta (W) to the Coronary Artery, One Artery (Ø) using the harvested saphenous vein, represented by device value Autologous Venous Tissue (9). The second code represents the Bypass (1) to the Coronary Artery, One Artery (Ø) from the Internal Mammary, Left (9) with No Device (Z) since the internal mammary artery graft remained attached at its origin.

The left greater saphenous vein harvested is considered a free graft and is coded separately as stated in guideline B3.9. Only a portion of the Saphenous Vein, Left (Q) found in the Lower Veins (6) body system was harvested, meeting the definition of root operation Excision (B). The approach was Open (Ø) and since the vein was used for therapeutic purpose, No Qualifier (Z) is coded.

Root Operation		
Excision (B)	Definition:	Cutting out or off, without replacement, a portion of a body part
	Explanation:	The qualifier DIAGNOSTIC is used to identify excision procedures that are biopsies

The index listing for Bypass, cardiopulmonary lists the complete code 5A1221Z.

Case Study 4.59. Repair, Deviated Nasal Septum Using Ear Cartilage

The patient was taken to the operating room and placed in supine position. The appropriate level of general endotracheal anesthesia was induced. The procedure began with an inverted incision and elevation of the skin of the nose in the submucoperichondrial plane over the medial crural footplates and lower lateral cartilages and up over the dorsum. The septal angle was approached and submucoperichondrial flaps were elevated. There was evidence of an old fracture with severe nasal septal deviation to the right hand side. Separate alignment of the cartilaginous nose from the bony nose was encountered. The upper laterals were divided and medial and lateral osteotomies were carried out. There was inadequate septal cartilage to be used as spreader graft so instead the decision was made to use the patient's left ear cartilage. A left postauricular incision was made, and the conchal bowl cartilage graft was harvested. The defect was closed with 3-0 running locking chromic and a sterile pressure dressing applied. The ear cartilage graft was placed to put two spreader grafts on the left and one spreader graft on the right. The two on the left extended all the way up to the caudal tip, the one on the right just primarily the medial wall. It was placed in such a way to correct a caudal dorsal deviation of the nasal tip septum. A middle crus stitch was used to unite the domes, and the nose was projected by suturing the medial crural footplates of the caudal septum in deep projected fashion. Crushed ear cartilage was placed in the pockets above the spreader grafts in the area of the deficient dorsal nasal height and the lateral nasal sidewall height. The spreader brought an excellent aesthetic appearance to the nose. Mucoperichondrial flaps were closed. The skin was closed with 5-0 chromic and 6-0 fast absorbing gut. Doyle splints were placed on each side of the nasal septum and secured and a Denver splint was applied. The patient was awakened in the operating room and taken to the recovery room in good condition.

Code(s):

09SM0ZZ	**Reposition Nasal Septum, Open Approach**
09UM07Z	**Supplement Nasal Septum with Autologous Tissue Substitute, Open Approach**
09B1XZZ	**Excision of Left External Ear, External Approach**

Rationale:

The deviated nasal septum was realigned or repositioned, correcting the deviation of the nasal septum. This meets root operation definition Reposition (S). In addition to the repositioning, ear cartilage was placed as a spreader graft to supplement the repositioning and keep the nasal passages unobstructed. Supplement (U) is the root operation used to capture this portion of the procedure.

Root Operation		
Reposition (S)	Definition:	Moving to its normal location, or other suitable location, all or a portion of a body part
	Explanation:	The body part is moved to a new location from an abnormal location, or from a normal location where it is not functioning correctly. The body part may or may not be cut out or off to be moved to the new location.
Supplement (U)	Definition:	Putting in or on biological or synthetic material that physically reinforces and/or augments the function of a portion of a body part
	Explanation:	The biological material is non-living, or is living and from the same individual. The body part may have been previously replaced, and the SUPPLEMENT procedure is performed to physically reinforce and/or augment the function of the replaced body part.

The use of a Reposition (S) code and a Supplement (U) code is supported by multiple procedure guideline B3.2c, which follows, as there is a separate objective for each procedure—one to realign the septum and one to reinforce the septum—even though both are performed on the same body part Nasal Septum (M).

PCS Guideline
Multiple procedures
B3.2   During the same operative episode, multiple procedures are coded if:
c. Multiple root operations with distinct objectives are performed on the same body part.
Example: Destruction of sigmoid lesion and bypass of sigmoid colon are coded separately.

An Open (Ø) approach is reported for both codes. The device character for the Supplement (U) portion of the procedure is Autologous Tissue Substitute (7) since the patient's own tissue was used for the graft.

The Excision (B) of the ear cartilage used to facilitate the Supplement (U) procedure is also separately reportable. The ear cartilage, a free graft from a different body part, exemplifies the B3.9 guideline. Anatomical term concha is not found in the Body Part Key; however, based on its anatomical location in relation to anatomical terms that are classified to the external ear body part, such as the tragus, fourth character External Ear, Left (1) is the most appropriate.

Figure 4.20. External Ear

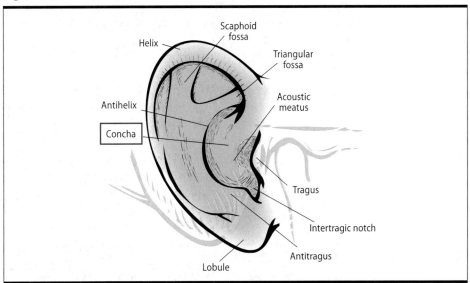

Removal of the ear cartilage takes place directly on the surface of the external ear meeting the approach definition of External (X). No Qualifier (Z) is used for the qualifier since the ear cartilage was removed for therapeutic, not diagnostic, reasons.

The preprocedural plan was to use the patient's septal cartilage as grafting material. Due to the lack of septal cartilage, however, ear cartilage was used instead. Had the septal cartilage been used, it would not have been appropriate to assign a separate code for excision of the septal cartilage. This would have been considered a local graft harvest, which does not comply with the stipulation in the B3.9 guideline, which states that the graft is obtained from a different body part.

Case Study 4.60. Split Thickness Skin Graft (STSG) for Third Degree Arm Burn

The patient was taken to the operating room and placed supine on the operating table. After adequate sedation was provided, the right upper extremity was prepped and draped in sterile fashion. The upper arm wound was sharply debrided. It was approximately 4 x 5 cm in area. A 4 x 5 cm split-thickness skin graft was harvested from the upper aspect of the left thigh. The graft was meshed and applied to the arm wound. The graft was secured with running suture. Attention was turned to the donor site, which was dressed with Xeroform and gauze. The arm was wrapped in Kerlix dressing. The patient tolerated the procedure and was transported to recovery.

Code(s):

ØHRBX74   **Replacement of Right Upper Arm Skin with Autologous Tissue Substitute, Partial Thickness, External Approach**

ØHBJXZZ   **Excision of Left Upper Leg Skin, External Approach**

Rationale:

Replacement (R) of skin is the primary objective for this procedure. Before the skin graft was placed on the upper arm, the wound was debrided back to healthy tissue. The root operation Excision (B) is defined as "cutting off without replacement" and the Replacement explanation says the body part may have been taken out "during the Replacement procedure." These definitions explain why no code is needed for the debridement of the burned skin; only the root operation Replacement (R) is reported for the replacement of the skin. Split thickness and partial thickness are synonymous terms and are captured in the qualifier value Partial Thickness (4). External (X) approach is the only approach available for skin replacement procedures.

Root Operation		
Replacement (R)	Definition:	Putting in or on a biological or synthetic material that physically takes the place and/or function of all or a portion of a body part
	Explanation:	The body part may have been taken out or replaced, or may be taken out, physically eradicated, or rendered nonfunctional during the REPLACEMENT procedure. A REMOVAL procedure is coded for taking out the device used in a previous replacement procedure.
Excision (B)	Definition:	Cutting out or off, without replacement, a portion of a body part
	Explanation:	The qualifier DIAGNOSTIC is used to identify excision procedures that are biopsies

The split-thickness skin graft was created from the patient's own skin, and was a free graft taken from a separate body part other than where the primary wound was located, meeting the stipulations outlined in guideline B3.9. Therefore, a code for Excision (B) of Skin, Left Upper Leg (J), using an External (X) approach is applied.

Definitions
full-thickness skin graft. Epidermis and full dermis layers are harvested. These grafts are typically used when the skin loss is significant (e.g., injuries, burns, severe ulcers, etc.). The donor graft is harvested via a scalpel and, because of its thickness, the donor site usually takes a longer amount of time to heal.
split-thickness skin graft. Graft that involves harvesting of the epidermis (top layer of skin) and part of the dermis (middle layer of skin). A surgical instrument called a dermatome is often used to harvest the tissue and healing of the donor site takes little time.

Fusion Procedures of the Spine

Spinal fusions are complex procedures using a variety of surgical techniques and devices to achieve the procedural objective. ICD-10-PCS contains three guidelines specific to coding spinal fusions. The primary purpose of guideline B3.10a is to provide the objective of the root operation Fusion (G), as it relates specifically to the spine, and discusses the options available within the spinal body part values. The second guideline, B3.10b, offers guidance for coding multiple procedures in spinal fusions. Guideline B3.10c focuses on the types of devices that are used to complete the fusion with the hierarchy of these devices and their corresponding PCS values.

Guidelines B3.10a, B3.10b and B3.10c

B3.10a	**The body part coded for a spinal vertebral joint(s) rendered immobile by a spinal fusion procedure is classified by the level of the spine (e.g. thoracic). There are distinct body part values for a single vertebral joint and for multiple vertebral joints at each spinal level.** ***Example:*** **Body part values specify Lumbar Vertebral Joint, Lumbar Vertebral Joints, 2 or More and Lumbosacral Vertebral Joint.**
B3.10b	**If multiple vertebral joints are fused, a separate procedure is coded for each vertebral joint that uses a different device and/or qualifier.** ***Example:*** **Fusion of lumbar vertebral joint, posterior approach, anterior column and fusion of lumbar vertebral joint, posterior approach, posterior column are coded separately.**
B3.10c	**Combinations of devices and materials are often used on a vertebral joint to render the joint immobile. When combinations of devices are used on the same vertebral joint, the device value coded for the procedure is as follows:** • **If an interbody fusion device is used to render the joint immobile (alone or containing other material like bone graft), the procedure is coded with the device value Interbody Fusion Device** • **If bone graft is the *only* device used to render the joint immobile, the procedure is coded with the device value Nonautologous Tissue Substitute or Autologous Tissue Substitute** • **If a mixture of autologous and nonautologous bone graft (with or without biological or synthetic extenders or binders) is used to render the joint immobile, code the procedure with the device value Autologous Tissue Substitute** ***Examples:*** **Fusion of a vertebral joint using a cage style interbody fusion device containing morselized bone graft is coded to the device Interbody Fusion Device.** **Fusion of a vertebral joint using a bone dowel interbody fusion device made of cadaver bone and packed with a mixture of local morselized bone and demineralized bone matrix is coded to the device Interbody Fusion Device.** **Fusion of a vertebral joint using both autologous bone graft and bone bank bone graft is coded to the device Autologous Tissue Substitute**

AHA Coding Clinic

2018, 1Q, 8	Placement of Bone Morphogenetic Protein & Spinal Fusion Surgery
2018, 1Q, 22	Spinal Fusion Procedures without Bone Graft
2017, 2Q, 23	Decompression of Spinal Cord and Placement of Instrumentation
2017, 1Q, 21	Staged Scoliosis Surgery with Iliac Fixation and Spinal Fusion
2014, 3Q, 36	Lumbar Interbody Fusion of Two Vertebral Levels
2014, 2Q, 6	Composite Grafting (Synthetic versus Nonautologous Tissue Substitute)
2014, 2Q, 6	Posterior Lumbar Fusion with Discectomy
2013, 3Q, 25	360-Degree Spinal Fusion
2013, 1Q, 21	Spinal Fusion of Thoracic and Lumbar Vertebrae
2013, 1Q, 29	Cervical and Thoracic Spinal Fusion

Spinal Fusion Overview

Body System (Character 2)

The objective of a spinal fusion, also called spinal arthrodesis, is to render immobile one or more vertebral joints, which are the interspaces between the vertebral bones. Spinal levels as discussed in guideline B3.10a refer to the cervical (C1-C7), thoracic (T1-T12), and lumbar (L1-L5) levels. The ICD-10-PCS Upper Joints (R) body system includes the cervical and thoracic levels, while the lumbar level is located in Lower Joints (S) body system. The following table lists the Upper and Lower Joints body systems with their corresponding body part values, including joints that span more than one spinal level.

Table 4.4. Upper and Lower Joints

Upper Joints (ØRG)	Lower Joints (ØSG)
Ø Occipital-cervical Joint	Ø Lumbar Vertebral Joint
1 Cervical Vertebral Joint	1 Lumbar Vertebral Joints, 2 or more
2 Cervical Vertebral Joints, 2 or more	3 Lumbosacral Joint
4 Cervicothoracic Vertebral Joint	5 Sacrococcygeal Joint
6 Thoracic Vertebral Joint	6 Coccygeal Joint
7 Thoracic Vertebral Joints, 2 to 7	7 Sacroiliac Joint, Right
8 Thoracic Vertebral Joints, 8 or more	8 Sacroiliac Joint, Left
A Thoracolumbar Vertebral Joint	

Root Operation (Character 3)

The root operation definition of Fusion (G) refers to the joining of the **articular** part between the bones, which is the interspace that joins two bones together. For this reason, the root operation Fusion (G) is not found in the Upper or Lower Bone body system tables but instead is offered only in the Upper and Lower Joints body system tables.

Root Operation		
Fusion (G)	Definition:	Joining together portions of an articular body part, rendering the articular body part immobile
	Explanation:	The body part is joined together by fixation device, bone graft, or other means

Body Part (Character 4)

The body part values identify the location and number of vertebral joints that are being fused. Several specific body part values (character 4) are provided in the fusion tables in order to identify whether a single joint, multiple joints, or a single joint that spans two anatomically different spinal levels are fused.

Spotlight
The number of fusions is counted by the number of intervertebral joints, also called interspaces, fused, not the number of vertebrae involved. For example, a fusion that spans from T2 through T9 is considered seven joint interspaces, coded with body part value Thoracic Vertebral Joints, 2 to 7 (7).

The spine provides structural support for the head, neck, trunk, and pelvis; allows for mobility of the trunk; houses and protects the spinal cord; and protects the spinal nerve roots and internal organs. The spine is composed of cervical, thoracic, lumbar, sacral, and coccygeal vertebrae. The cervical, thoracic, and lumbar vertebrae are mobile joints while the sacral and coccygeal vertebrae are immobile.

Vertebrae in each of these spinal levels have slightly different appearances, but with the exception of the first two cervical vertebrae (C1 atlas, and C2 axis), the vertebrae in each of the regions consist of the same basic structures. The vertebrae are composed of an anterior and posterior arch with a hole in the center called the spinal foramen. The anterior portion of each vertebra is a large oval bony portion called the vertebral body. Two short cylinder-shaped pedicles with two flattened bones called lamina, along with the processes, make up the posterior arch. There are a number of projections on the lamina, called processes (articular, transverse, and spinous).

Definitions
anterior arch. Also called the vertebral body, discs that connect each vertebral body together and create the cushion that enables motion and weight bearing.
posterior arch. Made up of the pedicles, laminae, and spinal process, the pedicles are the stubs of bone that extend from the backside of the vertebral body. Nerve roots exit from the spinal canal to the body between the pedicles. Laminae are the flat plates that form the "roof" over the spinal canal and connect the pedicles to the spinous process. The spinal processes are the bony projections off of the lamina, which are the attachment point for muscles and ligament. In between each vertebral joint are two facet joints, which allow the movement and stability of the spinal column.

Figure 4.21. Spine and Vertebra

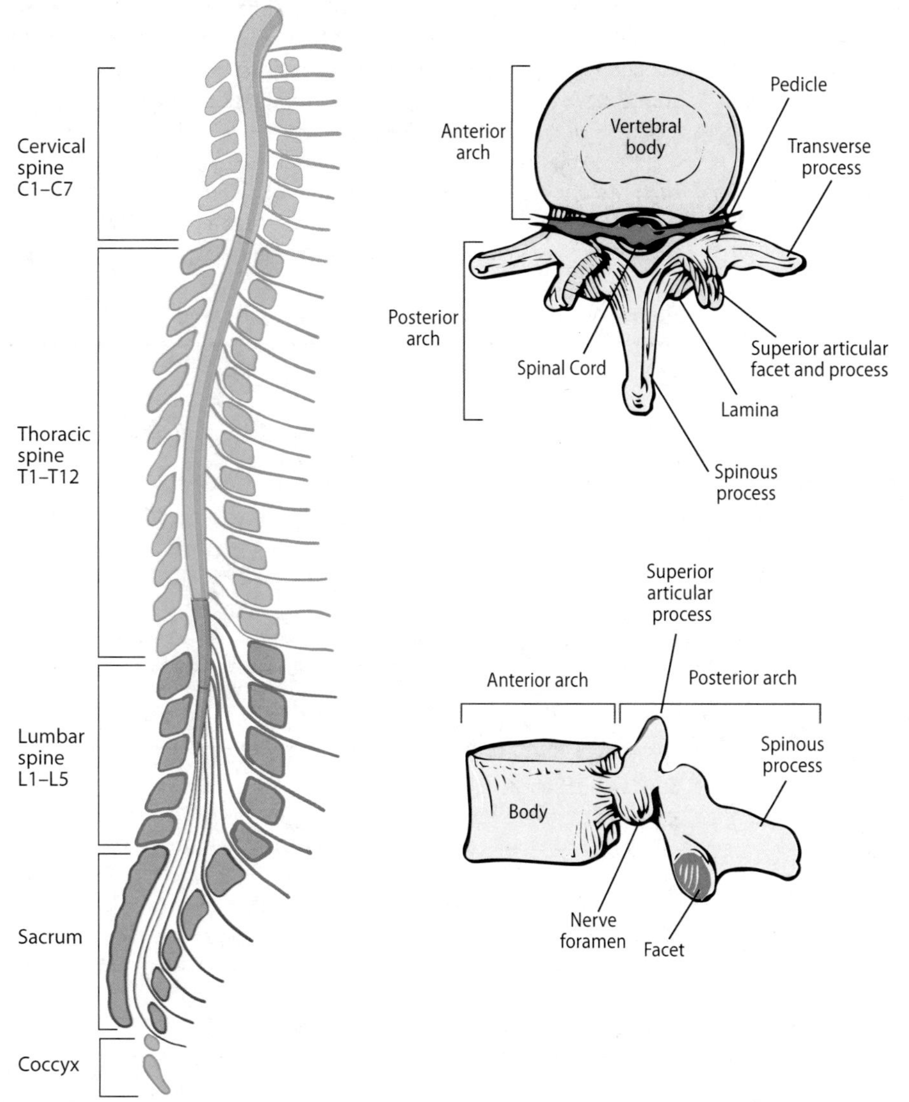

Approach (Character 5)

The word "approach" is used in two different contexts when coding spinal fusions, captured by the fifth and seventh characters. The approach value in the **fifth-character** position represents the method by which the vertebral joint was accessed and includes the choices of Open (Ø), Percutaneous (3), and Percutaneous Endoscopic (4). An Open (Ø) approach is defined as cutting through layers to access the site with the ability to visualize it without instrumentation. A Percutaneous (3) approach uses fluoroscopy to visualize the site and is performed through access tubes inserted into tiny incisions. Visualization for a Percutaneous Endoscope (4) approach is performed through scopes.

Spotlight
According to *AHA Coding Clinic,* 2013, 4Q, 108, the ICD-10-PCS guidelines do not directly address minimally invasive surgical procedures, and the operative report must be carefully reviewed to determine how the procedure site was visualized in order to apply the PCS approach definitions.

Device (character 6)

The device value supplies the type of device used to render the joint immobile. Because several different types of material can be used, alone or together, but only one device value per code can be assigned, guideline B3.10c provides a hierarchy of these materials to assist in proper code assignment. When an interbody fusion device is used in conjunction with other graft materials, it trumps all of the other graft materials including autologous (autograft) and nonautologous (allograft) with or without synthetic extenders or binders (BMP, etc.). If no interbody fusion device is used, autologous trumps the use of nonautologous graft when both are utilized. Nonautologous graft (with or without synthetic extenders or binders) is used as a device value if it is the only material applied to facilitate the fusion. There is no option for No Device for the spinal joint body parts in the Fusion tables as a spinal fusion requires graft material to be considered a fusion.

Figure 4.22. Fusion Device Hierarchy

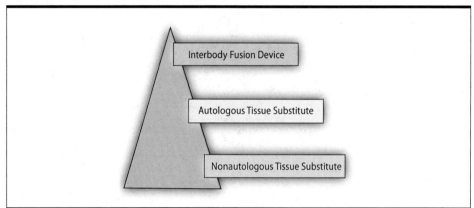

Device Values

Interbody Fusion Device (A): An implant that facilitates bone growth to fuse two or more vertebra. Interbody Fusion Devices are only used to fuse the anterior column but can be placed via anterior, lateral, or posterior approach. Some words to look for are metal or titanium cage (Ray Threaded, Zimmer, BAK), polyetheretherketone (PEEK) cage, polymer (Bengal), or threaded bone dowel. Although an Interbody Fusion Device is filled with autologous or nonautologous grafting material, only the device value for Interbody Fusion Device (A) is used. (See Fusion Device Hierarchy figure)

Figure 4.23. Interbody Fusion Device

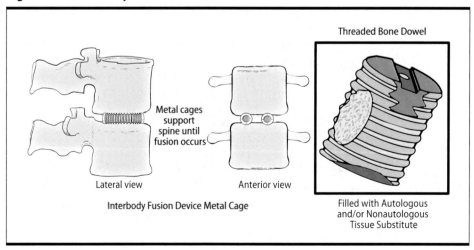

Spotlight
Two recently developed interbody fusion devices are the Nanotextured Surface and Radiolucent Porous devices. These devices are NOT coded in the Medical and Surgical (Ø) section and instead are coded from the New Technology (X) section. If either of these are mentioned in the operative report or listed in the devices used, table XRG should be used to report these spinal fusions. These devices, along with guidelines, are discussed in more detail in Chapter 9 New Technology Guidelines.

Autologous Tissue Substitute (7): Generally referred to as autograft, it is comprised from bone material taken from the patient's own body. Bone graft material may be bone chips obtained from the surrounding vertebra during the approach, also referred to as locally harvested bone graft. Alternatively, it may be harvested from a remote site, usually the iliac crest, through a separate incision. An additional code is necessary when the bone graft is obtained from a remote site (Guideline B3.9). No additional code is required for locally harvested graft material since obtaining this bone graft material is inherent to the approach.

Nonautologous Tissue Substitute (K): This tissue substitute is often referred to as an allograft, which is cadaver bone obtained from a tissue bank. It is often mixed with demineralized bone substitute or bone morphogenetic proteins (BMP). Allograft is only coded if used without any autograft or interbody fusion device.

Spotlight
If facilities choose to code the placement of bone morphogenic protein (BMP), assign code 3EØUØGB Introduction of recombinant bone morphogenic protein into joints, open approach.

Qualifier (Character 7)

The word "approach" is also used in the **seventh-character** qualifier value, referring to the anatomical access and fusion point. The qualifier values identify whether the anterior or posterior side of the spinal column was fused and whether the fusion was accomplished using an anterior or posterior approach. Fusion is typically performed on either the anterior column or the posterior column of the spine, although fusion of the anterior and posterior columns can also be performed in the same operative episode. When the access is performed laterally (on the side), it is considered an anterior approach.

Definitions
anterior column fusion. Fusing of the vertebral body of adjacent vertebra, often referred to as interbody fusion with access by anterior, posterior, or lateral incision.
posterior column fusion. Fusing of the adjacent posterior anatomy including laminae, pedicles, transverse process, and/or facets with access by posterior, posterolateral, or lateral transverse incision.

Knowledge of the different types of spinal fusions can assist in the appropriate choice of the qualifier value. Some of the more common acronyms that may be seen in a spinal fusion operative report are explained here along with their appropriate qualifier choice.

Figure 4.24. Supine, Lateral, and Prone Positions

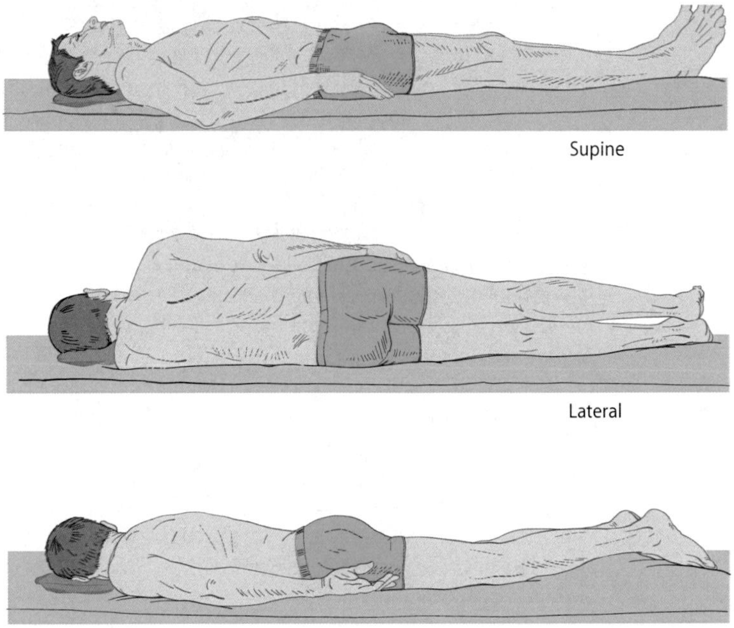

Supine

Lateral

Prone

Anterior Approach, Anterior Column (Ø)

Anterior lumbar interbody fusion (ALIF)

> The patient is placed in a *supine* position with the access made through the front or abdominal area to fuse the anterior spinal column. Although it involves retracting large blood vessels and intestines, there is less risk of spinal nerve injury.

Anteromedial (Smith-Robinson)

> This technique uses an approach through the front of the neck to fuse the anterior cervical column and is used mainly for C3 to T1 fusions.

Extreme lateral interbody fusion (XLIF), direct lateral interbody fusion (DLIF), transpsoas interbody fusion

> The three surgical techniques listed above (XLIF, DLIF, and transpsoas) use a minimally invasive approach to fuse the anterior column with access laterally (from the side) or through the psoas muscle. Although these techniques are minimally invasive, the operative report must be closely examined to determine the correct approach value. If the surgeon is opening the surgical site enough to visualize the site without instrumentation (i.e., endoscope or fluoroscopy) or uses a retractor to better visualize the area, then an Open (Ø) approach is the appropriate choice.

> However, some techniques involve visualizing the site using instrumentation percutaneously. The XLIF is the most likely candidate for Percutaneous (3) approach as fluoroscopy is often used to guide the probe, dilator, and retractor through two small incisions in the side. The disc particles are removed and the fusion device is inserted through these canals.

Spotlight
The insertion of screws and rods in the performance of Anterior Approach, Anterior Column techniques to stabilize the fusion is considered inherent to the fusion procedure and is not coded separately.

Posterior Approach, Posterior Column (1)

Posterior or posterolateral fusion

> The patient is in the *prone* position and the incision is made through the back. Graft material is placed along the sides or between the vertebra with titanium screws and rods typically inserted for stability in order to fuse the posterior column. Screws and rods are considered inherent to the fusion procedure and not coded separately.

Posterior Approach, Anterior Column (J)

Posterior lumbar interbody fusion (PLIF)

> This technique fuses the anterior column of the spine using an implant like a bone dowel; Ray threaded, PEEK, or other cage; with or without graft material. The approach is performed with the patient in the *prone* position with the incision made in the lower back. Instrumentation such as pedicle screws and rods are typically inserted for stability and are not coded separately.

Figure 4.25. Posterior Lumbar Interbody Fusion (PLIF)

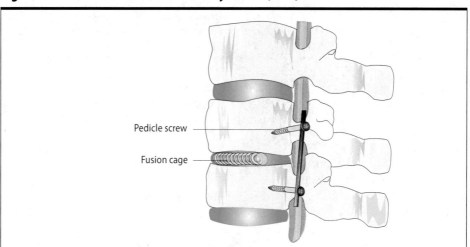

Transforaminal lumbar interbody fusion (TLIF)

> This approach from the back is performed with the removal of a facet joint to better access the disc space through the foramen. The disc is removed and replaced with an interbody fusion device to fuse the anterior column. **Note:** In a TLIF, the posterior column is often additionally fused through this same approach, using bone graft or synthetic grafting material such as BMP along with pedicle rods and screws. An additional procedure is reported to represent the qualifier value of the Posterior Column, Posterior Approach with the appropriate device value indicating the type of graft material used.

Axial lumbar interbody fusion (AxiaLIF)

> Performed on L5-S1, this technique is the least invasive approach for the sacral (transsacral) area. A small incision (1") is made next to the coccyx (tailbone) where a series of dilator tubes are inserted until the canal is large enough to perform the procedure. A drill is inserted through the dilator tube and guided by fluoroscopy into the disc space between L5 and the sacrum. The center of the disk is removed though the tube and replaced with bone growth material. A threaded rod is guided through the canal and implanted from the sacrum up through the center of the L5 vertebra above the disc. Pedicle screws may also be percutaneously inserted to stabilize the fusion but are not coded separately.

Multiple Procedures

A single code is used when the fusion uses the same device AND qualifier character for the same PCS body part. Multiple codes are assigned in the following situations:

- The fusion spans different spinal levels represented by distinct PCS body part values. For instance, fusion of C6 to T1 includes the cervical (C6-C7) and cervicothoracic (C7-T1) vertebral joints—two different body part character values in table ØRG.

- Different devices are used to fuse different vertebral joints. For instance, when an interbody fusion device is used for one vertebral joint in the lumbar spine and autologous bone graft is used at a different vertebral joint in the lumbar spine or other level in the spine.

- Different qualifiers are used to fuse different vertebral joints. For example, when one lumbar vertebral joint is fused via a posterior approach on the posterior column, while another lumbar or other vertebral joint is fused via a posterior approach but on the anterior column.

Spotlight
360° fusion refers to the fusion of the anterior and posterior column using an anterior and a posterior approach in the same operative session and requires a minimum of two codes.

Beyond the Guidelines

A number of separately reportable procedures follow that may be commonly performed in conjunction with spinal fusions or performed on their own.

Decompressive Laminectomy or Foraminotomy

AHA Coding Clinic

2017, 2Q, 23	Decompression of Spinal Cord and Placement of Instrumentation
2016, 2Q, 16	Decompressive Laminectomy/Foraminotomy and Lumbar Discectomy
2015, 2Q, 20	Cervical Laminoplasty
2015, 2Q, 21	Multiple Decompressive Cervical Laminectomies
2015, 2Q, 34	Decompressive Laminectomy
2013, 4Q, 116	Spinal Decompression

The terms laminectomy (complete removal of lamina) and laminotomy (partial removal of lamina) are often used interchangeably. Laminectomy is excision of the lamina, which is the bone on the backside of the spinal canal; foraminotomy is the removal of bone around the neural foramen, the space where the nerve root exits the spinal canal. Although part or all of the lamina is being excised, the actual objective of the procedure is to relieve the pressure from the spinal nerve roots or spinal cord by "releasing" the nerve roots or cord. The correct root operation is Release (N), which is coded as a separate procedure from table Ø1N.

Root Operation		
Release (N)	Definition:	Freeing a body part from an abnormal physical constraint by cutting or by use of force
	Explanation:	Some of the restraining tissue may be taken out but none of the body part is taken out

Spotlight
If the laminectomy is done solely to reach the site of the fusion and is NOT performed for decompression of the nerve root, it is inherent to the fusion procedure and is not coded separately. See guideline B3.1b.

Figure 4.26. Laminotomy with Decompression

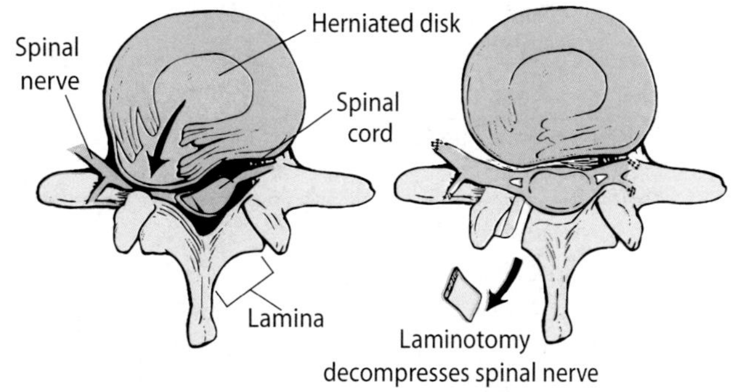

Figure labels: Spinal nerve, Herniated disk, Spinal cord, Lamina, Laminotomy decompresses spinal nerve

Discectomy (Diskectomy)

AHA Coding Clinic

2016, 2Q, 16   Decompressive Laminectomy/Foraminotomy and Lumbar Discectomy

2014, 2Q, 6   Posterior Lumbar Fusion with Discectomy

2014, 2Q, 7   Anterior Cervical Thoracic Fusion with Total Discectomy

A discectomy is often performed to facilitate a fusion and must be coded as a separate procedure. The operative report must be carefully scrutinized to determine if part (Excision (B)) or all (Resection (T)) of the disk was removed.

Root Operation		
Excision (B)	Definition:	Cutting out or off, without replacement, a portion of a body part
	Explanation:	The qualifier DIAGNOSTIC is used to identify excision procedures that are biopsies
Resection (T)	Definition:	Cutting out or off, without replacement, all of a body part
	Explanation:	None

Intraoperative Neuromonitoring

AHA Coding Clinic

2015, 1Q, 26   Intraoperative Monitoring Using Sentio MMG®

If a facility chooses to code intraoperative neuromonitoring, it is coded from the Measurement and Monitoring (4) section with body system Physiological Systems (A). It involves using one or more neurophysiologic testing techniques in real time in the operating room to assess the integrity of neural structures. It includes cranial nerve, peripheral nerve, and spinal cord testing performed intraoperatively. Commonly used modalities include electroencephalogram, somatosensory evoked potentials (SSEP), brainstem auditory evoked potentials, electromyogram, nerve conduction studies, motor evoked potentials, and transcranial Doppler. Upper and lower extremity SSEP, which monitors the spinal cord function via stimulation of the peripheral nerves, is a common monitoring technique used. It monitors the electrical activity of the peripheral nervous system via external electrodes attached to specific areas of the body and requires only one code (4A11X4G). Other techniques may be used, represented by different codes. It is recommended that each facility work with the surgeon to determine which type is routinely used in their specific facilities.

Root Operation		
Measurement and Monitoring Section (4)		
Monitoring (1)	Definition:	Determining the level of a physiological or physical function repetitively over a period of time
Measurement (Ø)	Definition:	Determining the level of a physiological or physical function at a point in time

Disc Replacement

Recently, disc replacement with an artificial disc rather than spinal fusion has shown favorable clinical outcomes. These are performed on cervical or lumbar discs at this time. Some of the current FDA approved brands include Prestige™, PRODISC®, BRYAN®, SECURE®, PMC®, and Mobi-C® for cervical spine; Charite® and ProDisc® for lumbar spine. Since the objective of this procedure is to replace the entire disc, the appropriate root operation is Replacement (R). Replacement (R) includes the removal of the body part, so a separate code is not assigned for the resection of the disc.

Root Operation		
Replacement (R)	Definition:	Putting in or on a biological or synthetic material that physically takes the place and/or function of all or a portion of a body part
	Explanation:	The body part may have been taken out or replaced, or may be taken out, physically eradicated, or rendered nonfunctional during the REPLACEMENT procedure. A REMOVAL procedure is coded for taking out the device used in a previous replacement procedure.

Figure 4.27. Lumbar Artificial Disc Replacement

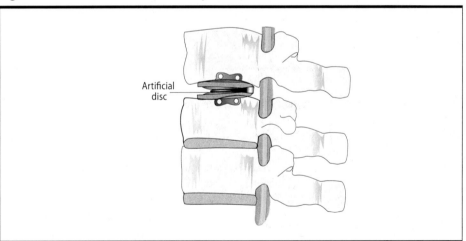

Artificial disc

Spinal Stabilization Devices

The use of pedicle rods and screws to **augment** a spinal fusion is not coded separately and is different from the insertion of a spinal stabilization device, which are all relatively new technologies and are constantly being updated. These devices are found in the Upper Joints (ØRH) and Lower Joints (ØSH) Insertion (H) root operation tables and have various values for the device character to identify the specific type of spinal stabilization device. These procedures can be performed in lieu of or in conjunction with spinal fusions.

Root Operation		
Insertion (H)	Definition:	Putting in a nonbiological appliance that monitors, assists, performs, or prevents a physiological function but does not physically take the place of a body part
	Explanation:	None

There are three different types of spinal stabilization devices:

- Interspinous Process (IPD) (B)

  Also known as decompression or distraction devices, these are still in early stages of use and are used for decompression of spinal stenosis in lieu of spinal fusion. Some of the brand names are X-STOP, Wallis, DIAM, and CoFlex.

- Pedicle-Based (C)

  These are derived from the use of pedicle screws and rods used in spinal surgery but are newer devices that are being tested in standalone procedures, as well as in conjunction with spinal fusions or artificial disc replacements. Instead of rigid rods they use flexible, movable, and even inflatable rods. Some brand names are Graf, Dynesys, IsoBar, and Dynamic Soft System.

- Facet Replacement (D)

  These are designed to replace facet joints while maintaining spinal movement for use primarily for pain from the degeneration of facet joints. This should not be confused with the root operation Replacement (R) as it should appropriately be coded as an Insertion (H) of a facet replacement stabilization device. These are also relatively new to the market. Some brand names are Anatomic Facet Replacement System (AFRS), Total Facet Arthroplasty System (TFAS), and Total Posterior System (TOPS).

Practical Application for Guidelines B3.10a, B3.10b, and B3.10c and Beyond the Guidelines

Case Study 4.61. Fusion, Cervicothoracic

The patient was put into the supine position. Dissection was performed to C6 where anterior portions of the discs were removed between C6, C7, and T1. Two titanium cages packed with demineralized bone matrix (DBM) were inserted into C6-C7 and C7 to T1 spaces.

Code(s):

0RG10A0	**Fusion of Cervical Vertebral Joint with Interbody Fusion Device, Anterior Approach, Anterior Column, Open Approach**
0RG40A0	**Fusion of Cervicothoracic Vertebral Joint with Interbody Fusion Device, Anterior Approach, Anterior Column, Open Approach**
0RB30ZZ	**Excision of Cervical Vertebral Disc, Open Approach**
0RB50ZZ	**Excision of Cervicothoracic Vertebral Disc, Open Approach**

Rationale:
Although the Upper Joints (R) body system includes a body part value for two or more joints, multiple codes must be used for this fusion to indicate the distinctly separate body parts according to guideline B3.10a. The fusion of C6 to C7 is considered one cervical joint represented by the body part Cervical Vertebral Joint (1). The fusion of C7 to T1 is also one joint that crosses separate spinal levels (cervical and thoracic) and is reported with a different body part value of Cervicothoracic Vertebral Joint (4), also found in the Upper Joints (R) body system.

The cages used to facilitate the fusion are represented by the sixth character, device. Because only one device value for each code can be assigned, Interbody Fusion Device (A) is always the applicable device value when used along with autologous bone graft, nonautologous material, or synthetic substitute.

The patient was in the supine position, which denotes that an anterior approach was used. The use of an interbody fusion device indicates that the fusion was performed on the anterior spinal column. The qualifier Anterior Approach, Anterior Column (Ø) is the correct value for both of the fusion codes.

AHA Coding Clinic, 2014, 2Q, 7, instructs that the discectomy is reported separately when performed with a spinal fusion. Since only partial discs in C6-C7 and C7-T1 were removed, Excision (B) is the appropriate root operation. The Excision table in the Upper Joints body system (ØRB) includes body part values for the Cervical Vertebral Disc (3) and the Cervicothoracic Vertebral Disc (5). Since these body parts are represented by different body part values, the discectomy procedures are reported with two codes.

An Open (Ø) approach was used to access the vertebral interspace to perform all procedures.

Case Study 4.62. Fusion, Posterior Lumbar Interbody Fusion (PLIF)

From prone position, an incision was made and a laminectomy performed from L4-L5. BAK cages filled with allograft and BMP were placed at L4-L5 and L5-S1. Pedicle screws and rods were inserted to further stabilize the fusion. SSEP intraoperative neurophysiologic monitoring was performed.

Code(s):

ØSGØØAJ	**Fusion of Lumbar Vertebral Joint with Interbody Fusion Device, Posterior Approach, Anterior Column, Open Approach**
ØSG3ØAJ	**Fusion of Lumbosacral Joint with Interbody Fusion Device, Posterior Approach, Anterior Column, Open Approach**
4A11X4G	**Monitoring of Peripheral Nervous Electrical Activity, Intraoperative, External Approach**

Rationale:
Two codes must be used for the fusion to indicate separate body parts as defined by guideline B3.10a. Multiple codes are necessary to specify each different vertebral level fused: one code for L4-L5, Lumbar Vertebral Joint (Ø), and another code for L5-S1, Lumbosacral Joint (3). Both body part values are located in the Lower Joints (3) body system in the Fusion root operation table (ØSG).

A BAK cage was used in this fusion procedure and is captured by the device value Interbody Fusion Device (A). The BAK cage described in the body of the report trumps the allograft, which includes BMP, according to the hierarchy outlined in guideline B3.10c.

The presence of an Interbody Fusion Device (A), which is used to fuse the vertebral body, indicates that the anterior column was fused. The patient's prone position signifies that a posterior approach was used. This supplies the necessary information to indicate that the correct qualifier is Posterior Approach, Anterior Column (J). With no mention of small incisions, tubes, or retractors, this was clearly an Open (Ø) approach.

The intraoperative neuromonitoring is coded from the Measurement and Monitoring (4) section of PCS with body system Physiological Systems (A). Electrodes were placed via an External (X) approach on the extremities to monitor the Electrical Activity (4) of the Peripheral Nervous (1) body system during the surgery.

The laminectomy is not coded separately as there was no indication that a decompression procedure was performed, which implies that a laminectomy was only done to reach the operative site.

Pedicle screws and rods are not coded separately as they are inherent in the fusion procedure.

Case Study 4.63. Fusion, Axial Lumbar Interbody Fusion (AxiaLIF)

The patient was admitted for an AxiaLIF procedure for treatment of L5-S1 degenerative disc disease. The patient was placed prone with a 1 inch incision made trans-sacrally. Using a guide pin and fluoroscopy, the surgeon accessed the top of the sacrum. Dilators were inserted and a transosseous working canal created. Through the canal, the surgeon removed enough of the disc to make room for the threaded cage filled with allograft and BMP.

Code(s):

ØSG33AJ   **Fusion of Lumbosacral Joint with Interbody Fusion Device, Posterior Approach, Anterior Column, Percutaneous Approach**

ØSB43ZZ   **Excision of Lumbosacral Disc, Percutaneous Approach**

Rationale:

The AxiaLIF procedure is a minimally invasive technique used to fuse L5 and S1, which involves the Lumbosacral Joint (3) body part in the Lower Joints (S) body system. When determining the appropriate code for the technique, it is helpful to check the qualifier choices first. This one was done with a posterior approach near the sacrum using an interbody fusion device to fuse the anterior spine, so the qualifier value is Posterior Approach, Anterior Column (J).

The surgeon visualized the site with fluoroscopy and performed the fusion through a working canal through which tubes were passed, which is considered a Percutaneous (3) approach.

Even though an interbody fusion device and allograft were used for the fusion, the hierarchy guidelines in B3.10c indicate that only the Interbody Fusion Device (A) is coded.

In ICD-10-PCS, partial discectomies are coded separately with root operation Excision (3). This is supported by *AHA Coding Clinic,* 2014, 2Q, 7. The Lumbosacral Disc (4) is found in the Lower Joints (S) body system and was removed percutaneously through the canal.

Case Study 4.64. Fusion, Posterior Lumbar and Direct Lateral Interbody Fusion (DLIF)

Procedures: Posterior arthrodesis L3-5; direct lateral lumbar interbody fusion (DLIF) L4-5.

At the start of the procedure, an incision was made in the left iliac crest to obtain bone graft. With the patient prone, the back was prepped and draped. A midline incision was made, carried down through the subcutaneous tissues to the fascial layer. The routine technique for identification and cannulation of the L3 pedicle was performed and 45 mm x 6.5 mm diameter screws from the Theken system were used through L3 to L5. Good fixation was obtained. A rod was bent to appropriate contours and placed into the caps of the pedicle screws and the cap screws tightened down firmly over the rod and a mixture of harvested bone graft and cadaver graft was placed into this prepared area. The patient was turned on his side and a small left-sided incision was made lateral to the disk space. The fibers of the psoas muscle were gently separated without cutting. The space from L4 to L5 was entered and an 11 mm x 25 mm PEEK intervertebral biomechanical device was placed, packed with Progenix and autologous bone across the midline with good purchase of the endplates.

Code(s):

ØSG1Ø71   **Fusion of 2 or more Lumbar Vertebral Joints with Autologous Tissue Substitute, Posterior Approach, Posterior Column, Open Approach**

ØSGØØAØ   **Fusion of Lumbar Vertebral Joint with Interbody Fusion Device, Anterior Approach, Anterior Column, Open Approach**

ØQB3ØZZ   **Excision of Left Pelvic Bone, Open Approach**

Rationale:

Interspaces L3 to L4 and L4 to L5, represented by body part value Lumbar Vertebral Joints, 2 or More (1), were fused using local bone graft mixed with cadaver bone. The device hierarchy dictates that Autologous Tissue Substitute (7) trumps the cadaver bone. The qualifier provides additional specificity related to the approach and site of the fusion, which in this case is Posterior Approach, Posterior Column (1). The screws and rods are inherent to the fusion and are not coded.

Fusion (G) of anterior column L4-L5 was also performed, which is represented by a different qualifier than that of the posterior column and necessitates an additional code. It is called a DLIF because of the approach method (direct lateral) and use of an Interbody Fusion Device (A). Even though the DLIF was done from the side (lateral), it is still considered an anterior technique. For this additional code, only one body part value, Lumbar Vertebral Joint (Ø), was fused using the qualifier Anterior Approach, Anterior Column (Ø).

According to guideline B3.10c, when an interbody fusion device and bone graft are used in one fusion, the interbody fusion device overrides the bone graft; when autologous and nonautologous (allograft) bone graft are both used, only the autologous bone graft is coded.

Based on guideline B3.10b, one code is used for the posterior column for both levels from L3-L5 using the autologous bone graft, with the other code indicating only the level L4-L5 anterior fusion with an interbody fusion device and autologous bone graft.

Harvest of the bone graft from the iliac crest is coded separately with root operation Excision (B) and body part Pelvic Bone, Left (3) from the Lower Bones (Q) body system in accordance to guideline B3.9.

All procedures were performed via an Open (Ø) approach. Although the DLIF documented that a "small" incision was made, there is no indication that visualization of the site was performed with any scope or fluoroscopy but rather by direct visualization.

PCS Guideline
Excision for Graft
B3.9   If an autograft is obtained from a different procedure site in order to complete the objective of the procedure, a separate procedure is coded.   *Example:* Coronary bypass with excision of saphenous vein graft, excision of saphenous vein is coded separately.

Case Study 4.65. Fusion, Cervical

Procedures Performed: Anterior interbody fusion at C4-C5, C5-C6, and C6-C7 utilizing Bengal cages times three; Anterior instrumentation for stabilization by Slim-LOC plate C4, C5, C6, and C7; Anterior cervical discectomy at C4-C5, C5-C6, and C6-C7.

The patient was brought into the operating room, placed in a supine position, and general anesthesia was administered. The anterior aspect of the neck was prepped and draped in a routine sterile fashion. A linear skin incision was made in the skin fold line from just to the right of the midline to the leading edge of the right sternocleidomastoid muscle and taken sharply to platysma, which was dissected in a subplatysmal manner, and then the prevertebral space was encountered. A #11 blade was used with discectomies being performed removing grossly and very degenerated discs at C4-C5, C5-C6, and C6-C7. Appropriate size Bengal cages were filled with the patient's own bone elements and countersunk into position, filled along with fusion putty, and once these were quite tightly applied and checked, further stability was added by the placement of a Slim-LOC plate of appropriate size with appropriate size screws, and a post placement x-ray showed well-aligned elements.

Code(s):

ØRG2ØAØ	**Fusion of 2 or more Cervical Vertebral Joints with Interbody Fusion Device, Anterior Approach, Anterior Column, Open Approach**
ØRT3ØZZ	**Resection of Cervical Vertebral Disc, Open Approach**

Rationale:

Even though root operation Fusion (G) was performed on three interspaces of the cervical spine, all were accomplished with the same device Interbody Fusion Device (A), same qualifier Anterior Approach, Anterior Column (Ø), and same Open (Ø) approach. Since the body part value Cervical Vertebral Joints, 2 or more (2) represents all three joints, only one code is needed to capture the fusion.

A secondary code is reported to denote the root operation Resection (3) of the discs. Only one code is needed for the resection, even though three discs were completely removed. The Resection table ØRT does not have a separate value for C4-C5 disc, C5-C6 disc, and C6-C7 disc. Instead, only body part value Cervical Vertebral Disc (3), located in the Upper Joints (R) body system, is provided to represent all discs in the cervical region. Since the same root operation was performed on three discs represented by the same body part character, only one code should be applied. A query should be considered to ensure that the three discs were, in fact, completely removed (resected) rather than partially removed, which is coded with Excision (B).

Case Study 4.66. Fusion, Lumbar with Decompression and Discectomy

The patient was placed prone on the Jackson's spinal table with all bony prominences well padded. His lumbar spine was sterilely prepped and draped in the usual fashion. A previous midline incision was extended from approximate level of L3 to S1. A laminotomy was meticulously performed around the L4 nerve root until wide decompression was obtained. The nerve roots were individually inspected and additional decompression was extended from the level of the inferior half of L3 to the superior half of S1. Once this was identified, lamina was shaved with a rongeur and foraminotomies were created to allow additional mobility. Posterior pieces of damaged disc from L4-L5 were removed.

Carbon fiber cages 11 mm in height x 9 mm in width x 25 mm in length were packed with local bone graft and allograft. These were impacted at the interspace of L4-L5 under direct image intensification. Permanent screws were placed at L4, L5, and S1 bilaterally. This was performed under direct image intensification. The position was verified in AP and lateral images. Once this was completed, the posterolateral gutters were decorticated with an AM2 Midas Rex burr down to bleeding subchondral bone. The wound was copiously irrigated with antibiotic solution and suctioned dried. The morcellized allograft and local bone graft were mixed and packed copiously from the transverse processes of L4-S1 bilaterally. A 0.25 inch titanium rod was contoured of appropriate length to span from L4-S1. Appropriate cross connecters were applied and the construct was placed over the pedicle screws.

Code(s):

ØSGØØAJ	**Fusion of Lumbar Vertebral Joint with Interbody Fusion Device, Posterior Approach, Anterior Column, Open Approach**
ØSGØØ71	**Fusion of Lumbar Vertebral Joint with Autologous Tissue Substitute, Posterior Approach, Posterior Column, Open Approach**
ØSG3Ø71	**Fusion of Lumbosacral Joint with Autologous Tissue Substitute, Posterior Approach, Posterior Column, Open Approach**
Ø1NBØZZ	**Release Lumbar Nerve, Open Approach**
ØSB2ØZZ	**Excision of Lumbar Vertebral Disc, Open Approach**

Rationale:

Two different levels of the vertebral spine were fused: L4 to L5 represented by body part value Lumbar Vertebral Joint (Ø) and L5 to S1 represented by body part value Lumbosacral Joint (3). According to guideline B3.2a, multiple procedure codes are assigned when the same root operation is performed on different body parts as defined by distinct body part values.

PCS Guideline
Multiple procedures
B3.2　　During the same operative episode, multiple procedures are coded if: a. The same root operation is performed on different body parts as defined by distinct values of the body part character. *Examples:* Diagnostic excision of liver and pancreas are coded separately. Excision of lesion in the ascending colon and excision of lesion in the transverse colon are coded separately.

The device and qualifier value also influence code selection based on guideline B3.10b. Both of the fusions were performed via a posterior approach; however, the L4-L5 joint involved fusion of both sides of the spinal column, the Posterior Approach, Anterior Column (J) using an Interbody Fusion Device (A) and the Posterior Approach, Posterior Column (1) using Autologous Tissue Substitute (7). Because two different qualifiers are used, two codes are needed for this one vertebral joint to capture fusion of the anterior and posterior columns.

Selection of the appropriate device character is based on a hierarchy established by guideline B3.10c. If an interbody fusion device is used, regardless of whether local bone and/or allograft material was also used, only Interbody Fusion Device (A) is coded.

At the L5-S1 level, only the posterior column was fused using autologous/allograft bone mixture, so only one code is needed. When Autologous Tissue Substitute (7) is used along with Nonautologous Tissue Substitute (K), only the Autologous Tissue Substitute (7) device value is used. A Nonautologous Tissue Substitute (K) device value would only be chosen if that was the only material used to fuse the vertebral joint(s).

It is not appropriate to code a separate procedure for the insertion of screws, rods, plates, or other fixation devices used in a fusion procedure. *AHA Coding Clinic,* 2014, 3Q, 30, indicates that these materials are integral to the fusion procedure.

A code for partial discectomy was reported based on guidance from *AHA Coding Clinic,* 2014, 2Q, 6. When a disc is removed as part of a fusion procedure, the disc removal is coded in addition to the fusion. The root operation depends on whether only part of the disc was removed (Excision) or the entire disc was removed (Resection). As with the fusion code, Upper or Lower Joints is the appropriate body system for the Excision (B) or Resection (T) of a vertebral disc.

An additional code should also be included for the decompression procedure performed. The objective of this procedure is to remove enough bony (lamina) material to decompress or "release" the nerve roots from impingement. Release (N) is the correct root operation choice according to *AHA Coding Clinic,* 2015, 2Q, 30.

Root Operation		
Release (N)	Definition:	Freeing a body part from an abnormal physical constraint by cutting or by use of force
	Explanation:	Some of the restraining tissue may be taken out but none of the body part is taken out

The nerve being freed or released is the lumbar spinal nerve. The Body Part Definition Key (excerpt following) includes the lumbar spinal nerve in Lumbar Nerve (B) body part value, which is in the Peripheral Nervous System (1).

ICD-10-PCS Value	Definition
Lumbar Nerve	**Includes:** Lumbosacral trunk Spinal nerve, lumbar Superior clunic (cluneal) nerve

---

Case Study 4.67. Disk Replacement

The patient was placed in the supine position and an incision made in the low abdomen. Careful dissection was made around organs and vessels to reach the area of L4-L5. A discectomy was performed, removing the collapsed and herniated disc between L4 and L5, and a Charite replacement was inserted with excellent placement and fit.

Code(s):

ØSR2ØJZ   Replacement of Lumbar Vertebral Disc with Synthetic Substitute, Open Approach

Rationale:

In this example, no fusion was performed. Instead, root operation Replacement (R) is used for this newer technology of disc replacement using an artificial Charite disc. This three-piece device is made from metal and medical grade plastics and is coded as Synthetic Substitute (J). The explanation for root operation Replacement (R) clarifies that the removal of the body part is included, thus eliminating the need to use an additional code for the discectomy. The body part Lumbar Vertebral Disc (2) is located in the Lower Joints (S) body system.

Root Operation		
Replacement (R)	Definition:	Putting in or on a biological or synthetic material that physically takes the place and/or function of all or a portion of a body part
	Explanation:	The body part may have been taken out or replaced, or may be taken out, physically eradicated, or rendered nonfunctional during the REPLACEMENT procedure. A REMOVAL procedure is coded for taking out the device used in a previous replacement procedure.

Inspection Procedures

The root operation Inspection (J) is used when the objective is to examine the body parts by direct visualization or with the use of instrumentation. It also applies when the purpose is to manually explore the body parts externally or through the body layers, such as through skin and subcutaneous tissue, to reach an organ. Inspections are often performed with an endoscope, which is a slender, optical instrument that can be a flexible illuminated tube or a rigid tube. Examples of inspections with the use of an endoscope include diagnostic endoscopy procedures such as:

- Arthroscopy: joint interior
- Bronchoscopy: lower respiratory tract
- Colonoscopy: large intestine
- Colposcopy: cervix
- Cystoscopy: urinary tract, bladder
- Esophagogastroduodenoscopy (EGD): esophagus, stomach, and duodenum
- Endoscopic retrograde cholangiopancreatography (ERCP): bile and pancreatic ducts
- Hysteroscopy: uterus
- Laparoscopy: abdominal or pelvic cavity
- Thoracoscopy: chest cavity

Manual inspections include procedures such as digital rectal exam, laparotomy with direct visualization, and palpation of intestines or other abdominal organs.

The root operation Inspection (J) is coded when the sole objective of the procedure is to examine a body part. A number of guidelines in PCS make reference to the root operation Inspection (J), such as B3.2d in the Multiple procedure guidelines, which indicates that if one approach is planned (e.g., laparoscopy) but the procedure is converted to another approach (e.g., open), the initial approach is coded separately using the root operation Inspection (J).

PCS Guideline
Multiple procedures
B3.2   During the same operative episode, multiple procedures are coded if: d. The intended root operation is attempted using one approach, but is converted to a different approach. *Example:* Laparoscopic cholecystectomy converted to an open cholecystectomy is coded as percutaneous endoscopic Inspection and open Resection.

Discontinued or incomplete procedures guideline B3.3 states that the root operation Inspection (J) should be assigned when a procedure is discontinued without any other root operation being performed.

PCS Guideline
Discontinued or incomplete procedures
B3.3   If the intended procedure is discontinued or not otherwise completed, code the procedure to the root operation performed. If a procedure is discontinued before any other root operation is performed, code the root operation Inspection of the body part or anatomical region inspected. *Example:* A planned aortic valve replacement procedure is discontinued after the initial thoracotomy and before any incision is made in the heart muscle, when the patient becomes hemodynamically unstable. This procedure is coded as an open Inspection of the mediastinum.

Guidelines covered here relate specifically to the root operation Inspection (J) and clarify the following circumstances:

- Whether to code Inspection (J) when it is done for the purpose of providing assistance, reaching the site, or supplying visual guidance to achieve another objective
- What determines the appropriate body part value when multiple tubular body parts are inspected
- What procedure is reported when an Inspection (J) is followed by another procedure during the same operative episode using different approach values

Root Operation		
Inspection (J)	Definition:	Visually and/or manually exploring a body part
	Explanation:	Visual exploration may be performed with or without optical instrumentation. Manual exploration may be performed directly or through intervening body layers.

Guideline B3.11a

B3.11a Inspection of a body part(s) performed in order to achieve the objective of a procedure is not coded separately.

Example: **Fiberoptic bronchoscopy performed for irrigation of bronchus, only the irrigation procedure is coded.**

AHA Coding Clinic

2015, 3Q, 9   Aborted Endovascular Stenting of Superficial Femoral Artery

2013, 4Q, 117   Percutaneous Endoscopic Placement of Gastrostomy Tube

If the inspection is being done on the same body part, for the purpose of guidance or assistance only, in order to perform the objective of the definitive root operation, it is considered inherent in the definitive procedure and is not reported separately. For example, an examination is often performed at the beginning of a procedure to ensure adequate access and at the end of the procedure to confirm proper completion. If the examination is done as guidance to facilitate completion of a procedure with a different objective, it is considered part of the definitive procedure and is not coded separately. This is consistent with the advice of general guideline B3.1b that explains that procedural steps necessary to reach the operative site and close the operative site are not coded separately.

PCS Guideline	
General guidelines	
B3.1b	Components of a procedure specified in the root operation definition and explanation are not coded separately. Procedural steps necessary to reach the operative site and close the operative site, including anastomosis of a tubular body part, are also not coded separately.
	Examples: Resection of a joint as part of a joint replacement procedure is included in the root operation definition of Replacement and is not coded separately.
	Laparotomy performed to reach the site of an open liver biopsy is not coded separately. In a resection of sigmoid colon with anastomosis of descending colon to rectum, the anastomosis is not coded separately.

Practical Application for Guideline B3.11a

Case Study 4.68. Percutaneous Endoscopic Gastrostomy (PEG) Tube Insertion

The gastrointestinal endoscope was introduced through the pharynx into the esophagus. The esophagus was normal to the level of the gastroesophageal junction. No significant ulcerations appreciated. The scope was advanced to the stomach where no gastritis was appreciated. The scope was retroflexed. No hiatal hernia was noted, no significant ulceration. The body of the stomach, cardia, and fundus were unremarkable. The antrum was within normal limits. The duodenum was intubated. The stomach was insufflated with the air channel on the endoscope.

Following this, the light was visualized on the anterior abdominal wall. The skin was anesthetized and appropriate entry location marked. A large gauge needle was used to enter the lumen of the stomach under visualization. After making a small incision, a dilator with break-away sheath was inserted over the guidewire until seen to enter the lumen of the stomach without difficulty. The wire was grasped with a snare and brought retrograde through the esophagus and through the mouth. The PEG tube was attached and brought back through the mouth and the esophagus to lie appropriately in the stomach. The endoscope was reintroduced. The lie of the bolster was appropriate and secured. Dry sterile dressing was applied.

Code(s):
ØDH63UZ   **Insertion of Feeding Device into Stomach, Percutaneous Approach**

Rationale:
A PEG tube is a means of supplying nutrition to the patient when oral intake is not possible or adequate. It consists of a tube that runs from the stomach to an external cutaneous opening in the abdominal wall where the nutritional substance is administered (see following illustration).

The endoscope is used as the guidance instrument needed to visualize the site of the insertion of the feeding tube and to assist in its placement. The objective of the procedure is not the inspection of the esophagus, even though it is visualized. This examination is done specifically to ensure the safe insertion of the feeding tube, which is brought though a percutaneous incision through the external abdominal wall into the stomach. This visualization or inspection is considered inherent to the Insertion (H) procedure and is not coded separately according to *AHA Coding Clinic,* 2013, 4Q, 117.

The endoscopic guidance component of the procedure uses an approach through the natural opening of the mouth; however, this approach was used only to assist with the procedure and is not the approach assigned for the definitive procedure. The definitive procedure is the insertion of the feeding tube, which is performed via a Percutaneous (3) approach through the abdominal wall. The tube was advanced into the Stomach (6), which is the body part value for the Insertion (H) root operation.

Root Operation		
Insertion (H)	Definition:	Putting in a nonbiological appliance that monitors, assists, performs, or prevents a physiological function but does not physically take the place of a body part
	Explanation:	None

The PCS index for PEG (percutaneous endoscopic gastrostomy) lists the full code ØDH63UZ. Although the index may be used to locate a table, the tables should always be consulted to find the appropriate code based on the objective of the procedure as documented in the operative report.

Figure 4.28. Percutaneous Endoscopic Gastrostomy (PEG) Tube Placement

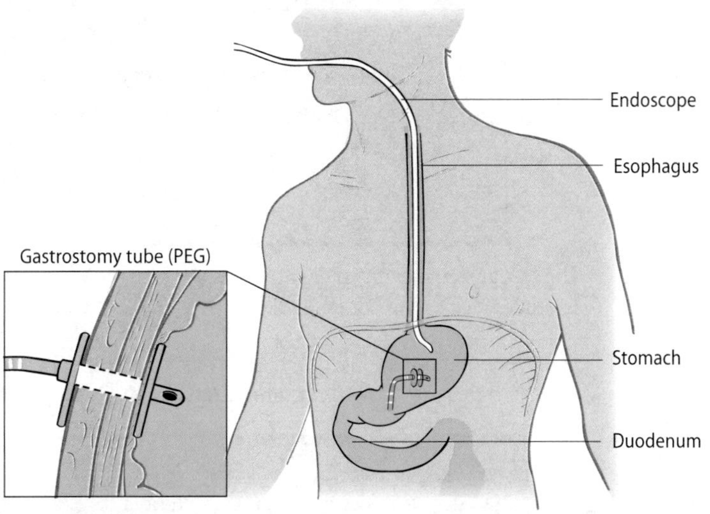

Case Study 4.69. ERCP with Removal of Known Stones

The scope was advanced into the esophagus to a normal major papilla in the descending duodenum without detailed examination of the upper GI tract. The bile duct was deeply cannulated with the short-nosed traction sphincterotome. Contrast was injected. The lower third of the main bile duct contained multiple stones. A 10 mm biliary sphincterotomy was made with a monofilament short-tip traction sphincterotome using ERBE electrocautery. There was no post-sphincterotomy bleeding. The common bile duct was swept with a balloon and all stones were removed. This was followed by placement of a stent to improve drainage.

Code(s):

ØFC98ZZ	**Extirpation of Matter from Common Bile Duct, Via Natural or Artificial Opening Endoscopic**
ØF798DZ	**Dilation of Common Bile Duct with Intraluminal Device, Via Natural or Artificial Opening Endoscopic**

Rationale:

Endoscopic retrograde cholangiopancreatography (ERCP) is a type of imaging used to diagnose conditions affecting the bile and pancreatic ducts. The same endoscopic imaging technique can also be used to visualize these ducts during the performance of therapeutic procedures, such as stone removal and stent insertion or removal. Because the intent of this procedure was for therapeutic intervention involving stone removal and stent placement, the ERCP is considered inherent to the procedure and is not coded as a separate root operation.

Spotlight
The root operation Inspection (J) is NOT used to report a diagnostic ERCP.
The alphabetic index under ERCP (endoscopic retrograde cholangiopancreatography) currently lists *see* Fluoroscopy, Hepatobiliary System and Pancreas BF1. An ERCP differs from other endoscopic procedures in that it uses a camera to send images to a monitor rather than just a scope that is used for direct visualization and is the reason for indexing ERCP to Fluoroscopy (F) in the Imaging (B) section instead of to Inspection (J) in the Medical and Surgical (Ø) section.

Because there are multiple root operations, each with distinct objectives, performed during this procedure on the same body part, two different codes must be reported according to Multiple procedures guideline B3.2c as shown in the following box.

PCS Guideline
Multiple procedures
B3.2   During the same operative episode, multiple procedures are coded if:
c. Multiple root operations with distinct objectives are performed on the same body part.
Example: Destruction of sigmoid lesion and bypass of sigmoid colon are coded separately.

The first objective of the procedure was removal of the stones, classified to root operation Extirpation (C) of the Common Bile Duct (9).

The intent of the stent insertion was to dilate the tubular body part. This second objective fits root operation Dilation (7) of the Common Bile Duct (9) with the use of an Intraluminal Device (D).

Root Operation		
Extirpation (C)	Definition:	Taking or cutting out solid matter from a body part
	Explanation:	The solid matter may be an abnormal byproduct of a biological function or a foreign body; it may be imbedded in a body part or in the lumen of a tubular body part. The solid matter may or may not have been previously broken into pieces.
Dilation (7)	Definition:	Expanding an orifice or the lumen of a tubular body part
	Explanation:	The orifice can be a natural orifice or an artificially created orifice. Accomplished by stretching a tubular body part using intraluminal pressure or by cutting part of the orifice or wall of the tubular body part.

Although not reported as a separate code, the ERCP was used as an instrument to facilitate the objective of Extirpation (C) of stones and Dilation (7) of the duct, captured in both procedures by the approach value Via Natural or Artificial Opening Endoscopic (8). Both of the procedures performed in the Common Bile Duct (9) body part are found in the Hepatobiliary System and Pancreas (F) body system.

Guideline B3.11b

B3.11b   If multiple tubular body parts are inspected, the most distal body part (the body part furthest from the starting point of the inspection) is coded. If multiple non-tubular body parts in a region are inspected, the body part that specifies the entire area inspected is coded.
Examples: **Cystoureteroscopy with inspection of bladder and ureters is coded to the ureter body part value.**
Exploratory laparotomy with general inspection of abdominal contents is coded to the peritoneal cavity body part value.

AHA Coding Clinic

2016, 2Q, 20   Capsule Endoscopy of Small Intestine

2015, 4Q, 16   Changes to the ICD-10-PCS Official Guidelines for Coding and Reporting

Tubular body parts transport solids, liquids, and gases throughout the body. They include the cardiovascular system and body parts such as those contained in the gastrointestinal tract, genitourinary tract, biliary tract, and respiratory tract.

An inspection of tubular body parts often includes examination of various body parts on the route to a distal point. As this guideline explains, rather than listing each individual site, only the most distal point needs to be coded. While the term **distal** in medical terms generally means the furthest point away from the body center, the term **distal** in this guideline refers to the furthest point reached from the insertion of the inspection instrument or the deepest location obtained from the starting point of the exam.

The body part value can often be easily determined due to the limited body part values offered in the root operation Inspection (J) tables in comparison to other root operation tables within each body system. For example, in the Respiratory (B) body system, for an inspection of the upper, middle, and lower bronchus, the only option is the Tracheobronchial Tree (Ø) rather than the more specific bronchial lobes. A colonoscopy in the Gastrointestinal (D) body system, performed only to the sigmoid colon, is reported with Lower Intestinal Tract (D) because no specific body part values such as sigmoid colon are available in that Inspection (J) table. Guideline B3.11b also clarifies that inspections of multiple non-tubular body parts can be grouped together when there is an all-inclusive body part value available that encompasses multiple, specific body part values. Some examples of larger non-tubular body part values that encompass several smaller individual body parts include Cranial Cavity (1), Pelvic Cavity (J), Peritoneal Cavity (G), and Oral Cavity and Throat (3), which can be found in the Anatomical Regions, General (W) body system.

Practical Application for Guideline B3.11b

Case Study 4.70. Bronchoscopy through Tracheostomy

Flexible bronchoscopy was performed with a 2.8 mm bronchoscope through the tracheostomy. The trachea, left mainstem bronchus, left upper lobe bronchus, lingula bronchus, and left lower lobe bronchus were widely patent and in normal anatomic position. The right mainstem bronchus, right upper lobe, right middle lobe, and right lower lobe were also in a normal position and clear of mucus.

Code(s):
ØBJØ8ZZ   Inspection of Tracheobronchial Tree, Via Natural or Artificial Opening Endoscopic

Rationale:
Bronchoscopy uses a slender optical instrument called a bronchoscope that is inserted into the nose, mouth, or a tracheal stoma. This approach value is Via Natural or Artificial Opening Endoscopic (8). Although multiple individual parts of the Respiratory System (B) were examined, it is only necessary to report one code. The root operation Inspection (J) was performed on the trachea, mainstem bronchi bilaterally, and the more distal portions of the bronchi in all lung lobes bilaterally. Even though individual bronchial body part values are available in other root operation tables, only the Tracheobronchial Tree (Ø) body part value is available in the Inspection (J) root operation table and this single body part value encompasses all of the body parts that were inspected during this procedure. The term Bronchoscopy in the alphabetic index gives the complete correct code ØBJØ8ZZ.

Figure 4.29. Tracheobronchial Tree

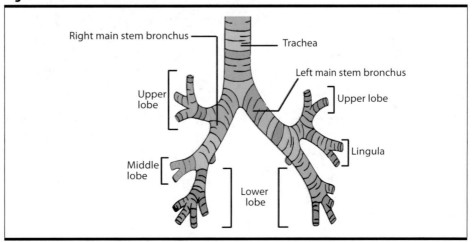

Case Study 4.71. Colposcopy and Hysteroscopy

Procedure: Colposcopy examination with diagnostic hysteroscopy.

The cervix, including the upper adjacent portion of the vagina, was examined through a colposcope. A speculum was inserted into the vagina to fully expose the cervix. The colposcope was withdrawn and exchanged for a hysteroscope, which was advanced through the vagina and into the cervical os to the uterine cavity. The uterine cavity was inspected with the fiberoptic scope for abnormalities.

Code(s):

ØUJD8ZZ   Inspection of Uterus and Cervix, Via Natural or Artificial Opening Endoscopic

Rationale:

Even though the colposcopy typically examines the vulva and vagina as well as the cervix, and the hysteroscopy examines the uterus, only Inspection (J) of the Uterus and Cervix (D) body part is reported because the uterus was the most distal body part inspected. The instruments used for visualization were inserted through the vagina for an approach of Via Natural or Artificial Opening Endoscopic (8). Since the term inspection indicates that the procedure is diagnostic, it is redundant to include a separate qualifier for Diagnostic (X) for the root operation Inspection (J); therefore, only No Qualifier (Z) is available.

Definitions
colposcopy. Procedure in which the physician views the cervix and vagina through a colposcope, a binocular microscope used for direct visualization of the vagina, ectocervix, and endocervix.
hysteroscopy. Visualization and inspection of the uterus using a fiberoptic endoscope inserted through the vagina and cervical os into the uterine cavity. This procedure may be performed for diagnostic purposes only or included with therapeutic procedures performed at the same time.

Figure 4.30. Colposcopy

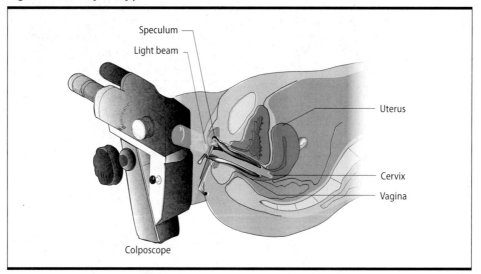

Figure 4.31. Hysteroscopy

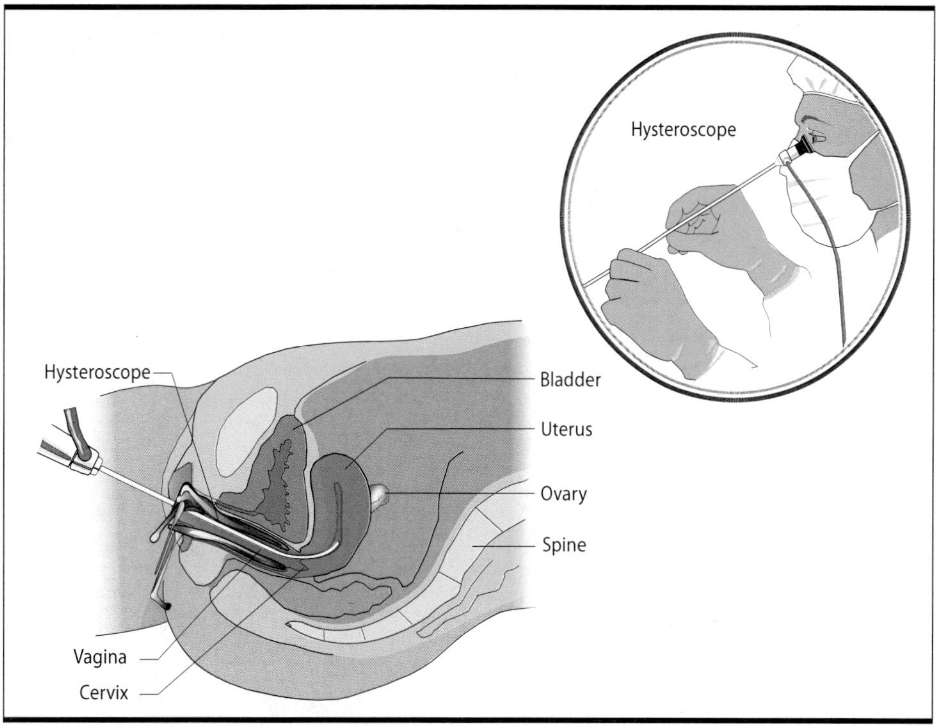

Case Study 4.72. Exploratory Laparotomy for Cancer Staging

With the patient supine and under endotracheal anesthesia, the entire abdomen and lower chest were prepped with pHisoHex and saline and draped with sterile sheets in the usual manner. Through an upper midline incision, the peritoneal cavity was entered. Exploration revealed a huge mass posterior to the seventh rib, which was penetrating the stomach. This mass measured about 7 inches in diameter. It was fixed in the omentum and to part of the colon. It also ascended into the liver, and there were multiple liver metastases and multiple peritoneal metastases. Through the gastrohepatic ligament, the mass was further exposed. The patient was inoperable with metastatic carcinomatosis.

Code(s):
ØWJGØZZ   Inspection of Peritoneal Cavity, Open Approach

Rationale:
Terminology that can indicate an Inspection (J) procedure was performed includes words such as exploratory or diagnostic examination. A laparotomy is an Open (Ø) incision into the abdominal wall to gain access to the abdominal or peritoneal cavity. The peritoneum, omentum, and organs were inspected for extent of the malignancy. The body part Peritoneal Cavity (G), located in the Anatomical Regions, General (W) body system, is the only code needed because it is the whole body part, which includes the peritoneum and all of the contents contained within. The only qualifier choice for Inspection (J) is No Qualifier (Z) as the root operation Inspection (J) already implies a diagnostic procedure.

Definitions
peritoneal cavity. Potential space within the peritoneum membranes that includes the peritoneum plus all of the organs contained within, such as the stomach, liver, gallbladder, pancreas, spleen, and most of the intestines.
peritoneum. Serous membrane of the abdominal and pelvic cavity that includes the mesothelium and connective tissue that lines the walls and covers the viscera of the contents of the abdominal cavity. Includes the greater and lesser omentum, mesentery, mesocolon, and falciform ligament.

Guideline B3.11c

> **B3.11c** **When both an Inspection procedure and another procedure are performed on the same body part during the same episode, if the Inspection procedure is performed using a different approach than the other procedure, the Inspection procedure is coded separately.**
>
> *Example:* Endoscopic Inspection of the duodenum is coded separately when open excision of the duodenum is performed during the same procedural episode.

AHA Coding Clinic

2017, 2Q, 15	Low Anterior Resection with Sigmoidoscopy
2015, 3Q, 24	Esophagogastroduodenoscopy with Epinephrine Injection for Control of Bleeding
2015, 2Q, 27	Thoracoscopic Talc Pleurodesis
2015, 1Q, 33	Robotic-Assisted Laparoscopic Hysterectomy Converted to Open Procedure
2014, 1Q, 20	Fiducial Marker Placement
2013, 2Q, 36	Insertion of Ventriculoperitoneal Shunt with Laparoscopic Assistance

The differentiating condition in this guideline is the use of different approaches. When different approaches are used, the Inspection procedure is no longer considered inherent and needs to be coded separately.

Practical Application for Guideline B3.11c

Case Study 4.73. Sleeve Gastrectomy with EGD

The patient was draped and prepped in the normal sterile manner. The abdomen was entered using a 5-mm optical trocar 15 cm inferior to the xiphoid. A 5-mm left-sided port, a 5-mm right-sided port, and a 5- and 15-mm port were placed in the right upper midline. The pylorus was identified and transected to the greater curve mesentery about 4 to 5 cm from the pylorus, completely mobilizing the greater curve. The greater curve was longitudinally transected all the way along the mesentery and the greater curve border using a LigaSure device, completely mobilizing the fundus. Once the greater curvature and the fundus were mobilized in their entirety, the antrum of the stomach was partially transected 5 cm from the pylorus using a black buttressed Tri Staple stapling device and a 36-French bougie was inserted. The bougie was used as a template to longitudinally transect the stomach along the lesser curve using the 36-French bougie as a stylet using purple buttressed Tri Staple stapling devices. Once finished, an EGD was performed to check the duodenum; no obvious leaks or complications were found. Once it was noted that there were no obvious air leaks and nice patent anastomosis, the stomach was removed from the 15-mm port site and closed using a #1 Prolene suture. The skin was closed using 4-0 Monocryl and Dermabond skin glue.

Code(s):

ØDB64Z3	**Excision of Stomach, Percutaneous Endoscopic Approach, Vertical**
ØDJ08ZZ	**Inspection of Upper Intestinal Tract, Via Natural or Artificial Opening Endoscopic**

Rationale:
Two codes are required to capture the procedures performed. Both codes are located in the Gastrointestinal (D) body system tables.

Sleeve gastrectomy, also referred to as vertical gastrectomy, is the partial removal of the greater curvature of the stomach, after which the remnant looks like a tube or sleeve as shown in the following illustration. This procedure is performed to reduce stomach volume for morbidly obese patients. Since only part of the Stomach (6) was removed, the appropriate root operation is Excision (B). The qualifier Vertical (3), in the Excision (B) table, identifies this type of stomach excision. The excision of the stomach was performed by laparoscopy, which is considered a Percutaneous Endoscopic (4) approach.

Root Operation		
Excision (B)	Definition:	Cutting out or off, without replacement, a portion of a body part
	Explanation:	The qualifier DIAGNOSTIC is used to identify excision procedures that are biopsies

Because the excisional portion of the procedure was done via a different approach than the postprocedural inspection, the root operation Inspection (J) is coded separately. The inspection was performed with an EGD (esophagogastroduodenoscopy), which involves insertion of an endoscope through the mouth and advancement into the duodenum. This approach is classified as Via Natural or Artificial Opening Endoscopic (8). The Upper Intestinal Tract (Ø) body part value includes inspection through the duodenum, the most distal point examined. The difference between coding the use of the esophagogastroduodenoscopy in this procedure as compared to the PEG tube insertion is that in this procedure the EGD was not used to actually guide or perform the excision as in the PEG insertion, but rather had a separate objective of Inspection of the body part.

Figure 4.32. Sleeve Gastrectomy

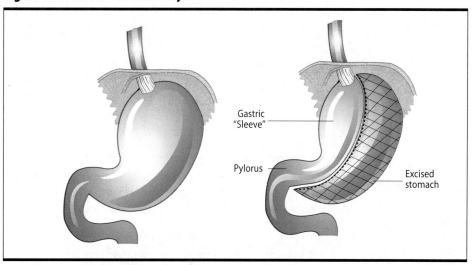

Gastric "Sleeve"

Pylorus

Excised stomach

Case Study 4.74. Arthroscopy with Knee Derangement Repair

Arthroscopic examination of the medial and lateral meniscus, tendons, bursa, ligaments, cartilage, and patella of the right knee was performed. All structures were normal with the exception of the patellar tendon, which was noted to be completely detached from the patella. The arthroscope was withdrawn and an incision was made followed by open repair of detached patellar tendon. Sutures were placed in the patellar tendon and threaded through drill holes in the kneecap. The sutures were tied at the top of the kneecap resulting in excellent reduction of the tendon to the patella.

Code(s):

ØLMQØZZ   **Reattachment of Right Knee Tendon, Open Approach**

ØSJC4ZZ   **Inspection of Right Knee Joint, Percutaneous Endoscopic Approach**

Rationale:

Two codes are needed to capture the different objectives performed in this example. A diagnostic arthroscopy was performed that identified the source of the problem within the knee, followed by Reattachment (M) of the patellar tendon. Since the Inspection (J) was performed using a Percutaneous Endoscopic (4) approach and Reattachment (M) was done via an Open (Ø) approach, guideline B3.11c states that the Inspection (J) is to be coded separately.

Multiple overlapping body layers were inspected, but only the Inspection (J) of the Knee Joint, Right (C) found in the Lower Joints (S) body system is coded as per the following guideline B3.5.

PCS Guideline
Overlapping body layers
B3.5   If the root operations Excision, Repair or Inspection are performed on overlapping layers of the musculoskeletal system, the body part specifying the deepest layer is coded.
Example: Excisional debridement that includes skin and subcutaneous tissue and muscle is coded to the muscle body part.

Note that guideline B3.5 only refers to procedures on the overlapping layers of the musculoskeletal system. In contrast, guideline B3.11b provides instruction regarding tubular and other non-musculoskeletal, non-tubular body parts. For instance, a diagnostic laparoscopy of multiple abdominal body parts (non-tubular) is not reported using each individual body part, or the deepest one; rather, a code from the Anatomical Regions, General (W), such as Peritoneal Cavity (G), is used to represent all of the body parts. An inspection on tubular body parts, such as the bladder and ureter, is coded to ureter to represent the most distal body part inspected.

Repairing the tendon is best captured by root operation Reattachment (M) since the sutures placed return the patellar tendon back to its normal location.

Root Operation		
Reattachment (M)	Definition:	Putting back in or on all or a portion of a separated body part to its normal location or other suitable location
	Explanation:	Vascular circulation and nervous pathways may or may not be reestablished

The Body Part Key (appendix D) lists Knee Tendon, Right (C) to be used for the anatomical term right patellar tendon. This body part value can be found in the Tendons (L) body system. An Open (Ø) approach was used; No Device (Z) and No Qualifier (Z) are the correct sixth and seventh characters, respectively.

Figure 4.33. Suture Reattachment of Patellar Tendon

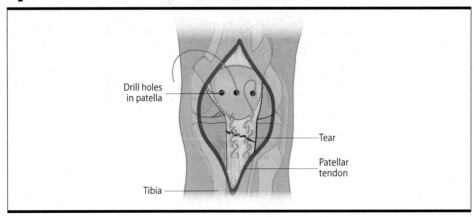

Case Study 4.75. Diagnostic Laparoscopy with Adhesiolysis

Indication: Intractable nausea and vomiting secondary to suspected bowel obstruction.

Procedures Performed:

1. Diagnostic laparoscopy

2. Exploratory laparotomy with extensive adhesiolysis

The patient was taken to the operating room and placed in a supine position. After anesthesia was administered, the patient's abdomen was prepped and draped in the usual sterile fashion. A Hasson trocar was inserted and secured with 0 Vicryl suture. The camera was inserted and the large bowel was visualized. Moving closer to the small bowel, multiple adhesions were noted, which appeared to obstruct the proximal jejunum. There was a particular area that was encased in a thick rind or membrane. It was evident upon entrance that this portion of the small bowel could not be accessed due to the amount of adhesions. The Hasson trocar was removed and the pneumoperitoneum decompressed. The incision was extended superiorly and inferiorly. The focus was to free the obstruction, which was noted on inspection of the small bowel and appeared to be in the proximal jejunum. The segments of the intestine were mobilized and the adhesions lysed, freeing up what appeared to be a chronic obstruction. The entire small bowel was mobilized on the left side of the abdomen, which was where the obstructions were noted. There was a portion of small bowel in the pelvis that was adhesed and unable to be safely mobilized. There did not appear to be any sign of obstructive process in this area. There did not appear to be any other remaining obstructive process. The lap and instrument counts were correct x2 at this juncture. The fascial defect was closed with running number 1 looped PDS suture. The skin was closed loosely with staples. Adaptic was placed over the incision, and VAC sponge was wound onto the Adaptic. An adhesive dressing was placed over the VAC sponge, followed by suction tubing. The VAC motor was then attached and there was no sign of leak noted. The patient tolerated the procedure well, was sent to the recovery room in stable but guarded condition. Plans were made for the patient to be extubated and eventually sent to the intensive care unit.

Code(s):

ØDNAØZZ	Release Jejunum, Open Approach
ØDJD4ZZ	Inspection of Lower Intestinal Tract, Percutaneous Endoscopic Approach

Rationale:

Two procedure codes are essential for describing this scenario since both procedures had specific objectives and were carried out with different approaches. The Inspection (J) was performed to locate and diagnose the obstruction. Because only specific body parts, the large intestine and jejunum, were evaluated during the laparoscopic portion of this procedure, the Inspection (J) table in the Gastrointestinal (D) body system was chosen. This is more appropriate than the Anatomical Regions, General (W) inspection table because not all organs or body parts within the peritoneal cavity were visualized.

The body part values for Inspection (J) in the Gastrointestinal (D) body system do not include specific values for all of the anatomical parts of the intestine, only upper or lower intestinal tract. Guideline B4.8 explains that the Lower Intestinal Tract (D) body part value includes the portion of the gastrointestinal tract from the jejunum down to and including the rectum and anus.

PCS Guideline
Upper and lower intestinal tracts
B4.8   In the Gastrointestinal body system, the general body part values Upper Intestinal Tract and Lower Intestinal Tract are provided as an option for the root operations Change, Inspection, Removal and Revision. Upper Intestinal Tract includes the portion of the gastrointestinal tract from the esophagus down to and including the duodenum, and Lower Intestinal Tract includes the portion of the gastrointestinal tract from the jejunum down to and including the rectum and anus.   *Example:* In the root operation Change table, change of a device in the jejunum is coded using the body part Lower Intestinal Tract.

Use of the trocars and camera indicate that the Inspection (J) was done laparoscopically, which is a Percutaneous Endoscopic (4) approach.

The adhesions were found to be the cause of the obstruction, thus it was necessary to free the Jejunum (A) from the adhesions, described with root operation Release (N). The Jejunum (A) is the appropriate body part used based on guideline B3.13.

PCS Guideline
Release procedures
B3.13   In the root operation Release, the body part value coded is the body part being freed and not the tissue being manipulated or cut to free the body part.   *Example:* Lysis of intestinal adhesions is coded to the specific intestine body part value.

Root Operation		
Release (N)	Definition:	Freeing a body part from an abnormal physical constraint by cutting or by use of force
	Explanation:	Some of the restraining tissue may be taken out but none of the body part is taken out

Although the original intent was to release the jejunum via the laparoscope, the extensive adhesions made it necessary to abandon this approach (percutaneous endoscopic) and instead reach and release the obstruction via an Open (Ø) approach.

Occlusion Versus Restriction for Vessel Embolization Procedures

Guideline B3.12

> **B3.12   If the objective of an embolization procedure is to completely close a vessel, the root operation Occlusion is coded. If the objective of an embolization procedure is to narrow the lumen of a vessel, the root operation Restriction is coded.**
>
> *Examples:* **Tumor embolization is coded to the root operation Occlusion, because the objective of the procedure is to cut off the blood supply to the vessel.**
>
> **Embolization of a cerebral aneurysm is coded to the root operation Restriction, because the objective of the procedure is not to close off the vessel entirely, but to narrow the lumen of the vessel at the site of the aneurysm where it is abnormally wide.**

AHA Coding Clinic

2017, 4Q, 31   Resuscitative Endovascular Balloon Occlusion of the Aorta

2017, 4Q, 34   Occlusion/Ligation of Pulmonary Trunk & Right Pulmonary Artery

2016, 2Q, 26   Embolization of Pulmonary Arteriovenous Fistula

2015, 2Q, 27   Uterine Artery Embolization Using Gelfoam

2014, 3Q, 26   Coil Embolization of Gastroduodenal Artery with Chemoembolization of Hepatic Artery

2014, 1Q, 24   Endovascular Embolization for Gastrointestinal Bleeding

Definition
embolization. Development or forming of a clot or embolus by natural or artificial means.

When the PCS alphabetic index is consulted for Embolization, it instructs *see* Occlusion and *see* Restriction. The purpose of this guideline is to further explain the difference between the intent of the root operation Restriction (V) in contrast with root operation Occlusion (L) as it relates to embolization procedures. In an embolization procedure, substances or synthetic materials called embolic agents are instilled with a catheter to form a blockage or clot within the tubular body part. Catheter embolization is a minimally invasive procedure that is often performed to:

- Reduce or cut off blood supply to tumors or fibroids
- Eliminate abnormal growths, such as arteriovenous malformations (AVM) or fistulas (AVF)
- Stop internal bleeding, as in the gastrointestinal tract or liver
- Treat aneurysms to avoid rupture by partially or totally occluding the weak bulge within the artery wall

Root Operation		
Occlusion (L)	Definition:	Completely closing an orifice or lumen of a tubular body part
	Explanation:	The orifice can be a natural orifice or an artificially created orifice
Restriction (V)	Definition:	Partially closing an orifice or the lumen of a tubular body part
	Explanation:	The orifice can be a natural orifice or an artificially created orifice

Restriction (V) procedures involve narrowing the diameter of a tubular body part, but not closing it completely. The restriction process may involve intraluminal (from within the tubular body part) or extraluminal (from outside the tubular body part) methods. Occlusion (L) procedures involve completely closing off a tubular body part or orifice. Tubular body parts transport solids, liquids, and gases throughout the body and include blood vessels, intestines, bronchus, fallopian tubes, bile ducts, and ureters. The similarities between Restriction (V) and Occlusion (L) include the fact that they are only performed on tubular body parts and that intraluminal and extraluminal methods may be used to accomplish the objective.

Spotlight
Embolic agents are represented by the device character Intraluminal Device (D) and include plastic or gelatin particles such as microspheres or beads, liquid agents such as cyanoacrylates (glue), Ethylene Vinyl Alcohol Copolymer (Onyx), Sclerosant, or Ethiodol (inert oil based). Also included in this device category are small soft metal coils, plugs (e.g., Amplatzer), and powder or sponge Gelfoam. Although not considered an embolization, stents such as the Pipeline™ device (braided, cylindrical mesh) are also considered intraluminal devices that can be used to partially (restrict) or fully occlude the flow of contents within a tubular body part.

Practical Application for Guideline B3.12

Case Study 4.76. Embolization, Cerebral Arteriovenous Malformation (AVM)
A small incision was made over the femoral artery and a catheter was inserted into the vessel and manipulated using fluoroscopic guidance through the vascular system to the cerebral AVM site. A HydroCoil 14 was threaded through the catheter and into the AVM. The coil continued to be introduced into the defect until the entire defect was filled and confirmed under fluoroscopy. Acrylic glue was injected into the smaller feeding branch. An injection of contrast was applied and it was ensured that the coiling was successful in blocking the blood flow to the AVM entirely, thereby closing the hemorrhage site. The catheter was removed.

Code(s):

Ø3LG3DZ   **Occlusion of Intracranial Artery with Intraluminal Device, Percutaneous Approach**

Rationale:
A brain arteriovenous malformation (AVM), as shown in the following illustration, is an abnormal connection between the arteries and veins in the brain that usually forms before birth. This defect disrupts the normal vascular process since blood flows directly from the arteries to veins without passing through the capillaries. Over time, the abnormal blood vessels may weaken and bleeding in the brain may occur if the vessels rupture. An arteriovenous malformation can develop anywhere in the body but is most often found in the brain or spine. Although the cause of AVMs is unclear, most people are born with them. Once diagnosed, an AVM can usually be treated in order to prevent complications.

To eliminate the AVM, coils and glue were used together as the Intraluminal Device (D) to completely close off the abnormal blood supply in the feeding intracranial artery to the AVM rather than just to restrict the flow. Since the objective was to completely stop the flow, Occlusion (L) is the appropriate root operation. The only information provided for the body part treated was the cerebral artery, which is captured by the body part Intracranial Artery (G) in the Upper Arteries (3) body system. The coils and glue were instilled with a catheter, which is considered a Percutaneous (3) approach. Even though both coils and glue were instilled, only one code is necessary because the same root operation (objective) was performed on the same body part with the same device character and approach.

Figure 4.34. Ateriovenous Malformation (AVM)

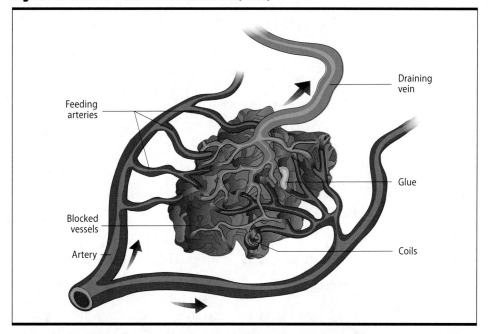

Case Study 4.77. Embolization, Tumor

A liver cancer patient, with a tumor too large for surgery, underwent embolization of the feeding branch of the hepatic artery with polymer beads. A catheter was inserted into the femoral vein and advanced to the hepatic artery proper, the branch of the hepatic artery that is feeding the tumor. Polymer beads were instilled through the catheter into the branch shutting off the blood supply to the tumor.

Code(s):

Ø4L33DZ   Occlusion of Hepatic Artery with Intraluminal Device, Percutaneous Approach

Rationale:

In this procedure, a catheter was passed through the femoral artery into the hepatic artery branch, which was feeding the tumor. The small particles or beads, which are coded as Intraluminal Device (D), were injected through the catheter and plugged the branch, completely cutting off the blood supply to the tumor in hopes of shrinking or killing it. Occlusion (L) is the appropriate root operation with a Percutaneous (3) approach. The body part being occluded was a branch of the left hepatic artery, which based on guideline B4.2 codes to the Hepatic Artery (3), found in the Lower Arteries (4) body system.

PCS Guideline
Branches of body parts
B4.2   Where a specific branch of a body part does not have its own body part value in PCS, the body part is typically coded to the closest proximal branch that has a specific body part value. In the cardiovascular body systems, if a general body part is available in the correct root operation table, and coding to a proximal branch would require assigning a code in a different body system, the procedure is coded using the general body part value.
Examples: A procedure performed on the mandibular branch of the trigeminal nerve is coded to the trigeminal nerve body part value.
Occlusion of the bronchial artery is coded to the body part value Upper Artery in the body system Upper Arteries, and not to the body part value Thoracic Aorta, Descending in the body system Heart and Great Vessels.

Case Study 4.78. Embolization, Intrauterine

Procedure: Intrauterine embolization for uterine fibroids.

A catheter was inserted in the right internal iliac artery. Small pledgets of Gelfoam and microspheres were inserted into a syringe and injected through the catheter into the right uterine artery.

Code(s):

Ø4LE3DT   **Occlusion of Right Uterine Artery with Intraluminal Device, Percutaneous Approach**

Rationale:

The root operation Occlusion (L) is correct because the objective of the procedure was to completely block the blood supply to the uterine fibroids by obstructing the feeding uterine artery with Gelfoam and microspheres, which are coded as Intraluminal Device (D). Because there is no body part for uterine artery included in the body part character values, the Body Part Key in appendix D was consulted. The Body Part Key indicates that the uterine artery is included in the values for Internal Iliac Artery, Left or Right. The occlusion was performed on the right uterine artery so the correct body part is Internal Iliac Artery, Right (E). In table Ø4L a seventh-character qualifier is available for Uterine Artery, Right (T) to more specifically identify the artery in which the occlusion procedure was performed. This qualifier value is found in the row containing the body part Internal Iliac Artery, Right (E). Note that a separate row is available for body part Internal Iliac Artery, Left (F) with a qualifier value for Uterine Artery, Left (U). All of these arteries are contained in the Lower Arteries (4) body system. Documentation indicates an approach using a catheter inserted into the artery, which is a Percutaneous (3) approach.

Case Study 4.79. Embolization, Aneurysm Coiling

A patient with a brain aneurysm was admitted for endovascular coiling. The physician inserted a catheter into the femoral artery and guided it to the site of the aneurysm in the left posterior cerebral artery. Next, the physician placed a Cerecyte® bioactive microcoil through the catheter into the aneurysm, which disrupted the flow of blood into the aneurysm and prevented rupture of the aneurysm.

Code(s):

Ø3VG3BZ   **Restriction of Intracranial Artery with Bioactive Intraluminal Device, Percutaneous Approach**

Rationale:

An aneurysm is formed by a weakened area in a vessel that protrudes and engorges with blood and may pose a risk of bursting. The objective of aneurysm coiling is to block blood flow to the aneurysm but keep the blood flowing through the vessel (see following illustration). Restriction (V) is the correct root operation for this procedure as the coils are wound into the bulging area until it is closed off, thereby allowing blood flow to the normal lumen only. The coils may be bare platinum or have a bioactive coating (hydrogel) made from bioabsorbable polymer, which induces an inflammatory response to promote faster filling and healing. Since the device values include Intraluminal Device, Bioactive (B) and a separate value for (nonbioactive) Intraluminal Device (D), it is important to discern whether the coils had a bioactive coating or were bare metal. Some terms that indicate the use of bioactive coils are Matrix, Cerecyte, and Nexus. This example specifically states bioactive microcoil. Therefore, the correct device value is Intraluminal Device, Bioactive (B).

According to the Body Part Key in appendix D, the posterior cerebral artery is included in the Intracranial Artery (G) body part value, which is located in the Upper Arteries (3) body system. Since the site was accessed via a catheter inserted into the femoral artery and guided up to the aneurysm, the approach is Percutaneous (3).

Figure 4.35. Aneurysm Embolization with Coils

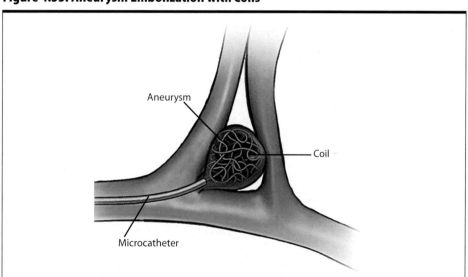

Spotlight
Aneurysms can be treated from outside of the vessel rather than with embolization and are also reported with Restriction (V). When a clip or other device is placed on the outside of the blood vessel, the appropriate device character is Extraluminal Device (C).

Beyond the Guidelines

Use of Restriction or Occlusion

The following case studies go beyond the embolization guideline and investigate other examples using Restriction (V) or Occlusion (L). These procedures partially or entirely prevent contents from flowing freely through tubular body parts using methods other than embolization of the lumen. These methods may use intraluminal devices (stents), extraluminal devices (clips), or they may not use a device (sutures, staples, cautery).

AHA Coding Clinic

2018, 2Q, 18	Transverse Rectus Abdominis Myocutaneous (TRAM) Delay
2018, 1Q, 10	Revision of Transjugular Intrahepatic Portosystemic Shunt
2018, 1Q, 23	Tubal Ligation Procedure
2017, 4Q, 31	Resuscitative Endovascular Balloon Occlusion of the Aorta
2017, 4Q, 36	Alfieri Stitch Procedure
2017, 4Q, 57	Transorifice Esophageal Vein Banding
2017, 3Q, 22	Laparoscopic Esophagomyotomy (Heller Type) and Toupet Fundoplication
2016, 4Q, 89-94	Branched and Fenestrated Endograft Repair of Aneurysms
2016, 2Q, 30	Clipping (Occlusion) of Cerebral Artery, Decompressive Craniectomy and Storage of Bone Flap in Abdominal Wall
2015, 3Q, 30	Insertion of Cervical Cerclage
2014, 3Q, 28	Laparoscopic Nissen Fundoplication and Diaphragmatic Hernia Repair
2014, 1Q, 9	Endovascular Repair of Abdominal Aortic Aneurysm
2013, 4Q, 112	Endoscopic Banding of Esophageal Varices

Case Study 4.80. Aneurysm Clipping

Under general anesthesia, small burr holes were made for the craniotome, a bone window was cut, and the flap removed. The brain was gently retracted to locate and isolate the arterial aneurysm. A small titanium clip was placed at the base of the bulge. The skull flap was replaced.

Code(s):

Ø3VGØCZ   Restriction of Intracranial Artery with Extraluminal Device, Open Approach

Rationale:

The small burr holes were made to allow for the use of the craniotome, which is a small saw used by the surgeon to connect the burr holes and cut out a bone flap. This bone flap was removed to visualize and reach the site of the aneurysm via Open (Ø) approach and was replaced at the end of the procedure. Replacement of the flap, when done during the same operative episode, is inherent in the closure and is not coded separately.

The aneurysm clips are placed on the external part of the vessel at the base of the bulge with the intention of narrowing the lumen and blocking the blood supply into the weakened bulge. This clip is considered an Extraluminal Device (C).

Figure 4.36. Aneurysm Clipping

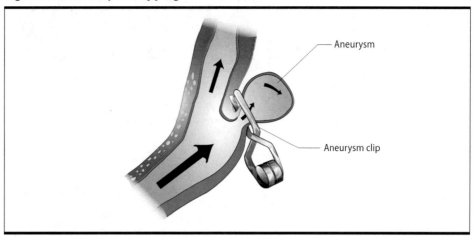

While the blood is restricted from the bulging area, it still flows freely though the vessel, which is the objective of root operation Restriction (V). The documentation stated that this vessel was located in the brain, thus the appropriate body part is Intracranial Artery (G) located in the Upper Arteries (3) body system.

Spotlight
• Burr holes into the skull can be used for open or percutaneous procedures. One or more burr holes can be used to make an opening large enough for a small saw to cut a bone flap for an open approach. A small burr hole can also be used as an insertion point for instrumentation used percutaneously. The operative report must be carefully read to determine the proper approach value.
• Bone flaps may not be immediately replaced; instead, the wound may be left open to allow for brain swelling. If the bone flap is placed into the patient's abdominal wall for storage, root operation Reposition (S) is reported for the placement. If the bone flap is kept frozen in a bone bank, it is considered integral and not coded separately (*AHA Coding Clinic,* 2016, 2Q, 29-30). If a separate operative encounter is performed for the sole purpose of replacing the bone flap, the following root operations are used:
- If the patient's own bone flap is used and stored in the abdominal wall, the appropriate root operation for removing it from the abdominal wall is Extirpation (C) and Reposition (S) with internal fixation device for replacement into the skull using titanium plates and screws (*AHA Coding Clinic,* 2017, 3Q, 22).
- If a synthetic plate (e.g., metal or plastic) is used to replace the skull, the root operation is Replacement (R) with the appropriate device character because a synthetic material is physically taking the place/function of the previously removed skull bone.
- If a partial plate is used in conjunction with the patient's own bone, the root operation is Supplement (U) because the partial plate is used to reinforce and/or augment the function of the skull.

Figure 4.37. Open Approach Using Burr Hole and Craniotome

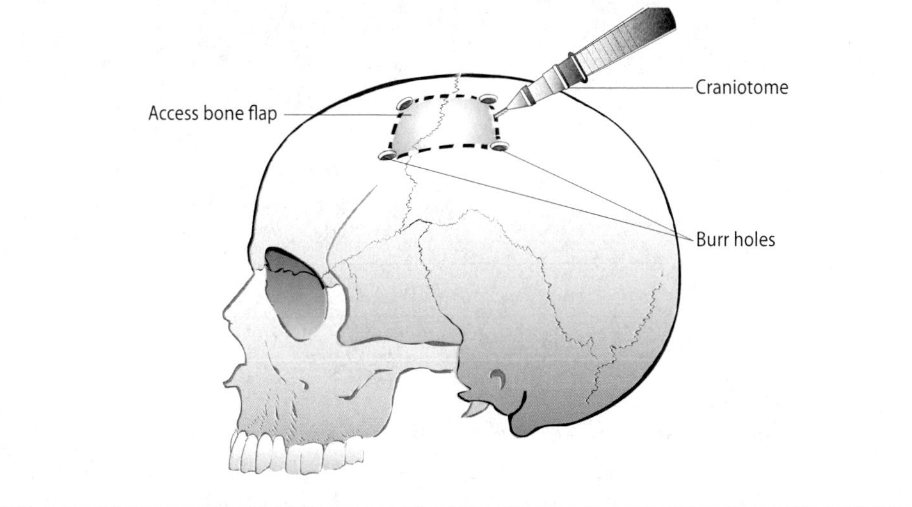

Case Study 4.81. Endovascular Repair of Abdominal Aortic Aneurysm

The patient was brought to the operating room with a known 4 cm infrarenal abdominal aortic aneurysm. With the patient in supine position under general anesthesia, the abdomen and lower extremities were prepped and draped in sterile fashion. Bilateral groin incisions were made and the patient was heparinized. Each component of the GORE ® EXCLUDER ® AAA fenestrated stent-graft was advanced through the access sheaths. The components were deployed, placement confirmed, and adequate sealing noted.

Code(s):

Ø4VØ3E6   **Restriction of Abdominal Aorta, Bifurcation, with Branched or Fenestrated Intraluminal Device, One or Two Arteries, Percutaneous Approach**

Rationale:

The device used to facilitate the restriction procedure in this example is the GORE® EXCLUDER® AAA Endoprosthesis. This device is comprised of two components: a main trunk that bifurcates into two legs, one short and one long (trunk-ipsilateral component), and the contralateral leg component, which resembles a typical stent device. The two components are inserted into the patient, one via the right sided femoral access the other via the left sided femoral access, and connected to each other inside the patient. The device is placed with the main trunk at the head of the aorta with the bifurcated legs, which act as landing zones, extended into the common iliac arteries, one in the right and one in the left. The device is expanded and angiography performed to ensure the device is stable and a proper seal obtained, with adequate blood flow through all sections of the device and no leaking outside of the device (endoleaks).

Repair of the infrarenal abdominal aorta, the part of the aorta directly under the renal arteries, is reported with Abdominal Aorta (Ø) body part included in the Lower Arteries (4) body system. The Artery and Vein Table in chapter 3 Body Systems is useful in determining the correct body system. The qualifier value Bifurcation (6) identifies that the procedure was performed to restrict the lumen of the abdominal aorta at the bifurcation. The device value Intraluminal Device, Branched or Fenestrated, One or Two Arteries (E), captures the fenestrated stent-graft. A Percutaneous (3) approach was used in this example; however, aortic aneurysm repairs with stent-grafts are also often performed using an Open (Ø) approach so care must be taken when reviewing the operative report to capture the correct approach character.

Although the landing zones may involve crossing anatomic boundaries into another body part, a code is not assigned for the landing zone even if it is in a different body part unless it is also treating another aneurysm at that site.

Definitions
fenestrated. Pierced or perforated with one or more openings to ensure that the blood flow is preserved from the side branch arteries into the main stented artery.

Root Operation		
Restriction (V)	Definition:	Partially closing an orifice or the lumen of a tubular body part
	Explanation:	The orifice can be a natural orifice or an artificially created orifice

Figure 4.38. Abdominal Aorta Stent Graft

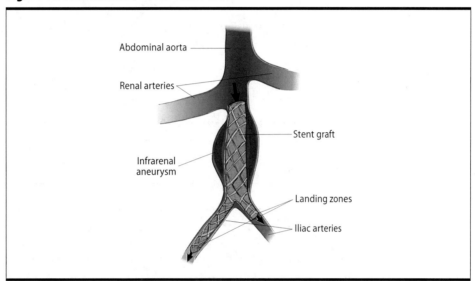

Case Study 4.82. Tubal Ligation
Procedure: Laparoscopic ligation of the right and left fallopian tubes with clips. Anesthesia was administered, infraumbilical and suprapubic 5 mm incisions made, and the abdomen insufflated. A 5 mm laparoscopic trocar and sleeve was inserted in the patient's abdominal cavity and the laparoscope used to visualize the pelvic organs. The patient was placed in the Trendelenburg position. A second 5 mm trocar and sleeve were placed through the suprapubic incision under direct visualization. At this time, using the laparoscope, clips were placed on the left and right fallopian tubes resulting in sterilization.

Code(s):
ØUL74CZ   **Occlusion of Bilateral Fallopian Tubes with Extraluminal Device, Percutaneous Endoscopic Approach**

Rationale:
According to the alphabetic index, the term Ligation directs the user to *see* Occlusion.

Root Operation		
Occlusion (L)	Definition:	Completely closing an orifice or the lumen of a tubular body part
	Explanation:	The orifice can be a natural orifice or an artificially created orifice

The left and right fallopian tubes are included in body part value Fallopian Tubes, Bilateral (7), located in the Female Reproductive System (U) body system. This follows the advice of guideline B4.3, which specifies that if a bilateral body part value exists, only one code is needed to capture the right and left body parts.

PCS Guideline
Bilateral body part values
B4.3   Bilateral body part values are available for a limited number of body parts. If the identical procedure is performed on contralateral body parts, and a bilateral body part value exists for that body part, a single procedure is coded using the bilateral body part value. If no bilateral body part value exists, each procedure is coded separately using the appropriate body part value. *Example:* The identical procedure performed on both fallopian tubes is coded once using the body part value Fallopian Tube, Bilateral. The identical procedure performed on both knee joints is coded twice using the body part values Knee Joint, Right and Knee Joint, Left.

A laparoscopic procedure is considered a Percutaneous Endoscopic (4) approach. The device is placed on the outside of the fallopian tubes, clamped shut, and held in place by spring clips and is reported with the device value Extraluminal Device (C).

Spotlight
When a ligation is followed by excision of the fallopian tube(s), root operation Excision (B) should be used.

Case Study 4.83. Cervical Cerclage

A pregnant patient presented at 14-weeks gestation for a cervical cerclage using the McDonald technique. The patient was taken to the operating room and epidural anesthesia administered. She was draped and prepped in the usual sterile fashion. A weighted speculum was placed in the posterior vaginal wall and the right-angle retractor used to visualize the cervix. The cervix was grasped by Allis forceps. Mersilk on a Mayo needle was used to insert a purse string suture high around the cervix opening and five more passes of the needle were performed until the opening was tight enough.

Code(s):
ØUVC7ZZ   **Restriction of Cervix, Via Natural or Artificial Opening**

Rationale:
A cervical cerclage is typically performed during weeks 12 to 16 to prevent premature labor. In the McDonald technique, a purse string suture is placed in the upper cervix to restrict the opening of the cervix. The PCS index for Cerclage directs the user to *see* Restriction. The sutures are being placed in the Cervix (C), which is found in the Female Reproductive System (U) body system. An approach of Via Natural or Artificial Opening (7) is used since the speculum is placed directly through the vaginal opening. No Device (Z) is appropriate as sutures are not considered a device based on guideline B6.1b.

PCS Guideline
General guidelines
B6.1b   Materials such as sutures, ligatures, radiological markers and temporary post-operative wound drains are considered integral to the performance of a procedure and are not coded as devices.

Case Study 4.84. Nissen Fundoplication

A patient with severe GERD undergoes a laparoscopic gastroesophageal fundoplication. The patient was prepped and draped after general anesthesia was administered. The abdomen was insufflated with CO_2 and the Optiview and other trocars placed in a standard fashion. The operation was begun by elevating the liver and placing it in a self-retaining retractor holder. The omentum was dissected off the greater curvature of the stomach from approximately the midbody of the stomach up to the peritoneal attachment at the angle of HIS to the left crus of the diaphragm. The lesser omentum was opened using a Harmonic scalpel. The right crus and the left crus of the diaphragm were identified and dissected from the apices to the base. The phrenicoesophageal ligament was divided using the Harmonic scalpel.

Once complete, circumferential mobilization of the gastroesophageal junction was accomplished. The mediastinal dissection was carried out using blunt dissection. Once adequate dissection was achieved, the closure was carried out using two interrupted 2-0 Surgidac sutures using the Endo Stitch device. Once this was completed, the fundoplication was carried out in standard fashion after placing the fundus through the retroesophageal window. There was good and easy passage of the fundus and it stayed in place without any tension. The fundoplication was carried out in standard fashion using two interrupted 2-0 Surgidac sutures to create the fundoplication. Both sutures incorporated a small bite of the esophageal muscular wall.

Once this was completed, hemostasis was assured and the skin incisions were closed.

Code(s):

ØDV44ZZ   Restriction of Esophagogastric Junction, Percutaneous Endoscopic Approach

Rationale:

During this procedure, the fundus (curved part) of the stomach was wrapped around the lower esophagus, tightening and strengthening the esophageal sphincter to help prevent acid reflux. The root operation Restriction (V) best describes this objective. The body part that was tightened or restricted was the Esophagogastric Junction (4), located in the Gastrointestinal (D) body system. Insertion of the Optiview and other trocars indicate that this was a laparoscopic or Percutaneous Endoscopic (4) approach. There are No Devices (Z) and No Qualifiers (Z) used in this procedure.

Figure 4.39. Nissen Fundoplication

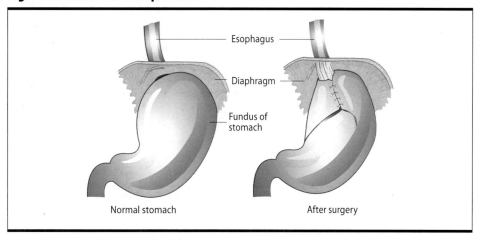

Esophagus

Diaphragm

Fundus of stomach

Normal stomach   After surgery

Release Procedures

Guideline B3.13

> **B3.13** **In the root operation Release, the body part value coded is the body part being freed and not the tissue being manipulated or cut to free the body part.**
>
> *Example:* **Lysis of intestinal adhesions is coded to the specific intestine body part value.**

AHA Coding Clinic

2018, 2Q, 22	Excision of Synovial Cyst
2017, 4Q, 35	Release of Myocardial Bridge
2017, 3Q, 10	Repair of Chiari Malformation
2017, 2Q, 23	Decompression of Spinal Cord and Placement of Instrumentation
2017, 1Q, 35	Lysis of Omental and Peritoneal Adhesions
2016, 3Q, 32	Rotator Cuff Repair, Tenodesis, Decompression, Acromioplasty and Coracoplasty
2016, 2Q, 16	Decompressive Laminectomy/Foraminotomy and Lumbar Discectomy
2016, 2Q, 17	Removal of Longitudinal Ligament to Decompress Cervical Nerve Root
2016, 2Q, 23	Thoracic Outlet Syndrome and Release of Brachial Plexus
2016, 2Q, 29	Decompressive Craniectomy with Cryopreservation and Storage of Bone Flap
2015, 3Q, 15	Vascular Ring Surgery with Release of Esophagus and Trachea
2015, 3Q, 16	Vascular Ring Surgery and Double Aortic Arch
2015, 2Q, 18	Cervical Laminoplasty
2015, 2Q, 19	Multiple Decompressive Cervical Laminectomies
2015, 2Q, 20	Arthroscopic Release of Shoulder Joint
2015, 2Q, 20	Arthroscopic Subacromial Decompression
2015, 2Q, 22	Penetrating Keratoplasty and Anterior Segment Reconstruction
2015, 2Q, 30	Decompressive Laminectomy
2014, 4Q, 39	Abdominal Component Release with Placement of Mesh for Hernia Repair
2014, 3Q, 33	Radial Fracture Treatment with Open Reduction Internal Fixation, and Release of Carpal Ligament
2014, 1Q, 3-6	Lysis of Adhesions

Root Operation		
Release (N)	Definition:	Freeing a body part from an abnormal physical constraint by cutting or by use of force
	Explanation:	Some of the restraining tissue may be taken out but none of the body part is taken out

The root operation Release (N) is coded when a procedure is performed with the objective of freeing a body part from abnormal restraints created by another body part. Some diagnostic terms that may indicate an abnormal constraint include adhesions, synechiae, or contracture. Additionally, surgical terms that might indicate a release include procedures with the suffix -lysis or -otomy. Guideline B3.13 defines the body part value to be used when coding Release (N) specifically as the body part that is being freed, not the body part being cut and/or manipulated during the procedure. Common release procedures include carpal tunnel release, adhesiolysis, excision of contracture, frenulotomy for treatment of tongue-tie syndrome, tendon release, and freeing of abdominal adhesions.

Spotlight
A Release (N) root operation procedure may include cutting into the surrounding tissues and attachments.

Practical Application for Guideline B3.13

Case Study 4.85. Carpal Tunnel Release

After adequate anesthesia was obtained, the patient's right arm was prepped and draped in the usual sterile fashion. An incision was made from the level of the distal palmar crease and in line with the flexion crease. It was carried down to the subcutaneous tissue. The transverse carpal ligament was identified and incised. A hemostat was placed on the ulnar side of the carpal canal. The transverse carpal ligament was lysed from proximal to distal. The forearm fascia was split proximally. The median nerve was neurolysed in its entirety. The floor of the carpal canal was inspected and noted to be free of osteophytes and tumors. The wound was irrigated out and was infiltrated with Marcaine. The skin was closed with 5-0 nylon sutures.

Code(s):

Ø1N5ØZZ   **Release Median Nerve, Open Approach**

Rationale:

Carpal tunnel release procedures are commonly performed by cutting the transverse carpal ligament in order to relieve pressure on the median nerve, which runs through the carpal tunnel. It is the pressure on the median nerve that results in the symptoms of carpal tunnel syndrome.

The median nerve was released from a physical constraint so root operation Release (N) captures this procedure. Although the ligament was cut, guideline B3.13 instructs that the body part being released is coded, which is the Median Nerve (5), found in the Peripheral Nervous (1) body system. The same body part value Median Nerve (5) is assigned regardless of whether the release was performed on the right or left side. The approach is Open (Ø) and there are No Device (Z) and No Qualifier (Z) choices listed in table Ø1N.

Figure 4.40. Carpal Tunnel Release

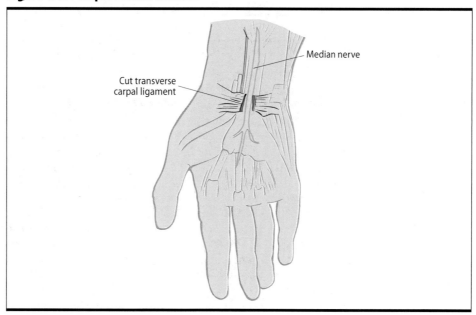

Median nerve

Cut transverse
carpal ligament

Case Study 4.86. Lysis, Adhesions, Pelvic

A laparoscope was inserted into the patient's abdomen. Upon inspection of the pelvic organs, it was apparent that the patient's right ovary and fallopian tube were grossly adherent to the pelvic sidewall. Using a scalpel, the adhesions between the ovary and sidewall were cut, as were the adhesions between the fallopian tube and the pelvic sidewall. The ovary and fallopian tube looked intact at the end of the dissection. The laparoscope was removed and all sites closed. The patient tolerated the procedure and was in stable condition.

Code(s):

ØUNØ4ZZ　　Release Right Ovary, Percutaneous Endoscopic Approach

ØUN54ZZ　　Release Right Fallopian Tube, Percutaneous Endoscopic Approach

Rationale:

The pelvic adhesions were the physical constraints cut in this example, meeting the root operation definition of Release (N). The ovary and fallopian tube were restrained by these pelvic adhesions, and although no manipulation, cuts, etc. were performed on the Ovary, Right (Ø) and Fallopian Tube, Right (5), they were the body parts being freed. The ovaries and fallopian tubes are part of the Female Reproductive (U) body system. Two different body parts, each having their own unique body part value, were released, so two codes are needed based on the following multiple procedure guideline B3.2a. Percutaneous Endoscopic (4) approach is appropriate because a laparoscope was used to visualize the body parts, as well as to carry out the adhesiolysis.

PCS Guideline
Multiple procedures
B3.2　　During the same operative episode, multiple procedures are coded if: a. The same root operation is performed on different body parts as defined by distinct values of the body part character.   *Examples:* Diagnostic excision of liver and pancreas are coded separately.   Excision of lesion in the ascending colon and excision of lesion in the transverse colon are coded separately.

Case Study 4.87. Lysis, Adhesions for Hip Impingement

The left hip was prepped and draped in normal sterile fashion. Preoperative time out confirmed the operative site and antibiotic infusion. Traction was applied to the left lower extremity. An anterolateral portal was established and a camera introduced followed by portal creation and camera insertion in the midanterior position with adequate visualization of the hip capsule.

The two portal sites were enlarged slightly for mobilization. The patient had adhesions of the capsule down to the labrum, which were released utilizing a Beaver blade. At that point, the traction was released. The patient had the above stated adhesions within the extra-articular compartment. A combination of a shaver as well as a burr was utilized to remove the adhesions and any residual bone along the femoral head neck junction. Very minimal to no resection was needed of the bone itself, although an additional amount of bone in the far lateral portion of the femoral neck was removed. The retinacular vessels were identified and protected. The hip was placed through a range of motion. The hip was felt to be free of impingement. The instruments were then removed from the hip. The portals were irrigated and closed with a 2-0 Vicryl followed by 3-0 nylon in the skin. They were infused with approximately 10 mL of Marcaine without epinephrine. The patient tolerated the procedure well.

Code(s):

ØSNB4ZZ　　Release Left Hip Joint, Percutaneous Endoscopic Approach

Rationale:

The focus of this procedure was the Release (N) of the hip joint. Adhesions in the capsule, as well as adhesions and residual bone along the femoral head/neck junction, were impinging on the joint reducing range of motion and causing pain. By cutting into and/or removing the adhesions and bone not typically found in the joint area, the Hip Joint, Left (B) found in body system Lower Joints (S) was released from this constraint. A Percutaneous Endoscopic (4) approach was used with No Device (Z) and No Qualifier (Z).

Case Study 4.88. Decompressive Laminectomy

Having obtained proper consent, the patient was taken to the operative suite where general endotracheal anesthesia was induced by the anesthesia team. The patient was positioned prone on the open OSI table. The upper thoracic region of his back was prepped and draped in the usual sterile fashion. Intraoperative fluoroscopy was brought into the operative field and used to localize the T1-T2 level. The skin overlying this level was infiltrated with 0.25% Marcaine with epinephrine. A number 10 blade skin knife was used to make an incision in the skin and dissection was carried down through the deep dermis and subcutaneous tissue with monopolar cautery. The spinous processes were encountered deep.

The laminae were exposed. There was a self-retaining retractor that was placed into the wound for retraction. Location was confirmed with fluoroscopy. The T1 and T2 levels were once again localized. Once the muscle had been removed off the lamina in subperiosteal fashion, a Leksell rongeur, a high-speed drill, and a 2 mm Kerrison punch were used to perform a wide decompressive laminectomy involving T1 and T2. Abnormal-appearing bone and some soft tissue surrounding the bone were noted. Findings within the bone were certainly suspicious for a neoplastic process. The left lamina, particularly at T1, appeared to be moth eaten. The bone was soft and friable. The thoracic cord at the T1-T2 level was widely and completely decompressed posteriorly using a series of Kerrison punches and pituitary pullers. A 2 mm Kerrison punch was used predominantly. A 3 mm Kerrison punch was used widely in order to resect the majority of the neoplastic appearing process at T1. This was all collected as specimen and sent to pathology for further study.

With good decompression at T1-T2, attention was turned to closing. Bone wax was used to wax the bony edges and hemostasis was achieved with bipolar cautery and with FloSeal. The wound was irrigated with copious amounts of saline solution. A number 10 French round fluted Blake drain was left in the epidural space and tunneled out through the skin with a trocar. The wound was closed in layers with interrupted 0 and 2-0 Vicryl pop-off sutures. The skin edges were reapproximated with staples. A sterile dressing was applied.

Code(s):

00NX0ZZ	Release Thoracic Spinal Cord, Open Approach
0PB40ZX	Excision of Thoracic Vertebra, Open Approach, Diagnostic

Rationale:

Two codes are required because two surgical objectives are described. The first objective was to release the thoracic spinal cord at the T1-T2 level. The second objective was to evaluate the excised bone to determine if the abnormal appearing bone was the result of a neoplastic process.

Spotlight
A decompressive laminectomy or laminotomy is frequently performed to free a spinal nerve root, reported with one of the nerve body parts from the Peripheral Nervous System (1) instead of the spinal cord body part from the Central Nervous System and Cranial Nerves (0). The documentation in the operative report must be closely reviewed to ensure proper body part and body system selection.

In this operative report, a portion of the Thoracic Spinal Cord (X) from the Central Nervous System and Cranial Nerves (Ø) at level T1-T2 was compressed by the abnormal bone and soft tissue. The removal of this bone and tissue with subsequent freeing of the cord is coded using Release (N) as the root operation. An Open (Ø) approach was used.

The biopsy was a separate objective performed on the same body part necessitating a second code based on Multiple procedures guideline B3.2c.

PCS Guideline
Multiple procedures
B3.2   During the same operative episode, multiple procedures are coded if: c. Multiple root operations with distinct objectives are performed on the same body part.   *Example:* Destruction of sigmoid lesion and bypass of sigmoid colon are coded separately.

A portion of the Thoracic Vertebra (4) found in the Upper Bones (P) body system was sampled, meeting the root operation of Excision (B). An Open (Ø) approach was used and the qualifier is Diagnostic (X), since the sample was sent to pathology for further study.

Release Versus Division

Guideline B3.14

B3.14	**If the sole objective of the procedure is freeing a body part without cutting the body part, the root operation is Release. If the sole objective of the procedure is separating or transecting a body part, the root operation is Division.** *Examples:* **Freeing a nerve root from surrounding scar tissue to relieve pain is coded to the root operation Release.** **Severing a nerve root to relieve pain is coded to the root operation Division.**

AHA Coding Clinic

2017, 3Q, 11   Bilateral Escharotomy of Leg, Thigh and Foot

2017, 3Q, 22   Laparoscopic Esophagomyotomy (Heller Type) and Toupet Fundoplication

2017, 3Q, 23   Laparoscopic Pyloromyotomy

2017, 2Q, 12   Compartment Syndrome and Fasciotomy of Foot

2017, 2Q, 13   Compartment Syndrome and Fasciotomy of Leg

2015, 3Q, 16   Vascular Ring Surgery and Double Aortic Arch

There are two root operations that have the sole objective of cutting or separating body tissue. The two root operations are differentiated by whether the body part itself is cut into, transected, or separated, or whether the body part is being freed from an abnormal physical constraint. For Division (8) procedures, the body part that is being cut into or transected is coded; in Release (N) procedures, the body part value being freed is used.

Root Operation		
Release (N)	Definition:	Freeing a body part from an abnormal physical constraint by cutting or by use of force
	Explanation:	Some of the restraining tissue may be taken out but none of the body part is taken out
Division (8)	Definition:	Cutting into a body part, without draining fluids and/or gases from the body part, in order to separate or transect a body part
	Explanation:	All or a portion of the body part is separated into two or more portions

Practical Application for Guideline B3.14

Case Study 4.89. Achilles Tendon Release

A patient was admitted to undergo surgical release of the left Achilles tendon. A small open incision was made above the calcaneus, and the Achilles tendon was identified. A sharp incision was made into the Achilles tendon to facilitate dorsiflexion of the foot.

Code(s):

ØL8PØZZ   Division of Left Lower Leg Tendon, Open Approach

Rationale:

Although documentation may state that a release operation was performed, the coder must consult the operative report to confirm surgical technique. A Division (8) is defined as cutting into a body part in order to separate or transect a body part, whereas a Release (N) is the freeing of a body part by cutting an abnormal constraint, such as an adhesion.

In this case, the Achilles tendon itself was transected rather than a body part constricting the Achilles tendon, meeting the root operation definition of Division (8). The Body Part Key (appendix D) directs the user to Lower Leg Tendon, Left (P) as the body part value for the Achilles tendon, which can be found in the Tendons (L) body system. An incision was made in order to complete the procedure so the approach is Open (Ø).

Case Study 4.90. Episiotomy and Delivery

A 26-year-old female was admitted in labor at 39.5 weeks. The patient's labor was uneventful and the patient went on to deliver over a midline episiotomy, which was repaired with sutures.

Code(s):

ØW8NXZZ	Division of Female Perineum, External Approach
1ØEØXZZ	Delivery of Products of Conception, External Approach

Rationale:

During an episiotomy, the perineum is cut into or transected. The root operation Division (8) is used to capture the perineal incision done for the episiotomy. The PCS index for Episiotomy also directs the user to *see* Division, Perineum, Female ØW8N. A review of this table confirms that body system Anatomical Regions, General (W) and body part Perineum, Female (N) are correct. The incision was made directly on the skin for an External (X) approach. No additional code is required for the repair or suturing of the episiotomy as it is considered closure and is inherent to the procedure.

A code for the delivery, from the Obstetrics (1) section, is also needed in this example. The full code, 1ØEØXZZ, is found in the alphabetic index under Delivery, Manually assisted or Delivery, Products of Conception.

Root Operation		
Medical and Surgical Section (Ø)		
Division (8)	Definition:	Cutting into a body part, without draining fluids and/or gases from the body part, in order to separate or transect a body part
	Explanation:	All or a portion of the body part is separated into two or more portions
Obstetrics Section (1)		
Delivery (E)	Definition:	Assisting the passage of the products of conception from the genital canal

---

Case Study 4.91. Fasciotomy for Acute Compartment Syndrome

The patient was brought to the operating room and general anesthetic administered. The right leg and hemipelvis were prepped and draped in the usual sterile fashion for surgery. Anterior and posterior compartments of the right thigh were firm, as were the compartments of the lower leg. The medial compartment of the right thigh was easily compressible. After prepping and draping the right leg, an incision was made over the anterolateral aspect of the leg. The fascia was dissected down and incised of the anterior and lateral compartments. All muscle was viable. The four Cs (contractility, capacity to bleed, consistency, and color) were used to assess viability. There was no evidence of significant muscle ischemia, although the compartment was definitely under pressure. An incision was made just off the posteromedial border of the tibia and the superficial and deep posterior compartments were released. Similarly, all muscle looked viable. There was good hemostasis. Attention was turned to the thigh. An incision was made over the thigh from the lateral epicondyle to just below the greater trochanter and the anterior compartment released. The vastus lateralis was dissected off the intermuscular septum and released. Again, all muscle appeared viable. Hemostasis was good. All wounds were packed with saline-soaked Kerlix rolls, followed by Kerlix fluffs, ABDs, and a double 6-inch Ace from the toes proximally. The patient was taken to the recovery room, having tolerated the procedure well.

Code(s):

ØKNSØZZ	**Release Right Lower Leg Muscle, Open Approach**
ØKNQØZZ	**Release Right Upper Leg Muscle, Open Approach**

Rationale:

A fasciotomy procedure for compartment syndrome consists of cutting the fascia with the objective of relieving tension or pressure to an area of muscle. The root operation Release (N) should be assigned for the fasciotomies performed for the release of compartment syndrome because the fascia was incised, freeing the muscles. The Lower Leg Muscle, Right (S) and Upper Leg Muscle, Right (Q) were released from an abnormal physical constraint. An Open (Ø) approach was used and there was No Qualifier (Z) and No Device (Z).

Definitions
compartment syndrome. Compromised blood flow to the muscles and nerves within a closed anatomical space due to increased interstitial pressure buildup that has nowhere to go. Compartment syndrome is marked by pain, loss of sensation, and palpable tenseness in the compartment region. The resulting ischemia can cause necrosis and loss of myoneural function or even loss of the limb. Sometimes the compartment must be surgically opened by emergency fasciotomy to allow for release of the pressure and return of arterial blood flow.

The index lists fasciotomy to be coded using the root operations Division (8), Drainage (9), or Release (N), the full intent of the procedure must be understood to apply the correct root operation (*AHA Coding Clinic*, 2017, 2Q,13). In this case, the fasciotomy was performed in order to release the constrained leg muscles. Therefore, guideline B3.14 states that Release (N) is the correct root operation.

Spotlight
The ICD-10-PCS Index can be used to access the tables. It is organized alphabetically by the root operation (third character) or by common procedural terms. The index is a frame of reference only and the full intent of a procedure must be understood in order to assign the appropriate root operation. Convention A7 states, "It is not required to consult the index first before proceeding to the tables to complete the code. A valid code may be chosen directly from the tables." Common terms such as fasciotomy, osteotomy, and laminectomy may be assigned to additional root operations other than those identified in the index. The root operation assigned should be based on the procedure performed as described in the complete documentation contained in the operative report and not simply on a single descriptive term in the operative report.

Reposition for Fracture Treatment

Reposition of a fracture, also called reduction or manipulation, is used to treat most displaced fractures. However, fractures may also be treated using other surgical and nonsurgical techniques. The type of treatment depends on a number of factors, including:

- Type of fracture
- Location of fracture
- Presence or absence of displacement
- Severity of any displacement
- Whether the fracture is closed or open
- Extent of any soft tissue or nerve damage

Guideline B3.15

B3.15	**Reduction of a displaced fracture is coded to the root operation Reposition and the application of a cast or splint in conjunction with the Reposition procedure is not coded separately. Treatment of a nondisplaced fracture is coded to the procedure performed.**
	***Examples*: Casting of a nondisplaced fracture is coded to the root operation Immobilization in the Placement section.**
	Putting a pin in a nondisplaced fracture is coded to the root operation Insertion.

AHA Coding Clinic

2015, 2Q, 35	Application of Tongs to Reduce and Stabilize Cervical Fracture
2014, 4Q, 29	Rotational Osteosynthesis
2014, 4Q, 31	Reposition of Femur for Correction of Valgus and Recurvatum Deformities
2014, 4Q, 32	Open Reduction Internal Fixation of Fracture with Debridement
2014, 3Q, 33	Radial Fracture Treatment with Open Reduction Internal Fixation, and Release of Carpal Ligament
2013, 2Q, 39	Application of Cervical Tongs for Reduction of Cervical Fracture

Displaced and Nondisplaced Fractures

A displaced fracture is one in which the broken bones have moved such that the ends are no longer in alignment. Primary treatment for a displaced fracture requires that the bones are "repositioned" or put back to their normal location. Therefore, the root operation Reposition (S) is used. The use of external or internal fixation devices to maintain alignment of the fracture fragments are captured by the device value in the Reposition (S) table, so insertion of a fixation device is not reported with a separate PCS code. In addition, guideline B3.15 specifies that the application of a splint or sling is not coded separately when Reposition (S) of the displaced fracture is performed.

Root Operation		
Reposition (S)	Definition:	Moving to its normal location, or other suitable location, all or a portion of a body part
	Explanation:	The body part is moved to a new location from an abnormal location, or from a normal location where it is not functioning correctly. The body part may or may not be cut out or off to be moved to the new location.

When using the root operation Reposition (S), the ICD-10-CM diagnosis code should also reflect the presence of a displaced fracture. However, the diagnosis code alone cannot be used to determine the correct PCS code because ICD-10-CM diagnosis code guidelines specify that when a fracture has not been identified as displaced or nondisplaced, the default is to code the fracture as displaced. This means that a diagnosis code of displaced could be assigned without any actual displacement being documented. In addition, displaced fractures are sometimes treated by other methods, such as traction or temporary immobilization, especially when surgery needs to be delayed temporarily due to swelling of the fracture site or due to the patient's medical condition. Therefore, when coding fracture care, only the documentation related to the actual procedure should be used to assign the procedure code. A physician query may be needed to resolve any conflicts in the documentation.

With a nondisplaced fracture, the broken bones may have shifted but maintain proper alignment. Therefore, no repositioning is needed and the root operation performed is the one coded. Internal or external fixation devices may be used to treat nondisplaced fractures and when fixation devices are used without any repositioning of the fracture, the root operation is Insertion (H), which is found in the Medical and Surgical Section (Ø). Alternatively, a nondisplaced fracture may be immobilized using a cast or splint. When casting or splinting is the only procedure performed to treat the fracture, a code from the Placement (2) section is reported and the root operation value for Immobilization (3) is assigned.

Root Operation		
Medical and Surgical Section (Ø)		
Insertion (H)	Definition:	Putting in a nonbiological appliance that monitors, assists, performs, or prevents a physiological function but does not physically take the place of a body part
	Explanation:	None
Placement Section (2)		
Immobilization (3)	Definition:	Limiting or preventing motion of a body region

Fixation Devices for Fractures

The ICD-10-PCS classification system specifies the type of fixation device used in treating displaced fractures in the sixth character. A thorough understanding of each type of device is needed in order to code the correct character.

Internal fixation devices are implants (e.g., wires, pins, screws, plates) used to stabilize or join ends of fractured bones. These are placed in or on the bone with minimal potential protrusion of wire or pin above the skin surface. There are three PCS device characters for internal devices:

- Internal Fixation Device, Rigid Plate (Ø), only found in Table ØPS for body part Sternum (Ø)

Figure 4.41. Internal Fixation Device, Rigid Plate

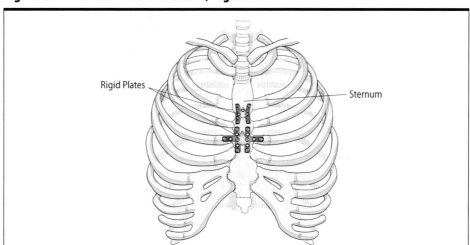

- Internal Fixation Device (4), including screws, plates, wires, or other implants other than intramedullary

Figure 4.42. Internal Fixation Device

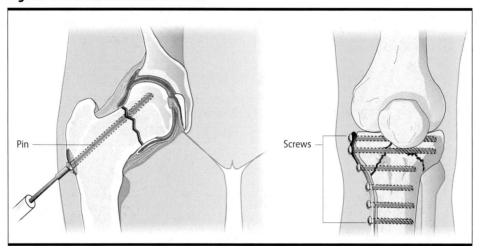

- Internal Fixation Device, Intramedullary (6), which is a long rod or nail used to stabilize the long bones

Figure 4.43. Internal Fixation Device, Intramedullary

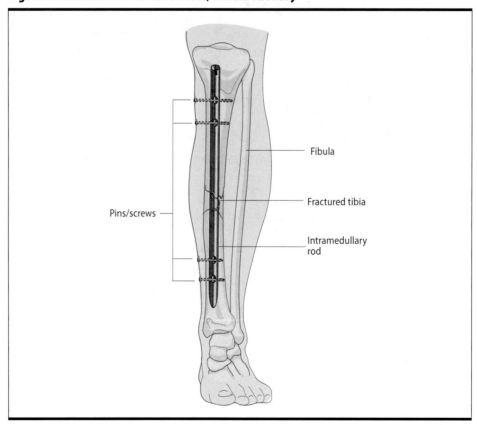

External fixation devices, although placed externally, are affixed directly to the bone by pins and screws through small incisions into the skin. The pins and screws are attached to a device outside of the skin, where it can be adjusted for proper bone alignment. The PCS device characters for external devices are:

- External Fixation Device (5), other than those following that have specific characters
- External Fixation Device, Monoplanar (B), a long rod inserted proximal and distal to the fracture that goes into the bone and is connected to a bar on the outside of the body in a single plane
- External Fixation Device, Ring (C), uses frames (rings) with wires, rods, clamps, and hinges or motors
- External Fixation Device, Hybrid (D), combines rings with planar frames

Figure 4.44. External Fixator Devices

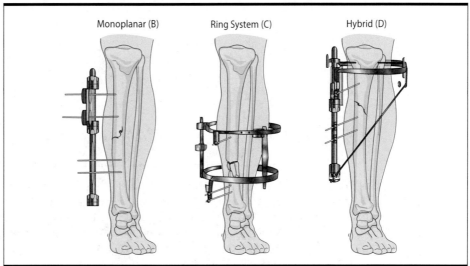

Monoplanar (B)   Ring System (C)   Hybrid (D)

Practical Application for Guideline B3.15

Case Study 4.92. Open Reduction Internal Fixation (ORIF) Ankle

Procedure: Open reduction, internal fixation of lateral and posterior malleolus for trimalleolar ankle fracture involving the posterior malleolus, lateral malleolus, and medial malleolus.

The patient was placed in the supine position and placed under general anesthesia with the right lower leg prepped and draped in the normal fashion. A lateral incision was made through the skin and subcutaneous tissue. The fibular fracture was recognized and a clamp applied until anatomically reduced. A single 2.7 mm lag screw was placed from A to P and a laterally-based periarticular Synthes plate positioned over the lateral malleolus. A proximal 3.5 mm cortical screw was placed into the diaphysis in order to fit the plate down to the bone. Five 2.7 mm screws were deployed distally into the lateral malleolus. These were placed using a standard Synthes technique. Excellent fixation was achieved in the lateral malleolus. The medial malleolus was not displaced and did not require fixation.

Attention was then turned to the posterior malleolus. A posterior malleolar plate with three holes distally was used. These holes were used in a lag mode under compression with 3.5 mm cortical screws, gaining excellent compression and anatomic articular reduction. Thorough irrigation was performed and the subcutaneous tissue and skin were closed.

Code(s):

ØQSJØ4Z   **Reposition Right Fibula with Internal Fixation Device, Open Approach**

ØQSGØ4Z   **Reposition Right Tibia with Internal Fixation Device, Open Approach**

Rationale:

Root operation Reposition (S) captures the intent of this procedure, which was to reduce or reposition the displaced bones of the lateral and posterior malleolus back into their original alignment with the use of internal fixation.

Two separately reportable procedures were performed during this operation, which follows the direction of guideline B3.2a. The medial malleolus fracture was not displaced and did not require fixation.

PCS Guideline
Multiple procedures
B3.2   During the same operative episode, multiple procedures are coded if:
a. The same root operation is performed on different body parts as defined by distinct values of the body part character.
Examples: Diagnostic excision of liver and pancreas are coded separately.
Excision of lesion in the ascending colon and excision of lesion in the transverse colon are coded separately.

The bones that form the ankle can be found in body system Lower Bones (Q). A review of table ØQS does not list body part characters for lateral or posterior malleolus. The right posterior malleolus is anatomically part of the Right Tibia (G), located behind the medial malleolus. According to the ICD-10-PCS Body Part Key, the right lateral malleolus is part of Fibula, Right (J). An Open (Ø) approach was used to access the fracture site and the Internal Fixation Device (4) consisted of plates and screws to hold the repositioned bones in place.

Figure 4.45. Lateral/Medial Malleolus

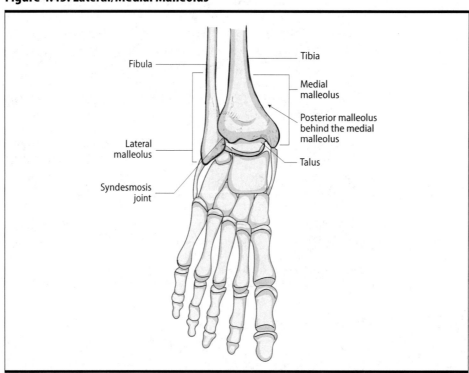

Case Study 4.93. Open Reduction Internal Fixation (ORIF) Hip

Procedure: Open reduction and internal fixation of right intertrochanteric hip fracture.

The right hip was prepped and draped in the usual sterile fashion. Next, a guidepin was placed over the hip and an AP fluoroscopic view taken. The proposed skin incision of approximately 12 cm in length was marked on the skin. The skin incision was made with a #10 blade, going down through the skin and subcutaneous tissue. Hemostasis was achieved with electrocautery. The IT-band was split longitudinally with electrocautery.

Next, the vastus lateralis was elevated and the posterior one-third was split longitudinally with electrocautery, also with use of a Key elevator, followed by placement of a Bennett leg loose retractor. The vastus lateralis was further developed with electrocautery at this time to expose the lateral femoral shaft. Next, the 135-degree guide with the pin was placed on the lateral femoral shaft and the guidepin was advanced through the lateral cortex into the femoral neck and checked under the lateral view, found to be in good position, and advanced into the head region, again checked under AP view, and advanced into the subcapital bone, again checked on the lateral view, and found to be in good position. This was then measured. It measured 90 mm. The decision was made to triple ream to 80 mm and place an 80 mm hip screw. Triple reaming was performed under AP fluoroscopic guidance. The 80-mm hip screw was placed, again under fluoroscopic guidance, and once felt to be in the correct position, it was checked again under the lateral view and found to be within the femoral head nicely. Back to the AP view, it was again visualized. The fracture was well reduced. The four-hole, 135-degree plate was advanced over the connector onto the screw and gently seated against the lateral femoral cortex. The connectors and guidepin were removed. The plate was gently impacted with a plastic impactor and mallet. Once fully seated, it was manually held in this position. The most distal hole in the plate was filled by drilling through both cortices, followed by depth gauge tapping, and placement of a propylene fully-threaded 4.5 cortical screw. The remainder of the holes in the plate were filled in a similar manner by drilling through both cortices, followed by depth gauge, and placement of the appropriate length 4.5, fully-threaded self-tapping screws. All screws were again securely tightened. The locking nut/screw was placed into the hip screw portion and was fully tightened. The entire contents were again checked under AP and lateral fluoroscopic views with hard copies printed off the C-arm. The site was again copiously irrigated with normal saline solution. The IT-band was closed with 0-Vicryl figure-of-eight interrupted sutures. The subcutaneous tissue was again irrigated with normal saline solution and the subcutaneous tissue was closed with 2-0 Vicryl interrupted sutures and the skin was closed with staples, followed by placement of Adaptic, 4x4s, ABD dressing, and elastic tape. The patient was gently transferred back to the hospital bed and transferred to recovery without difficulty.

Code(s):

0QS604Z   Reposition Right Upper Femur with Internal Fixation Device, Open Approach

Rationale:

Hip fracture is a commonly used term denoting a bone fracture involving the articular surface of the hip joint. Hip fractures may involve the acetabulum and/or the femur. In this case, the fracture occurred in the intertrochanteric area, which is located in the upper aspect of the femur between the greater and lesser trochanters and just below the femoral head, as shown in the following illustration. Intertrochanteric fractures are the most common type of hip fracture. Since the femur bone was repositioned and stabilized with a fixation device, as opposed to the hip joint, the correct body system is Lower Bones (Q). According to the Body Part Definitions listed in appendix E, the body part value Upper Femur, Right (6) includes the trochanter, femoral head, and femoral neck.

An Open (0) approach was used as evidenced by the 12 cm incision made into the skin and subcutaneous tissue. The correct root operation for reduction of a displaced fracture is Reposition (S). The Reposition was performed with the assistance of the hip screw, which was held in place with the plate and screws that were placed along the lateral side of the femoral cortex. These screws and plate are captured by a device value assignment of Internal Fixation Device (4).

Figure 4.46. Intertrochanteric Fracture

Intertrochanteric fracture

Femur

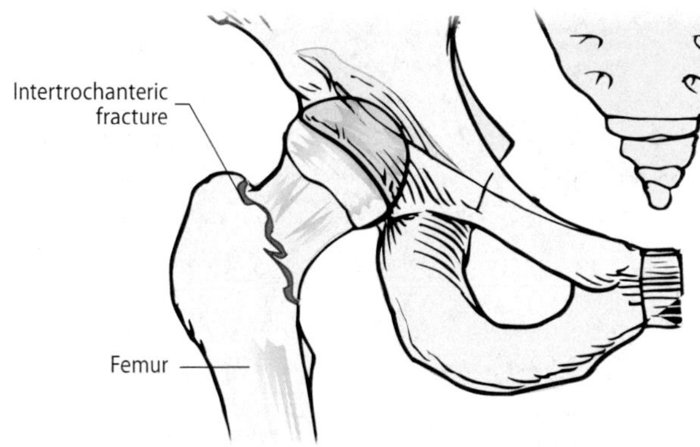

Case Study 4.94. Open Reduction Internal Fixation (ORIF) Hip with Intramedullary Rod

The left hip and left lower extremity were prepped and draped in the usual sterile manner. A guidewire was placed percutaneously into the tip of the greater trochanter and a small incision of 2.5 cm was made overlying the guidewire. An overlying drill was inserted to the proper depths. A Synthes 11 x 130 degrees trochanteric fixation was placed into the intramedullary canal to the proper depth. Proper rotation was obtained and the guide for the helical blade was inserted. A small incision was made for this as well. A guidewire was inserted and felt to be in proper position, in the posterior aspect of the femoral head, lateral, and the center position on AP. This placed the proper depths and lengths better. The outer cortex was enlarged and an 85-mm helical blade was attached to the proper depths and proper fixation was done. An appropriate size screw was tightened down. At this point, a distal guide was placed and drilled across both the cortices. Length was better. Appropriate size screw was inserted. Proper size and fit of the distal screw was also noted. At this point, on fluoroscopic control, it was confirming in AP and lateral direction. A near anatomical alignment was achieved to the fracture site and all hardware was properly fixed. Proper size and fit was noted. Excellent bony approximation was noted. At this point, both wounds were thoroughly irrigated, hemostasis confirmed, and closure was begun.

The fascial layers were reapproximated using #1 Vicryl in a figure-of-eight manner, the subcutaneous tissues were reapproximated in layers using #1 and 2-0 Vicryl sutures, and the skin was reapproximated with staples. The area was infiltrated with a mixture of a 0.25% Marcaine with Epinephrine and 1% plain lidocaine. Sterile dressing was applied. No complication was encountered throughout the procedure. The patient tolerated the procedure well. The patient was taken to the recovery room in stable condition.

Code(s):

0QS736Z   **Reposition Left Upper Femur with Intramedullary Internal Fixation Device, Percutaneous Approach**

Rationale:

This scenario provides a side-by-side comparison to the preceding example with the same intertrochanteric hip fracture but using a different surgical technique. The fracture fixation was performed in the same intertrochanteric location in the Lower Bones (Q) body system, captured by the Upper Femur, Left (7).

This Percutaneous Approach (3) uses a more minimally invasive technique with a small 2.5 cm incision made over the top of the greater trochanter where the guidewire and drill were used to insert the Synthes trochanteric fixation rod, which goes down into the medullary canal of the femur. This rod is represented by the device character Internal Fixation Device, Intramedullary (6). Another small incision was made over the lateral side of the femur and with a guidewire and drill, a screw was inserted across the cortex and through the rod to hold the intramedullary rod in place. Another screw was percutaneously placed further down the femur also across the cortex to help secure the rod in place (See the following illustration).

Figure 4.47. Intramedullary Hip Rod

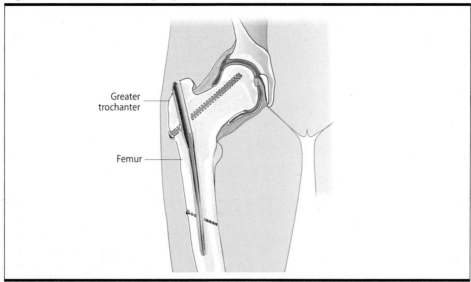

Greater trochanter

Femur

Case Study 4.95. External Fixation and Closed Reduction

Procedures: External fixation of left pilon fracture and closed reduction of left great toe.

Intraoperative fluoroscopy was used to identify the fracture site, as well as the appropriate starting point in the calcaneus for a transcalcaneal cross stent and in the proximal tibia with care taken to leave enough room for later plate fixation without contaminating the future operative site. A single centrally threaded calcaneal cross tunnel was placed across the calcaneus parallel to the joint surface followed by placement of two Schanz pins in the tibia. A frame-type external fixator was applied in traction with attempts to get the fracture fragments out to length, but not overly distract the fracture and restore coronal and sagittal alignment as much as possible. When this was adequate, the fixator apparatus was locked in place, and x-ray images were taken verifying correct placement of the hardware and adequate alignment of the fracture. Attention was turned to the left great toe, where a reduction of the proximal phalanx fracture was performed along with and buddy taping as this provided good stability and was least invasive. X-rays were taken showing good reduction of the base of the proximal phalanx of the great toe fracture. At this point, the pins were cut short and capped to protect the sharp ends. The stab wounds for the Schanz pin and cross pin were covered with gauze with Betadine followed by dry gauze, and the patient was awakened from anesthesia and transferred to the progressive care unit in stable condition.

Code(s):

ØQSH35Z   **Reposition Left Tibia with External Fixation Device, Percutaneous Approach**
ØQSRXZZ   **Reposition Left Toe Phalanx, External Approach**

Rationale:

Two PCS codes are needed to appropriately represent this procedure. Even though the same root operation Reposition (S) was performed on the same body system Lower Bones (Q), two separate fracture sites were treated as represented by two distinct body part values. In addition, two different approaches were required for the two separate fracture sites.

A pilon fracture, also called a plafond fracture, involves the articular surface of the tibia at the ankle joint so it is classified as a distal tibial fracture. In this case, it is the left pilon that is fractured so the body part is Tibia, Left (H). Although the screws were inserted into the calcaneus and the tibia, the objective of the procedure was to restore alignment or Reposition (S) of the fractured tibia, which determines the appropriate body part value. The approach used for the pilon fracture is

Percutaneous (3) since the pins needed to go through skin and soft tissue layers in order to reach the bone. Since the only description of the device was frame type, the fixator apparatus and pins are captured by the device value External Fixation Device (5).

The proximal phalanx of the left great toe is captured by the body part Toe Phalanx, Left (R). The toe fracture was reduced by force applied directly through the skin, meeting the definition of Reposition (S) by External (X) approach. Only buddy taping was used to stabilize the fracture so the device value is No Device (Z).

Spotlight
Often pins or screws used to apply an external fixation device are inserted above and below the fracture line, into different bones than the fractured body part. When using the root operation Reposition with a device character for External Fixation Device, the body part value is determined by the intent of the root operation and is coded to the body part being repositioned or reduced.

Case Study 4.96. Open Reduction Internal Fixation (ORIF) Mandibular Fracture

Procedures: Open treatment of mandibular fracture on the left and right sides using internal fixation.

The patient was admitted after sustaining an injury to the maxillofacial area. Based on the clinical and radiological examination results, the patient was diagnosed with a fracture in the right angle and a contralateral fracture through the left body of the mandible. Reduction of the left body fracture was completed followed by insertion of a large profile locking plate. Attention was then directed to the right angle fracture, which was reduced and treated with a miniplate.

Code(s):

ØNST04Z   **Reposition Right Mandible with Internal Fixation Device, Open Approach**

ØNSV04Z   **Reposition Left Mandible with Internal Fixation Device, Open Approach**

Rationale:

The mandible is U shaped and multiple fracture sites are common. Whenever one fracture of the mandible is identified, one or more additional fractures are usually found.

This case study does not specify if the fractures are displaced or nondisplaced. ICD-10-CM Guideline I.C.19.c directs the coder to use displaced when not further specified.

ICD-10-PCS guideline B3.15 states that reduction of a displaced fracture is coded to the root operation Reposition (S). There is no single body part character to represent both sides of the mandible in the Head and Facial Bones (N) body system. Two procedure codes are needed to represent the two sides treated. The right angle is coded as body part Mandible, Right (T) and the left body as Mandible, Left (V).

The approach character Open (Ø) is chosen based on the information stating that the procedure was performed as open. Both the profile locking plate and miniplate are Internal Fixation Devices (4).

Figure 4.48. Mandible Fracture

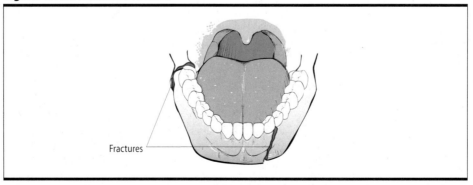

Fractures

Transplantation Versus Administration

Guideline B3.16

> **B3.16** **Putting in a mature and functioning living body part taken from another individual or animal is coded to the root operation Transplantation. Putting in autologous or nonautologous cells is coded to the Administration section.**
>
> *Example:* **Putting in autologous or nonautologous bone marrow, pancreatic islet cells or stem cells is coded to the Administration section.**

AHA Coding Clinic

2016, 4Q, 112 Transplantation
2016, 4Q, 113 Bone Marrow and Stem Cell Transfusion (Transplantation)
2014, 3Q, 13 Orthotopic Liver Transplant with End to Side Cavoplasty
2013, 3Q, 18 Heart Transplant Surgery

Traditionally, the term transplant has been used to describe transplantation of part or all of a living body part, such as a lobe of the liver or an entire kidney, as well as putting in cells such as stem cells, bone marrow, or pancreatic islet cells. In PCS, these two different types of transplants are reported with codes from different sections. Transplantation of living body parts are coded in the Medical and Surgical (Ø) section with the root operation Transplantation (Y). When stem cells, bone marrow, and pancreatic islet cells are transplanted, the procedure is coded in the Administration (3) section with one of two root operations: Transfusion (2) or Introduction (Ø).

Transplantation (Y)—Medical and Surgical (Ø) and Obstetrics (1) Sections

The root operation Transplantation (Y) represents a relatively small number of procedure codes performed on a limited number of body parts in ICD-10-PCS. In the Medical and Surgical section and the Obstetrics section, the definition and explanation are the same.

Root Operation		
Transplantation (Y)	Definition:	Putting in or on all or a portion of a living body part taken from another individual or animal to physically take the place and/or function of all or a portion of a similar body part
	Explanation:	The native body part may or may not be taken out, and the transplanted body part may take over all or a portion of its function

Transplantation procedures coded to the Medical and Surgical (Ø) section can involve a variety of different sources, including organs or portions of organs from other individuals or from animals. Coders should understand the different definitions related to the tissue type for transplantation organs. This information is used in the selection of the seventh-character Qualifier.

Definitions
allogeneic. Taken from different individuals of the same species.
syngeneic. Having to do with individuals or tissues that have identical genes, such as identical twins.
zooplastic. Tissue obtained from an animal.

The operative report for an organ transplant may include a detailed description of the work done to obtain the donor organ, as well as procedures performed on the donor organ itself. However, only those procedures performed on the recipient are coded.

Introduction (Ø), Transfusion (2)—Administration (3) Section

Transplantation of bone marrow, stem cells, and pancreatic islet cells involves transfusion or introduction of autologous or nonautologous cells into the body. Bone marrow obtained by bone marrow extraction, usually from the iliac crest, and stem cells obtained from cord blood or peripheral blood are classified as blood or blood products. Administration of bone marrow and stem cells (excluding embryonic stem cells) are reported with root operation Transfusion (2). Pancreatic islet cells are not classified as blood or blood products and are reported with the root operation Introduction (Ø); however, pancreatic islet cell transplantation is considered experimental and is only performed on a limited basis in facilities approved for this clinical trial.

Root Operation		
Introduction (Ø)	Definition:	Putting in or on a therapeutic, diagnostic, nutritional, physiological, or prophylactic substance except blood or blood products
Transfusion (2)	Definition:	Putting in blood or blood products

Practical Application for Guideline B3.16

Case Study 4.97. Transplant, Kidney

A 48-year-old female with a history of hypertensive chronic kidney disease that has progressed to stage V presented for right kidney transplant; the donor was her 35-year-old sister. The transplant procedure was accomplished without complications.

Code(s):

ØTYØØZØ   Transplantation of Right Kidney, Allogeneic, Open Approach

Rationale:

The ICD-10-PCS index lists Transplantation, Kidney, Right as ØTYØØZ, which includes all of the character values for the code except for the qualifier. The case above lists the donor as the recipient's sister. Since the recipient is 48 and the sister is 35, they cannot be identical twins and the appropriate qualifier is Allogeneic (Ø).

Case Study 4.98. Transplant, Bone Marrow

In a sterile environment, nonautologous bone marrow was delivered into the patient's bloodstream through a central venous catheter.

Code(s):

30243G4   Transfusion of Allogeneic Unspecified Bone Marrow into Central Vein, Percutaneous Approach

Rationale:

Although the title Bone Marrow Transplant may initially lead the user to the root operation tables for Transplantation, this is actually a transfusion procedure. It should be coded to the Administration (3) section of PCS and Circulatory (Ø) body system, using root operation Transfusion (2).

The character assignments in the Administration (3) section differ from those in the Medical and Surgical (Ø) section. This section represents codes for procedures that put in or on a therapeutic, prophylactic, protective, diagnostic, nutritional, or physiological substance.

The fourth character Central Vein (4) is the site where the substance was administered. When catheters are used to introduce substances into the circulatory system, the approach is Percutaneous (3).

Sixth-character values include broad categories of substances that can be transfused or introduced; Bone Marrow (G) was the substance transfused. Since the bone marrow substance was further identified as nonautologous, indicating that the bone marrow was from another individual, the correct seventh-qualifier character is Allogeneic, Unspecified (4) since no further information was given as to the relationship of the donor.

Transfer Procedures using Multiple Tissue Layers

Guideline B3.17

> **B3.17**   **The root operation Transfer contains qualifiers that can be used to specify when a transfer flap is composed of more than one tissue layer, such as a musculocutaneous flap. For procedures involving transfer of multiple tissue layers including skin, subcutaneous tissue, fascia or muscle, the procedure is coded to the body part value that describes the deepest tissue layer in the flap, and the qualifier can be used to describe the other tissue layer(s) in the transfer flap.**
>
> *Example:* **A musculocutaneous flap transfer is coded to the appropriate body part value in the body system Muscles, and the qualifier is used to describe the additional tissue layer(s) in the transfer flap.**

AHA Coding Clinic

2018, 1Q, 10	Complex Wound Closure Using Pericranial Flap
2017, 4Q, 67	New Qualifier Values - Pedicle Flap Procedures
2017, 2Q, 18	Esophagectomy and Esophagogastrectomy with Cervical Esophagogastrostomy
2016, 3Q, 30	Resection of Femur with Interposition Arthroplasty
2015, 3Q, 33	Cleft Lip Repair Using Millard Rotation Advancement
2015, 2Q, 26	Pharyngeal Flap to Soft Palate
2014, 4Q, 41	Abdominoperineal Resection (APR) with Flap Closure of Perineum and Colostomy
2014, 3Q, 18	Placement of Reverse Sural Fasciocutaneous Pedicle Flap
2014, 2Q, 10	Transverse Abdominomyocutaneous (TRAM) Breast Reconstruction
2014, 2Q, 12	Pedicle Latissimus Myocutaneous Flap with Placement of Breast Tissue Expanders
2013, 4Q, 109	Separating Conjoined Twins

Transfer (X) procedures use grafted tissue to replace or take over the function of all or a portion of a body part. Unlike the root operation Replacement (R), the grafting tissue used in Transfer (X) procedures maintain their original vascular and nervous connections. The term graft is rarely used when describing transfer procedures. The more commonly used term is flap, denoting that not all of the tissue is freed. Common procedural descriptions that may be encountered include advancement flap, rotational flap, or pedicle flap.

Root Operation		
Replacement (R)	Definition:	Putting in or on a biological or synthetic material that physically takes the place and/or function of all or a portion of a body part
	Explanation:	The body part may have been taken out or replaced, or may be taken out, physically eradicated, or rendered nonfunctional during the REPLACEMENT procedure. A REMOVAL procedure is coded for taking out the device used in a previous replacement procedure.
Transfer (X)	Definition:	Moving, without taking out, all or a portion of a body part to another location to take over the function of all or a portion of a body part
	Explanation:	The body part transferred remains connected to its vascular and nervous supply

Spotlight
Because transferred tissue is a part of and still connected to the patient (autologous), synthetic tissue or tissue from another person or animal (nonautologous) would not be found in the operative reports for transfer procedures. The use of synthetic or nonautologous grafts would be another clue in determining the appropriate root operation of Replacement (R) versus Transfer (X).

Although Transfer tables are found in many PCS body systems, this guideline provides advice on how to appropriately code transfer procedures that involve multiple layers of tissue. This guideline is similar to and consistent with overlapping body layers guideline B3.5, which specifically addresses Excision, Inspection, and Repair procedures, stipulating that only the deepest layer of body tissue is coded. This maintains consistency of data reporting within the PCS coding system.

PCS Guideline
Overlapping body layers
B3.5   If the root operations Excision, Repair or Inspection are performed on overlapping layers of the musculoskeletal system, the body part specifying the deepest layer is coded.
Example: Excisional debridement that includes skin and subcutaneous tissue and muscle is coded to the muscle body part.

The integumentary and musculoskeletal systems of the body are composed of multiple layers of tissue, captured in PCS by multiple body systems with multiple body part characters. The layers most often used in transfer procedures are skin, subcutaneous tissue, fascia, and muscles. For the root operation Transfer, the body system and body part value assigned is the deepest layer transferred (e.g., muscle). Because the flap (graft) is not completely freed from the patient, the only sixth-character Device value available is No Device (Z). The seventh character Qualifier provides additional detail by identifying any other layers (e.g., skin, subcutaneous tissue) that were transferred along with the deepest layer.

Practical Application for Guideline B3.17

Case Study 4.99. Flap, Gluteus Musculocutaneous
Procedure: Wound closure with left gluteus musculocutaneous flap.
A patient with a previous sacral pressure ulcer debridement presented for flap closure. General endotracheal anesthesia was given without any complications. All of the previous necrotic soft tissue, fascia, and muscle had been earlier excised and the wound was prepared for final closure. The physician incised into the deep dermis. Electrocautery was used to dissect down to the lateral edge. The flap was elevated in a lateral to medial direction. The gluteus muscle was divided down by its insertion and the physician elevated the muscle and skin and subcutaneous paddle. Once mobilized, a Doppler was used to identify the superior and inferior gluteal arteries and they were marked. Additional muscle division was completed along the edge of the sacrum, taking care to preserve the blood supply. Once adequate mobilization was achieved, the flap was rotated across the sacral wound and approximated to the contralateral gluteus muscle. The physician used 0 Vicryl sutures to inset the muscle, sewing it to the contralateral side. A 15 French Blake drain was left underneath the flap, which was brought out laterally and secured to the skin with 3-0 Nylon. Once the muscle was inset with 0 Vicryl, the physician used 2-0 Vicryl to complete closure of the superficial fascia and some of the deep dermis. The skin was stapled shut. The patient tolerated the procedure well.

Code(s):

ØKXPØZ2   Transfer Left Hip Muscle with Skin and Subcutaneous Tissue, Open Approach

Rationale:

In this example, a portion of the gluteal muscle, along with the skin and subcutaneous tissue, was transferred to the open sacral wound, while a portion of the flap remained connected to its vascular and nervous supply. The body system Muscles (K) is assigned as it is the deepest layer involved. Since the vascular connections were maintained, the root operation Transfer (X) is appropriate. The body part is the muscle that was transferred, which was the left gluteal muscle. According to the body part key, the left gluteal muscle is included in the PCS body part value Hip Muscle, Left (P).

The procedure was performed using an Open (Ø) approach with No Device (Z) inserted. The qualifier identifies the other body parts that were transferred with the muscle flap; in this case, the Skin and Subcutaneous Tissue (2) were transferred.

Spotlight
Although the tissue used in the transfer procedure may come from a different body site, a code for Excision (B) should not be reported separately. Only when the grafting tissue used for a procedure is completely freed from its original site can a separate excision code be reported.

Chapter 5. Body Part Guidelines

Body Part Overview

Body Part: Character 4

Character 1	Character 2	Character 3	Character 4	Character 5	Character 6	Character 7
Section	Body System	Root Operation	Body Part	Approach	Device	Qualifier

The body part, specified in the fourth character, indicates the specific part of the body system on which the procedure was performed. The body part value works in combination with the body system value (character 2) to define the precise location of the procedure. PCS provides information and tools to assist in appropriate body part selection, including the Body Part Key and Definitions Tables, alphabetical index, guidelines, and conventions.

Body Part Key and Body Part Definitions

There are only 34 possible character values for any PCS character field. Some cases require that specific anatomical sites be grouped together under more general sites. The Body Part Key provides information that routes the user from a more specific anatomical body part (when known) to the more general PCS term. Arranged in alphabetical order by the specific body part, the Body Part Key is found in appendix D in this book.

The following table represents an entry in the Body Part Key. Specific body part sites are listed, along with the most appropriate PCS body part to be assigned.

Term	ICD-10-PCS Value
Ascending pharyngeal artery	External Carotid Artery, Right
	External Carotid Artery, Left

Conversely, the Body Part Definitions, found in appendix E, are alphabetized by the more general PCS term with the inclusive specific body parts listed under each general term. In some circumstances, it may be useful to reference the Body Part Definitions to understand which separate body sites are mapped to a certain PCS value. For instance, if a procedure is performed on several arteries of the head and neck, the user may find it helpful to determine whether they are all classified to the External Carotid Artery body part.

ICD-10-PCS Value	Definition
External Carotid Artery, Left **External Carotid Artery, Right**	**Includes:** Ascending pharyngeal artery Internal maxillary artery Lingual artery Maxillary artery Occipital artery Posterior auricular artery Superior thyroid artery

The ICD-10-PCS official coding guidelines related to body part are discussed in this chapter.

General Guidelines

Guidelines B4.1a, B4.1b, and B4.1c apply to all body parts, providing instruction on proper body part value assignment when specific body parts named in an operative report do not have a body part value in ICD-10-PCS, when the term "peri" is used in the body part description, or when a procedure is performed on a continuous section of a tublular body part.

Guideline B4.1a

B4.1a	**If a procedure is performed on a portion of a body part that does not have a separate body part value, code the body part value corresponding to the whole body part.**
	Example: **A procedure performed on the alveolar process of the mandible is coded to the mandible body part.**

AHA Coding Clinic

2017, 2Q, 16	Excision of Floor of Mouth
2017, 2Q, 16	Incision and Drainage of Floor of Mouth
2016, 4Q, 86	Coronary and Peripheral Artery Bifurcation
2016, 4Q, 95	Intracardiac Pacemaker
2016, 3Q, 28	Lingual Tonsillectomy, Tongue Base Excision and Epiglottopexy
2016, 2Q, 18	Amygdalohippocampectomy
2016, 1Q, 19	Biopsy of Neobladder Malignancy
2016, 1Q, 23	Endoscopic Ultrasound with Aspiration Biopsy of Common Hepatic Duct
2015, 1Q, 22	Incision and Drainage of Abscess of Femoropopliteal Bypass Site
2015, 1Q, 22	Incision and Drainage of Groin Abscess
2015, 1Q, 31	Bilateral Browpexy
2014, 3Q, 31	Closure of Paravalvular Leak Using Amplatzer® Vascular Plug
2014, 1Q, 8	Diagnostic Lumbar Tap

There are many distinct body parts that do not have their own specific body part value in PCS. The whole body part value is used if the part documented is a specific portion of a whole body site; if not, the Body Part Key (appendix D) should be referenced to determine the most appropriate body part value. For example, a procedure performed on a sweat gland is, for PCS coding purposes, coded to body part Skin.

Term	ICD-10-PCS Value
Sweat gland	Skin

Similarly, a procedure performed on the mastoid process is coded to body part Temporal Bone.

Term	ICD-10-PCS Value
Mastoid Process	Temporal Bone, Right Temporal Bone, Left

Practical Application for Guideline B4.1a

Case Study 5.1. Parietal Lobe Resection

A patient was admitted for open resection of a primary malignancy of the parietal lobe of the brain. The patient was placed in the prone position after general endotracheal anesthesia was administered. The scalp was prepped and draped in the usual fashion. The BrainLab was brought in to supplement the use of an operating microscope, which was used to localize the tumor. A transverse linear incision was made, the scalp galea was reflected, and the quadrilateral bone flap was removed after placing burr holes in the midline and over the parietal areas directly over the tumor. The bone flap was elevated. The interhemispheric space was entered after incising the dura in an inverted U fashion based on the superior side of the sinus. Using the operating microscope, the resection was gradually completed by debriding all the directions with the help of image guidance to make sure that total removal of the large metastatic tumor involving the parietal lobe was obtained. After gross total removal of the tumor, irrigation was used to wash the tumor bed and a meticulous hemostasis was obtained using bipolar cautery. The dura was closed with 4-0 Nurolon in a watertight fashion. DuraGen was applied over the dura, the bone flap was replaced and secured with miniplate, and the Jackson-Pratt was left in the subgaleal space. The scalp was closed with 2-0 Vicryl and staples for the skin.

Code(s):

00B70ZZ	**Excision of Cerebral Hemisphere, Open Approach**
8E09XBZ	**Computer Assisted Procedure of Head and Neck Region**

Rationale:

A portion of the parietal lobe containing the malignancy was removed in this procedure. Since only a portion (and not the entire lobe) was removed, Excision (B) is the correct root operation. The PCS index does not contain a listing for Excision, Parietal lobe. Consulting the Body Part Key, users are instructed to use Cerebral Hemisphere (7), found in Central Nervous System and Cranial Nerves (0).

Figure 5.1. Brain

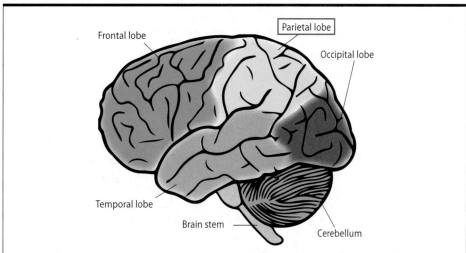

An Open (0) approach was stated, No Device (Z) is the only sixth-character choice, and since the objective of this procedure was to remove the already diagnosed malignancy, the appropriate seventh character is No Qualifier (Z).

Most neurosurgeries involve computer-assisted imaging and navigation. An additional code is reported to represent the use of the BrainLab System. The BrainLab, like Stealth, is a frameless stereotaxy imaging and navigational system. This is reported with a Computer Assisted Procedure (B) code, which is found in the Other Procedures (8) section with a body part for Head and Neck Region (9). No other imaging, such as fluoroscopy, MRI, or CT, was mentioned so No Qualifier (Z) is used for the qualifier.

Case Study 5.2. Strabismus Surgery

The patient was taken to the operating suite. After induction of general anesthesia, the patient was prepped and draped. A speculum was placed in the left eye. An incision was made in the conjunctiva at the limbus. The medial rectus muscle was isolated with a muscle hook. The medial muscle was resected and reattached to the sclera by adjustable sutures. Attention was turned to the lateral rectus muscle. The procedure was repeated. A single 10-0 Nylon suture was placed. TobraDex ointment was instilled into the left conjunctival sac and a firm patch placed on the left eye. The patient tolerated the procedure well and was sent to recovery in satisfactory condition.

Code(s):

Ø8SMØZZ   **Reposition Left Extraocular Muscle, Open Approach**

Ø8SMØZZ   **Reposition Left Extraocular Muscle, Open Approach**

Rationale:

The intent of the procedure was to move the position of the medial and lateral rectus muscles; root operation Reposition (S) is assigned.

Definition
strabismus. Misalignment of the eyes due to an imbalance in extraocular muscles.

Root Operation		
Reposition (S)	Definition:	Moving to its normal location, or other suitable location, all or a portion of a body part
	Explanation:	The body part is moved to a new location from an abnormal location, or from a normal location where it is not functioning correctly. The body part may or may not be cut out or off to be moved to the new location.

Figure 5.2. Extraocular Muscles

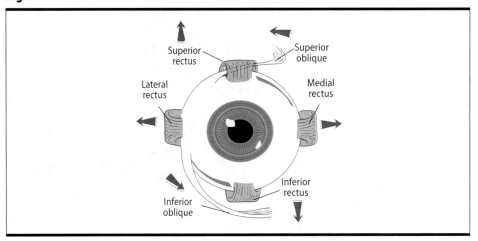

The ICD-10-PCS index does not list body part values for medial or lateral rectus muscles under Reposition (S). Consulting the Body Part Key, the medial and lateral rectus muscles direct the coder to use Extraocular Muscle, Left (M) and Extraocular Muscle, Right (L), which are located in the Eye (8) body system rather than the Muscle (K) body system. PCS body part values Extraocular Muscle, Left (M) and Extraocular Muscle, Right (L) include all six of the muscles that comprise the extraocular muscle as shown in the following excerpt from the Body Part Definitions (appendix E).

ICD-10-PCS Value	Definition
Extraocular Muscle, Left **Extraocular Muscle, Right**	**Includes:** Inferior oblique muscle Inferior rectus muscle Lateral rectus muscle Medial rectus muscle Superior oblique muscle Superior rectus muscle

Two codes are needed to correctly capture this procedure as stated in multiple procedures guideline B3.2b. The left medial and left lateral rectus muscles are coded using the body part Extraocular Muscle, Left (M); however, since both muscles are separate and distinct body parts, two codes are needed. The left and right distinction for extraocular muscles applies to the left and right eye, not the location of the muscles within the eye.

The approach is Open (Ø) and No Device (Z) and No Qualifier (Z) applies.

PCS Guideline
Multiple procedures   B3.2   During the same operative episode, multiple procedures are coded if: b. The same root operation is repeated in multiple body parts, and those body parts are separate and distinct body parts classified to a single ICD-10-PCS body part value.   *Example:* Excision of the sartorius muscle and excision of the gracilis muscle are both included in the upper leg muscle body part value, and multiple procedures are coded.   Extraction of multiple toenails are coded separately.

Case Study 5.3. Drainage, Psoas Muscle Abscess

A patient had an abscess of the right psoas muscle that needed to be surgically drained. The patient was placed in a right semilateral position and prepped and draped in the usual fashion. A long incision was made at the flank to locate and drain 300 ml pus from all of the abscess pockets in the psoas. The patient tolerated the procedure and was sent home on oral antibiotics.

Code(s):
ØK9NØZZ   Drainage of Right Hip Muscle, Open Approach

Rationale:
The psoas muscles originate in the trunk on each side of the lumbar vertebrae and cross the respective ilium to insert in the lesser trochanters of the femurs, which is depicted in the following illustration. The anatomical position of this muscle is classified as Hip Muscle, Right (N) or Hip Muscle, Left (P) according to the Body Part Key found in appendix D.

Guideline B4.1a states that since the psoas muscle is not listed as a separate body part value, it is coded using the whole body part as indicated in the Body Part Key.

Figure 5.3. Psoas Muscle

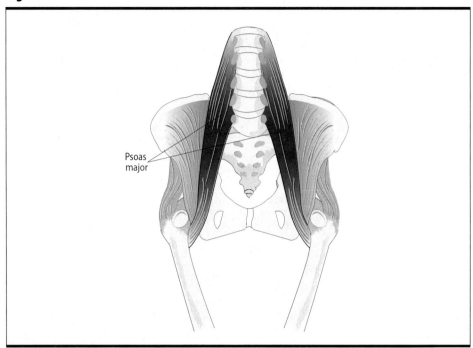

Psoas major

In this example, fluid was being removed, meeting the root operation definition of Drainage (9). The body part value Hip Muscle, Right (N) is found in the Muscles (K) body system. An Open (Ø) approach was stated, No Device (Z) is used, and since this scenario did not indicate that the fluid being drained was for diagnostic purposes, No Qualifier (Z) is the appropriate seventh character.

Root Operation		
Drainage (9)	Definition:	Taking or letting out fluids and/or gases from a body part
	Explanation:	The qualifier DIAGNOSTIC is used to identify drainage procedures that are biopsies

Case Study 5.4. Excision, Foot Dorsal Venous Arch Aneurysm

The patient was brought to the surgical suite and placed in the supine position. Cardiopulmonary monitoring was initiated and sedation performed. The area of the left dorsal foot venous arch aneurysm was prepped and draped in typical sterile fashion. The skin overlying the abscess was anesthetized with 1% lidocaine mixed with 0.5% Marcaine. The skin was opened with a #15 blade overlying the abnormal vasculature. All abnormal venous structures and branches were ligated with 2-0 and 3-0 silk and excised. Hemostasis was complete. The skin was closed and the wound dressed.

Code(s):
Ø6BVØZZ   Excision of Left Foot Vein, Open Approach

Rationale:
The dorsal venous arch of the foot is a superficial vein that connects the lesser saphenous vein and the greater saphenous vein, as shown in the following illustration.

Figure 5.4. Dorsal Venous Arch

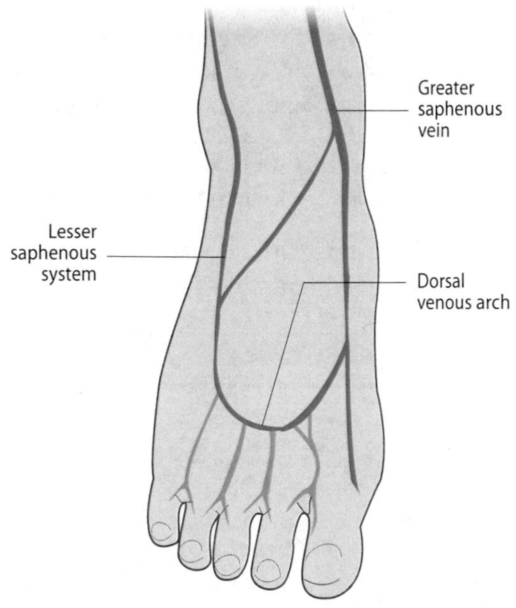

In this example, the aneurysm was isolated and excised. Only the abnormal vasculature was removed, meeting the root operation of Excision (B). It should also be noted that there is not a Resection (T) table in the Lower Veins (6) body system.

Root Operation		
Excision (B)	Definition:	Cutting out or off, without replacement, a portion of a body part
	Explanation:	The qualifier DIAGNOSTIC is used to identify excision procedures that are biopsies

The Body Part Key (appendix D) indicates that Foot Vein, Left (V) is used for the left dorsal venous arch. An Open (Ø) approach was used as evidenced by the skin being opened with a blade. No Device (Z) and No Qualifier (Z) are used for the sixth and seventh characters, respectively.

Guideline B4.1b

> **B4.1b** If the prefix "peri" is combined with a body part to identify the site of the procedure, and the site of the procedure is not further specified, then the procedure is coded to the body part named. This guideline applies only when a more specific body part value is not available.
>
> *Examples:* A procedure site identified as perirenal is coded to the kidney body part when the site of the procedure is not further specified.
>
> A procedure site described in the documentation as peri-urethral, and the documentation also indicates that it is the vulvar tissue and not the urethral tissue that is the site of the procedure, then the procedure is coded to the vulva body part.

AHA Coding Clinic

2018, 1Q, 25	Periacetabular Osteotomy for Repair of Congenital Hip Dysplasia
2016, 2Q, 31	Periacetabular Ostectomy for Repair of Congenital Hip Dysplasia
2015, 4Q, 16	Changes to the ICD-10-PCS Official Guidelines for Coding and Reporting
2014, 4Q, 18	Obstetrical Periurethral Laceration
2014, 4Q, 47	Catheter Ablation of Peripulmonary Veins
2013, 2Q, 38	Catheter Ablation to Treat Atrial Fibrillation

Many physicians provide documentation that includes the prefix "peri-," which means "around" or "in the region of." For instance, "periauricular" means around the external ear area. The body part value of the site included in the word with "peri-" is assigned unless documentation specifically refers to another distinct site. For example, although a physician may describe a catheter ablation as around the pulmonary veins or peripulmonary, in reality, the pulmonary vein is not the body part destroyed. Instead, the ablation is actually performed on the hearts "conduction mechanism." When the word "peri" is used, it is important to review the operative report carefully for the actual objective of the procedure and compare it with the surrounding anatomical structures to ensure selection of the appropriate body part (*AHA Coding Clinic*, 2014, 4Q, 47).

Practical Application for Guideline B4.1b

> **Case Study 5.5. Fistulectomy**
>
> **Procedure:** Excision of perianal fistula.
>
> The patient was placed in the supine position under general LMA anesthesia. The patient was placed in the lithotomy position, and the perianal area was prepped and draped in the usual sterile manner. The opening to the exterior had closed, and using a scalpel, it was opened. There was some fluid and pus that drained. The lacrimal duct probe was placed into the tract and it easily went through the internal opening of the fistula. Both ends of the lacrimal duct probe were held, and the perianal fistula was excised with cautery. Hemostasis was achieved with cautery. The patient tolerated the procedure well and was taken to the recovery room in good condition.

Code(s):
0DBQ0ZZ   Excision of Anus, Open Approach

Rationale:
Fistulectomy is a surgical procedure in which a fistulous tract is excised (cut out) completely. Only the fistula tract was removed, so the appropriate root operation is Excision (B). This example highlights the use of guideline B4.1b in that no additional information was given regarding the body part excised; therefore, the body part named, Anus (Q) found in the Gastrointestinal (D) body system, is coded. A scalpel was used for an Open (0) approach. No Device (Z) is used and No Qualifier (Z) is the appropriate seventh character as the removal of the fistula was for therapeutic purposes.

Definition
fistula. Abnormal tube-like passage between two body cavities or organs or from an organ to the outside surface.

Root Operation		
Excision (B)	Definition:	Cutting out or off, without replacement, a portion of a body part
	Explanation:	The qualifier DIAGNOSTIC is used to identify excision procedures that are biopsies

Figure 5.5. Anal Fistula

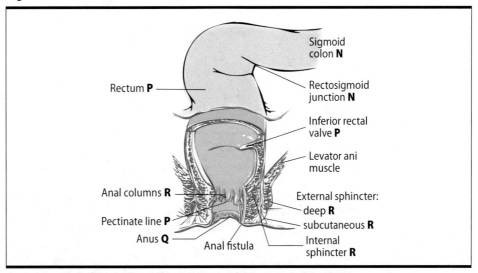

Sigmoid colon **N**

Rectosigmoid junction **N**

Rectum **P**

Inferior rectal valve **P**

Levator ani muscle

Anal columns **R**

External sphincter: deep **R**

Pectinate line **P**

subcutaneous **R**

Anus **Q**

Anal fistula

Internal sphincter **R**

Case Study 5.6. Drainage, Peritonsillar Abscess
An 18-gauge needle was inserted into the peritonsillar abscess and 2 cc of pus was aspirated. The patient tolerated the procedure well and was sent home on oral antibiotics.

Code(s):

ØC9P3ZZ   Drainage of Tonsils, Percutaneous Approach

Rationale:

A peritonsillar abscess is a common deep neck infection that results from a collection of pus located between the capsule of the palatine tonsil and the pharyngeal muscles.

Drainage (9) is the appropriate root operation to use since fluid was taken out. There is no peritonsillar body part value listed in the Mouth and Throat (C) body system. Guideline B4.1b instructs that the body part named be coded when "peri" is used as a prefix and no further specificity is available. Tonsils (P) is the correct body part value in this example. Only one body part value is listed for Tonsils (P) so laterality is not captured in the code. A needle was used for the drainage, meeting the approach definition of Percutaneous (3). No Device (Z) was used and there was no indication that the fluid was being studied further, so No Qualifier (Z) is used as the seventh character.

Root Operation		
Drainage (9)	Definition:	Taking or letting out fluids and/or gases from a body part
	Explanation:	The qualifier DIAGNOSTIC is used to identify drainage procedures that are biopsies

Figure 5.6. Tonsillar Abscess

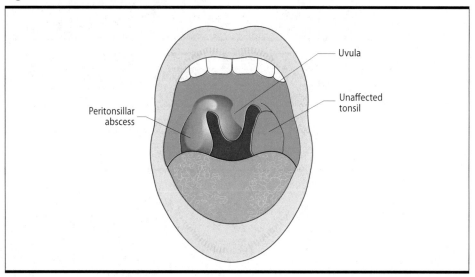

Uvula

Unaffected tonsil

Peritonsillar abscess

Case Study 5.7. Drainage, Periparotid Abscess

The patient was brought to the operating room and placed on the operating table in the supine position. General endotracheal anesthesia was administered without any difficulty. A modified Blair incision was marked starting at a right preauricular crease and coursing behind the right ear lobule into a skin crease behind the angle of mandible. A 15 blade was used to make the modified Blair incision, which was carried down to the level of the sternocleidomastoid muscle in the neck and the tragal cartilage anterior to the auricle. The intervening tissue was carefully dissected to the periparotid area until the large abscess cavity was located anterior to the parotid. Cultures were taken and a copious amount of purulent material was drained. When this was completed, a .025 inch Penrose drain was inserted and the incision closed in a two-layer fashion with 4-0 Vicryl and interrupted 5-0 nylon. A small part of the posterior aspect of the incision was left open where the drain was sutured in place. A compression dressing was applied and the patient was awakened, extubated, and transferred to recovery.

Code(s):

ØW96ØØZ   Drainage of Neck with Drainage Device, Open Approach

Rationale:

Periparotid refers to the area around the parotid gland, which includes one of the salivary glands and the parotid lymph nodes. Although guideline B4.1b states that the prefix "peri" combined with a body part can be used to identify the site of the procedure, it also adds that if the site is further specified, this guideline does not apply. In this case, the Drainage (9) was not performed on the Parotid Gland, Right (8) or Left (9), which is in the Mouth and Throat (C) body system, **or** on the parotid lymph nodes, which are in the Lymphatic and Hemic Systems (7) body system. The Drainage (9) was performed in a cavity of the neck "anterior to the parotid," which is reported with body part Neck (6) from the Anatomical Regions, General (W) body system. An incision was made and the tissues dissected down to reach the abscess, which is classified as an Open (Ø) approach. The Penrose drain was inserted and left in place so the device value of (Ø) Drainage Device is appropriate. The only qualifier option in the row with Drainage Device (Ø) is No Qualifier (Z).

A secondary code for taking cultures is unnecessary. The objective was to drain the abscess with the cultures an inherent part of the procedure. Since Drainage (9) was the only root operation performed, and no additional body parts or approaches were involved, multiple procedure guidelines do not apply.

Guideline B4.1c

B4.1c	**If a procedure is performed on a continuous section of a tubular body part, code the body part value corresponding to the furthest anatomical site from the point of entry.** ***Example:*** **A procedure performed on a continuous section of artery from the femoral artery to the external iliac artery with the point of entry at the femoral artery is coded to the external iliac body part.**

AHA Coding Clinic

2017, 1Q, 51   Bronchoalveolar Lavage

2016, 3Q, 31   Iliofemoral Endarterectomy with Patch Repair

This guideline is similar to and consistent with the instruction given in Guideline B3.11b, located in the root operation section, and specifically discusses Inspection procedures. Guideline B4.1c expands on and clarifies this advice by including all procedures performed on continuous sections of tubular body parts. An important distinction when determining the furthest point of the procedure is that it is the most distal from the point where the body was initially entered. Tubular body parts transport solids, liquids, and gases throughout the body. They include the cardiovascular system and body parts such as those contained in the gastrointestinal tract, genitourinary tract, biliary tract, and respiratory tract. Some procedures that may be affected by this guideline include thrombectomies, enterectomies, bronchoscopies, and arteriectomies.

PCS Guideline
Inspection procedures
B3.11b   If multiple tubular body parts are inspected, the most distal body part (the body part furthest from the starting point of the inspection) is coded. If multiple non-tubular body parts in a region are inspected, the body part that specifies the entire area inspected is coded. *Examples:* Cystoureteroscopy with inspection of bladder and ureters is coded to the ureter body part value. Exploratory laparotomy with general inspection of abdominal contents is coded to the peritoneal cavity body part value.

Practical Application for Guideline B4.1c

Case Study 5.8. Atherectomy, Lower Arteries
Indication: Occluded right superficial femoral artery (SFA), right popliteal artery, and proximal occlusion of the right anterior tibial artery causing critical limb ischemia.
Details: After obtaining informed consent, the patient was brought to the cath lab and prepped and draped. The right groin was anesthetized with 1% lidocaine. The right common femoral artery was cannulated using a modified Seldinger technique with a micropuncture kit upgraded to a 6-French sheath. A catheter was placed into the proximal right common femoral artery and the occlusion was crossed using a V-18 wire. At the anterior tibial artery level, a Treasure Floppy wire was used to cross the proximal vessel and exchanged over the catheter for a Pathway wire. Atherectomy was performed on the plaque using the 2.1 mm Pathway catheter with the blade down. The angiography showed flow from the proximal SFA all the way down to the foot. After flow was established, the proximal anterior tibial artery was dilated using a 3.5 mm balloon, which was exchanged for a 4 mm drug-coated balloon. The balloon was deflated and removed. Angiography was performed and showed 0% residual and TIMI-3 flow distally all the way down to the foot.

Code(s):

Ø4CP3ZZ	**Extirpation of Matter from Right Anterior Tibial Artery, Percutaneous Approach**
Ø47P3Z1	**Dilation of Right Anterior Tibial Artery using Drug-Coated Balloon, Percutaneous Approach**
B41FYZZ	**Fluoroscopy of Right Lower Extremity Arteries using Other Contrast**

Rationale:

Blood flow to the foot was obstructed from continuous plaque in the SFA through the popliteal artery and ending in the proximal anterior tibial artery. Plaque removal is reported with root operation Extirpation (C) and, based on advice from Guideline B4.1c, the appropriate body part value is Anterior Tibial Artery, Right (P) since it is the most distal point of the procedure.

After the matter was removed, Dilation (7) was performed using an inflated balloon to flatten any remaining plaque against the artery walls. Guideline B4.1c still applies, and body part Anterior Tibial Artery, Right (P) is reported. Since the balloon was removed after the procedure, it is not considered a device; sixth-character No Device (Z) is reported. The first balloon was exchanged for a second balloon, reported with seventh-character qualifier Drug-Coated Balloon (1). This balloon was left in for a designated amount of time to release antiproliferative medication to the arteries, which assists in limiting restenosis. This balloon was also removed. All of the procedures were accomplished using a Percutaneous (3) approach.

Definition
drug-coated balloons. Newer addition to the treatment of peripheral vascular disease, these balloons are currently coated with paclitaxel along with different types of carriers or excipients that complete the drug transfer to the vessel wall. They have shown significant reduction in restenosis rates and can be used in place of a chronically implanted stent.

This procedure also meets coding advice given in guideline B3.2c, which states that during the same operative episode, multiple procedures are coded if multiple root operations with distinct objectives are performed on the same body part. Removal of plaque by Extirpation, followed by Dilation of the artery with the balloon, represents two distinct objectives.

Root Operation		
Extirpation (C)	Definition:	Taking or cutting out solid matter from a body part
	Explanation:	The solid matter may be an abnormal byproduct of a biological function or a foreign body; it may be imbedded in a body part or in the lumen of a tubular body part. The solid matter may or may not have been previously broken into pieces.
Dilation (7)	Definition:	Expanding an orifice or the lumen of a tubular body part
	Explanation:	The orifice can be a natural orifice or an artificially created orifice. Accomplished by stretching a tubular body part using intraluminal pressure or by cutting part of the orifice or wall of the tubular body part.

Angiography is reported with a code from the Imaging (B) section. Fluoroscopy (1) is used to visualize endovascular procedures. Since there is no unspecified value for contrast type, facilities reporting this imaging are urged to work with their radiologists to determine the type of contrast media used and develop internal, facility-specific guidelines identifying the contrast type. Most use low or other contrast—this example assumes a default of Other Contrast (Y).

Case Study 5.9. Enterectomy, Left Carotid Arteries

Description of operation: The left side of the neck was prepped in the usual sterile fashion and the incision site was infiltrated with 1% Xylocaine with epinephrine.

A skin incision was made with a scalpel along the anterior border of the left sternocleidomastoid muscle. Subcutaneous tissues, platysma, and deep cervical fascia along the anterior border of the sternocleidomastoid muscle were divided. The common facial vein was ligated, clipped, and divided. The common, internal, and external carotid arteries were dissected out and surrounded with vessel loops.

Eight thousand (8,000) units of heparin were administered intravenously and allowed to circulate for three minutes. The internal carotid artery was occluded followed by occlusion of the common and external carotid arteries. A #11 blade was used to make an arteriotomy in the common carotid artery. The arteriotomy was extended with scissors through the bulb and up the internal carotid artery to a point beyond the distal extent of disease. A shunt was inserted and held in place with clamps.

Standard endarterectomy was then performed. Eversion technique was used to facilitate the endarterectomy in the external carotid artery. The distal endpoint feathered smoothly at the proximal internal carotid artery level. Any remaining loose debris was removed with plaque forceps. The surface of the artery was irrigated with copious amounts of heparinized saline. The arteriotomy was closed with a Dacron patch using running 6-0 Prolene suture.

Code(s):

Ø3CLØZZ	**Extirpation of Matter from Left Internal Carotid Artery, Open Approach**
Ø3ULØJZ	**Supplement Left Internal Carotid Artery with Synthetic Substitute, Open Approach**

Rationale:

In an endarterectomy, the vessel is incised and opened. The plaque is peeled away from the wall of the artery, which is reported with root operation Extirpation (C). The left common carotid artery originates from the aorta, just above the heart, and runs up the left side of the neck where it divides (bifurcates) into the left internal and external carotid arteries. According to guideline B4.1c, the most distal site of the tubular body part is reported for this procedure, which is the Internal Carotid Artery, Left (L). This case didn't clearly specify if the occlusion removed was in the bifurcation so No Qualifier (Z) was used. A patch graft was used, which is coded as a separate procedure using root operation Supplement (U). An Open (Ø) approach was used to access the site and perform the arteriotomy, which is an incision through the arterial wall and is inherent in the procedure as part of accessing the site.

AHA Coding Clinic, 2016, 2Q, 11, discusses the separate reporting of the Dacron® patch graft using Supplement (U) with Synthetic Substitute (J). *AHA Coding Clinic,* 2014, 4Q, 37 and 2016, 1Q, 31, instruct that a bovine patch artery repair is reported with root operation Supplement (U) with device value Nonautologous Tissue Substitute (K).

This procedure also meets the coding advice given in guideline B3.2c, which states that during the same operative episode multiple procedures are coded if multiple root operations with distinct objectives are performed on the same body part. Removal of the plaque by Extirpation, followed by Supplement of artery with patch graft, represents two distinct objectives.

Root Operation		
Extirpation (C)	Definition:	Taking or cutting out solid matter from a body part
	Explanation:	The solid matter may be an abnormal byproduct of a biological function or a foreign body; it may be imbedded in a body part or in the lumen of a tubular body part. The solid matter may or may not have been previously broken into pieces.
Supplement (U)	Definition:	Putting in or on biological or synthetic material that physically reinforces and/or augments the function of a portion of a body part
	Explanation:	The biological material is non-living, or is living and from the same individual. The body part may have been previously replaced, and the Supplement procedure is performed to physically reinforce and/or augment the function of the replaced body part.

Spotlight
These examples are supported and explained by *AHA Coding Clinic,* 2016, 3Q, 31, which states that the appropriate body part value reported for procedures performed on overlapping or continuous lesions in a tubular body part is the most distal site from the entry point.

Case Study 5.10. Bronchoalveolar Lavage (BAL)

The physician inserted a flexible bronchoscope into the mouth and advanced past the larynx to inspect the bronchus, through the right main, the middle lobe, to the right lower lobe. After visualization of the bronchus, the alveolar lung tissue was sampled by irrigating with saline in small amounts. This was followed by carefully suctioning the fluid. The bronchoscope was removed.

Code(s):

ØB9F8ZX   **Drainage of Right Lower Lung Lobe, Via Natural or Artificial Opening Endoscopic, Diagnostic**

Rationale:

Bronchoscopy with alveolar lavage, or bronchoalveolar lavage, is a diagnostic procedure that uses repeated instillation and aspiration of lavage fluid to target specific smaller alveolar airways, which are lung tissue. The intent is to obtain cells and noncellular components such as airway secretions from the epithelial surface of the lower respiratory tract for microbiological, cytological, or immunological analysis.

Bronchoalveolar lavage can be found in the ICD-10-PCS Index to Procedures under the main term Lavage, subterm bronchial alveolar, diagnostic see Drainage, Respiratory System 0B9. Alternatively, it can also be found at the main term BAL (bronchial alveolar lavage), diagnostic see Drainage, Respiratory System ØB9.

Root Operation		
Drainage (9)	Definition:	Taking or letting out fluids and/or gases from a body part
	Explanation:	The qualifier DIAGNOSTIC is used to identify drainage procedures that are biopsies

Refer to ICD-10-PCS table 0B9 to complete the code. As BAL involves washing out and sampling alveoli of the lung, the lung body part values capture the objective of the procedure. In this case, the furthest anatomical site reached is the body part alveolar (lung) tissue of the Lower Lung Lobe, Right (F), and is consistent with ICD-10-PCS guideline B4.1c, which states: "If a procedure is performed on a continuous section of a tubular body part, code the body part value corresponding to the furthest anatomical site from the point of entry."

The procedure is performed via a bronchoscope inserted through the nose or oral cavity, so the approach is Via Natural or Artificial Opening Endoscopic (8). Sixth character Z is assigned for the device value, as no devices remain at the end of the procedure. Seventh-character qualifier Diagnostic (X) is required, as the intent of the BAL is diagnostic, obtained for microbiological, cytological, or immunological analysis.

Branches of Body Parts

Guideline B4.2

B4.2	Where a specific branch of a body part does not have its own body part value in PCS, the body part is typically coded to the closest proximal branch that has a specific body part value. In the cardiovascular body systems, if a general body part is available in the correct root operation table, and coding to a proximal branch would require assigning a code in a different body system, the procedure is coded using the general body part value.
	Examples: A procedure performed on the mandibular branch of the trigeminal nerve is coded to the trigeminal nerve body part value.
	Occlusion of the bronchial artery is coded to the body part value Upper Artery in the body system Upper Arteries, and not to the body part value Thoracic Aorta, Descending in the body system Heart and Great Vessels.

AHA Coding Clinic

2018, 2Q, 18   Transverse Rectus Abdominis Myocutaneous (TRAM) Delay

2017, 4Q, 46-55 New and Revised Body Part Values

2016, 4Q, 86   Coronary and Peripheral Artery Bifurcation

2016, 4Q, 97   Phrenic Neurostimulator

2016, 4Q, 134   Changes to the ICD-10-PCS Official Guidelines for Coding and Reporting

2016, 1Q, 23   Endoscopic Ultrasound with Aspiration Biopsy of Common Hepatic Duct

2015, 3Q, 28   Bilateral Renal Artery Bypass

2015, 1Q, 35   Evacuation of Hematoma for Control of Postprocedural Bleeding

Many branches of body parts, such as nerves, arteries, and veins do not have specific PCS body part values assigned to them. A thorough understanding of anatomy is needed in order to pair the closest proximal branch with a specific body part value. The Body Part Key (appendix D) and Body Part Definitions (appendix E) are useful resources for body part identification.

Practical Application for Guideline B4.2

Case Study 5.11. Open Reduction Internal Fixation (ORIF) and Repair of Digital Nerve Laceration

Preoperative Diagnosis: Closed intraarticular fracture of the right proximal 5th metatarsal head.

Postoperative Diagnosis: Closed intraarticular fracture of the right proximal 5th metatarsal head and partially transected dorsal digital nerve, right great toe.

Procedure Note: The patient was placed on the fracture table and all extremities were well padded, including all bony prominences. The right leg was prepped and draped in usual sterile fashion. A dorsal incision was made just distal to the right metatarsal head. This was carried down sharply through the skin to the metatarsal joint. The fracture was reduced and alignment confirmed by C-arm image followed by placement of two interfragmentary screws.

After repairing the metatarsal head fracture, the surgical wound was extended and explored to examine the foot for any additional injuries not seen on the x-rays. All tendons and muscles were intact; however, a partial transection of the right great toe dorsal digital nerve was identified. This transection was approximately 1.5 cm in length with jagged edges from what appeared to be a tearing motion. The cleaned edges were debrided, irrigated, and repaired nicely without creating tension on the nerve itself. The nerve was repaired with five sutures of self-absorbing Lycra with overlaid mattress sutures for extra stability. All wounds were irrigated with saline and the patient's wounds approximated, soft dressings applied, and the patient transferred to the recovery area.

Code(s):

0QSN04Z	Reposition Right Metatarsal with Internal Fixation Device, Open Approach
01QH0ZZ	Repair Peroneal Nerve, Open Approach

Rationale:

Two codes are needed to capture the full extent of this procedure. The fracture was reduced, meeting the root operation definition of Reposition (S), and the nerve was repaired, which meets the root operation definition of Repair (Q).

Root Operation		
Reposition (S)	Definition:	Moving to its normal location, or other suitable location, all or a portion of a body part
	Explanation:	The body part is moved to a new location from an abnormal location, or from a normal location where it is not functioning correctly. The body part may or may not be cut out or off to be moved to the new location.
Repair (Q)	Definition:	Restoring, to the extent possible, a body part to its normal anatomic structure and function
	Explanation:	Used only when the method to accomplish the repair is not one of the other root operations

The Metatarsal, Right (N) bone found in the Lower Bones (Q) body system was reduced, which meets the root operation Reposition (S) as outlined in the following guideline B3.15. An Open (0) approach was used since an incision was made through many layers. The screws that were placed meet the definition of an Internal Fixation Device (4).

PCS Guideline
Reposition for fracture treatment
B3.15   Reduction of a displaced fracture is coded to the root operation Reposition and the application of a cast or splint in conjunction with the Reposition procedure is not coded separately. Treatment of a nondisplaced fracture is coded to the procedure performed. *Example:* Casting of a nondisplaced fracture is coded to the root operation Immobilization in the Placement section. Putting a pin in a nondisplaced fracture is coded to the root operation Insertion.

The second code needed is for the Repair (Q) of the dorsal digital nerve. No body part value exists for dorsal digital nerve so the user must consult foot anatomy to determine the closest nerve branch that does have a body part value. PCS includes two main body part values for foot nerves: Tibial Nerve (G) and Peroneal Nerve (H). According to PCS Body Part Definitions, found in appendix E, the following nerves are included in each body part value:

Tibial Nerve (G)	Peroneal Nerve (H)
Lateral plantar nerve	Common fibular nerve
Medial plantar nerve	Common peroneal nerve
Medial popliteal nerve	External popliteal nerve
Medial sural cutaneous nerve	Lateral sural cutaneous nerve

Since dorsal digital nerve is not listed in the Body Part Definitions or Body Part Key, the user must refer to anatomical knowledge or references to differentiate between these two body part values. Anatomically, the tibial nerve supplies sensation to the plantar (sole) side while the peroneal provides sensation to the dorsal side of the foot. In this example, the Peroneal Nerve (H) from the Peripheral Nervous (1) body system is the appropriate body part value as it provides sensation to the dorsal side of the great toe.

Spotlight
A solid knowledge of anatomy and access to accurate anatomy references are important in applying ICD-10-PCS codes. This is especially vital in understanding guidelines B4.1b and B4.2, which relate to the concepts of "peri" and "branches" of body parts.

Case Study 5.12. Digital Nerve Repair

The right palmar index finger laceration was opened and extended proximally and distally in a zig-zag manner to facilitate wound exposure. The skin flaps were dissected with a #15 blade and were held in position with interrupted 4-0 nylon sutures. The subcutaneous tissues were gently dissected and the proximal and distal aspects of the palmar nerve were identified. There was found to be a 100 percent transection of this nerve.

At this point, the operating room microscope was brought into the field, and the remaining portion of the operation was performed under the microscope. Proximal and distal nerve ends were identified and released from all adjacent soft tissue structures. The proximal and distal ends were subsequently transected to create fresh edges for suturing. A primary end-to-end epineurial repair was performed at the nerve utilizing interrupted 9-0 nylon suture. At the end of the repair, the nerve was found to be in excellent approximation. Two small pieces of Gelfoam were placed around the nerve coaptation site.

The tourniquet was deflated. Bleeding points were controlled with direct pressure and hand elevation. The skin was closed in one layer with interrupted 5-0 Prolene suture. Antibiotic ointment was applied to the incision line.

Code(s):

Ø1Q5ØZZ   Repair Median Nerve, Open Approach

Rationale:

The palmar nerve of the right index finger was sutured in this example. The root operation definitions table shown after the illustration confirms that Repair (Q) is the correct root operation since no other root operation is appropriate to reflect the objective of this procedure. Since no body part value exists for palmar nerve, the user must find the closest proximal branch with a defined body part value. The median nerve contains the palmar cutaneous branch, which provides cutaneous innervation to the palmar aspect of the thumb, index and middle fingers, and the radial half of the ring finger. Therefore, the Median Nerve (5), found in the Peripheral Nervous (1) body system, is coded. The approach is Open (Ø); No Device (Z) and No Qualifier (Z) are the only options listed in the Repair (Q) table.

Figure 5.7. Palmar Nerve Branches

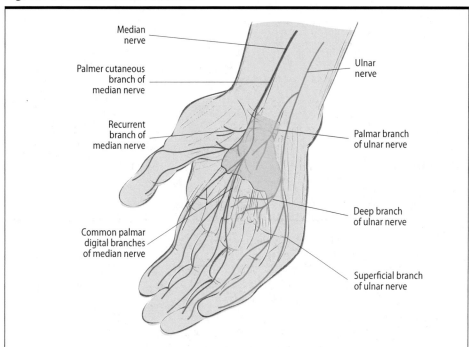

Root Operation		
Repair (Q)	Definition:	Restoring, to the extent possible, a body part to its normal anatomic structure and function
	Explanation:	Used only when the method to accomplish the repair is not one of the other root operations

Case Study 5.13. Nerve Graft

Indication: Lingual nerve transection that occurred during third molar surgery performed three months ago that did not respond to primary lingual nerve repair.

Procedure: Using a paralingual mucosal incision, the lingual nerve was explored and a symptomatic neuroma was identified and resected resulting in a 9 mm nerve gap. An interpositional graft was performed with harvest of the medial sural nerve. Tension-free repair was completed. The patient tolerated the procedure well.

Code(s):

ØØBKØZZ	**Excision of Trigeminal Nerve, Open Approach**
ØØUKØ7Z	**Supplement Trigeminal Nerve with Autologous Tissue Substitute, Open Approach**
Ø1BGØZZ	**Excision of Tibial Nerve, Open Approach**

Rationale:

Third molar (wisdom tooth) surgery is the most common cause of lingual nerve injuries. The injuries are usually transient; however, if no improvement is noted within a few months, surgical options may be considered.

Figure 5.8. Lingual Nerve

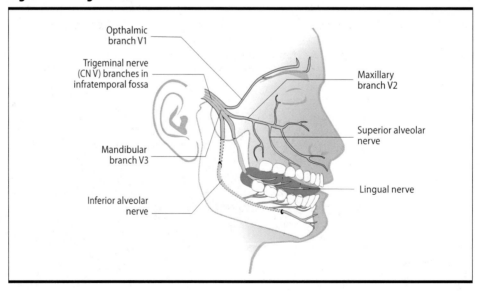

Opthalmic branch V1

Trigeminal nerve (CN V) branches in infratemporal fossa

Maxillary branch V2

Superior alveolar nerve

Mandibular branch V3

Lingual nerve

Inferior alveolar nerve

In this example, a symptomatic neuroma was also noted and removed. Excision (B) is the appropriate root operation since only a portion of the lingual nerve was removed. The PCS Index for Excision, Nerve does not list an option for lingual nerve. Additionally, the Body Part Key (appendix D) does not have a listing. Guideline B4.2 says to use the closest proximal branch that has a body part value. The lingual nerve is a branch of the mandibular division of the Trigeminal Nerve (K) found in the Central Nervous System and Cranial Nerves (Ø) body system. An incision was made in order to perform the procedure, which meets the approach definition of Open (Ø). There was no indication that the neuroma was removed for diagnostic purposes, so No Device (Z) is the appropriate seventh character.

Definition
neuroma. Any type of tumor growing from a nerve or comprised of nerve cells and fibers.

A second code is needed to capture the graft procedure. There is no option currently for Replacement (R) in the Central Nervous System and Cranial Nerves (Ø) body system presumably because the whole nerve can't be replaced. There is an option for Repair (Q), however, Supplement (U) is the appropriate root operation. The root operation Supplement (U) contains a specific device value for the autologous tissue graft making it a more appropriate choice. In addition, the examples provided for Supplement (U) in the root operation definitions (see appendix C) refer to a free nerve graft.

Spotlight
AHA Coding Clinic, 2017, 2Q, 21 and 2015, 1Q, 28 both state, "In ICD-10-PCS, the root operation 'Supplement' can function where needed as a 'Repair with device NEC' option, when a more specific code is not available."

A graft involves putting in biological or living material to reinforce or augment a body part or, according to the ICD-10-PCS definitions, Supplement (U). The graft is used to reinforce or augment the lingual nerve, which is coded as Trigeminal Nerve (K) contained in the Central Nervous System and Cranial Nerves (Ø) body system. The medial sural nerve harvested from the patient is an Autologous Tissue Substitute (7).

A third code is required for the harvesting of the medial sural nerve. According to guideline B3.9, if an excision is performed to obtain an autograft, a separate procedure is reported.

PCS Guideline
Excision for graft
B3.9 If an autograft is obtained from a different procedure site in order to complete the objective of the procedure, a separate procedure is coded. *Example:* Coronary bypass with excision of saphenous vein graft, excision of saphenous vein is coded separately.

The appropriate root operation is Excision (B) since only a portion of the medial sural nerve is harvested. The medial sural nerve is a branch off the tibial nerve, originating just below the knee and extending down the back of the leg and is commonly used for grafting procedures. Along with the lateral sural nerve, which branches off the peroneal nerve, these nerves provide sensation to the lateral portion of the calf, ankle, foot, and heel. In the Peripheral Nervous System (1) table for Excision (B), there is no specific character for the medial sural nerve. Guideline B4.2 directs the user to select Tibial Nerve (G) as the body part value since the medial sural nerve is a branch of the tibial nerve. This can also be determined by using the ICD-10-PCS Body Part Key found in appendix D.

Root Operation		
Supplement (U)	Definition:	Putting in or on biological or synthetic material that physically reinforces and/or augments the function of a portion of a body part
	Explanation:	The biological material is non-living, or is living and from the same individual. The body part may have been previously replaced, and the SUPPLEMENT procedure is performed to physically reinforce and/or augment the function of the replaced body part.
Excision (B)	Definition:	Cutting out or off, without replacement, a portion of a body part
	Explanation:	The qualifier DIAGNOSTIC is used to identify excision procedures that are biopsies

Beyond the Guidelines

Body Parts Nearby Other Body Parts

Documentation may contain a certain portion of a body part using terminology related to another nearby body part. For example, the documentation may specify the "prostatic urethra," meaning the portion of the urethra that is near/through the prostate, not a portion of the prostate itself. Refer to the illustration below of the male urinary system. The prostatic urethra is that portion of the urethra that passes through the prostate.

Figure 5.9. Prostatic Urethra

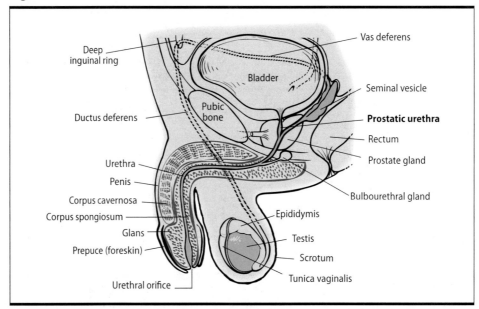

Case Study 5.14. Repair, Prostatic Urethra Stricture

Indications: Prostatic urethra stricture due to fibrosis from past history of radiotherapy.

The patient was placed in the high lithotomy position and a midline perineal incision was made. The bulbospongiosus muscle was dissected away from the corpus spongiosum. Dissection was completed to the urethra. The fibrotic column of the strictured urethra was followed as far as possible. The urethra was marked at the distal level of the defect and transected. The transected distal part of the urethra was spatulated after removal of all fibrosis. The residual fibrosis at the proximal (prostatic) end of the urethra was removed layer by layer with curved scissors until the open, healthy urethra was reached. A spatulated end-to-end anastomosis was made with eight interrupted polyglycolic 3x0 sutures between the prostatic urethra and the proximal bulbar urethra.

Code(s):

ØTBDØZZ   Excision of Urethra, Open Approach

Rationale:

The objective of the procedure was to remove the area of the urethra that was strictured due to fibrotic blockage and to reconnect it. Only a portion of the prostatic urethra was removed, not the full urethra, making Excision (B) rather than Resection (T) the correct root operation.

Root Operation		
Excision (B)	Definition:	Cutting out or off, without replacement, a portion of a body part
	Explanation:	The qualifier DIAGNOSTIC is used to identify excision procedures that are biopsies
Resection (T)	Definition:	Cutting out or off, without replacement, all of a body part
	Explanation:	None

The body part is referred to as the prostatic urethra because this part of the urethra passes through the prostate. The appropriate body part value is still part of the Urethra (D) in the Urinary System (T). An Open (Ø) approach was used with No Device (Z) and No Qualifier (Z). According to guideline B3.1b, the anastomosis is considered inherent to the procedure and is not coded separately.

PCS Guideline
General guidelines
B3.1b   Components of a procedure specified in the root operation definition and explanation are not coded separately. Procedural steps necessary to reach the operative site and close the operative site, including anastomosis of a tubular body part, are also not coded separately.
Example: Resection of a joint as part of a joint replacement procedure is included in the root operation definition of Replacement and is not coded separately.
Laparotomy performed to reach the site of an open liver biopsy is not coded separately. In a resection of sigmoid colon with anastomosis of descending colon to rectum, the anastomosis is not coded separately.

Bilateral Body Part Values

Guideline B4.3

B4.3	**Bilateral body part values are available for a limited number of body parts. If the identical procedure is performed on contralateral body parts, and a bilateral body part value exists for that body part, a single procedure is coded using the bilateral body part value. If no bilateral body part value exists, each procedure is coded separately using the appropriate body part value.**
	Example: **The identical procedure performed on both fallopian tubes is coded once using the body part value Fallopian Tube, Bilateral.**
	The identical procedure performed on both knee joints is coded twice using the body part values Knee Joint, Right and Knee Joint, Left.

AHA Coding Clinic

2017, 1Q, 18	Sutureless Repair of Pulmonary Vein Stenosis
2017, 1Q, 20	Preparatory Nasal Adhesion Repair Before Definitive Cleft Palate Repair
2017, 1Q, 21	Staged Scoliosis Surgery with Iliac Fixation and Spinal Fusion
2016, 3Q, 20	Excisional Debridement of Sacrum

PCS recognizes that there are many procedures that are routinely performed on bilateral body parts. For those procedures (and their corresponding root operations), bilateral body part values were developed. In most cases, a single body part value is also available when the procedure is performed unilaterally. Refer to table ØTM below; body part values are available for Right, Left, and Bilateral Kidneys and Right, Left, and Bilateral Ureters.

Ø	**Medical and Surgical**		
T	**Urinary System**		
M	**Reattachment**	Definition: Putting back in or on all or a portion of a separated body part to its normal location or other suitable location	

Body Part Character 4	Approach Character 5	Device Character 6	Qualifier Character 7
Ø Kidney, Right 1 Kidney, Left 2 Kidneys, Bilateral 3 Kidney Pelvis, Right 4 Kidney Pelvis, Left 6 Ureter, Right 7 Ureter, Left 8 Ureters, Bilateral B Bladder C Bladder Neck D Urethra	Ø Open 4 Percutaneous Endoscopic	Z No Device	Z No Qualifier

Guideline B4.3 states that when a bilateral body part value is available, the single bilateral value should be coded. However, it is necessary to report two codes if the procedure is performed on both sides and a bilateral option is not available.

Practical Application for Guideline B4.3

Case Study 5.15. Ligation, Vas Deferens, Bilateral

A male patient was admitted for a percutaneous bilateral ligation of the vas deferens. Using a percutaneous puncture approach, the bilateral vas deferens was isolated and ligatures applied.

Code(s):

ØVLQ3ZZ   **Occlusion of Bilateral Vas Deferens, Percutaneous Approach**

Rationale:

The vas deferens is a muscular tube in the male reproductive system that carries sperm from the epididymis to the urethra. Although many procedures can be performed on tubular body parts, there are four root operations that, by definition, can only be performed on tubular body parts: Bypass (1), Dilation (7), Occlusion (L), and Restriction (V).

Root Operation		
Bypass (1)	Definition:	Altering the route of passage of the contents of a tubular body part
	Explanation:	Rerouting contents of a body part to a downstream area of the normal route, to a similar route and body part, or to an abnormal route and dissimilar body part. Includes one or more anastomoses, with or without the use of a device.
Dilation (7)	Definition:	Expanding an orifice or the lumen of a tubular body part
	Explanation:	The orifice can be a natural orifice or an artificially created orifice. Accomplished by stretching a tubular body part using intraluminal pressure or by cutting part of the orifice or wall of the tubular body part
Occlusion (L)	Definition:	Completely closing an orifice or lumen of a tubular body part
	Explanation:	The orifice can be a natural orifice or an artificially created orifice
Restriction (V)	Definition:	Partially closing an orifice or the lumen of a tubular body part
	Explanation:	The orifice can be a natural orifice or an artificially created orifice

In this example, the vas deferens was completely closed off with the ligatures, so Occlusion (L) is the appropriate root operation to use. The PCS index lists Occlusion, Vas Deferens with three options: Bilateral (ØVLQ), Left (ØVLP), and Right (ØVLN). Since bilateral was stated in the case study and a body part value for bilateral exists, only the one code should be reported. Review of code ØVLQ found in the Male Reproductive (V) body system confirms the body part Vas Deferens, Bilateral (Q). A Percutaneous (3) approach was used along with No Device (Z) as per guideline B6.1b and No Qualifier (Z).

PCS Guideline
General Guidelines
B6.1b   Materials such as sutures, ligatures, radiological markers and temporary post-operative wound drains are considered integral to the performance of a procedure and are not coded as devices.

Case Study 5.16. Removal, Ureteral Stones

The patient was given a general laryngeal mask anesthetic and prepped and draped in the lithotomy position. A semirigid ureteroscope was passed through the bladder and into the right ureter to the level of the obstructing stone. The stone in the distal ureter was targeted and engaged with the holmium laser and a 20-micrometer fiber with a maximum energy of 5 watts. The stone was fragmented and retrieved using a stone basket. A similar procedure was carried out on the left side with the stone in the ureter fragmented and removed with a basket. The ureteroscope was removed and the patient was transferred to the recovery room in good condition.

Code(s):

0TC68ZZ	Extirpation of Matter from Right Ureter, Via Natural or Artificial Opening Endoscopic
0TC78ZZ	Extirpation of Matter from Left Ureter, Via Natural or Artificial Opening Endoscopic

Rationale:

Ureteroscopes are used to look inside the ureters and kidneys. It has an eyepiece at one end, a rigid or flexible tube in the middle, and a tiny lens and light at the other end of the tube. Additionally, small instruments can be inserted through the ureteroscope to treat problems in the ureter or kidney or to perform a biopsy.

Figure 5.10. Ureteroscope

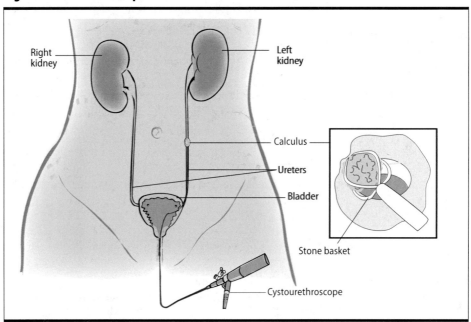

In this example, stones in both the right and left ureter were fragmented with a laser and removed with a stone basket. *AHA Coding Clinic,* 2015, 2Q, 7 provides guidance as to the appropriate root operation to use, stating that Extirpation (C) is coded when solid matter has been removed and that fragmentation is inherent to the Extirpation (C).

Root Operation		
Extirpation (C)	Definition:	Taking or cutting out solid matter from a body part
	Explanation:	The solid matter may be an abnormal byproduct of a biological function or a foreign body; it may be imbedded in a body part or in the lumen of a tubular body part. The solid matter may or may not have been previously broken into pieces.

Ureter, Right (6) and Ureter, Left (7) are found in the Urinary (T) body system. Although Ureters, Bilateral (8) is available in other tables in the Urinary System body system, no bilateral body part value exists in table ØTC, so a code for each ureter needs to be reported. The ureteroscope was inserted directly through the urethra and since the scope allows for visualization of the ureters, Via Natural or Artificial Opening Endoscopic (8) is the appropriate approach to use. No Device (Z) and No Qualifier (Z) are the only options available for the sixth and seventh characters, respectively.

Case Study 5.17. Orchiopexy

Procedure: Bilateral orchiopexy performed for undescended testicles.

The patient was placed in the supine position and prepped and draped in the usual manner. A 0.25% Marcaine was infiltrated subcutaneously in the skin crease in the left groin in the area of the intended incision. An inguinal incision was made through this area, carried through the subcutaneous tissues to the anterior fascia. The left testicle was isolated and found in a superficial pouch of the inguinal canal. Adequate length was achieved without causing too much tension on the spermatic vessels. Using blunt and sharp dissection, a tunnel was made down into the scrotum. An incision was made in the scrotal wall and a dartos pouch was developed. A straight clamp was passed retrograde with one finger guiding the point up into the inguinal incision. A 3-0 Prolene suture was placed through the testicle and used to draw the testicle down through the scrotal pouch outside the scrotum. The inguinal incision was closed in layers and 0.25% Marcaine was infiltrated around the incision, 3-0 chromic catgut was used to close the incision in layers without difficulty, and the skin was closed with interrupted sutures of 4-0 chromic catgut. The scrotal incision was closed with interrupted sutures of 4-0 chromic catgut and a benzoin-soaked bolster was tied to the Prolene sutures that had been placed through the scrotal wall with separate Keith needles. Attention was turned to the right side, where an orchiopexy was performed in a similar fashion. The right testicle was located in a superficial pouch of the inguinal canal and there was adequate length on the spermatic cord. The sub dartos pouch was created in a similar fashion and the wounds were closed similarly as well. At the end of the procedure, collodion was applied over the abdominal incision. The patient was sent to the recovery room in stable condition.

Code(s):

ØVSCØZZ　　**Reposition Bilateral Testes, Open Approach**

Rationale:

Orchiopexy is the surgical fixation of an undescended testicle into the scrotum. This procedure is most often performed in male infants or very young children. In adults, orchiopexy is most often done to treat testicular torsion. A thorough review of the operative report is needed in order to assign the correct root operation. Reposition (S) is used when undescended testicles are moved into the scrotum; Repair (Q) is used when the procedure is done to prevent torsion.

Root Operation		
Reposition (S)	Definition:	Moving to its normal location, or other suitable location, all or a portion of a body part
	Explanation:	The body part is moved to a new location from an abnormal location, or from a normal location where it is not functioning correctly. The body part may or may not be cut out or off to be moved to the new location.
Repair (Q)	Definition:	Restoring, to the extent possible, a body part to its normal anatomic structure and function
	Explanation:	Used only when the method to accomplish the repair is not one of the other root operations

In this example, Reposition (S) is the correct root operation since the testes were moved into the scrotum. The Male Reproductive (V) body system contains values for Testis, Right (9), Testis, Left (B), and Testes, Bilateral (C). When assigning the fourth character identifying the body part, the user must note the laterality. Because the same root operation was performed on the right and left side, and a bilateral value exists, one code using Testes, Bilateral (C) is correct rather than two separate codes identifying the right and left sides.

Incisions were made in the groin for an Open (Ø) approach. No Device (Z) and No Qualifier (Z) are used.

Case Study 5.18. Blepharoplasty, Cosmetic

Procedure: Bilateral cosmetic blepharoplasty.

With the patient in the supine position, the eyelid region to be resected was identified and marked in an elliptical fashion with a sterile marking pen. Lidocaine and epinephrine were injected into each upper eyelid. A #15 blade was used to cut through the skin of the eyelid tissue to be removed in the right eye. The surgical calipers were used to measure the supratarsal incisions so that the incision was symmetrical from the ciliary margin bilaterally. The previously outlined excessive skin of the right upper eyelid was excised with blunt dissection. Hemostasis was obtained with a bipolar cautery.

A thin strip of orbicularis oculi muscle was excised in order to expose the orbital septum on the right. Herniated orbital fat was exposed. The protruding fat in the medial pocket was carefully excised and the stalk meticulously cauterized with the bipolar cautery unit. Excess orbicularis oculi was resected.

The lateral aspect of the upper eyelid incision was closed utilizing interrupted 6-0 Prolene sutures by incorporating skin and orbicularis on the inferior portion and skin on the superior portion of the interrupted suture. A simple running suture was passed through skin, utilizing a 6-0 Prolene suture.

The same procedure was performed for the patient on the left eye, removing skin and taking care of the herniated fat. Careful hemostasis was obtained on the upper lid areas. At the end of the operation, the patient's vision and extraocular muscle movements were checked and found to be intact.

Code(s):
Ø8ØNØZZ   **Alteration of Right Upper Eyelid, Open Approach**

Ø8ØPØZZ   **Alteration of Left Upper Eyelid, Open Approach**

Rationale:
Blepharoplasty, also known as eyelid lift, is a plastic surgery of the eyelids to remove excess fat and redundant skin weighing down the lid. The eyelid is pulled tight and sutured to support sagging muscles. It is most often done for cosmetic reasons, but may also be done to improve the sight of patients whose sagging upper eyelids obscure their vision.

The PCS index for Blepharoplasty lists *see* Repair, Eye Ø8Q; *see* Replacement, Eye Ø8R; *see* Reposition, Eye Ø8S; and *see* Supplement, Eye Ø8U. In this case, however, the procedure was done for a cosmetic reason, which meets the root operation definition of Alteration (Ø).

Spotlight
The ICD-10-PCS Index can be used to access the tables. It is organized alphabetically by the root operation (third character) or by common procedural terms. The index is a frame of reference only and the full intent of a procedure must be understood in order to assign the appropriate root operation. Convention A7 states, "It is not required to consult the index first before proceeding to the tables to complete the code. A valid code may be chosen directly from the tables." Common terms such as fasciotomy, osteotomy, and laminectomy may be assigned to additional root operations other than those identified in the index. The root operation assigned should be based on the procedure performed as described in the complete documentation contained in the operative report and not simply on a single descriptive term in the operative report.

Alteration (Ø) is the correct root operation for all procedures performed solely to improve appearance. All methods, approaches, and devices used for the objective of improving appearance are coded here. Therefore, only one root operation is coded.

Root Operation		
Alteration (Ø)	Definition:	Modifying the anatomic structure of a body part without affecting the function of the body part
	Explanation:	Principal purpose is to improve appearance

The Eye (8) body system does not list a bilateral upper eyelid value; therefore, two codes are needed to capture this procedure: one for Upper Eyelid, Right (N) and one for Upper Eyelid, Left (P). The approach is Open (Ø) with No Device (Z) and No Qualifier (Z).

Spotlight
Because some surgical procedures can be performed for medical or cosmetic purposes, coding for Alteration (Ø) requires diagnostic confirmation that the surgery was in fact performed to improve appearance.

Coronary Arteries

Guideline B4.4

B4.4	**The coronary arteries are classified as a single body part that is further specified by number of arteries treated. One procedure code specifying multiple arteries is used when the same procedure is performed, including the same device and qualifier values.**

Examples: **Angioplasty of two distinct coronary arteries with placement of two stents is coded as Dilation of Coronary Artery, Two Arteries with Two Intraluminal Devices.**

Angioplasty of two distinct coronary arteries, one with stent placed and one without, is coded separately as Dilation of Coronary Artery, One Artery with Intraluminal Device, and Dilation of Coronary Artery, One Artery with no device.

AHA Coding Clinic

2018, 2Q, 24	Coronary Artery Bifurcation
2017, 4Q, 35	Release of Myocardial Bridge
2016, 4Q, 82	Coronary Artery, Number of Arteries
2016, 4Q, 84	Coronary Artery, Number of Stents
2016, 4Q, 86	Coronary and Peripheral Artery Bifurcation

Note: The following were written before the phrase "number of sites" was replaced with "number of arteries."

2016, 3Q, 36	Type of Contrast Medium for Angiography (High Osmolar, Low Osmolar, and, Other)
2016, 1Q, 27	Aortocoronary Bypass Graft Utilizing Y-Graft
2015, 3Q, 9	Failed Attempt to Treat Coronary Artery Occlusion
2015, 3Q, 10	Coronary Angioplasty with Unsuccessful Stent Insertion
2015, 2Q, 3	Coronary Artery Intervention Site
2014, 2Q, 4	Coronary Angioplasty of Bypassed Vessel

Beginning with the FY 2017 version of ICD-10-PCS, the coronary body part values and guideline B4.4 were reworded with a very important distinction, changing the focus from the number of sites treated to the number of **arteries** treated. This change in wording impacts all previous instructions that were released prior to the third quarter of 2016, including *AHA Coding Clinic.* Since much of the advice contained within the *AHA Coding Clinic* is still relevant, they are still listed in this chapter. Users should take care to use the advice of the newly worded guideline when applying these *AHA Coding Clinic.*

New device values indicating the number of stents placed were also added for FY 2017. This change, in addition to counting the number of arteries rather than sites, offers more accurate data collection. The number of distinctly separate arteries that are included in the coronary artery body parts plus the number of stents used to treat those arteries are now accounted for.

Root Operation (Character 3)

Coronary artery body part values in PCS are offered in a limited number of root operation tables. The tables include Bypass, Dilation, Extirpation, Replace, Repair, and Reposition in the Medical Surgical section and Extirpation in the New Technology section. **Note:** Reposition only offers Coronary Artery, One Artery (Ø) and Coronary Artery, Two Arteries (1).

Root Operation		
Bypass (1)	Definition:	Altering the route of passage of the contents of a tubular body part
	Explanation:	Rerouting contents of a body part to a downstream area of the normal route, to a similar route and body part, or to an abnormal route and dissimilar body part. Includes one or more anastomoses, with or without the use of a device.
Dilation (7)	Definition:	Expanding an orifice or the lumen of a tubular body part
	Explanation:	The orifice can be a natural orifice or an artificially created orifice. Accomplished by stretching a tubular body part using intraluminal pressure or by cutting part of the orifice or wall of the tubular body part.
Extirpation (C)	Definition:	Taking or cutting out solid matter from a body part
	Explanation:	The solid matter may be an abnormal byproduct of a biological function or a foreign body; it may be imbedded in a body part or in the lumen of a tubular body part. The solid matter may or may not have been previously broken into pieces.
Release (N)	Definition:	Freeing a body part from an abnormal physical constraint by cutting or by the use of force
	Explanation:	Some of the restraining tissue may be taken out but none of the body part is taken out
Repair (Q)	Definition:	Restoring, to the extent possible, a body part to its normal anatomic structure and function
	Explanation:	Used only when the method to accomplish the repair is not one of the other root operations
Reposition (S)	Definition:	Moving to its normal location, or other suitable location, all or a portion of a body part
	Explanation:	The body part is moved to a new location from an abnormal location, or from a normal location where it is not functioning correctly. The body part may or may not be cut out or off to be moved to the new location.

Guideline B4.4 focuses on Dilation procedures that are interchangeably documented as percutaneous transluminal coronary angioplasty (PTCA) or percutaneous coronary intervention (PCI). PTCA or PCI refers to the treatment of stenosed or blocked coronary arteries using arterial catheters that deliver balloons and/or stents to the site of the culprit lesions to dilate the lumen of the artery and restore blood flow.

Definition
lumen. Interior space of a tubular body part such as an artery or intestine.

Body Part (Character 4)

The coronary artery body part values in PCS are listed by the number of coronary arteries treated instead of by individual coronary arteries.

PCS Coronary Artery Body Part Values
0 Coronary Artery, One Artery
1 Coronary Artery, Two Arteries
2 Coronary Artery, Three Arteries
3 Coronary Artery, Four or More Arteries

When counting the number of arteries treated, each individual artery of the coronary anatomy is considered a distinctly separate entity.

All coronary artery body part values are inclusive of main arteries such as:

- Left main coronary artery (LMCA) which divides into:

    - left anterior descending (LAD)

    - circumflex artery

    - also included are smaller branches such as:

        - left (obtuse) marginal (OM)

        - septal branch (SP)

        - left diagonal

- Right coronary artery (RCA) including:

    - right posterior descending

    - right posterolateral branch

    - right marginal

Figure 5.11. Coronary Arteries

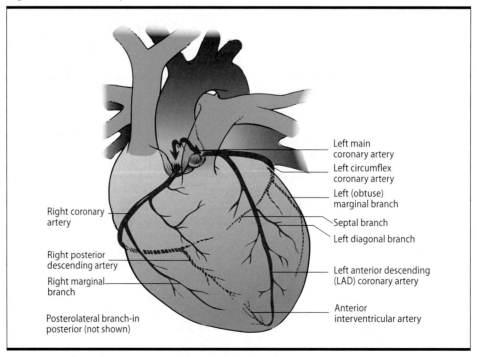

Device (Character 6)

Stents are represented as Intraluminal Devices in the sixth-character device value and are categorized in PCS by three types:

- Bare metal stent (BMS) is simply called Intraluminal Device, specified by the number of stents

- Drug-eluting stent (DES) is Intraluminal Device, Drug-eluting, specified by the number of stents

- Radioactive-eluting stent (Brachytherapy) is Intraluminal Device, Radioactive

The two types that are most commonly used are bare metal and drug-eluting. Radioactive stents were largely discontinued with the improvement of drug-eluting stents, although there is still research being conducted to determine any advantages or benefits of this technology.

Because it may be difficult to differentiate between bare metal and drug-eluting stents, two tables have been provided: one listing bare metal stents (BMS) and the other drug-eluting stents (DES) by common name, composition (material/drug type), and company (manufacturer).

Bare Metal Stent (BMS)

The first stents, referred to as bare metal stents (BMS), were approved in the mid-1990s. Since then, more than 25 different companies have developed and introduced bare metal stents using a variety of materials, such as nitinol, stainless steel, and cobalt chromium, with countless designs and sizes. Although still in use, bare metal stents comprise only a limited amount of the stents inserted today. Because it is necessary to adhere to a longer regiment of dual antiplatelet therapy with drug-eluting stent (DES) in comparison to the bare metal stent, it is reasonable to use the BMS in circumstances such as:

- Patients who are likely to be noncompliant with dual antiplatelet therapy

- Patients who require a noncardiac surgery within four to six weeks of implementation

- Patients with active bleeding or history of bleeding problems

Table 5.1. Intraluminal Device, Bare Metal

Name	Material	Company
Multi-link, Multi-link Vision, Multi-link Mini Vision	Cobalt Chromium	Abbott Vascular
Multi-link Ultra, Multi-Link Zeta	Stainless Steel	Abbott Vascular
Coroflex Blue, Coroflex Blue Ultra, Coroflex Blue Neo	Cobalt Chromium	B. Braun Melsungen AG
Coroflex	Stainless Steel	B. Braun Melsungen AG
Veriflex BMS	Stainless Steel	Boston Scientific
REBEL	Platinum Chromium	Boston Scientific
Integrity BMS	Cobalt Alloy	Medtronic Inc.
Driver BMS	Cobalt Chromium	Medtronic Inc.
MicroDriver BMS	Cobalt Chromium	Medtronic Inc.

Drug-Eluting Stent (DES)

The first drug-eluting stents, the Sirolimus-eluting stent (SES) and the Paclitaxel-eluting stent (PES), were approved in the USA in 2003 and 2004, respectively. Referred to as "first generation," the PES is no longer in use and the SES is rarely used in the United States. They have been replaced by thinner, more deliverable, and more biocompatible "second generation" stents: Everolimus-eluting stent (EES) and most recently Zotarolimus-eluting stent (ZES). The "second generation" stents cause less inflammation and promote more rapid healing than their predecessors.

Table 5.2. Intraluminal Device, Drug-eluting

Name	Drug Type	Company
Second Generation 2008-		
Xience Alpine, Xience Prime, Xience Xpedition	Everolimus (EES)—Cobalt Chromium	Abbott Vascular
SYNERGY™	Everolimus (EES) Platinum Chromium	Boston Scientific
Promus Element™ Plus, PREMIER™	Everolimus (EES) Platinum Chromium	Boston Scientific
ENDEAVOR®	Zotarolimus (E-ZES)	Medtronic Inc.
Resolute	Zotarolimus (R-ZES)	Medtronic Inc.
First Generation 2003-		
TAXUS (infrequently used in U.S.)	Paclitaxel (PES)	Boston Scientific
ION (infrequently used in U.S.)	Paclitaxel (PES)	Boston Scientific
Cypher (no longer avail in U.S.)	Sirolimus (SES)	Cordis/Johnson & Johnson

Figure 5.12. Coronary Artery Stent

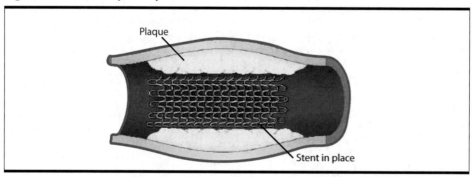

Plaque

Stent in place

Spotlight

The value No Device (Z) is used when balloon angioplasty is performed with no stent placement, often referred to as POBA (plain old balloon angioplasty).

Qualifier (Character 7)

The seventh-character qualifier offers the option of Bifurcation (6) for use when a treatment spans the area where two arteries join together. For PCS coding purposes, treatment on a single lesion spanning two arteries (bifurcation), such as a main and a branch of the main, is recognized as treating two separate arteries. The number of codes used to capture the treatment varies depending on whether the same root operation and device is used in both arteries. (*AHA Coding Clinics,* 2018, 2Q, 24; 2016, 4Q, 86-89)

Only one code is reported for treatment of a single lesion spanning two arteries if the procedure (e.g., dilation) and device type (e.g., drug-eluting stents) is the same in both arteries.

Example:

Dilation is performed on a lesion that extends from the LAD through the diagonal branch, with two drug-eluting stents, one in each artery. In this example, only one code is assigned:

0271356   **Dilation of Coronary Artery, Two Arteries, Bifurcation, with Two Drug-eluting Intraluminal Devices, Percutaneous Approach**

Two codes are reported for treatment of a single lesion spanning two arteries if a different device type is used in each artery.

Example:

The main LAD is treated with dilation with a drug-eluting stent and only balloon dilation (No Device) is performed in the diagonal branch. In this example, two codes are assigned:

0270346   **Dilation of Coronary Artery, One Artery, Bifurcation, with Drug-eluting Intraluminal Device, Percutaneous Approach**

02703ZZ   **Dilation of Coronary Artery, One Artery, Percutaneous Approach**

Guideline B4.4 provides advice to assist in the determination of how many codes to report depending on the number of arteries treated (fourth character) and types of devices used (sixth character). The following decision tree and examples with codes and rationales are provided to further clarify the advice.

Figure 5.13. Coronary Artery Dilation Decision Tree

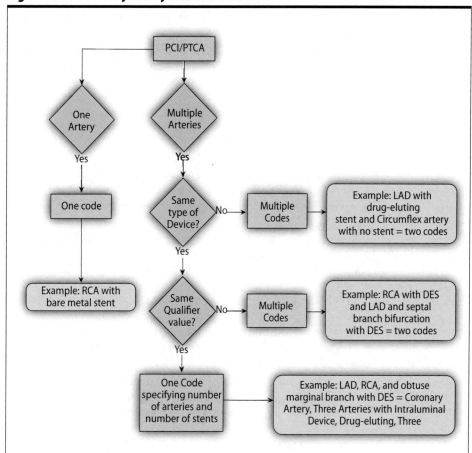

PCI/PTCA Examples for Guideline B4.4

Case Study 5.19. PTCA: One Coronary Artery, Multiple Stents

Procedure Note:
Right coronary artery treated with three bare metal stents.

Code(s):

02703FZ   **Dilation of Coronary Artery, One Artery with Three Intraluminal Devices, Percutaneous Approach**

Rationale:
One code is needed to report this procedure since only the right coronary artery was treated. The correct body part is Coronary Artery, One Artery (0) with device value Intraluminal Device, Three (F) for the placement of three bare metal stents.

Case Study 5.20. PTCA: Two Coronary Arteries, Single Stent

Procedure Note:
Left anterior descending artery (LAD) treated with a Medtronic Resolute stent and circumflex artery with plain old balloon angioplasty (POBA) and no stent.

Code(s):

027034Z   **Dilation of Coronary Artery, One Artery with Drug-eluting Intraluminal Device, Percutaneous Approach**

02703ZZ   **Dilation of Coronary Artery, One Artery, Percutaneous Approach**

Rationale:
Two codes are needed since the type of device or lack of device is different for each of the separate coronary arteries treated. Even though two specific arteries were treated, the body part value for Coronary Artery, One Artery (0) is reported twice: one coronary artery with the Intraluminal Device, Drug-eluting (4), which represents only one stent used, and one coronary artery treated with No Device (Z).

Consulting Table 5.2 shows that the Resolute stent by Medtronic is a Zotarolimus drug-eluting stent. Bifurcation is not mentioned and not reported.

Case Study 5.21. PTCA: Coronary Arteries with Bifurcation and Multiple Stents

Procedure Note:
Right coronary artery (RCA) treated with a drug-eluting stent (DES); bifurcation of the LAD and septal branch treated with two drug-eluting stents.

Code(s):

027034Z   **Dilation of Coronary Artery, One Artery with Drug-eluting Intraluminal Device, Percutaneous Approach**

0271356   **Dilation of Coronary Artery, Two Arteries, Bifurcation, with Two Drug-eluting Intraluminal Devices, Percutaneous Approach**

Rationale:
Even though the same device, drug-eluting stent, was used in all three arteries, qualifier value Bifurcation (6) was different, requiring the use of two codes. The first code represents one Intraluminal Device, Drug-eluting (4) placed into the RCA, Coronary Artery, One Artery (0). The second code includes a device value for the Intraluminal Device, Drug-eluting, Two (5) for the two stents placed into the Bifurcation (6), which is a different qualifier value requiring the additional code. Two arteries were involved in the stenting of the bifurcation, which is specified by Coronary Artery, Two Arteries (1).

Case Study 5.22. PTCA: Multiple Coronary Arteries and Stents

Procedure Note:
Left anterior descending (LAD), obtuse marginal branch of left coronary artery and right coronary artery (RCA) each treated with a drug-eluting stent.

Code(s):

0272360Z   **Dilation of Coronary Artery, Three Arteries with Three Drug-eluting Intraluminal Devices, Percutaneous Approach**

Rationale:
One code captures the three distinct arteries in the one body part value, Coronary Artery, Three Arteries (2) and all of the stents in the device value Intraluminal Device, Drug-eluting, Three (6).

Case Study 5.23. PTCA: Multiple Coronary Arteries, Different Treatments

Procedure Note:
Two bare metal stents placed in the RCA, the distal LAD treated with one drug-eluting stent, the diagonal branch treated with one drug-eluting stent, and plain old balloon angioplasty (POBA) performed on the distal septal branch.

Code(s):

02703EZ   **Dilation of Coronary Artery, One Artery with Two Intraluminal Devices, Percutaneous Approach**

0271355Z   **Dilation of Coronary Artery, Two Arteries with Two Drug-eluting Intraluminal Devices, Percutaneous Approach**

02703ZZ   **Dilation of Coronary Artery, One Artery, Percutaneous Approach**

Rationale:
Three codes are needed because there are three different device values used: Intraluminal Device, Two (E) for the bare metal stents; Intraluminal Device, Drug-eluting, Two (5) for the drug-eluting stents; and No Device (Z) for the POBA. Each different device value must be reported with the body part value that describes the number of arteries treated. Reporting these three codes indicates that four total arteries (RCA, LAD, diagonal branch, and distal septal branch) were treated and four stents used: two in the RCA, one each in the LAD and diagonal branch, and one artery did not use a device.

Case Study 5.24. PTCA: Two Coronary Arteries, Multiple Stents

Procedure Note:
Three drug-eluting stents placed into the mid left anterior descending artery (LAD) and another two DES placed into the mid circumflex artery.

Code(s):

0271377Z   **Dilation of Coronary Artery, Two Arteries with Four or More Drug-eluting Intraluminal Devices, Percutaneous Approach**

Rationale:
The body part Coronary Artery, Two Arteries (1) represents the two different arteries treated. Since all five drug-eluting stents placed in both arteries are the same PCS device type, the device value is reported as Intraluminal Device, Drug-eluting, Four or More (7). Only one code is necessary since it includes the number of arteries treated and the number of stents used.

Beyond the Guidelines

Other Cardiac Diagnostic and Interventional Procedures

AHA Coding Clinic

2018, 2Q, 24   Coronary Artery Bifurcation

2018, 1Q, 12   Percutaneous Balloon Valvuloplasty & Cardiac Catheterization with Ventriculogram

2016, 4Q, 86   Coronary and Peripheral Artery Bifurcation

2016, 4Q, 114   Fluorescence Vascular Angiography

2016, 3Q, 36   Type of Contrast Medium for Angiography (High Osmolar, Low Osmolar, and Other)

2016, 3Q, 37   Fractional Flow Reserve

Angiography using fluoroscopy is a procedure that is generally performed in conjunction with coronary artery dilation. This imaging procedure, coded using tables from the Imaging (B) section, assists with the diagnosis of stenosis or lesions, as well as safely guides the guidewires and catheters to the appropriate treatment site(s). Contrast agent, dye, or medium is injected into the arteries to enhance the visibility by delineating borders of the substances and matter within the arteries. Various types of contrast agents are used to enhance all types of X-rays, CT, and MR imaging. For coronary arteries, intra-arterial injections of contrast are used with fluoroscopy and require a higher rate of contrast administration.

Spotlight
Osmolality is the measure of how many particles are in a solution. High osmolar contrast agents are ionic compounds that dissociate (separate) in solution and have an osmolality that is five to eight times that of blood. Low osmolar contrast agents are nonionic compounds that are water soluble but do not separate, resulting in fewer particles in solution. Iso-osmolar contrasts have an osmolality equal to that of blood.

Contrast agents are classified by their osmolality: high, low, or iso-osmolar. High osmolar iodine (HOCM) as a radiocontrast agent was accidentally discovered in the 1920s when it was used to treat syphilis. Although it was widely used, it caused many side effects such as nausea, itching, and warmth. In the 1950s it was ascertained to cause acute kidney injury in some patients. The development of low osmolar (LOCM) in the 1980s and iso-osmolar (IOCM) in the 1990s diminished some of these adverse effects. High osmolar, although still used for some imaging, is not currently recommended for intravenous use due to its high risk of adverse effects. Contrast-induced nephropathy (CIN) is still a concern with all contrast mediums particularly when administered intra-arterially. Research suggests that certain patient populations are at higher risk, and best practice indicates use of lowest possible doses. The following table lists common contrast mediums along with the appropriate PCS value.

Table 5.3. Contrast

Scientific Name	Trade Name	Osmolality	PCS Value
iodixanol	Visipaque	Iso-osmolar	Other Contrast (Y)
iotrolan	Isovist	Iso-osmolar	Other Contrast (Y)
iohexol	Omnipaque	Low Osmolar	Low Osmolar (1)
iomeprol	Iomeron	Low Osmolar	Low Osmolar (1)
iopamidol	Isovue/Iopamiro	Low Osmolar	Low Osmolar (1)
iopromide	Ultravist	Low Osmolar	Low Osmolar (1)
ioversol	Optiray	Low Osmolar	Low Osmolar (1)
ioxaglate	Hexabrix	Low Osmolar	Low Osmolar (1)
ioxilan	Oxilan	Low Osmolar	Low Osmolar (1)
*diatrizoate	Hypaque	High Osmolar	High Osmolar (Ø)
*metrizoate	Isopaque	High Osmolar	High Osmolar (Ø)
*No longer used for coronary angiography.			

Case Study 5.25. PTCA: Percutaneous Transluminal Coronary Angioplasty

Findings:

Right coronary artery with some minimal disease in the midportion, but with a long segment 95 to 99 percent lesion in the distal portion and 90 percent in the midposterior descending branch of right coronary artery.

Left main coronary artery had no significant lesion.

Left anterior descending was 100 percent chronically occluded proximally after the first and second septal and first diagonal branch, status post single left internal mammary graft to left anterior descending.

Procedure:

1.   Left heart catheterization and coronary angiography.

2.   Left ventriculography.

3.   Placement of two sequential stents: 2.5 x 23-mm stent proximally with minimal overlap of a distal 2.5 x 18-mm long stent to RCA.

4.   POBA to midposterior descending branch of right.

The patient was brought to the cardiac catheterization laboratory and right groin prepped and draped in usual sterile manner. Femoral artery was punctured and with guidewire and fluoroscopy, a #6 French sheath advanced. French coronary Judkins diagnostic catheter was advanced to the aorta. The ostium of the right coronary artery was cannulated and three injections of 8 mL to 10 mL of Visipaque contrast were administered. The right coronary system was visualized and recorded. This catheter was replaced with a #6 French left coronary Judkins diagnostic catheter. Ostium of left coronary artery was selectively cannulated and several injections of 8 mL to 10 mL of contrast were given. Left coronary system was visualized and recorded. This catheter was replaced again by a #6 French right coronary Judkins catheter, which advanced easily to the left subclavian artery and selective cannulation of left internal mammary artery graft was done. Multiple injections with multiple views of the left internal mammary artery and insertion site to LAD and distal LAD were obtained. This catheter was removed and replaced by a #6 French pigtail catheter, which was advanced to the left ventricular cavity. Pressure tracings were recorded and left ventriculography obtained by injection of 36 mL of contrast in three seconds. This catheter was removed with pullback and pressure tracing recorded. It was determined that a balloon angioplasty and stent placement of right coronary artery was needed. A French 6 right coronary Judkins guiding catheter was advanced to the aorta and the ostium of the right coronary artery cannulated. A 0.014-inch wire was advanced with some difficulty across this high-grade subtotal long lesion to the distal right coronary artery. Angiomax for anticoagulation according to protocol based on the patient's body weight was given. A 2.5 x 20-mm long balloon was advanced across the lesion where multiple dilatations were performed, and the balloon was removed. Initially, a 2.5 x 23-mm and subsequently a 2.5 x 18-mm long ZES stents were placed in the area of lesion with minimal overlap and dilatation with maximum pressure of 14 atmospheres in both the stents, making the diameter of the stent to about 2.75 mm. The midposterior descending branch was deemed too small for stenting so POBA was performed with multiple inflations until the lumen was adequately dilated. The balloon was deflated and removed. Final injection showed excellent result with no residual lesion. The catheter was removed and the arterial puncture was sealed off with the use of Angio-Seal device.

Code(s):

027035Z	Dilation of Coronary Artery, One Artery with Two Drug-eluting Intraluminal Devices, Percutaneous Approach
02703ZZ	Dilation of Coronary Artery, One Artery, Percutaneous Approach
B211YZZ	Fluoroscopy of Multiple Coronary Arteries using Other Contrast
B212YZZ	Fluoroscopy of Single Coronary Artery Bypass Graft using Other Contrast
B215YZZ	Fluoroscopy of Left Heart using Other Contrast
4A023N7	Measurement of Cardiac Sampling and Pressure, Left Heart, Percutaneous Approach
3E03317	Introduction of Other Thrombolytic into Peripheral Vein, Percutaneous Approach

Rationale:

The objective of this procedure was to restore the blood flow through the lumen of the right coronary artery and its posterior descending branch. Because different device values were used, based on the advice of guideline B4.4, multiple codes are needed to report the Dilation (7) portion of this procedure, the root operation for the opening of the lumen of these two arteries. The correct body system and root operation table can be located by consulting PTCA (percutaneous transluminal coronary angioplasty) in the index, which states *see* Dilation, Heart and Great Vessels 027.

Root Operation		
Dilation (7)	Definition:	Expanding an orifice or the lumen of a tubular body part
	Explanation:	The orifice can be a natural orifice or an artificially created orifice. Accomplished by stretching a tubular body part using intraluminal pressure or by cutting part of the orifice or wall of the tubular body part.

The body part values for coronary arteries are listed by the number of arteries treated, **not** individual artery names or number of sites treated. Although two arteries were treated, because two different device values were used, the body part value Coronary Artery, One Artery (0) must be reported twice, each with its unique device value.

In the right coronary artery (RCA), a balloon was inflated in the artery to push the plaque up against the arterial walls opening the lumen, which is considered inherent in the dilation. Two stents, both described as ZES or Zotarolimus eluting, were inserted to hold the artery open, reported with one device value Intraluminal Device, Drug-eluting, Two (5).

POBA is often used for "plain old balloon angioplasty," which means only balloon dilation was performed. Since no stents were used in the Dilation (7) of the posterior descending branch, No Device (Z) is the appropriate device value. The approach method for both was Percutaneous (3) with No Qualifier (Z) because the procedure was not performed on the bifurcation of the arteries.

Angiography (angiogram), the visualization of the arteries using contrast and fluoroscopy, was performed. Also performed was ventriculography (ventriculogram), the visualization of the right or most typically the left heart ventricle and its contractions.

Both of these procedures can be located in the index using Angiography, or Ventriculogram, cardiac, which lead to the same table Fluoroscopy, Heart B21. Since the imaging was performed on several different body part values, multiple codes from this table are reported. The angiogram with fluoroscopy was performed on Coronary Arteries, Multiple (1) and Coronary Artery Bypass Graft, Single (2) for the internal mammary bypass graft. Additionally, the ventriculogram was performed in the left heart ventricle reported with body part value Heart, Left (5). All of this imaging used contrast referred to as Visipaque, which is an iso-osmolar contrast and is not considered high or low but rather is coded as Other Contrast (Y) (see Contrast Table 5.3).

The ventriculogram was performed with a left heart catheterization (left heart cath/LHC), which is a diagnostic procedure that measures pressures and collects blood samples. This procedure can also be located in the index under Catheterization, Heart *see* Measurement, Cardiac 4A02. This table is located in the Measurement and Monitoring (4) section. The body system is Cardiac (2), approach Percutaneous (3), Function/Device is Sampling and Pressure (N), and the qualifier specifies the Left Heart (7).

Some facilities capture the injection of Angiomax, a thrombin inhibitor, which is located in the Administration (3) section. It is intravenously injected and reported with Peripheral Vein (3), Percutaneous (3) approach, Thrombolytic (1) substance, and Other Thrombolytic (7) as the qualifier.

Atherectomy

AHA Coding Clinic

2016, 4Q, 86   Coronary and Peripheral Artery Bifurcation
2015, 4Q, 8   New Section X Codes—New Technology Procedures

An atherectomy is performed to remove plaque from coronary arteries and can be used in conjunction with coronary artery dilation and stent placement.

There are four types of atherectomy devices: laser, directional, transluminal, and rotational.

- **Laser:** Used only to remove enough plaque for the performance of a balloon angioplasty procedure. Since the angioplasty is the objective, the laser is an inherent step in the balloon Dilation (7) procedure.

- **Directional:** Uses a catheter with a cup-shaped blade and container. The blade cuts the plaque from the artery, where it is deposited into the container and removed from the artery. This is reported as Extirpation (C), as the objective is to cut and remove the solid matter from the body.

- **Transluminal:** A hollow tube catheter with rotating blade is used to cut and suction the plaque from the artery. Extirpation (C) is appropriate since the objective is to cut and remove the solid matter.

- **Rotational:** Used for chronic, longer, calcified, or solid blockages or in-stent restenosis. The objective is to remove plaque and is reported with Extirpation (C). One type of rotational atherectomy called **orbital atherectomy** is a newer procedure and is reported in the New Technology Section (X). See the following illustration.

Root Operation		
Dilation (7)	Definition:	Expanding an orifice or the lumen of a tubular body part
	Explanation:	The orifice can be a natural orifice or an artificially created orifice. Accomplished by stretching a tubular body part using intraluminal pressure or by cutting part of the orifice or wall of the tubular body part.
Extirpation (C)	Definition:	Taking or cutting out solid matter from a body part
	Explanation:	The solid matter may be an abnormal byproduct of a biological function or a foreign body; it may be imbedded in a body part or in the lumen of a tubular body part. The solid matter may or may not have been previously broken into pieces.

Figure 5.14. Rotational Atherectomy

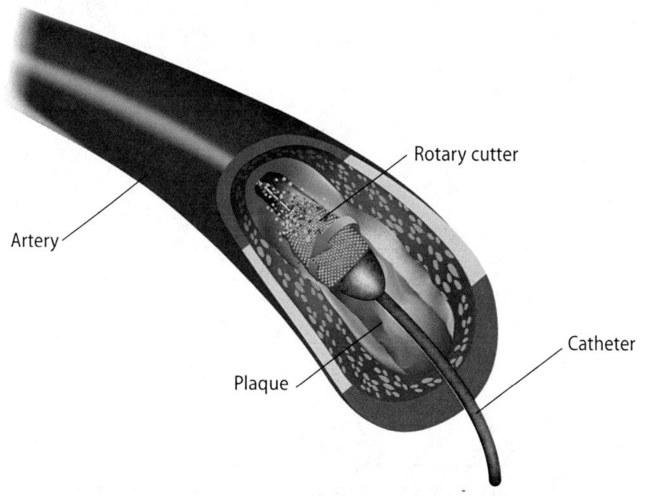

Spotlight

Documentation that states Orbital Atherectomy System (OAS), Diamondback 360®, or diamond coated crown indicates that the procedure is likely reported in the New Technology Section (X) and NOT the Medical Surgical Section (Ø).

Intravascular Ultrasonography (IVUS) and Fractional Flow Reserve (FFR)

AHA Coding Clinic

2016, 3Q, 37   Fractional Flow Reserve

Intravascular ultrasonography (IVUS)

The IVUS device consists of a miniature sound probe (transducer) on the tip of a coronary catheter that is threaded through the coronary arteries. Using ultrasound high-frequency sound waves, detailed images of the interior walls of the arteries are produced. In contrast to angiography, which shows a two-dimensional silhouette of the interior of the coronary arteries, IVUS shows a cross-section of the interior and the layers of the artery walls. The PCS table for IVUS is found in the Imaging (B) section, Heart (2), Ultrasonography (4) with a body part value of Coronary Artery, Single (Ø) or Coronary Artery, Multiple (1), contrast None (Z), sixth-character qualifier None (Z), and seventh-character qualifier Intravascular (3).

Code(s) for IVUS:

B24ØZZ3   **Ultrasonography of Single Coronary Artery, Intravascular**

B241ZZ3   **Ultrasonography of Multiple Coronary Arteries, Intravascular**

Fractional Flow Reserve (FFR)

FFR uses a guidewire to accurately measure blood pressure and flow through a coronary artery, determining the ratio between the maximum achievable blood flow in a diseased artery to the theoretical maximum flow in a normal artery. This enhances the ability to discern between potential myocardial infarction (MI) causing lesions that need to be revascularized with angioplasty and inconsequential lesions that may be medically treated. The acceptance of FFR has seen dramatic increase since the positive results of outcome-based studies called FAME and FAME II. Usage of FFR will likely increase as technological innovations in equipment are made. The code for Fractional Flow Reserve (FFR) is located in the Measurement and Monitoring (4) section, Physiological Systems (A), Measurement (Ø) with body system of Arterial (3), Percutaneous (3) approach, function value of Pressure (B), and qualifier value Coronary (C).

Code for FFR:
4AØ33BC   Measurement of Arterial Pressure, Coronary, Percutaneous Approach

Spotlight
Technically, a fractional flow reserve study measures blood pressure and flow within the arterial walls. Current *AHA Coding Clinic* advice lists only 4AØ33BC Measurement of Arterial Pressure, Coronary, Percutaneous Approach as the code to report when FFR is performed.

Figure 5.15. Fractional Flow Reserve

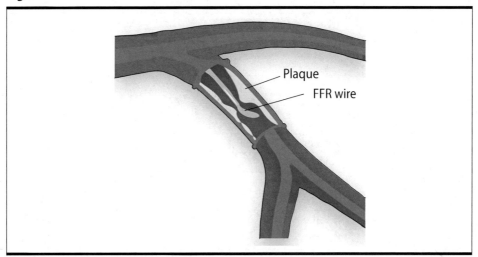

Unless the physician clearly documents that intravascular ultrasound imaging (IVUS) and/or fractional flow reserve (FFR) was performed, they can be tricky to recognize in the operative report. Oftentimes, indications that one of the procedures has been performed are found in the "Findings or Conclusions" section of the report.

Example:

Findings: Resting FFR was measured at 0.50, consistent with underperfused myocardium, despite robust collateralization from the LAD.

It is still necessary to locate the performance of the actual procedure in the operative report, and the only clue may be in the type of equipment used, such as a sentence stating that the physician exchanged one type of guidewire or catheter for another type. The following table can provide terms to look for, such as a Verrata™ guidewire indicating that a FFR is being performed, or the statement "Judkins catheter was exchanged for an Eagle Eye® catheter" which points to IVUS.

Example:

A Volcano Verrata™ wire was advanced first into the EBU guide in the left coronary system to equalize pressures, and subsequently into the distal RPDA and the distal reconstituted RCA perfused by collateral blood flow.

See table 5.4 for common manufacturer and device names of FFR and IVUS systems that may be noted in the patient's chart.

Root Operation		
Measurement and Monitoring Section (4)		
Measurement (0)	Definition:	Determining the level of a physiological or physical function at a point in time
Imaging Section (B)		
Ultrasonography (4)	Definition:	Real time display of images of anatomy or flow information developed from the capture of reflected and attenuated high frequency sound waves

Table 5.4. FFR and IVUS

Equipment/Function	Name	Manufacturer
FFR Guidewire	COMET™	Boston Scientific
FFR Guidewire	Verrata™	Volcano/Phillips
FFR Guidewire	ComboWire	Volcano/Phillips
FFR Guidewire	Pressurewire™Aeris	St. Jude Medical
FFR Guidewire	Pressurewire™Certus	St. Jude Medical
FFR Guidewire	Navvus™	ACIST/Medtronic
FFR Guidewire	Optowire®	Opsens
FFR/IVUS Guidewire	PrimeWire Prestige Plus	Volcano/Phillips
IVUS Catheter	Eagle Eye®	Volcano/Phillips
IVUS Catheter	Revolution®	Volcano/Phillips
IVUS Catheter	OptiCross®	Boston Scientific
IVUS Catheter	Kodama®	ACIST/Medtronic
FFR System	ILUMIEN system	St Jude Medical
FFR System	RXi Rapid Exchange	ACIST/Medtronic
IVUS System	ACIST HDi®	ACIST/Medtronic
FFR/IVUS System	Polaris	Boston Scientific
FFR/IVUS System	iFR®	Volcano/Phillips

Case Study 5.26. Atherectomy, Bifurcation with Stent Placement and IVUS

Indications: A 75-year-old male was admitted for unstable angina, with angina at rest for the past week. A coronary angiogram was performed earlier in the week and showed a calcified lesion involving the bifurcation of the LAD and the ostium of the left circumflex. Because of the severity of the patient's symptoms, he was brought back for intervention.

Procedure performed: The patient's left radial artery was prepped and draped in a sterile fashion. The left radial artery was accessed with a 6 French Terumo Glidesheath. IVUS with Polaris system was performed to evaluate the complexity of the lesion. Due to the Y shape of the bifurcation, "culotte" stenting was performed. The preparation of the lesion used rotational atherectomy, due to the level of calcification. With a 1.75 burr, two passes were made in the ostium of the LAD and then two passes in the ostium of the circumflex (CX). This was followed by a kissing balloon dilatation that predilated the LAD at 10 atm, then went over the Runthrough wire and predilated the CX at 10 atm. A 3.0 x 18 Promus stent was implanted into the LAD and a 3.0 x 18 Promus stent into the CX, bringing them back into the left main to create a carina. Post-kissing balloon dilation was performed. The intravascular ultrasound (IVUS) catheter was taken into the LAD and into the CX, and demonstrated that the stents were well apposed, without any evidence of edge dissection, and appropriately sizing the left main, which was approximately 5.5 mm. The guide was removed and a TR Band (Terumo) was placed over the radial artery.

Definitions
bifurcation. Division of an artery into two branches.
culotte stenting. One of several techniques developed for inserting stents into bifurcations of arteries that uses two stents. Both branches are predilated, the main vessel stented, and the side vessel stented by accessing through the stent struts of the main vessel overlapping the main vessel stent. Both vessels are postballoon dilated, which creates a flaring effect.
patent. Open and unobstructed.

Code(s):

02C13Z6	**Extirpation of Matter from Coronary Artery, Two Arteries, Bifurcation, Percutaneous Approach**
0271356	**Dilation of Coronary Artery, Two Arteries, Bifurcation, with Two Drug-eluting Intraluminal Devices, Percutaneous Approach**
B241ZZ3	**Ultrasonography of Multiple Coronary Arteries, Intravascular**

Rationale:

Two separate objectives were accomplished in this operative session. The first objective was to remove the plaque with the rotational atherectomy device, represented by root operation Extirpation (C). The second objective was to dilate and insert the stents that keep the lumen patent, reported with root operation Dilation (7). They were both performed in the bifurcation of two coronary arteries, from the left anterior descending (LAD) artery down through the left circumflex (CX), reported with body part value Coronary Artery, Two Arteries (1). Both were also performed using guidewires and catheters inserted through the radial artery. In ICD-10-PCS, there are not separate values to differentiate between radial or femoral technique; both are reported as Percutaneous (3). The Dilation (7) procedure device value of Intraluminal Device, Drug-Eluting, Two (5) is coded to indicate the type and number of stents used. The preceding Intraluminal Device, Drug-eluting stent table (table 5.2) can assist with the correct value for the Promus stents. The qualifier value in the seventh character represents the Bifurcation (6).

Root Operation		
Dilation (7)	Definition:	Expanding an orifice or the lumen of a tubular body part
	Explanation:	The orifice can be a natural orifice or an artificially created orifice. Accomplished by stretching a tubular body part using intraluminal pressure or by cutting part of the orifice or wall of the tubular body part.
Extirpation (C)	Definition:	Taking or cutting out solid matter from a body part
	Explanation:	The solid matter may be an abnormal byproduct of a biological function or a foreign body; it may be imbedded in a body part or in the lumen of a tubular body part. The solid matter may or may not have been previously broken into pieces.

Intravascular ultrasonography (IVUS) was performed prior to and after the procedure and is additionally coded. This is found in the Imaging (B) section, Heart (2) body system, Ultrasonography (4) table. Coronary Arteries, Multiple (1) is the body part value reported, None (Z) is reported for the fifth and sixth character, with Intravascular (3) as the qualifier value in the seventh-character position.

Case Study 5.27. Angiography Diagnostic, Fractional Flow Reserve (FFR) and Intravascular Ultrasonography (IVUS)

Procedure performed: An 86-year-old patient with chest pain was admitted for diagnostic imaging. The right femoral area was prepped and draped in usual sterile fashion. Lidocaine 2 mL was administered locally. The right femoral artery was cannulated with an 18-guage needle followed by a 6-French vascular sheath. A guiding catheter XB 3.5 was advanced and manipulated to cannulate the left and right coronary artery and angiography using Isovist was obtained. Minimal occlusion in the LAD with approximately 60 to 65 percent occlusion was noted in the septal and diagonal branches and also chronic total occlusion of the right coronary artery, which is well collateralized. Intracoronary nitroglycerin (200 µg) was administered and the catheter was exchanged for an OptiCross® catheter and advanced into the left and right coronary arteries. Following the IVUS, the catheter was exchanged and FFR was measured with a 0-014" Optowire®. FFR value on the left side was measured at 0.80. Based on the patient's age and health status, along with the FFR value, well-developed collaterals, size and location of lesions, it was determined that PCI was not recommended at this time and the patient be medically managed.

Code(s):

B211YZZ	**Fluoroscopy of Multiple Coronary Arteries using Other Contrast**
B241ZZ3	**Ultrasonography of Multiple Coronary Arteries, Intravascular**
4A033BC	**Measurement of Arterial Pressure, Coronary, Percutaneous Approach**

Rationale:

Three different types of diagnostic procedures were performed during this episode. The angiography, which is located in the Imaging (B) section, is a visualization of the Coronary Arteries, Multiple (1) using Fluoroscopy (1) enhanced with contrast. Isovist, the contrast mentioned, is an iso-osmolar contrast that is not classified to high or low contrast and is thus reported with Other Contrast (Y). This information may not always be supplied in the operative report and may need to be discovered in supporting documentation listed by brand and manufacturer.

The second imaging performed was an intravascular ultrasonography (IVUS), which uses Ultrasonography (4) of Coronary Arteries, Multiple (1) to produce detailed images of the arterial walls. The fifth and sixth characters are both reported with the value None (Z) and the seventh character Intravascular (3) as the appropriate qualifier.

The last diagnostic procedure was the fractional flow reserve study (FFR), which measures blood pressure and flow through coronary arteries. This is coded in the Measurement and Monitoring (4) section, table 4A0. The body part value is Arterial (3) and approach Percutaneous (3). The sixth character describes the function that is being measured, which is Pressure (B). The seventh-character qualifier specifies the arterial system, which is Coronary (C).

Root Operation		
Measurement (0)	Definition:	Determining the level of a physiological or physical function at a point in time

Tendons, Ligaments, Bursae, and Fascia Near a Joint

Guideline B4.5

> **B4.5**   Procedures performed on tendons, ligaments, bursae and fascia supporting a joint are coded to the body part in the respective body system that is the focus of the procedure. Procedures performed on joint structures themselves are coded to the body part in the joint body systems.
>
> *Example:* Repair of the anterior cruciate ligament of the knee is coded to the knee bursa and ligament body part in the bursae and ligaments body system.
>
> Knee arthroscopy with shaving of articular cartilage is coded to the knee joint body part in the Lower Joints body system.

AHA Coding Clinic

2017, 2Q, 21	Arthroscopic Anterior Cruciate Ligament Revision using Autograft with Anterolateral Ligament Reconstruction
2016, 3Q, 32	Rotator Cuff Repair, Tenodesis, Decompression, Acromioplasty and Coracoplasty
2016, 1Q, 30	Thermal Capsulorrhaphy of Shoulder
2015, 3Q, 14	Endoprosthetic Replacement of Humerus and Tendon Reattachment
2015, 2Q, 11	Repair of Patellar and Quadriceps Tendons with Allograft
2015, 1Q, 34	Arthroscopic Meniscectomy with Debridement and Abrasion Chondroplasty
2014, 4Q, 25	Femoroacetabular Impingement and Labral Tear with Repair
2014, 3Q, 9	Interspinous ligamentoplasty
2013, 3Q, 20	Superior Labrum Anterior Posterior (SLAP) Repair and Subacromial Decompression

Tendons are bands of dense fibrous tissue that connect muscle to bone. Procedures performed on tendons include tenotomies, reattachments of tendons, or tendon releases. When a procedure is performed on a tendon that is supporting a joint, because PCS has a separate body system value for Tendons (L), the procedure is reported using a code from the Tendon (L) body system rather than a joint body system. The body part values specified in the tendon tables detail the various locations of tendons throughout the body. One way to determine the accurate body part value within a tendon table is to use the Body Part Key (appendix D) or Body Part Definitions (appendix E) for muscles, as many tendons have the same name as the muscle it is connecting. This can assist in finding the most appropriate general grouping and a corresponding PCS character value for a particular tendon. For example, extensor digitorum longus, extensor hallucis longus, fibularis brevis, and tibialis anterior are all muscles classified to the Lower Leg Muscle body part; these same body part names are used for tendons and can be coded using the Lower Leg Tendon body part value.

Example: Lower Leg Muscle/Tendons

Muscle, Lower Leg	Tendon, Lower Leg
Extensor digitorum longus	Extensor digitorum longus
Extensor hallucis longus	Extensor hallucis longus
Fibularis brevis	Fibularis brevis
Tibialis anterior	Tibialis anterior

Ligaments are fibrous tissue that bind joints together and connect articular bones and cartilages. A bursa is a sac between a tendon and the bone beneath it that can act as a cushion. Procedures performed on bursae and ligaments may include bursectomy, bursotomy, repair, reconstruction, and suturing. Bursae and Ligaments (M) also have a specified body system in PCS. Therefore, any procedure on a bursa or ligament supporting a joint is coded using the Bursae and Ligaments (M) body system instead of a joint body system.

Conversely, PCS does not contain a body system or body part for cartilage. Cartilage that is found in the articulating surfaces of the joints is coded to the respective joint body system. For example, cartilage that provides cushioning in the knee joint is referred to as the meniscus and is found in the Lower Joints (S) body system under the Knee Joint, Right (C), or Knee Joint, Left (D) body part.

Spotlight
Applying this guideline can often be confusing. Identifying the correct body part that was the focus of a procedure can be difficult with incomplete documentation. It is important to not only understand anatomy but to consult references such as the *AHA Coding Clinics* for guidance. The *AHA Coding Clinics* applicable to guideline B4.5 are listed at the beginning of this section.

This guideline provides another example of why a good understanding of anatomy and the use of the Body Part Key and Body Part Definitions is so important for appropriate PCS coding. A review of the following Body Part Definitions table reveals that identification of the precise location of a knee procedure is necessary to ensure correct coding.

Example: Locate the lateral collateral ligament (LCL) and the lateral meniscus in the following table and illustration.

ICD-10-PCS Value	Definition
Knee Bursa and Ligament, Left **Knee Bursa and Ligament, Right**	**Includes:** Anterior cruciate ligament (ACL) Lateral collateral ligament (LCL) Ligament of head of fibula Medial collateral ligament (MCL) Patellar ligament Popliteal ligament Posterior cruciate ligament (PCL) Prepatellar bursa
Knee Joint, Femoral Surface, Left **Knee Joint, Femoral Surface, Right**	**Includes:** Femoropatellar joint Patellofemoral joint
Knee Joint, Left **Knee Joint, Right**	**Includes:** Femoropatellar joint Femorotibial joint Lateral meniscus Medial meniscus Patellofemoral joint Tibiofemoral joint
Knee Joint, Tibial Surface, Left **Knee Joint, Tibial Surface, Right**	**Includes:** Femorotibial joint Tibiofemoral joint
Knee Tendon, Left **Knee Tendon, Right**	**Includes:** Patellar tendon

Figure 5.16. Knee Meniscus

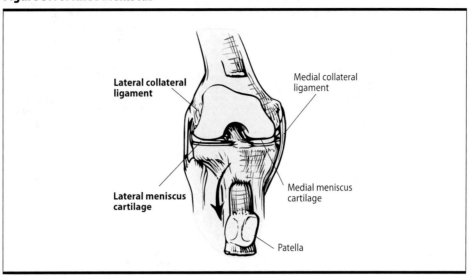

Practical Application for Guideline B4.5

Case Study 5.28. Repair, Anterior Talofibular Ligament

General anesthesia was administered and, intending on using a modified Broström technique, a curvilinear incision was made over the joint on the outside of the right ankle. The incision was opened down to the ankle joint where the anterior talofibular ligament (ATLF) was identified. The ATLF was found to be torn from the fibula. Small drill holes were made in the fibula and sutures were passed through the proximal edges of the ATLF through the drill holes and tied securely.

Code(s):
ØMMQØZZ   Reattachment of Right Ankle Bursa and Ligament, Open Approach

Rationale:
When an ankle sprain occurs, the ligament itself can be torn or it can be torn from the bone. If the tear is extensive, a Broström technique can be performed by anchoring the ligament back to the bone or replacing the ligament with a tendon. In this case, the ATLF was torn from the fibula and with string running though drill holes in the fibula the ligament was tied back onto the bone. The objective of the procedure was met as defined by the root operation Reattachment (M). The body part that was the focus of the procedure was the right ATLF, which is Ankle Bursa and Ligament, Right (Q) in the Bursae and Ligaments (M) body system. A curvilinear (C or J shaped) incision was made over the ankle joint and opened down through layers to visualize and reach the site, which is an Open (Ø) approach. See the following illustration for the ankle ligaments.

Root Operation		
Reattachment (M)	Definition:	Putting back in or on all or a portion of a separated body part to its normal location or other suitable location
	Explanation:	Vascular circulation and nervous pathways may or may not be reestablished

Figure 5.17. Ankle Ligament

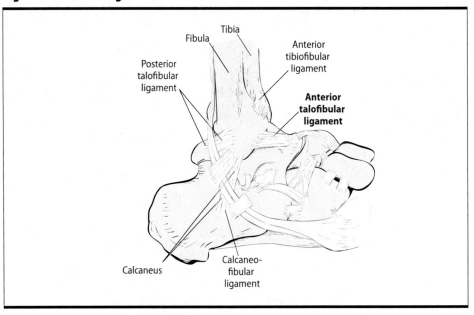

Case Study 5.29. Repair, Syndesmosis

A live stress x-ray was taken of the left syndesmosis. There was subtle but persistent instability of the syndesmosis ligaments with a little bit of talar tilt. The syndesmosis was manually reduced and with a small incision, a quadricortical 3.5 mm screw was placed across the fibula to tibia to stabilize the syndesmosis. This was done without complication.

Code(s):

ØSSG34Z   Reposition Left Ankle Joint with Internal Fixation Device, Percutaneous Approach

Rationale:

Some ankle fractures or sprains include the tearing of the ligament structure called the syndesmosis that holds together the tibia and fibula at the ankle socket. Since this unstable syndesmosis is not properly holding these bones together, the ankle joint is forced apart increasing potential for arthritis or chronic disability and must be repaired. To repair this, it is not enough to merely suture the ligaments, rather the fibula and tibia bones need to be correctly reduced and stabilized with syndesmotic screws. The objective of this procedure was to reduce and secure the displaced, unstable joint making Reposition (S) the appropriate root operation. Even though the ligaments were torn, the focus of the treatment was the Ankle Joint, Left (G) rather than the ligament. A small incision was made in order to place the screw, which meets the approach definition of Percutaneous (3). The screw is represented by Internal Fixation (4) as the device character.

Root Operation		
Reposition (S)	Definition:	Moving to its normal location, or other suitable location, all or a portion of a body part
	Explanation:	The body part is moved to a new location from an abnormal location, or from a normal location where it is not functioning correctly. The body part may or may not be cut out or off to be moved to the new location.

Case Study 5.30. Meniscectomy, Partial

The patient was placed in supine position. After general anesthesia was administered, the right lower leg was prepped and draped in the usual sterile fashion. A small stab incision was made inferolateral to the patella. The arthroscopic camera was introduced. The medial compartment was then entered. A needle was inserted inferomedial to the patella for localization in the anteromedial portal. Once this position was confirmed, another small stab incision was made. An arthroscopic probe was introduced. The anterior middle third of the medial meniscus appeared to be pristine. However, beginning at the junction of the mid-posterior third of the meniscus, extending back to the posterior root, there was noted to be a superior leaf flap, which was a large tear, that had flipped superiorly up onto itself. Upon probing, it was easily displaceable into the joint. Given these findings, a decision was made to proceed with partial medial meniscectomy. Using a combination of arthroscopic biters and arthroscopic shavers, this large superior flap tear was excised, taking great care in preserving as much normal cartilage as possible. The portals were closed using buried simple interrupted stitches of 4-0 Monocryl. Steri-Strips were applied. Sterile dressings were applied.

Code(s):

ØSBC4ZZ   **Excision of Right Knee Joint, Percutaneous Endoscopic Approach**

Rationale:

The medial meniscus is a semicircular pad of cartilage in the inside of the knee between the medial condyles of the femur and tibia and acts as a shock absorber between the tibia and femur. Acute tears often occur due to forceful twisting or bending, such as in sports injuries. Degenerative tears are more common in people 65 years and older because the meniscus loses elasticity and strength with age. Because it is cartilage rather than tendon, bursa, or ligament, it does not have its own body system and instead is considered part of the Knee Joint, Right (C) or Left (D) body part in the Lower Joints (S) body system. Only part of the meniscus was removed in this case, as it is best to retain as much cartilage as possible to avoid future arthritic conditions. This meets the definition of the root operation Excision (B). The procedure was done arthroscopically, which is a Percutaneous Endoscopic (4) approach. No Qualifier (Z) is used for the seventh character since no indication was given that the procedure was performed for diagnostic purposes.

Root Operation		
Excision (B)	Definition:	Cutting out or off, without replacement, a portion of a body part.
	Explanation:	The qualifier DIAGNOSTIC is used to identify excision procedures that are biopsies

---

Case Study 5.31. Drainage, Infected Bursa

Operative Procedure: The patient was placed supine on the operating table and given a local anesthetic. The right leg was prepped sterilely and draped in the usual sterile manner. There was a small 2 mm to 3 mm transverse abrasion over the top of the patella, which was draining serous fluid. This fluid was growing out Staph aureus preoperatively. The prepatellar bursa, which was inflamed, was carefully entered 3 mm below the midpoint of the lateral border of the patella and aspirated with an 18 gauge needle. 50 mL of fluid was drained and a pressure dressing applied.

Code(s):

ØM9N3ZZ   **Drainage of Right Knee Bursa and Ligament, Percutaneous Approach**

Rationale:

The objective of this procedure was to remove the infected serous fluid from the patella region, reported with root operation Drainage (9). The body part that contained the fluid was the prepatellar bursa which, according to the Body Part Key, is Knee Bursa and Ligament, Right (N) body part in the Bursae and Ligaments (M) body system. The Drainage (9) was performed with a needle, which is a Percutaneous (3) approach. According to this short op note, the infection had been diagnosed preoperatively. No drainage device was left in the knee and no further diagnostics performed, which makes No Device (Z) and No Qualifier (Z) the appropriate selections.

Root Operation		
Drainage (9)	Definition:	Taking or letting out fluids and/or gases from a body part
	Explanation:	The qualifier DIAGNOSTIC is used to identify drainage procedures that are biopsies

Figure 5.18. Knee Bursa

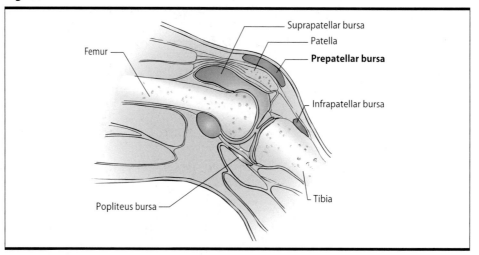

Case Study 5.32. Reconstruction, Right AC Joint with Hamstring Allograft

The patient is a 25-year-old male that fell from height a few months ago and sustained an AC separation. Nonoperative treatment was attempted; however, it has failed and he is still complaining of significant pain and inability to go back to work. He presented for operative fixation of his right AC joint.

Description of Procedure: The patient was brought to the operating room and placed in supine position. He was moved in the beach chair position using a McDonald head holder. All bony prominences were well padded. Ancef was given within one hour of incision time. The right arm was prepped and draped in a normal sterile fashion. A time out was performed per the standard protocol. Saber incision was made approximately 10 cm in length from the posterior aspect of the clavicle distally toward the coracoid process. Dissection was carried down through subcutaneous tissues to the delta trapezial fascia. This was incised with electrocautery longitudinally along the length of the clavicle. This was carried distally to expose the AC joint. The disk and the AC joint were excised with the rongeur. The clavicle was skeletonized. Dissection was carried down reflecting the deltoid inferiorly to expose the coracoid process. Careful dissection was taken to form a trough underneath the coracoid for passage of the grafts. Approximately 1 cm of the distal clavicle was excised using a sagittal saw. The edges of the bone cover were smoothed using a bur. Landmarks for the tunnel were marked approximately 4.5 cm from the AC joint. The most medial tunnel was 4.5 cm proximal to the AC joint and the lateral tunnel was 3 cm proximal to the AC joint. A guidewire was placed and a 5.5 mm hole was drilled at each tunnel site. The semi-tendinosis allograft was prepared on the back table for implantation. A suture passer was used to pass the hamstring allograft underneath the coracoid process and through the bone tunnels in the clavicle. A 5 mm interference screw was used to fix the medial tunnel. Once stable fixation was achieved, the fiber wire tape was tied over the top of the clavicle and the other end of the graft was passed through the lateral tunnel. This was also fixed with a 5 mm interference screw. After fixation of the graft, fluoro images were taken and confirmed adequate reduction of the AC joint. The wound was then thoroughly irrigated with normal saline. Vancomycin power was placed deep in the wound. The deltoid trapezial fascia was closed with #2 fiber wire. The deep dermal layer was closed with 2-0 Vicryl suture followed by a 3-0 Monocryl in a subcuticular fashion. Dermabond was placed followed by 4 x 4's and Tegaderm. A sling was also placed while the patient was in the operating room. The patient was able to be awakened in the operating suite and taken to postanesthesia care unit in stable condition.

Code(s):

ØRSGØZZ	**Reposition Right Acromioclavicular Joint, Open Approach**
ØRUGØKZ	**Supplement Right Acromioclavicular Joint with Nonautologous Tissue Substitute, Open Approach**

Rationale:

Two codes are required to capture the repair of the AC joint. The objective of the first procedure was to realign the AC joint to its natural position to the clavicle. This was accomplished by the root operation Reposition (S). The focus of the reposition was the separated Acromioclavicular Joint, Right (G) body part located in the Upper Joints (R) body system. The excision of the AC joint is inherent to the repositioning and is not coded separately as per the following guideline B3.1b. The screws and fiber wire were actually used to attach the allograft, not as a fixation device for the reposition, thus the No Device (Z) value is used for the sixth character.

PCS Guideline
Multiple procedures
B3.1b Components of a procedure specified in the root operation definition and explanation are not coded separately. Procedural steps necessary to reach the operative site and close the operative site, including anastomosis of a tubular body part, are also not coded separately.
Example: Resection of a joint as part of a joint replacement procedure is included in the root operation definition of Replacement and is not coded separately.
Laparotomy performed to reach the site of an open liver biopsy is not coded separately. In a resection of sigmoid colon with anastomosis of descending colon to rectum, the anastomosis is not coded separately.

The application of the hamstring allograft to this site can be coded separately with the root operation Supplement (U) since the following multiple procedure guideline B3.2c states that during the same operative episode, multiple procedures are coded if multiple root operations with distinct objectives are performed on the same body site. This was performed not to reposition the joint, but to reinforce the realignment. The same Acromioclavicular Joint, Right (G) body part, Upper Joints (R) body system, and Open (Ø) approach are reported. The hamstring allograft from a cadaver donor rather than harvested from the patient is considered a Nonautologous Tissue Substitute (K) device value.

PCS Guideline
Multiple procedures
B3.2 During the same operative episode, multiple procedures are coded if:
c. Multiple root operations with distinct objectives are performed on the same body part.
Example: Destruction of sigmoid lesion and bypass of sigmoid colon are coded separately.

Root Operation		
Reposition (S)	Definition:	Moving to its normal location, or other suitable location, all or a portion of a body part
	Explanation:	The body part is moved to a new location from an abnormal location, or from a normal location where it is not functioning correctly. The body part may or may not be cut out or off to be moved to the new location.
Supplement (U)	Definition:	Putting in or on biological or synthetic material that physically reinforces and/or augments the function of a portion of a body part
	Explanation:	The biological material is non-living, or is living and from the same individual. The body part may have been previously replaced, and the SUPPLEMENT procedure is performed to physically reinforce and/or augment the function of the replaced body part.

The following illustration indicates the anatomical location of the acromioclavicular joint.

Figure 5.19. Shoulder Joint

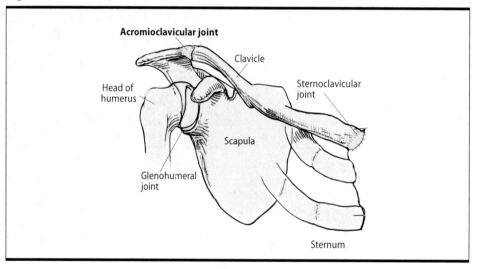

Skin, Subcutaneous Tissue, and Fascia Overlying a Joint

Guideline B4.6

B4.6	If a procedure is performed on the skin, subcutaneous tissue or fascia overlying a joint, the procedure is coded to the following body part:
	• **Shoulder is coded to Upper Arm**
	• **Elbow is coded to Lower Arm**
	• **Wrist is coded to Lower Arm**
	• **Hip is coded to Upper Leg**
	• **Knee is coded to Lower Leg**
	• **Ankle is coded to Foot**

AHA Coding Clinic

2014, 3Q, 14   Application of Thera Skin® and Excisional Debridement

There are no body part values in the Skin and Breast or Subcutaneous Tissue and Fascia body systems that use specific joint terminology, such as knee or shoulder, to describe the location of a procedure performed. When the procedure is performed on tissue that does not actually represent joint tissue but instead the surrounding tissue, such as skin or subcutaneous tissue, the information provided in the guideline above should be followed when assigning body part values. Note that skin and subcutaneous tissue and fascia overlying the elbow and wrist joints are **both** reported with lower arm. In contrast, knee is represented by lower leg and ankle by foot.

Table 5.5. Skin, Subcutaneous Tissue, and Fascia Overlying a Joint

Anatomical	PCS body part value	Anatomical	PCS body part value
Skin overlying:		Subcutaneous Tissue and Fascia overlying:	
Shoulder Joint	Skin, Right Upper Arm (B) Skin, Left Upper Arm (C)	Shoulder Joint	Subcutaneous Tissue and Fascia, Right Upper Arm (D) Subcutaneous Tissue and Fascia, Left Upper Arm (F)
Elbow Joint	Skin, Right Lower Arm (D) Skin, Left Lower Arm (E)	Elbow Joint	Subcutaneous Tissue and Fascia, Right Lower Arm (G) Subcutaneous Tissue and Fascia, Left Lower Arm (H)
Wrist Joint	Skin, Right Lower Arm (D) Skin, Left Lower Arm (E)	Wrist Joint	Subcutaneous Tissue and Fascia, Right Lower Arm (G) Subcutaneous Tissue and Fascia, Left Lower Arm (H)
Hip Joint	Skin, Right Upper Leg (H) Skin, Left Upper Leg (J)	Hip Joint	Subcutaneous Tissue and Fascia, Right Upper Leg (L) Subcutaneous Tissue and Fascia, Left Upper Leg (M)
Knee Joint	Skin, Right Lower Leg (K) Skin, Left Lower Leg (L)	Knee Joint	Subcutaneous Tissue and Fascia, Right Lower Leg (N) Subcutaneous Tissue and Fascia, Left Lower Leg (P)
Ankle Joint	Skin, Right Foot (M) Skin, Left Foot (N)	Ankle Joint	Subcutaneous Tissue and Fascia, Right Foot (Q) Subcutaneous Tissue and Fascia, Left Foot (R)

Practical Application for Guideline B4.6

Case Study 5.33. Punch Biopsy of Nevus

Operation: Punch biopsy of nevus, right elbow.

The right elbow was prepped with Betadine. A local anesthetic was injected around the area. A 4 mm skin punch was inserted into nevus, and a piece of the nevus was removed and sent to pathology. Minor bleeding was stopped by placing a 4 x 4 dressing over the site and applying pressure to the area. Once hemostasis was achieved, the area was cleaned with normal saline and a Band-Aid was applied.

Code(s):

ØHBDXZX   **Excision of Right Lower Arm Skin, External Approach, Diagnostic**

Rationale:

The small amount of tissue removed with the skin punch is reported with root operation Excision (B). Based on guideline B4.6, the appropriate body part excised was Skin, Right Lower Arm (D) of the Skin and Breast (H) body system since the nevus was located on the skin overlying the elbow joint. For the majority of skin body part values, External (X) approach is the only choice offered for excision procedures because these sites are visualized and accessed externally. The qualifier is Diagnostic (X) because the objective of the excision was to determine the pathology of the nevus. Minor bleeding is not considered a complication. It is inherent in the procedure and not coded separately.

Root Operation		
Excision (B)	Definition:	Cutting out or off, without replacement, a portion of a body part.
	Explanation:	The qualifier DIAGNOSTIC is used to identify excision procedures that are biopsies

---

Case Study 5.34. Foreign Body, Removal

Procedures:

1.   Debridement of gunshot wound of the left shoulder.

2.   Removal of foreign body from the left upper back-trapezius muscle.

A 19-year-old female was shot this evening in a drive-by shooting. According to police, she was mistaken for a gang member. She was brought by ambulance to the emergency room and stabilized, then brought to the operating room for surgery to remove the bullets or bullet fragments.

The patient was placed supine on the operating table and general anesthesia was induced. The patient was then placed in the right lateral decubitus position with the left side up. The shoulder, posterior neck, and back were prepped and draped in the usual sterile fashion. Starting with the left shoulder gunshot tract, an elliptical incision was made around the wound, and using a scalpel, devitalized tissue was cut out up to and including the deltoid fascia. It was decided that the bullet could be better accessed posteriorly. The subcutaneous cavity was also debrided, and hemostasis was achieved using electrocautery and clamps. After achieving hemostasis, the cavity was packed with Betadine dressings, and sterile dressings applied over the wound.

Next, the patient was rotated to expose the upper back area. A transverse incision was made over the palpable foreign body in the upper-back area. Using blunt and sharp dissection, this foreign body was removed from the trapezius muscle tissue. It looked like a solid bullet with slight deformity. After removing the bullet, the cavity was irrigated and hemostasis was achieved using electrocautery. The wound was closed with layered suture.

Code(s):

ØJBFØZZ   **Excision of Left Upper Arm Subcutaneous Tissue and Fascia, Open Approach**

ØKCGØZZ   **Extirpation of Matter from Left Trunk Muscle, Open Approach**

Rationale:

Accessing the word debridement in the alphabetic index leads to Excisional *see* Excision or Non-excisional *see* Extraction. The gunshot wound tract was cleaned and the damaged tissues cut out (excised) with the use of a scalpel, which fits the description of an excisional debridement. The use of a sharp instrument alone does not determine whether Excision (B) or Extraction (D) is used. Documentation must contain terminology to indicate that tissue was "cut out" or "excised" with an instrument such as scalpel, scissors, or electrocautery tip. The use of the terminology "excisional debridement was performed" is also acceptable if it is denoted in the description of the procedure as noted in *AHA Coding Clinic,* 2015, 3Q, 3. In this operative report, the correct root operation for the debridement is Excision (B).

Based on guideline B3.5, the location of the debridement is determined by the deepest layer of tissue removed, in this example the deltoid fascia. The deltoid fascia, located in the shoulder area, is reported with Subcutaneous Tissue and Fascia, Left Upper Arm (F) in the Subcutaneous Tissue and Fascia (J) body system. Using the Body Part Key (appendix D) is an efficient way to locate the correct PCS body part value for deltoid fascia. Since the incision cut through layers of skin and subcutaneous tissue to reach the deltoid fascia, it is reported by an Open (Ø) approach.

PCS Guideline
Overlapping body layers
B3.5   If the root operations Excision, Repair or Inspection are performed on overlapping layers of the musculoskeletal system, the body part specifying the deepest layer is coded.   *Example:* Excisional debridement that includes skin and subcutaneous tissue and muscle is coded to the muscle body part.

The second code, ØKCGØZZ, describes the removal or Extirpation (C) of the bullet from within the trapezius muscle. Extirpation is a term rarely documented by physicians but according to Convention A11 it is the coder's responsibility to know and understand these PCS terms. Based on this convention, the coder can use the root operation definition and explanation to determine that Extirpation (C) is the appropriate root operation without having to query the physician.

PCS Guideline
Convention
A11   Many of the terms used to construct PCS codes are defined within the system. It is the coder's responsibility to determine what the documentation in the medical record equates to in the PCS definitions. The physician is not expected to use the terms used in PCS code descriptions, nor is the coder required to query the physician when the correlation between the documentation and the defined PCS terms is clear.   *Example:* When the physician documents "partial resection" the coder can independently correlate "partial resection" to the root operation Excision without querying the physician for clarification.

According to the Body Part Key (appendix D), the trapezius muscle is reported with Trunk Muscle, Left (G) of the Muscles (K) body system. No Device (Z) and No Qualifier (Z) are reported as the sixth and seventh characters for both of the codes in this case. Both codes in this example demonstrate the importance of consulting the Body Part Key.

Term	ICD-10-PCS Value
Trapezius muscle	Trunk Muscle, Right
	Trunk Muscle, Left

Root Operation		
Excision (B)	Definition:	Cutting out or off, without replacement, a portion of a body part.
	Explanation:	The qualifier DIAGNOSTIC is used to identify excision procedures that are biopsies
Extirpation (C)	Definition:	Taking or cutting out solid matter from a body part
	Explanation:	The solid matter may be an abnormal byproduct of a biological function or a foreign body; it may be imbedded in a body part or in the lumen of a tubular body part. The solid matter may or may not have been previously broken into pieces.
Extraction (D)	Definition:	Pulling or stripping out or off all or a portion of a body part by the use of force
	Explanation:	The qualifier DIAGNOSTIC is used to identify extraction procedures that are biopsies

Figure 5.20. Deltoid/Trapezius Muscles

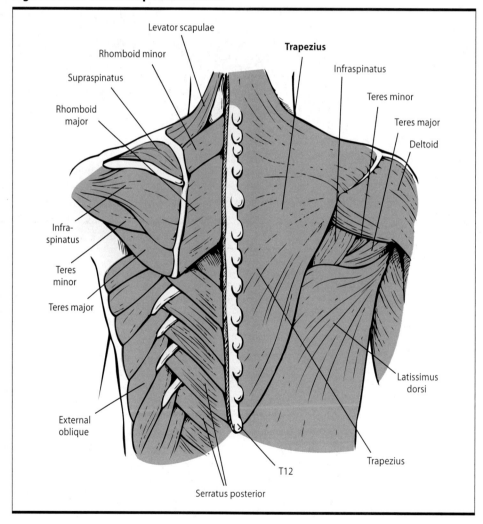

Case Study 5.35. Debridement, Excisional

Procedure: Debridement of stage III necrotic iliac decubitus ulcer, concern for hip joint osteomyelitis.

Operative Procedure: The patient was properly prepped and draped under local sedation. The ulcer over the hip joint appeared necrotic. A 0.25% Marcaine was injected circumferentially around the left hip necrotic decubitus ulcer. A wide excision and debridement of the necrotic decubitus ulcer taken down to the iliac fascia and all necrotic tissue was removed using electrocautery. There was no sign of deeper necrosis into the joint. All bleeding was cauterized with electrocautery, a Kerlix stack was placed, and a pressure dressing applied. The patient was sent to recovery in satisfactory condition.

Code(s):

ØJBMØZZ   Excision of Left Upper Leg Subcutaneous Tissue and Fascia, Open Approach

Rationale:

Based on ICD-10-CM, a stage III decubitus or pressure ulcer is generally defined as full-thickness skin loss with damage or necrosis of subcutaneous tissue. This provides a hint about the possible depth of the debridement. If muscle or bone was removed, the ulcer stage would have been more likely described as a stage IV ulcer. However, the documentation of the operative report must match the procedure coded. If there is doubt, query the physician.

Root operation Excision (B) is reported because the documentation was clear that Excision (B) rather than Extraction (D) of the necrotic tissue was performed. The use of an electrocautery tip to excise necrotic tissue is an accepted method of excisional debridement.

Spotlight
Excision may be accomplished by use of any of the following sharp instruments (not an all-inclusive list): • Scalpel • Scissors • Wire • Bone saw • Electrocautery tip

Documentation states excision of the iliac fascia of the hip; however, consulting the Excision table in the Subcutaneous Tissue and Fascia body system (ØJB) for the body part value may incorrectly lead to Subcutaneous Tissue and Fascia, Pelvic Region. Guideline B4.6 specifically addresses procedures performed on the skin, subcutaneous tissue, and fascia overlying joints. This guideline advises that those procedures performed over the hip are coded to Subcutaneous Tissue and Fascia, Right Upper Leg (L) or Left Upper Leg (M). This information is confirmed in the Body Part Key, which also reports Iliac fascia as Subcutaneous Tissue and Fascia, Right Upper Leg and Left Upper Leg.

In this example, iliac fascia, which is part of the hip, is coded with body part value Subcutaneous Tissue and Fascia, Left Upper Leg (M) located in the Subcutaneous Tissue and Fascia (J) body system. The debridement was an Open (Ø) procedure with No Device (Z) and No Qualifier (Z) indicated.

Case Study 5.36. Aspiration, Knee

Operation: Puncture aspiration of postoperative seroma of the lateral right knee.

Anesthesia: 5 cc 1% lidocaine with epinephrine.

A 38-year-old woman S/P excision of melanoma of the right knee nine days ago returned today for follow-up. The patient has developed a postoperative seroma that warrants drainage.

The risks and benefits of the procedure were explained to the patient. The patient elected to proceed with the procedure.

The area on the side of the knee was prepped and draped in the usual sterile fashion. Five ccs of lidocaine with epinephrine was injected in the area of the seroma. The seroma was punctured into the subcutaneous tissue with a 16-gauge needle and 30 ccs of fluid aspirated. A pressure dressing was applied to the wound.

Code(s):

0J9N3ZZ   **Drainage of Right Lower Leg Subcutaneous Tissue and Fascia, Percutaneous Approach**

Definition
seroma. Swelling caused by the collection of serum, or clear fluid, in the tissues.

Rationale:

A needle was used to perform a Percutaneous (3) aspiration of a seroma on the lateral knee, which is reported with the root operation Drainage (9). The seroma was located in the subcutaneous aspect of the knee, not the knee joint itself. This is reported with Subcutaneous Tissue and Fascia, Right Lower Leg (N) body part in the Subcutaneous Tissue and Fascia (J) body system. There is no verbiage indicating that this procedure was performed for diagnostic purposes and no drainage tube was placed, so No Device (Z) and No Qualifier (Z) are reported.

Root Operation		
Drainage (9)	Definition:	Taking or letting out fluids and/or gases from a body part
	Explanation:	The qualifier DIAGNOSTIC is used to identify drainage procedures that are biopsies

Spotlight
An attempted aspiration that results in the removal of no fluid is coding using Inspection as the appropriate root operation (*AHA Coding Clinic*, 2017, 1Q, 50).

Fingers and Toes

Guideline B4.7

> **B4.7** **If a body system does not contain a separate body part value for fingers, procedures performed on the fingers are coded to the body part value for the hand. If a body system does not contain a separate body part value for toes, procedures performed on the toes are coded to the body part value for the foot.**
>
> *Example:* **Excision of finger muscle is coded to one of the hand muscle body part values in the Muscles body system.**

This guideline communicates the correct reporting for procedures performed on specific anatomy of the fingers and toes located in body systems that do not contain these individual body part values. The following body systems do not include body part values for fingers or toes and necessitate the use of the body part value for hand or foot:

- Upper Arteries
- Lower Arteries
- Upper Veins
- Lower Veins
- Skin and Breast (except finger or toe nails)
- Subcutaneous Tissue and Fascia
- Muscles
- Tendons
- Bursae and Ligaments

Note that the body systems of upper and lower bones and joints **do** contain body part values for fingers and toes.

The tendons and ligaments of the fingers have no distinct PCS value assigned to them. The appropriate PCS character value for hand tendon or hand ligament should be assigned as shown in the following table.

Anatomical Term	PCS Body System	PCS Body Part Value
Extensor tendon	Tendons (L)	Hand Tendon, Right (7), Left (8)
Flexor digitorum superficialis tendon	Tendons (L)	Hand Tendon, Right (7), Left (8)
Flexor digitorum profundus tendon	Tendons (L)	Hand Tendon, Right (7), Left (8)
Collateral ligament	Bursae and Ligaments (M)	Hand Bursa and Ligament, Right (7), Left (8)

Practical Application for Guideline B4.7

Case Study 5.37. Tendon Laceration Repair

The oblique laceration of the distal aspect of the right distal phalanx, fifth finger, medial side was explored. The laceration was approximately 3 centimeters in length. The laceration was found to involve approximately two-thirds of the extensor tendon. Repair of the tendon was accomplished using interrupted 4-0 Vicryl suture.

Code(s):

ØLQ7ØZZ   **Repair Right Hand Tendon, Open Approach**

Rationale:

The root operation Repair (Q) is used as the default when the procedure does not fit any other root operation. Lacerations fixed with staples or sutures are reported with Repair (Q).

Root Operation		
Repair (Q)	Definition:	Restoring, to the extent possible, a body part to its normal anatomic structure and function
	Explanation:	Used only when the method to accomplish the repair is not one of the other root operations

The extensor tendon in the right little finger was repaired, which is identified with Hand Tendon, Right (7) in the Tendons (L) body system. An Open (Ø) approach was used to reach the tendon through the skin and subcutaneous layers. According to Guideline B6.1b, sutures are not considered a device so No Device (Z) is reported as well as No Qualifier (Z).

PCS Guideline	
B6.1b	Materials such as sutures, ligatures, radiological markers and temporary post-operative wound drains are considered integral to the performance of a procedure and are not coded as devices.

Case Study 5.38. Tendon Reattachment

A 23-year-old male slid from the roof and grasped shingles, lacerating the right little finger. He was sent to the operating room due to loss of flexion of the flexor digitorum profundus (FDP) tendon. He was placed supine and IV induction of anesthesia was performed. The little finger had a big U-shaped laceration to it that started between the MP and the PIP and went almost all the way up to the DIP on the outside. Looking inside, it was clear the sublimis was intact but the profundus was completely gone. Traveling through the sheath, the other end of it was found. The incision was extended on the ulnar side about half an inch at the most. It gave enough room to get up to the stub. Attention was turned to the proximal side. Looking down the sheath, the physician probed for the profundus using a tendon passer as far as possible, but could not find it. A chevron incision was made about an inch in length in the skin and subcutaneous tissue. The tendon was found. It had doubled over and was caught down just about that same area. It was grasped with a pickup and pulled out through the incision site. A 0 Vicryl was placed through it. The tendon passer was placed from the distal to the proximal side and the 0 Vicryl was tied to the tendon and the tendon pulled back to its normal position. A pullout wire was placed through the proximal side of the profundus tendon and taken through the distal side and out through the end of the tendon, through a drill hole in the distal phalanx and through the nail with a button at the end of it. Xeroform was placed underneath the button and the wire pulled tight. The sheath was closed as best as possible over the area and Xeroform placed over it.

Code(s):

ØLM7ØZZ   Reattachment of Right Hand Tendon, Open Approach

Rationale:
The flexor digitorum profundus (FDP) originates in the forearm at the medial condyle of the elbow and at its distal end attaches to the distal phalanx. It directly flexes the distal interphalangeal (DIP) joint and indirectly flexes the proximal interphalangeal (PIP) joint. The flexor digitorum superficialis (FDS) (superficial) and profundus (deep) run together through a sheath through each digit.

Figure 5.21. Flexor Tendons Inserting in the Finger

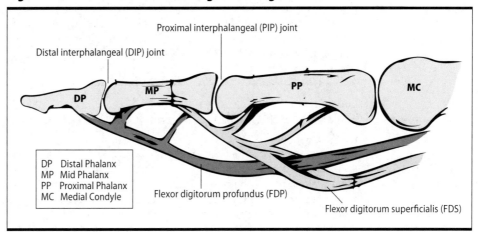

Unlike the previous example, this tendon was completely detached from the bone at the distal phalanx.

To repair this injury, it is necessary to retrieve the detached end of the tendon, pull it back through the sheath, and attach it to its normal or "other suitable" location, fitting the root operation of Reattachment (M). In this case, it is reattached through the bone and held taut with a suture to a button exteriorly on the fingernail. The button is generally removed in four to six weeks. There is no PCS body part value for finger tendon, so based on advice from guideline B4.7, the appropriate body part value is Hand Tendon, Right (7) in the Tendons (L) body system. The procedure was performed with an Open (Ø) approach and the only device and qualifier choice is No Device (Z) and No Qualifier (Z).

Figure 5.22. Reattachment of Tendon, Pullout Button Technique

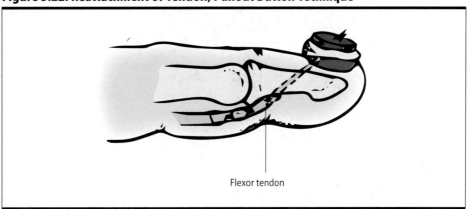

Flexor tendon

Root Operation		
Reattachment (M)	Definition:	Putting back in or on all or a portion of a separated body part to its normal location or other suitable location
	Explanation:	Vascular circulation and nervous pathways may or may not be reestablished

Case Study 5.39. Debridement, Cellulitis of Toe

A patient presented to her dermatologist's office with cellulitis of her left big toe caused by an unknown source, potentially a wood sliver. The dermatologist performed a 4 sq cm excisional debridement of the toe down into the level of the subcutaneous tissue. The wound was appropriately dressed, and the patient was told to follow up with the physician in one week to check the progress of the wound.

Code(s):

ØJBRØZZ   Excision of Left Foot Subcutaneous Tissue and Fascia, Open Approach

Rationale:

Accessing the word debridement in the alphabetic index leads to Excisional *see* Excision or Non-excisional *see* Extraction. In order to report excisional debridement, documentation must contain terminology to indicate that tissue was "cut out" or "excised" with an instrument such as a scalpel, scissors, or an electrocautery tip. According to *AHA Coding Clinic,* 2015, 3Q, 3, the use of terminology such as "excisional debridement was performed" is also acceptable if it is denoted in the description of the procedure. Based on this advice, the correct root operation for this debridement is Excision (B). If tissue was scraped, brushed, or minor trimming was performed, it is considered a nonexcisional debridement and is reported with the root operation of Extraction (D).

Root Operation		
Excision (B)	Definition:	Cutting out or off, without replacement, a portion of a body part
	Explanation:	The qualifier DIAGNOSTIC is used to identify excision procedures that are biopsies

Although the subcutaneous tissue was removed from the great toe, since there is no body part value of toe in the Subcutaneous Tissue and Fascia (J) body system, the correct PCS body part value is Subcutaneous Tissue and Fascia, Left Foot (R).

The site was accessed by cutting through the skin layer into the subcutaneous tissue, which is reported with an Open (Ø) approach. There was No Device (Z) used. Since the intent was to remove infected tissue rather than biopsy, the correct qualifier is No Qualifier (Z).

Case Study 5.40. Foreign Body, Removal from Toe

A patient stepped on broken glass on the beach. Due to pain when walking and concern for infection, she was advised to have it removed.

Procedure: Excision of broken glass deep in middle toe.

The patient was laid supine on the table and local anesthetic administered with 1% Xylocaine with epinephrine applied underneath the right 2nd toe at the distal tip. Using a 15 blade, the right toe was incised deep into the soft tissue and a large piece of dirty glass was removed. The wound was irrigated and cauterized. Silvadene and band-aid were applied.

Code(s):

ØJCQØZZ   Extirpation of Matter from Right Foot Subcutaneous Tissue and Fascia, Open Approach

Rationale:

Although the procedure title says "excision of …," according to convention A11, "It is the responsibility of the coder to determine what the documentation in the medical record equates to in the PCS definitions." When a foreign body such as glass is removed from a body part, the appropriate root operation is Extirpation (C). Since the glass was deep into the soft tissue but no muscle was mentioned, the correct body system is Subcutaneous Tissue and Fascia (J). Because there is no toe body part value, based on guideline B4.7, the correct body part value is Subcutaneous Tissue and Fascia, Right Foot (Q). The skin was incised with a blade into the soft tissues so it is an Open (Ø) approach. There is No Device (Z) and No Qualifier (Z).

Root Operation		
Extirpation (C)	Definition:	Taking or cutting out solid matter from a body part
	Explanation:	The solid matter may be an abnormal byproduct of a biological function or a foreign body; it may be imbedded in a body part or in the lumen of a tubular body part. The solid matter may or may not have been previously broken into pieces.

Upper and Lower Intestinal Tract

Guideline B4.8

B4.8	**In the Gastrointestinal body system, the general body part values Upper Intestinal Tract and Lower Intestinal Tract are provided as an option for the root operations Change, Inspection, Removal and Revision. Upper Intestinal Tract includes the portion of the gastrointestinal tract from the esophagus down to and including the duodenum, and Lower Intestinal Tract includes the portion of the gastrointestinal tract from the jejunum down to and including the rectum and anus.**
	Example: **In the root operation Change table, change of a device in the jejunum is coded using the body part Lower Intestinal Tract.**

AHA Coding Clinic

2018, 1Q, 18	Argon Plasma Coagulation of Duodenal Arteriovenous Malformation
2017, 4Q, 105	Control of Gastrointestinal Bleeding
2017, 2Q, 15	Low Anterior Resection with Sigmoidoscopy
2016, 2Q, 20	Capsule Endoscopy of Small Intestine
2015, 3Q, 24	Esophagogastroduodenoscopy with Epinephrine Injection for Control of Bleeding

The gastrointestinal (GI) system is composed of a series of anatomical structures that begin at the mouth and continue through the anus. The PCS classification divides the GI tract into upper and lower sections with the dividing line between the duodenum and jejunum. The specific anatomical structures of the upper and lower GI tract are illustrated in figure 5.23. and outlined in the following table.

Table 5.6. Components of Upper and Lower GI Tract

Upper GI Tract	Lower GI Tract
Upper esophagus	Jejunum
Middle esophagus	Ileum
Lower esophagus	Cecum
Esophagogastric junction	Ascending colon
Stomach	Transverse colon
Pylorus sphincter	Descending colon
Stomach, pylorus	Sigmoid colon
Duodenum	Rectum
	Anus

Figure 5.23. Upper Intestinal Tract (Ø) and Lower Intestinal Tract (D)

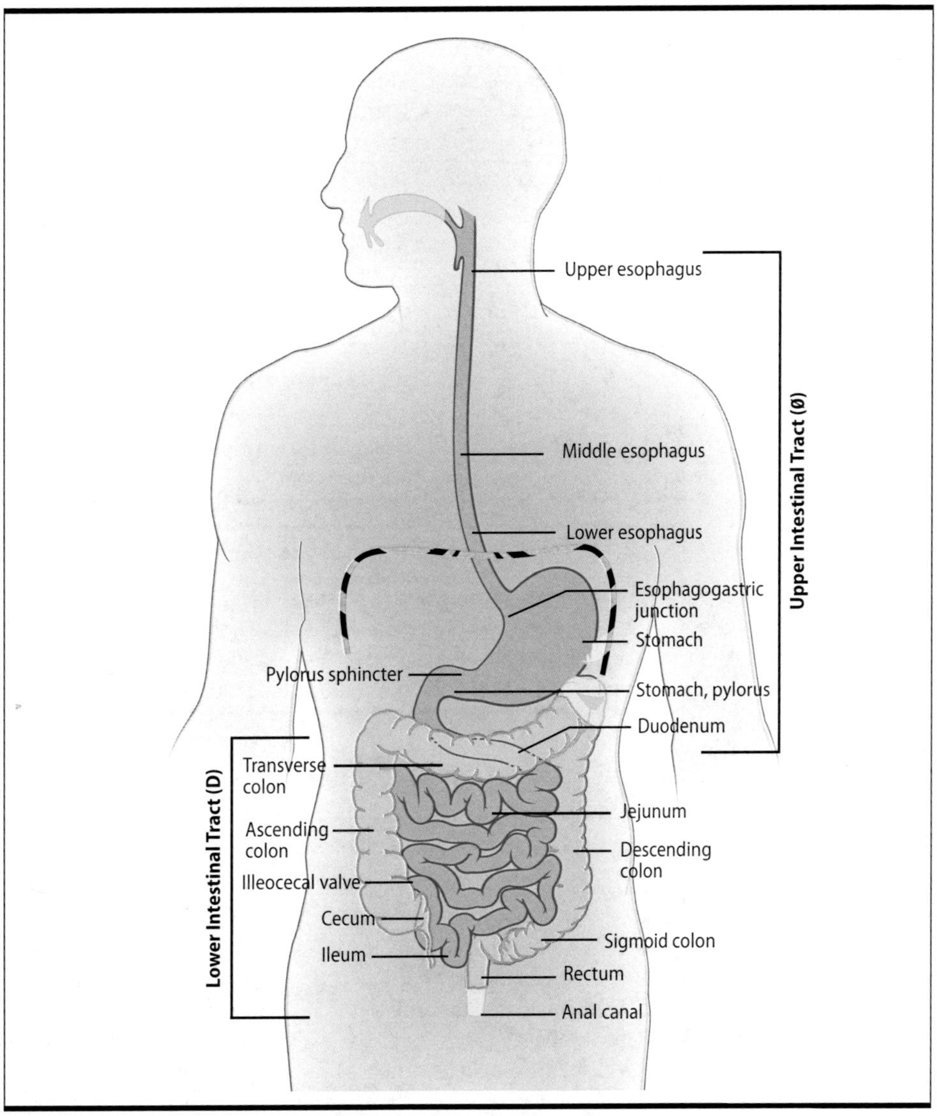

This guideline pertains to a very limited number of procedures within the Gastrointestinal (D) body system that are represented by root operations Change (2), Insertion (H), Inspection (J), Removal (P), and Revision (W). When specific body parts for the intestines such as sigmoid colon, duodenum, or jejunum are documented in an operative report using these root operations, the upper or lower intestinal tract body part values are used. In some of these root operations, specific values are available for body parts such as stomach, esophagus, anus, and rectum. The most specific body part documented should always be reported. Only default to upper and lower intestinal tract when a more specific option is not available or documentation is not further specified.

Root Operation		
Change (2)	Definition:	Taking out or off a device from a body part and putting back an identical or similar device in or on the same body part without cutting or puncturing the skin or a mucous membrane
	Explanation:	All CHANGE procedures are coded using the approach EXTERNAL
Insertion (H)	Definition:	Putting in a nonbiological appliance that monitors, assists, performs, or prevents a physiological function but does not physically take the place of a body part.
	Explanation:	None

Root Operation		
Inspection (J)	Definition:	Visually and/or manually exploring a body part
	Explanation:	Visual exploration may be performed with or without optical instrumentation. Manual exploration may be performed directly or through intervening body layers.
Removal (P)	Definition:	Taking out or off a device from a body part
	Explanation:	If a device is taken out and a similar device put in without cutting or puncturing the skin or mucous membrane, the procedure is coded to the root operation CHANGE. Otherwise, the procedure for taking out a device is coded to the root operation REMOVAL.
Revision (W)	Definition:	Correcting, to the extent possible, a portion of a malfunctioning device or the position of a displaced device
	Explanation:	Revision can include correcting a malfunctioning or displaced device by taking out or putting in components of the device such as a screw or pin

Spotlight
The body part value Gastrointestinal Tract (P) in the Anatomical Regions, General (W) body system includes all anatomical structures that comprise the upper and lower GI tracts. It is used for limited root operations when it is more appropriate to include the entire GI tract rather than just upper or lower.

Practical Application for Guideline B4.8

Case Study 5.41. Esophagogastroduodenoscopy (EGD)
The patient was placed in the left lateral decubitus position. Medications were given. After adequate sedation was achieved, the Olympus video endoscope was inserted into the mouth and advanced toward the duodenum. Mucosa appeared normal. The duodenum appeared normal. The scope was then brought back toward the stomach. The antrum and angularis appeared slightly erythematous. The scope was retroflexed to visualize the mucosa of rugal folds, the body, and fundus of the stomach. The scope was then anteflexed and brought back to the distal esophagus. All the esophageal mucosa appeared normal. The squamocolumnar junction appeared normal as well. The scope was removed and procedure terminated.

Code(s):

0DJ08ZZ   **Inspection of Upper Intestinal Tract, Via Natural or Artificial Opening Endoscopic**

Rationale:

The procedure performed is commonly referred to as an esophagogastroduodenoscopy or EGD. The EGD looks at the upper GI tract from the esophagus through the duodenum via a thin tube with a small light and camera (endoscope) inserted through the mouth. The correct root operation to describe an EGD is Inspection (J). Inspection (J) is one of the root operations that offers limited body part value choices. There is no option for esophagus or duodenum in the Inspection (J) table; however, according to guideline B4.8, body part Upper Intestinal Tract (0) includes the esophagus down through the duodenum. Since this one body part value includes all the parts visualized, only one code is needed to completely capture the Inspection (J). This guideline relates only to the Gastrointestinal (D) body system. Since the endoscope was inserted orally, the approach value is Via Natural or Artificial Opening Endoscopic (8). The values for No Device (Z) and No Qualifier (Z) are added as the sixth and seventh character.

Figure 5.24. Esophagogastroduodenoscopy (EGD)

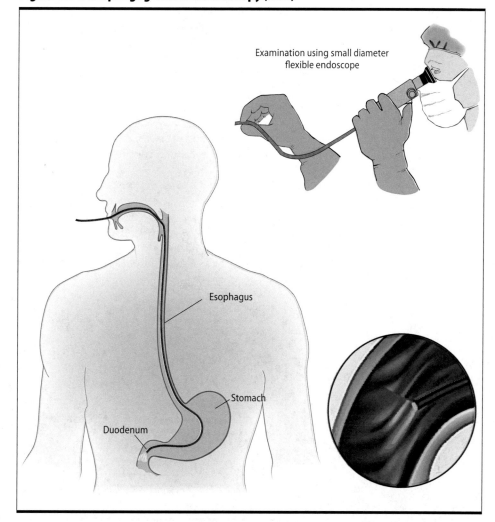

Examination using small diameter flexible endoscope

Esophagus

Stomach

Duodenum

Case Study 5.42. Colonoscopy

Description of procedure: After informed consent and sedation was given, the patient was placed in the left lateral decubitus position. A well-lubricated adult video colonoscope was advanced under direct vision from the rectum to the cecum without difficulty. The prep was found to be good. The mucosa was well seen. There were a few sigmoid diverticula, but other than that, the mucosa was unremarkable from the rectum to the cecum with no polyps, mass, or mucosal irregularity. The ileocecal valve and appendiceal orifice were clearly identified. No pathology was visualized at this level. The scope was fully withdrawn while examining the color, texture, anatomy, and integrity of the mucosa from the cecum to the anal canal. The patient tolerated the procedure well.

Code(s):

ØDJD8ZZ   **Inspection of Lower Intestinal Tract, Via Natural or Artificial Opening Endoscopic**

Rationale:

During a colonoscopy, a long flexible tube with a small video camera at the tip is used to examine the colon from the rectum to the cecum. This procedure is represented by root operation Inspection (J), which contains only a limited number of options for body part values. The body part value used in this example is Lower Intestinal Tract (D) because it includes any portion of the colon from the jejunum to the rectum. The colonoscope can only reach as far as the distal part of the ileum, which is why colonoscopies generally terminate at the ileocecal valve. Although the colonoscopy does not include the jejunum, this code still captures the rest of the colon that was examined. Since the colonoscope was inserted into the rectum and advanced through the colon, the correct approach value is Via Natural or Artificial Opening Endoscopic (8). Values No Device (Z) and No Qualifier (Z) are used as the sixth and seventh character.

Spotlight

If a polypectomy of the sigmoid is performed in the same episode as the examination of the entire colon, two codes are reported: one for the Excision (B) of the Sigmoid Colon (N) and a secondary code for the Inspection (J) of the Lower Intestinal Tract (D), which includes body parts from the rectum through the cecum.

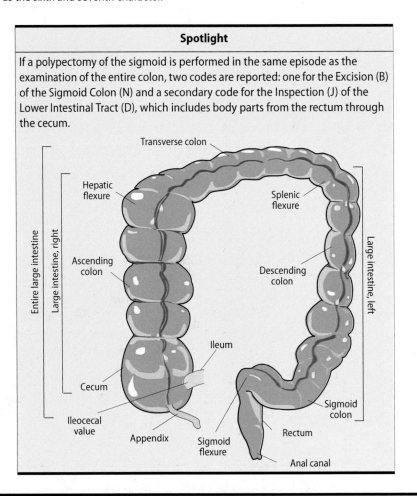

Case Study 5.43. Self-expanding Metal Stent (SEMS) Retrieval

Indications: A patient with malignant bowel stenosis presented with SEMS migration distally to blockage.

Procedure: Remove previously placed stent with possible replacement.

With the patient under sedation, the DBE probe was passed into the jejunum until the previous migrated stent was located. A 0.35-mm wire-guide was inserted through the working channel of the DBE probe into the distal small intestine under fluoroscopic guidance. The endoscope with the overtube was withdrawn, and the wire-guide was left across the stenosis. Forceps were introduced into the working channel of the scope. The migrated stent was grasped and pulled out. It was decided that the blockage was too extensive to deploy a replacement stent, so scope and guidewires were withdrawn and the procedure terminated.

Code(s):

ØDPD8DZ   **Removal of Intraluminal Device from Lower Intestinal Tract, Via Natural or Artificial Opening Endoscopic**

Rationale:

Self-expanding metal stents (SEMS) are used most often in patients with nonsurgical bowel blockages due to malignancies. A common complication is the migration of the stent, which can cause a bowel perforation. The SEMS in this case had migrated and was removed without replacement, reported with root operation Removal (P). If it had been possible to move the stent into its proper location without replacement, it would be coded with root operation Revision (W); if it had been removed and immediately replaced with the same or similar device, it would be reported with Change (2).

Root Operation		
Change (2)	Definition:	Taking out or off a device from a body part and putting back an identical or similar device in or on the same body part without cutting or puncturing the skin or a mucous membrane
	Explanation:	All CHANGE procedures are coded using the approach EXTERNAL
Removal (P)	Definition:	Taking out or off a device from a body part
	Explanation:	If a device is taken out and a similar device put in without cutting or puncturing the skin or mucous membrane, the procedure is coded to the root operation CHANGE. Otherwise, the procedure for taking out a device is coded to the root operation REMOVAL.
Revision (W)	Definition:	Correcting, to the extent possible, a portion of a malfunctioning device or the position of a displaced device
	Explanation:	Revision can include correcting a malfunctioning or displaced device by taking out or putting in components of the device such as a screw or pin

All of these root operations can **only** be used with a device. They are not used when reporting revisions of, changes to, or removal of a body part.

Although anatomically the jejunum is grouped with the small intestines, in the Gastrointestinal (D) body system in PCS it is reported as Lower Intestinal Tract (D) body part. Double balloon endoscopy (DBE) employs a technique in which a scope is passed through the mouth into the small intestine for a Via Natural or Artificial Opening Endoscopic (8) approach. The stent that was removed is considered an Intraluminal Device (D).

Case Study 5.44. Percutaneous Endoscopic Gastrojejunostomy (PEGJ) Tube Exchange

The malfunctioning GJ tube was removed. With lubrication, a 12 French red Robinson catheter was gently reinserted into the former J-tube tract without difficulty and was affixed to the skin temporarily. Tube placement confirmed that the feeding tube was in the jejunum, and the tube itself was affixed to the skin. The skin surrounding the J-tube was prepped and appropriately draped in a sterile fashion. The surrounding skin was infiltrated with 1% Lidocaine. A single suture of 2-0 nylon was placed in the skin and the drain was affixed without difficulty. The jejunostomy tube was easily flushed and drained. A dry sterile dressing was applied.

Code(s):

ØD2DXUZ **Change Feeding Device in Lower Intestinal Tract, External Approach**

Rationale:
When a device is exchanged for another device that is the same or similar in the same operative episode without making an incision or puncturing the skin or mucous membrane, the appropriate root operation is Change (2). Although the procedure was performed using an endoscope via the mouth versus a colonoscope via the rectum, the correct body part value is Lower Intestinal Tract (D) because it involves the jejunum, which based on guideline B4.8 is included in the Lower Intestinal Tract (D). The approach for a change procedure is always External (X). Feeding Device (U) is the appropriate device value for the GJ tube. No Qualifier (Z) value is assigned.

Chapter 6. Approach Guidelines

Approach Overview

Approach: Character 5

Character 1	Character 2	Character 3	Character 4	Character 5	Character 6	Character 7
Section	Body System	Root Operation	Body Part	Approach	Device	Qualifier

The fifth character in an ICD-10-PCS code represents the approach, the method or technique used to reach the procedure site. In the Medical and Surgical (Ø) section of PCS there are seven approach character values:

- Open (Ø)

- Percutaneous (3)

- Percutaneous Endoscopic (4)

- Via Natural or Artificial Opening (7)

- Via Natural or Artificial Opening Endoscopic (8)

- Via Natural or Artificial Opening with Percutaneous Endoscopic Assistance (F)

- External (X)

Approach Components
Correct approach assignment is determined by the following components:

- **Access location.** When procedures are performed on **internal** body sites, one of two general access locations is used: through the skin and mucous membranes or through an external orifice. The skin or mucous membrane can be punctured or cut to reach the site of the procedure. Every open and percutaneous approach falls into one of the following categories: Open (Ø), Percutaneous (3), or Percutaneous Endoscopic (4). A procedure site can also be reached via an external opening, which can be natural (e.g., the mouth) or artificial (e.g., a gastrointestinal stoma). External openings are represented in ICD-10-PCS as Via Natural or Artificial Opening (7), Via Natural or Artificial Opening Endoscopic (8), and Via Natural or Artificial Opening with Percutaneous Endoscopic Assistance (F).

- **Method.** The method specifies how the access location is entered for procedures performed on an internal body part. An Open (Ø) approach value indicates that the physician cut through the skin or mucous membrane and any other intervening body layers necessary to expose the procedure site. Instrumentation can also be introduced by insertion through an external opening or through a puncture or minor incision. This minor incision or puncture is not considered "open," because it does not expose the procedure site. A single approach value may contain more than one method, such as the Via Natural or Artificial Opening with Percutaneous Endoscopic Assistance (F) approach. This approach includes both the entry into an orifice to execute the actual procedure and the introduction of instrumentation by puncture or minor incision of skin, mucous membrane, and other body layers to provide visualization and assistance with the performance of the procedure, such as dissection to facilitate the removal of body parts.

- **Type of instrumentation.** Specialized equipment may be used for instrumentation on internal body parts. Instrumentation must be used for all approaches performed on internal body parts except the basic Open (Ø) approach. In some cases, instrumentation provides the ability to visualize the procedure site, such as a colonoscopy where the inside of the colon is viewed. In other cases, such as those related to needle biopsies, direct visualization is not used. The term *endoscopic* typically refers to instrumentation with internal visualization via a camera.

The last type of approach value is External (X). An external approach is performed directly on the skin or mucous membrane (such as a skin excision) or it may be performed indirectly by the application of external force through the skin (such as that used in a closed reduction of a fracture).

The following table provides a list of all seven approach values in PCS, along with their definitions, character values, access location, method, type of instrumentation (if any), and an example of each type of procedure.

Table 6.1. Approach Values

ICD-10-PCS Value	Definition	Access Location	Method	Instrumentation	Example
Open (Ø)	Cutting through the skin or mucous membrane and any other body layers necessary to expose the site of the procedure	Skin or mucous membrane, any other body layers	Cutting	None	Abdominal hysterectomy
Percutaneous (3)	Entry, by puncture or minor incision, of instrumentation through the skin or mucous membrane and any other body layers necessary to reach the site of the procedure	Skin or mucous membrane, any other body layers	Puncture or minor incision	Without visualization	Needle biopsy of liver, Liposuction
Percutaneous Endoscopic (4)	Entry, by puncture or minor incision, of instrumentation through the skin or mucous membrane and any other body layers necessary to reach and visualize the site of the procedure	Skin or mucous membrane, any other body layers	Puncture or minor incision	With visualization	Arthroscopy, Laparoscopic cholecystectomy
Via Natural or Artificial Opening (7)	Entry of instrumentation through a natural or artificial external opening to reach the site of the procedure	Natural or artificial external opening	Direct entry	Without visualization	Endotracheal tube insertion, Foley catheter placement
Via Natural or Artificial Opening Endoscopic (8)	Entry of instrumentation through a natural or artificial external opening to reach and visualize the site of the procedure	Natural or artificial external opening	Direct entry	With visualization	Sigmoidoscopy, EGD, ERCP
Via Natural or Artificial Opening with Percutaneous Endoscopic Assistance (F)	Entry of instrumentation through a natural or artificial external opening and entry, by puncture or minor incision, of instrumentation through the skin or mucous membrane and any other body layers necessary to aid in the performance of the procedure	Skin or mucous membrane, any other body layers	Direct entry with puncture or minor incision for instrumentation only	With visualization	Laparoscopic-assisted vaginal hysterectomy
External (X)	Procedures performed directly on the skin or mucous membrane and procedures performed indirectly by the application of external force through the skin or mucous membrane	Skin or mucous membrane	Direct or indirect application	None	Closed fracture reduction, Resection of tonsils

The following decision tree may be helpful in determining the correct approach value:

Figure 6.1. Approach Decision Tree

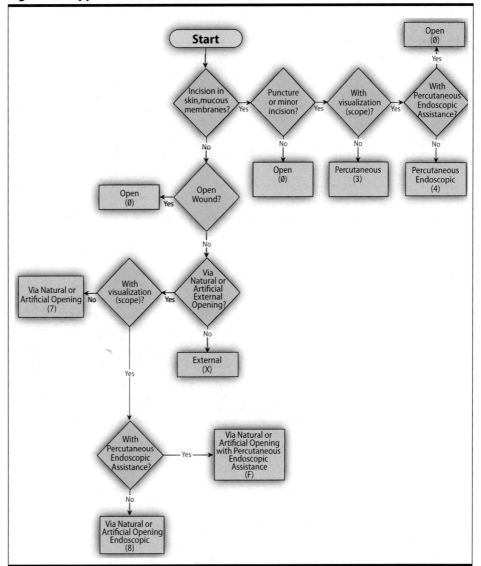

Coding guidelines help define which approach value should be selected when a combination of approaches are utilized. For instance, if a procedure is performed using a *laparoscopic-assisted open* approach, the procedure is coded to approach value Open (∅). Assigning the incorrect approach character value can easily result in an inappropriate MS-DRG assignment. The official coding guidelines related to PCS approaches are outlined in the following discussion.

Spotlight
ICD-10-PCS does not offer a separate approach value for minimally invasive approaches. The coder must choose the approach based on the ICD-10-PCS approach definitions and procedure documentation. For example, a percutaneous approach would not involve direct visualization while an open approach would (*AHA Coding Clinic,* 2013, 2Q, 108).

The following figures illustrate the approach techniques as described by ICD-10-PCS.

Figure 6.2. Open (Ø)

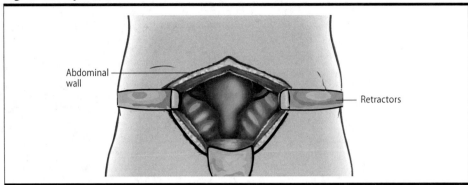

Figure 6.3. Percutaneous (3)

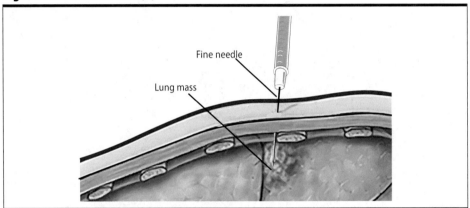

Figure 6.4. Percutaneous Endoscopic (4)

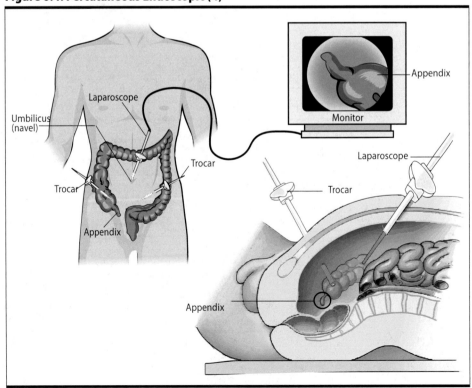

Figure 6.5. Via Natural or Artificial Opening (7)

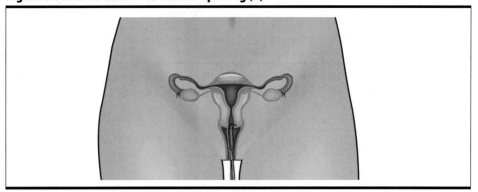

Figure 6.6. Via Natural or Artificial Opening Endoscopic (8)

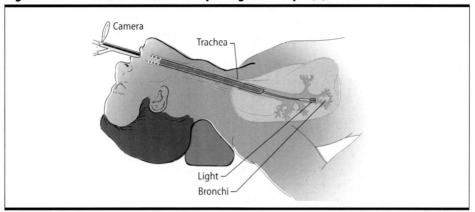

Figure 6.7. Via Natural or Artificial Opening with Percutaneous Endoscopic Assistance (F)

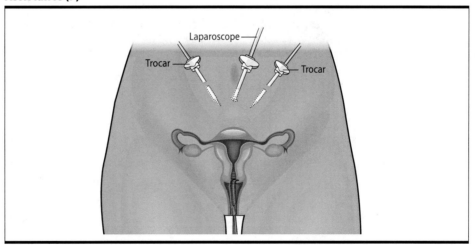

Figure 6.8. External (X)

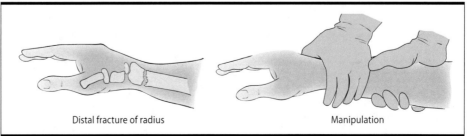

Open Approach with Percutaneous Endoscopic Assistance

Guideline B5.2

B5.2	**Procedures performed using the open approach with percutaneous endoscopic assistance are coded to the approach Open.**
	Example: **Laparoscopic-assisted sigmoidectomy is coded to the approach Open.**

AHA Coding Clinic

2014, 3Q, 16   Hand-Assisted Laparoscopy Nephroureterectomy

An endoscopically-assisted procedure is primarily accomplished through an incision, or open approach. In the case of a laparoscopic-assisted colectomy, the colon is visualized and can be mobilized and prepared for resection intracorporeally with the use of percutaneous ports and access instrumentation (Trocars); however, the actual resection and anastomosis is done extracorporeally through the mini laparotomy incision. This type of procedure is less disruptive and more accurate than a traditional open procedure as the laparoscope allows for visualization of areas that are difficult to see in an open procedure.

According to *AHA Coding Clinic,* 2014, 3Q, 16, a similar approach included in this guideline is referred to as a hand port laparoscopic-assisted (HAL) approach. HAL consists of creation of a 7 inch to 8 inch incision or hand port that allows the introduction of the surgeon's hand for assisting with the laparoscopic instruments, as well as exposing, retracting, dissecting, or maintaining hemostasis.

Regardless of whether the surgeon uses additional laparoscopic instrumentation to aid in the performance of the procedure, the Open (Ø) approach is assigned in PCS.

Definitions
extracorporeally (ECA). Situated or occurring outside of the body.
intracorporeally (ICA). Inside the body; situated or occurring within the body.

Practical Application for Guideline B5.2

Case Study 6.1. Laparoscopic-assisted Appendectomy

The patient was brought to the operating room and placed on the table in supine position. Endotracheal intubation and general anesthesia were obtained and the abdomen was prepped and draped in standard fashion. A longitudinal incision was made in the middle of the umbilicus and using blunt dissection, the anterior fascia was identified. The umbilicus was elevated with a Kocher clamp and stay sutures of 0 Vicryl were placed laterally along the midline. The fascia was opened using a 15 blade and the peritoneum was entered bluntly with a finger. A 12 mm Hassan trocar was placed along with two additional 5 mm trocars. An operative laparoscope was placed into the abdominal cavity after insufflation had been obtained. The appendix was easily identified, grabbed with graspers, and delivered into the umbilical wound after trocars were removed. The fascial incision was extended to allow evisceration of the cecum into the operative field. The mesoappendix was isolated off the appendix and tied with two silk sutures, cut between sutures. The base of the appendix was identified and an EndoGIA surgical stapler placed across it, transecting it. The cecum was delivered back into the abdominal cavity. Once hemostasis was achieved, the abdomen was deflated and the trocars removed. The umbilical wound was closed and sterile dressing applied. The patient tolerated the procedure without problems.

Code(s):
ØDTJØZZ   Resection of Appendix, Open Approach

Rationale:
The ICD-10-PCS index for Appendectomy lists *see* Excision, Appendix ØDBJ and *see* Resection, Appendix ØDTJ. In this example, the entire appendix was removed, since the operative report states that staples were placed at the base of the appendix, making root operation Resection (T) the correct choice. The Appendix (J) is part of the Gastrointestinal (D) system. Although a laparoscope was used in visualizing the appendix, the appendix was brought out through the incision in order to transect it. Therefore, this is coded as an Open (Ø) approach per guideline B5.2. No Device (Z) and No Qualifier (Z) are also reported..

Root Operation		
Resection (T)	Definition:	Cutting out or off, without replacement, all of a body part
	Explanation:	None

Spotlight
The operative report must be reviewed carefully to discern between a total laparoscopic procedure, reported as Percutaneous Endoscopic (4) approach, and an Open (Ø) procedure with laparoscopic assistance. If the procedure is performed entirely within the body with laparoscopy instruments and only small incisions made for the introduction of the instrumentation, the correct approach value is Percutaneous Endoscopic (4). If the incision is enlarged to allow a surgeon's hand to perform the procedure or to bring the body part outside of the body, Open (Ø) approach is appropriate.

Figure 6.9. Appendectomy

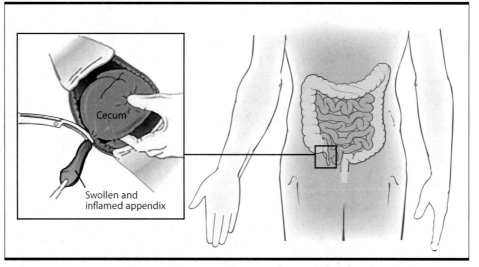

Cecum

Swollen and
inflamed appendix

Case Study 6.2. Laparoscopic-assisted Right Hemicolectomy

The patient was taken to the operating room and given general endotracheal anesthesia. He was placed in the supine position. A Foley catheter was placed. The abdomen was prepped and draped in the standard surgical fashion. Incision was carried down in the umbilicus approximately one half inch in length with the use of a scalpel. A Veress needle was introduced. The abdominal cavity was insufflated with CO2 gas.

A 12 mm bladeless trocar was introduced into the abdominal cavity with ease. The abdominal cavity was reinsufflated. A 10 mm, 30-degree scope was placed in the abdominal cavity. There was no evidence of any injury from the Veress needle or trocar. An additional 5 mm trocar was placed in the suprapubic position after a small stab incision was created with a 15 blade. This was placed under direct visualization and the exact same procedure was carried out with a 5 mm trocar in the left flank.

Using an additional 5 mm trocar, which was placed in the left upper quadrant after a small stab incision was created, the liver was retracted superiorly and the attachments of the transverse colon were taken down with use of sharp dissection. The omentum was taken off the transverse colon to the level of the midtransverse colon. The right colic artery was identified and taken with the use of the Ace Harmonic scalpel. The duodenum was identified and mobilized medially.

Once the colon was completely mobilized to the level of the mid to distal transverse colon, the 5 mm trocars were removed. The terminal ileum was grasped with a grasper, and the incision through the umbilicus was extended to approximately 3-1/2 inches in length with the use of cautery. A retractor was placed into the wound. The bowel, including the terminal ileum, right colon, and transverse colon were brought up through the incision. The terminal ileum, approximately 5 cm proximal to the ileocecal valve, was transected with a 75 GIA stapler and the midtransverse colon was transected in a similar fashion. The mesentery was taken with the use of Ace Harmonic scalpel. The specimen was passed off the field, labeled as right colon.

A functional side-to-side anastomosis was created with a 75 GIA stapler followed by closure with a TA60. The created anastomosis was reinforced with 3-0 Vicryl pop-off interrupted. The staple line was reinforced with 3-0 Vicryl pop-off interrupted in a Lembert fashion. The bowel was returned to the abdominal cavity. The omentum was draped over the bowel. The abdomen was copiously irrigated.

The fascia was approximated with #1 PDS in a running fashion. Subcutaneous tissue was copiously irrigated and the skin was approximated with staples. The trocar sites were approximated with staples as well. The abdomen was cleaned and dried. Dry sterile dressings were applied. The patient was transported to the recovery room in stable condition.

Code(s):

ØDTFØZZ   Resection of Right Large Intestine, Open Approach

Rationale:

In ICD-10-PCS, the right large intestine (colon) is assigned its own body part. Resection includes all of a body part, or any subdivision of a body part that has its own body part value in ICD-10-PCS, while Excision (B) includes only a portion of a body part. Because the surgeon removed the entire subdivision of the body part with its own body part value (the right half of the large intestine), the correct root operation is Resection (T).

Root Operation		
Resection (T)	Definition:	Cutting out or off, without replacement, all of a body part
	Explanation:	None

The Large Intestine, Right (F) body part value can be found in the Gastrointestinal (D) body system. Although a laparoscope was used to identify and mobilize the colon, the approach value is Open (Ø) as per guideline B5.2. Transection of the colon, as well as the anastomosis, was completed extracorporeally through the laparotomy incision.

Figure 6.10. Right Hemicolectomy

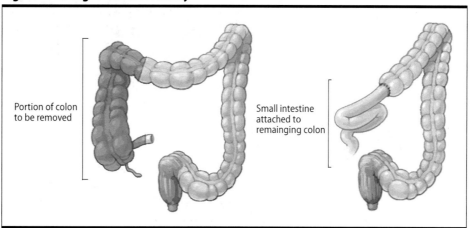

Portion of colon to be removed

Small intestine attached to remainging colon

According to ICD-10-PCS guideline B3.1b, the anastomosis, regardless of technique, is not reported separately. Therefore, only the resection code is assigned.

PCS Guideline
General Guidelines
B3.1b   Components of a procedure specified in the root operation definition and explanation are not coded separately. Procedural steps necessary to reach the operative site and close the operative site, including anastomosis of a tubular body part, are also not coded separately.
Example: Resection of a joint as part of a joint replacement procedure is included in the root operation definition of Replacement and is not coded separately.
Laparotomy performed to reach the site of an open liver biopsy is not coded separately. In a resection of sigmoid colon with anastomosis of descending colon to rectum, the anastomosis is not coded separately.

Case Study 6.3. Laparoscopic-assisted Myomectomy

The patient was taken to the operating room and placed in the dorsal lithotomy position after general anesthesia was administered. The patient was prepped and draped in the usual sterile fashion. Attention was turned to the patient's abdomen where a 5 mm incision was made in the umbilical fold, and a Veress needle introduced into the abdominal cavity and intraabdominal placement confirmed. The abdomen was insufflated with CO_2 gas and the Veress needle was removed with the 5 mm trocar introduced and appropriate intraabdominal placement confirmed by the 0-degree laparoscope. Two further incisions were made in the left lower quadrant and right lower quadrant to accommodate 10 mm trocars under direct visualization lateral to the inferior epigastric vessels.

An incision was made over the uterine serosa until the capsule of the leiomyoma was reached. Using a corkscrew manipulator, the uterus was elevated toward the midline suprapubic incision. With the trocar and manipulator attached to the myoma, the midline 5 mm incision was enlarged to a 4 cm to 5 cm transverse incision. After fascia was transversely incised at 4 cm to 5 cm, the rectus muscles were separated at the midline.

The peritoneum was entered transversely, and the leiomyomas were located and brought to the incision using the corkscrew manipulator; the uterus was raised with a uterine manipulator. The corkscrew manipulator was replaced with two Lahey tenacula. The uterus was brought to the skin through the minilaparotomy incision and two leiomyomas were excised.

The uterus was reconstructed in layers using 4-0 to 2-0 and 0-polydioxanone sutures and palpated to ensure that no small intramural leiomyomas were present. The uterus was returned to the peritoneal cavity, and the fascia and skin closed in layers. The laparoscope was used to evaluate the uterus and ensure final hemostasis. All equipment was removed. The patient tolerated the procedure well.

Code(s):

ØUB9ØZZ   Excision of Uterus, Open Approach

Rationale:

Myomectomy refers to the surgical removal of uterine fibroids (leiomyomas). Since only a portion of the uterus is removed, Excision (B) is the appropriate root operation. The ICD-10-PCS index for Myomectomy also directs a user to *see* Excision, Female Reproductive System ØUB.

Root Operation		
Excision (B)	Definition:	Cutting out or off, without replacement, a portion of a body part
	Explanation:	The qualifier DIAGNOSTIC is used to identify excision procedures that are biopsies

The Uterus (9) is part of the Female Reproductive (U) body system. Although two fibroids were excised, only one code is needed. *AHA Coding Clinic,* 2014, 4Q, 16, provides guidance stating that only one code is needed for the excision of multiple uterine fibroids because the excisions are being performed on only one body part value.

As per guideline B5.2, although laparoscope assistance was used, the correct approach is Open (Ø). No Device (Z) is the only option for the sixth character, and since there was no mention of further study being done, No Qualifier (Z) is used for the seventh character.

External Approach

Guideline B5.3a

General Guidelines

B5.3a   **Procedures performed within an orifice on structures that are visible without the aid of any instrumentation are coded to the approach External.**

Example: **Resection of tonsils is coded to the approach External.**

AHA Coding Clinic

2018, 1Q, 17	Repositioning of Impella Short-Term External Heart Assist Device
2017, 3Q, 5	Delivery of Placenta
2017, 2Q, 26	Exchange of Tunneled Catheter
2017, 1Q, 35	Epifix® Allograft
2016, 3Q, 19	Nonoperative Removal of Peripherally Inserted Central Catheter
2016, 2Q, 21	Laser Trabeculoplasty
2016, 2Q, 34	Assisted Vaginal Delivery
2016, 1Q, 9	Anteversion of Retroverted Pregnant Uterus
2015, 2Q, 12	Orbital Exenteration
2015, 2Q, 25	Penetrating Keratoplasty and Placement of Viscoelastic Eye with Paracentesis
2014, 4Q, 20	Control of Epistaxis
2014, 3Q, 12	Excision of Skin Tag from Labia Majora
2014, 3Q, 25	Excision of Soft Palate with Placement of Surgical Obturator

In order to assign an External approach value, the following should be considered:

- Did the procedure require incision into one or more body layers in order to visualize the site of the procedure?

- Was instrumentation required in order to visualize the site of the procedure?

There are some anatomical structures, such as those found within a body orifice (e.g., mouth, nose) that, although considered an internal body structure, do not require an incision through body layers OR instrumentation to visualize that structure in order to facilitate a procedure. When an anatomical structure can be directly visualized within a body orifice and does not require either of the above methods, the procedure may be coded with an External (X) approach.

Practical Application for Guidelines B5.3a

Case Study 6.4. Tonsillectomy with Fulguration of Adenoids

A 7-year-old female with chronic obstructive adenotonsillar hypertrophy presented for tonsillectomy and adenoidectomy (T&A). The patient was positioned, prepped, and anesthetized. Bilateral tonsils were identified in the oropharynx, dissected from the capsule, and removed. Bleeding vessels were controlled with electrocautery. A mirror was used to visualize the adenoid tissue, which upon identification was fulgurated.

Code(s):

ØCTPXZZ	Resection of Tonsils, External Approach
ØC5QXZZ	Destruction of Adenoids, External Approach

Rationale:

In this example, two codes are needed to capture the procedure because it was performed on two separate and distinct body part values: the Tonsils (P) and the Adenoids (Q). Additionally, two root operations were used.

Root Operation		
Resection (T)	Definition:	Cutting out or off, without replacement, all of a body part
	Explanation:	None
Destruction (5)	Definition:	Physical eradication of all or a portion of a body part by the direct use of energy, force, or a destructive agent
	Explanation:	None of the body part is physically taken out

Figure 6.11. Tonsils and Adenoids

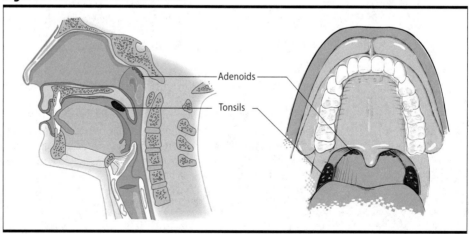

The tonsils were excised in their entirety meeting the root operation definition of Resection (T). Using the PCS index, the user is directed to ØCT for Tonsillectomy, *see* Resection, Mouth and Throat. There is no bilateral body part value for tonsils, nor body part values for right or left tonsils. Only one code is needed for the removal of both tonsils. The tonsils are removed directly through the mouth without any incision through other body layers to reach the excision site or visualization with instrumentation, for an External (X) approach. No Device (Z) and No Qualifier (Z) are the only sixth- and seventh-character options.

The adenoids were fulgurated, which in PCS terms meets the root operation definition of Destruction (5). Like tonsils, only one body part value exists for Adenoids (Q). The approach is External (X) since the procedure was performed through an orifice directly on the adenoidal surface, which was visible without the aid of instrumentation.

Definition
fulguration. Destruction of living tissue by using sparks from a high-frequency electric current.

Case Study 6.5. Control, Post-tonsillectomy Bleeding

The patient was placed supine after induction of general anesthesia was established. A mouth gag was placed. There was some oozing from the right inferior tonsillar fossa and the superior left tonsillar pole, which were easily controlled with suction cautery. The patient tolerated the procedure well and was transported to the recovery room.

Code(s):

ØW33XZZ   Control Bleeding in Oral Cavity and Throat, External Approach

Rationale:

The objective of this procedure was to stop postoperative bleeding, meeting the root operation definition of Control (3). The full explanation of the root operation Control (3) indicates that the body system for this procedure is found in the Anatomical Regions, General (W). There is no body part for Tonsils, so Oral Cavity and Throat (3) is the most appropriate. The approach is External (X) because the tonsillar area may be visualized and accessed externally without the use of instrumentation.

Root Operation		
Control (3)	Definition:	Stopping, or attempting to stop, postprocedural or other acute bleeding
	Explanation:	The site of the bleeding is coded as an anatomical region and not to a specific body part

---

Case Study 6.6. Excision, Soft Palate Tumor

Indications: The patient was diagnosed with squamous cell carcinoma of the soft palate two weeks ago.

Procedure: The patient was brought to the operating room and placed in supine position. General anesthesia was induced. The patient was intubated. The patient was prepped and draped in the usual sterile fashion, followed by a timeout to properly identify the patient and the procedure. 1% Lidocaine with 1:100,000 parts Epinephrine was locally infiltrated into the soft palate around the mass. The nasal surface of the soft palate was checked to ensure it would not be involved with the margins, and this was deemed to be true. Wide local excision of the soft palate mass was performed with 1 cm margins after which time the main specimen was sent to pathology for permanent specimen. Anterior, posterior, right lateral, and left lateral margins were taken and sent to pathology for frozen specimen, all of which returned negative for malignancy.

Code(s):

ØCB3XZZ   Excision of Soft Palate, External Approach

Rationale:

A portion of the soft palate was removed in this example, meeting the root operation definition of Excision (B).

Root Operation		
Excision (B)	Definition:	Cutting out or off, without replacement, a portion of a body part
	Explanation:	The qualifier DIAGNOSTIC is used to identify excision procedures that are biopsies

The Soft Palate (3) body part can be found in the Mouth and Throat (C) body system. Additionally, the ICD-10-PCS index for Excision, Palate, Soft directs the user to ØCB3.

The External (X) approach is used since the surgery was performed directly on the soft palate. No Device (Z) is the only option for the sixth character. Since the squamous cell carcinoma had been previously diagnosed, the removal of the tumor was for therapeutic reasons; No Qualifier (Z) is the appropriate seventh character.

Figure 6.12. Soft Palate

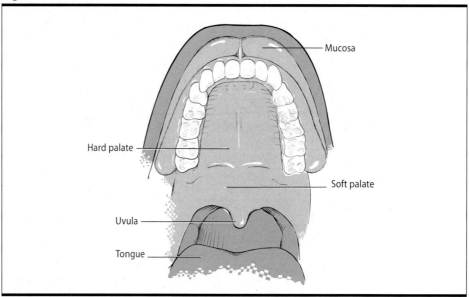

Guideline B5.3b

B5.3b	Procedures performed indirectly by the application of external force through the intervening body layers are coded to the approach External. *Example:* Closed reduction of fracture is coded to the approach External.

AHA Coding Clinic

2016, 1Q, 21   Elongation Derotation Flexion Casting

2014, 4Q, 32   Open Reduction Internal Fixation of Fracture with Debridement

2013, 4Q, 122   Extracorporeal Shock Wave Lithotripsy

2013, 2Q, 39   Application of Cervical Tongs for Reduction of Cervical Fracture

The second external approach guideline addresses the use of external force to accomplish the procedure. No visualization is used and no incision or puncture is necessary to complete the procedure. Rather, force is applied externally with the actual body part being manipulated underneath the surface. Some terms to look for that may indicate an External approach through body layers are closed reduction, flexing, using pressure, extracorporeal, manipulation, or manual reposition.

Practical Application for Guideline B5.3b

Case Study 6.7. Reduction, Nursemaid's Elbow

Beginning with the right elbow flexed, pressure was placed on the radial head. The wrist was supinated with the elbow still flexed and while moving the hand upward, the elbow was flexed. A faint click was heard and patient resumed use of limb.

Code(s):

ØRSLXZZ   **Reposition Right Elbow Joint, External Approach**

Rationale:

Nursemaid's elbow is a common injury most often found in children ages 1 to 4. Sometimes referred to as "pulled elbow," it occurs when a child's elbow is pulled and partially dislocated. Radial head subluxation is the medical term for this type of injury.

During a nursemaid's elbow reduction, the physician gently moves the joint back into normal position; Reposition (S) is the appropriate root operation to use. The Elbow Joint, Right (L) is found in the Upper Joints (R) body system. According to guideline B5.3b, the correct approach is External (X) since force was used to realign the joint. No Device (Z) was used and No Qualifier (Z) applies.

Root Operation		
Reposition (S)	Definition:	Moving to its normal location, or other suitable location, all or a portion of a body part
	Explanation:	The body part is moved to a new location from an abnormal location, or from a normal location where it is not functioning correctly. The body part may or may not be cut out or off to be moved to the new location.

Figure 6.13. Nursemaid's Elbow

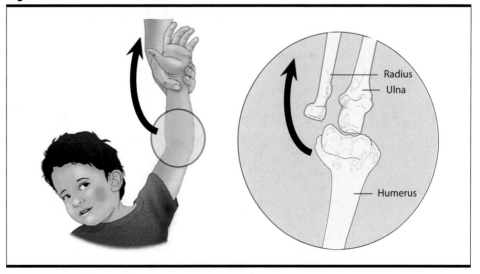

Case Study 6.8. Extracorporeal Shockwave Lithotripsy (ESWL)

After induction of general anesthesia, the patient was placed in the modified lithotomy position. Shock wave lithotripsy was started at a power setting of seven and eight, where a total of 2,000 shock waves were delivered to all areas of the stones in the left and right ureters. There appeared to be good fragmentation of the stones. The patient tolerated the procedure well and was sent to the recovery room in stable and satisfactory condition.

Code(s):

ØTF6XZZ   Fragmentation in Right Ureter, External Approach

ØTF7XZZ   Fragmentation in Left Ureter, External Approach

Rationale:

Physicians use extracorporeal shock wave lithotripsy (ESWL) to destroy calculi (stones) in the kidneys and ureters. The patient is placed on a special table with a fluid-filled cushion placed against the body. The physician uses fluoroscopic guidance to locate the calculus. Ultrasound shock waves are aimed at the stone(s), breaking up the calculus into small fragments that pass easily through the urinary system. ESWL is one of the most frequently performed procedures in urology practices and is an effective treatment for kidney and ureteral stones. Fragmentation (F) is coded for lithotripsy procedures when the solid matter is broken up but not removed.

Root Operation		
Fragmentation (F)	Definition:	Breaking solid matter in a body part into pieces
	Explanation:	Physical force (e.g., manual, ultrasonic) applied directly or indirectly is used to break the solid matter into pieces. The solid matter may be an abnormal byproduct of a biological function or a foreign body. The pieces of solid matter are not taken out.

There is no body part value for bilateral ureters in the Fragmentation (F) table of the Urinary (T) body system so separate values must be assigned for Ureter, Right (6) and Ureter, Left (7). The approach External (X) is assigned because ESWL is an externally applied, focused, high-intensity acoustic pulse that uses shock waves to break up the stones into smaller pieces.

Spotlight
When the fragments are broken up **and** removed, the correct root operation is Extirpation (C).

Case Study 6.9. Manipulation, Shoulder Joint

Indication: Frozen left shoulder.

Procedure: The patient was brought into the operating room and administered general anesthesia. The left shoulder was gently moved through a range of motions to separate adhesions. The patient tolerated the procedure well.

Code(s):

ØRNKXZZ   Release Left Shoulder Joint, External Approach

Rationale:

Frozen shoulder, also called adhesive capsulitis, is a condition that causes stiffness and pain in the shoulder joint and limits the shoulder's range of motion. In a frozen shoulder, the shoulder capsule thickens and stiff bands of tissue (adhesions) develop.

During the manipulation procedure, the physician forces the shoulder to move causing the adhesions to stretch or tear. This releases the tightening and increases range of motion. Therefore, the correct root operation for this procedure is Release (N) and the body part being released is the Shoulder Joint, Left (K) found in the Upper Joints (R) body system. The manipulation takes place by applying force through intervening body layers for an External (X) approach.

Root Operation		
Release (N)	Definition:	Freeing a body part from an abnormal physical constraint by cutting or by use of force
	Explanation:	Some of the restraining tissue may be taken out but none of the body part is taken out

---

Case Study 6.10. Reduction, Closed of Left Internal Hip Prosthetic

Indication: Patient with total hip arthroplasty presents to hospital after dislocating left hip.
Procedure: The patient was taken to the operating room, placed under general anesthesia, and laid supine on the operating table. Under fluoroscopy, in-line traction was applied to the left leg until the femoral head was perched on the acetabular liner. With internal rotation and pressure over the trochanter, the femoral head was reduced.

Code(s):
ØSWBXJZ   **Revision of Synthetic Substitute in Left Hip Joint, External Approach**
BQ11ZZZ   **Fluoroscopy of Left Hip**

Rationale:
A common complication with an internal hip prosthesis is the occasional movement of the device. To correct the device, the patient must undergo a procedure, coded using root operation Revision (W). In this example, the prosthetic hip device was reduced. Revision (W) is used since the device was being manipulated; this is in contrast to root operation Reposition (S), which is used for repositioning of a body part, as opposed to a device.

Root Operation		
Revision (W)	Definition:	Correcting, to the extent possible, a portion of a malfunctioning device or the position of a displaced device
	Explanation:	Revision can include correcting a malfunctioning or displaced device by taking out or putting in components of the device such as a screw or pin
Reposition (S)	Definition:	Moving to its normal location, or other suitable location, all or a portion of a body part
	Explanation:	The body part is moved to a new location from an abnormal location, or from a normal location where it is not functioning correctly. The body part may or may not be cut out or off to be moved to the new location.

The Hip Joint, Left (B) found in the Lower Joints (S) body system is coded using an External (X) approach since force was used through intervening body layers in order to complete the reduction. The sixth character for device is Synthetic Substitute (J) since the patient had a previous total hip arthroplasty and it is the device that was dislocated.

An additional code for fluoroscopy may be reported at some facilities.

Case Study 6.11. Reduction, Closed of Fourth and Fifth Metacarpals

Indication: Displaced fourth and fifth metacarpal fractures.

Procedure: After the establishment of successful anesthetic, IV antibiotics were given. The patient's right upper extremity was prepped and draped. At this time, the fourth metacarpal fracture was reduced with distraction and manipulation. Attention was turned to the fifth metacarpal. Following distraction and manipulation, it was decided that further augmentation was needed at which time an intramedullary retrograde pin was inserted. An ulnar gutter spica cast was applied. The patient tolerated the procedure well.

Code(s):

ØPSP34Z   **Reposition Right Metacarpal with Internal Fixation Device, Percutaneous Approach**

ØPSPXZZ   **Reposition Right Metacarpal, External Approach**

Rationale:

Two separate procedure codes are needed to capture the full intent of this procedure: one for the reduction of the fourth metacarpal fracture and another for the reduction and pinning of the fifth metacarpal. Guideline B3.15 instructs that Reposition (S) is the correct root operation to use for the reduction of a displaced fracture.

PCS Guideline
Reposition for fracture treatment
B3.15   Reduction of a displaced fracture is coded to the root operation Reposition and the application of a cast or splint in conjunction with the Reposition procedure is not coded separately. Treatment of a nondisplaced fracture is coded to the procedure performed. *Example:* Casting of a nondisplaced fracture is coded to the root operation Immobilization in the Placement section. Putting a pin in a nondisplaced fracture is coded to the root operation Insertion.

A reduction was performed on the fourth metacarpal, so correct coding includes root operation Reposition (S) and body part Metacarpal, Right (P) found in the Upper Bones (P) body system with an External (X) approach since force was applied externally. No Device (Z) and No Qualifier (Z) complete the code.

For the fifth metacarpal, Reposition (S) is the root operation along with Upper Bones (P) body system and body part Metacarpal, Right (P). A pin was inserted in addition to the reduction, which is captured with sixth-character Internal Fixation Device (4). Although an intramedullary pin was used, intramedullary is not offered as a device for the metacarpal body parts so the closest alternative is used. Even though an external reposition was performed, the procedure was ultimately accomplished with the pin that was inserted with a Percutaneous (3) approach.

The cast is not coded separately as stated in the previously shown guideline B3.15.

Root Operation		
Reposition (S)	Definition:	Moving to its normal location, or other suitable location, all or a portion of a body part
	Explanation:	The body part is moved to a new location from an abnormal location, or from a normal location where it is not functioning correctly. The body part may or may not be cut out or off to be moved to the new location.

Percutaneous Procedure via Device

Guideline B5.4

> **B5.4** **Procedures performed percutaneously via a device placed for the procedure are coded to the approach Percutaneous.**
>
> *Example:* **Fragmentation of kidney stone performed via percutaneous nephrostomy is coded to the approach Percutaneous.**

AHA Coding Clinic

2016, 1Q, 19 Embolization of Superior Hypophyseal Aneurysm Using Stent-Assisted Coil

2015, 3Q, 32 Approach Values for Repositioning and Removal of Cardiac Lead

2015, 2Q, 27 Uterine Artery Embolization Using Gelfoam

2014, 3Q, 19 Ablation of Ventricular Tachycardia with Impella® Support

2014, 1Q, 8 Lumbar Drainage Port Aspiration

This guideline provides coding direction when a device, such as a catheter, is used to access the surgical site in order to perform a procedure. The procedure does not take place on the device, but rather by means of the device. Percutaneous (3) approach should be assigned when entry is by a puncture or minor incision through the skin, mucous membrane, or any other body layers, whether or not a device is used to facilitate the percutaneous procedure.

Practical Application for Guideline B5.4

> **Case Study 6.12. Radiofrequency Ablation of Liver, Laparoscopic**
>
> A 60-year-old female with primary hepatocellular carcinoma presented for laparoscopic radiofrequency ablation. Under general anesthesia, laparoscopic ultrasound was performed and the lesion within the right lobe of the liver was located and mapped. The radiofrequency thermal ablation catheter was placed into the right lobe of the liver using ultrasound guidance. The tip of the probe was inserted into the center of the tumor and the prongs were deployed. Upon initiation of the ablation cycle, a target temperature was maintained for five minutes during each cycle. After completion of the cycle, the ablation device and laparoscope were removed. The patient tolerated the procedure and there were no complications.

Code(s):

ØF513ZZ **Destruction of Right Lobe Liver, Percutaneous Approach**

BF45ZZZ **Ultrasonography of Liver**

Rationale:

Radiofrequency ablation (RFA) is a minimally invasive technique used to treat cancer. RFA is performed using a needle electrode that is placed with the help of imaging directly into the cancerous tumor. High-frequency electrical current is passed through the electrode, destroying the cancer cells with the application of heat. Destruction (5) is the appropriate root operation because it fully captures the intent of RFA. In this example, the lesion in the right lobe of the liver is captured with body part Liver, Right Lobe (1) found in the Hepatobiliary System and Pancreas (F) body system. The needle electrode was inserted into the skin and advanced to the tumor site. Radiofrequency energy was applied through the electrode, which according to guideline B5.4 is captured as a Percutaneous (3) approach. No Device (Z) and No Qualifier (Z) are the only options for the sixth and seventh characters, respectively.

If reported, the ultrasound guidance is captured in the Imaging (B) section using body system Hepatobiliary System and Pancreas (F), Ultrasonography (4), and body part Liver (5).

Root Operation		
Destruction (5)	Definition:	Physical eradication of all or a portion of a body part by the direct use of energy, force, or a destructive agent
	Explanation:	None of the body part is physically taken out

Case Study 6.13. PTCA: Percutaneous Transluminal Coronary Angiography

Procedures: Selective coronary angiography, right and left coronary arteries; contrast left ventriculography with left heart catheterization; PTCA with Resolute stent of the right coronary artery.

Procedure description: The patient was brought to the catheterization suite and prepped and draped in the usual fashion and sedated using IV Versed and fentanyl. The skin and subcutaneous tissue overlying the right femoral artery was infiltrated with 1% lidocaine for local anesthesia. A 6-French sheath was placed in the right femoral artery. Diagnostic coronary angiography under fluoroscopy of the right and left coronary arteries using iso-osmolar contrast was performed with 6-French JL-4 and 6-French JR-4 diagnostic catheters, and a 6-French pigtail catheter was used to perform a left ventriculography, also under fluoroscopy with iso-osmolar contrast. It was determined that there was approximately 85 to 90 percent stenosis of the mid right coronary artery. A JR4 catheter was placed at the stenosis site, and the lesion was crossed with a guidewire. A 3.0 x 12 mm Resolute (R-ZES) stent was deployed to a total of 14 atmospheres. Follow-up angiography demonstrated 0 percent residual stenosis. The catheter and sheath were removed and Angio-Seal plug was deployed. The patient was transferred to the holding area in stable condition.

Code(s):

0270034Z   **Dilation of Coronary Artery, One Artery with Drug-eluting Intraluminal Device, Percutaneous Approach**

4A023N7   **Measurement of Cardiac Sampling and Pressure, Left Heart, Percutaneous Approach**

B211YZZ   **Fluoroscopy of Multiple Coronary Arteries using Other Contrast**

B215YZZ   **Fluoroscopy of Left Heart using Other Contrast**

Rationale:

The objective of a stent insertion is to open an abnormally closed blood vessel. This objective coincides with ICD-10-PCS root operation Dilation (7). ICD-10-PCS does not supply body part character values for individual coronary arteries but rather gives the option of one, two, three, or four or more coronary arteries. In this case, only one artery was expanded; body part Coronary Artery, One Artery (0) can be found in the Heart and Great Vessels (2) body system.

Root Operation		
Dilation (7)	Definition:	Expanding an orifice or the lumen of a tubular body part
	Explanation:	The orifice can be a natural orifice or an artificially created orifice. Accomplished by stretching a tubular body part using intraluminal pressure or by cutting part of the orifice or wall of the tubular body part.

Because the coronary artery was dilated and the stent inserted through a catheter, based on Guideline B5.4, this is considered a Percutaneous (3) approach because the objective was accomplished via a device (catheter) that was placed specifically to perform the procedure.

The Resolute (R-ZES) stent is drug-eluting and represented by Intraluminal Device, Drug-eluting (4). There was no mention of bifurcation so the seventh character is No Device (Z).

A diagnostic left heart catheterization was also performed, which according to the ICD-10 PCS index is reported as Measurement, Cardiac 4A02. The Sampling and Pressure (N) was performed using a Percutaneous (3) approach on the Left Heart (7).

Finally, the diagnostic coronary arteriography of multiple coronary arteries and left ventriculography via fluoroscopy with iso-osmolar contrast are captured with codes B211YZZ and B215YZZ, respectively.

For detailed information on coronary artery stents and contrast, see Chapter 5 Body Part Guidelines, guideline B4.4 Coronary Arteries.

Case Study 6.14. Aspiration, CSF from Lumbar Drainage Catheter Port

The tubing and lumbar drainage ports were secured with tape to stabilize the surface. The stopcocks to the transducer and drainage system were turned to off. A sterile environment was secured. Using a #25 gauge needle and 3 ml syringe, 0.5 ml was withdrawn from the previously placed port and discarded. Using another #25 gauge needle and 3 ml syringe, 2 ml of CSF was slowly aspirated from the port. The needle was removed from the syringe and capped with a blunt tip plastic cannula. The syringe was labeled and hand delivered to the laboratory. The stop cocks were reopened, tape removed from the port, and the transducer setup returned to preprocedural state.

Code(s):

009U3ZX   Drainage of Spinal Canal, Percutaneous Approach, Diagnostic

Rationale:

Aspiration is defined as removal of a sample of fluid through a needle, meeting the definition of root operation Drainage (9). The port from which the needle aspirates the cerebrospinal fluid (CSF) is in the lumbar spinal canal. The appropriate code can be found in table 009 in the Central Nervous System and Cranial Nerves (0) body system and body part Spinal Canal (U). The catheter was below the skin, so accessing the port via a needle qualifies as a Percutaneous (3) approach. This is further clarified in ICD-10-PCS guideline B5.4.

Since the device being accessed had been previously placed and no procedure was performed on or for the device specifically, No Device (Z) is the appropriate sixth-character assignment. As the aspiration was to sample CSF for microbes, the procedure is considered Diagnostic (X) for the seventh character (*AHA Coding Clinic*, 2014, 1Q, 8).

Root Operation		
Drainage (9)	Definition:	Taking or letting out fluids and/or gases from a body part
	Explanation:	The qualifier DIAGNOSTIC is used to identify drainage procedures that are biopsies

Case Study 6.15. Embolization, Left Uterine Artery Biosphere

With the patient in the supine position and after appropriate anesthetic, a one-quarter of an inch incision was made in the groin to access the femoral artery. A catheter was inserted into the artery and guided to the uterus with the aid of a fluoroscopic x-ray machine. With the catheter in the proper position, tiny, grain-sized plastic particles were injected into the left uterine artery cutting off the blood supply to the fibroids causing them to shrink.

Code(s):

Ø4LF3DU   **Occlusion of Left Uterine Artery with Intraluminal Device, Percutaneous Approach**

Rationale:

The intent of uterine artery embolization (UAE) is to block the blood supply to the uterine fibroids, meeting the root operation definition of Occlusion (L).

Root Operation		
Occlusion (L)	Definition:	Completely closing an orifice or lumen of a tubular body part
	Explanation:	The orifice can be a natural orifice or an artificially created orifice

According to guideline B5.4, the approach is Percutaneous (3) because the occlusion device was injected via a catheter and guided to the embolization site through a small sheath inserted into the groin.

The uterine artery is classified to Internal Iliac Artery, Left (F) according to the Body Part Key (appendix D). This can be found in the Lower Arteries (4) body system. In the seventh-character qualifier field, the Uterine Artery, Left (U) value is available, which is assigned since the Intraluminal Device (D), the biosphere material, was placed there.

Case Study 6.16. Ablation, AV Junction, Transcatheter

The patient was brought to the electrophysiology laboratory. Presenting rhythm was noted to be sinus rhythm with implantable cardioverter-defibrillator (ICD) diagnostic showing that this rhythm had been present for the last couple of days with atrial fibrillation, continuous, in the months preceding that. The patient's ICD was reprogrammed to backup VVI pacing at 40 beats per minute. The right groin was prepped and draped in the usual sterile fashion. Local anesthesia was achieved over the right femoral vessels using a combination of 1% lidocaine and 0.5% Marcaine. Using the Seldinger technique, an 8 French SRO guiding sheath was advanced over a long guidewire into the right atrium. Through the sheath, an EPT Chilli standard curve ablation catheter was advanced. Great care was taken throughout the procedure to avoid disruption of the ICD leads during catheter manipulation. The catheter was positioned across the tricuspid valve and the His bundle potential was located. The catheter was drawn back to a more proximal site with large atrial electrogram and barely visible His potential. At this site, radiofrequency energy was delivered. The patient developed immediate rapid junctional rhythm followed by development of complete heart block, which persisted throughout the ablation delivery. Two short ablation lesions were delivered as the rhythm was observed followed by 60-second energy delivery. All of these were delivered at the same site, constituting one lesion delivery; total ablation time was 82 seconds. Following the ablation delivery, which resulted in escape pacing at 40 beats per minute, the ICD was reprogrammed to DDD pacing at 90 beats per minute. The patient's rhythm was observed and no resumption of AV conduction was seen during a 30-minute waiting period. The electrode catheter was removed without disruption of the leads. The sheath was removed and digital pressure was applied until adequate hemostasis was achieved. The patient left the electrophysiology laboratory in stable condition.

Code(s):

Ø2583ZZ   **Destruction of Conduction Mechanism, Percutaneous Approach**

Rationale:

The heat from the radiofrequency energy destroys (ablates) the atrioventricular (AV) node that is responsible for the irregular impulses making Destruction (5) the appropriate root operation. The AV node is part of the Heart and Great Vessels (2) body system and captured with the body part value Conduction Mechanism (8). This can be found using the Body Part Key (appendix D). The catheter was placed percutaneously and the radiofrequency delivered via the catheter. Guideline B5.4 confirms that approach value Percutaneous (3) is appropriate. No Device (Z) and No Qualifier (Z) apply as the sixth and seventh characters, respectively.

Root Operation		
Destruction (5)	Definition:	Physical eradication of all or a portion of a body part by the direct use of energy, force, or a destructive agent
	Explanation:	None of the body part is physically taken out

Beyond the Guidelines

This section discusses a number of approach situations that are not covered in the guidelines that warrant additional mention.

Minimally Invasive Surgery

AHA Coding Clinic

2017, 1Q, 36   Approach value for Mini Thoracotomy

2013, 4Q, 123   Urolift® Procedure

2013, 4Q, 108   Minimally Invasive Surgical Approaches

2013, 3Q, 26   Transcatheter Replacement of Heart Valve (TAVR) with Measurements

A minimally invasive surgery is one in which small incisions are made in order to accommodate the insertion of instrumentation needed to complete the procedure. This technique allows for faster recovery and less scarring than traditional open procedures. Operative report documentation often refers to minimally invasive surgery; however, minimally invasive is not identified by a specific approach value in PCS. Documentation must be carefully reviewed with the correct assignment based on the definitions of each of the approach values using information such as method, visualization of the site, instrumentation used, and size of entry point.

Spotlight
The guidelines in ICD-10-PCS do not differentiate "minimally invasive approaches." Refer to the full definitions in ICD-10-PCS to determine the appropriate approach.

Case Study 6.17. Transapical Aortic Valve Replacement (TAVR)

Procedure performed: Transapical aortic valve replacement using a 20 mm Sapien 3 valve. A 3 cm incision was made through the sixth intercostal space on the right, exposing the apex. Aortography was performed for proper valve alignment. The patient was fully heparinized, and the apex was punctured with a Cook needle. A J-wire was placed across the aortic valve, directed around the aortic arch with a JR4 catheter, and placed into the descending thoracic aorta. This was replaced with an Amplatz wire and an ascender introducer was placed at the 3.5 cm mark and directed toward the valve. The Sapien valve was placed on the delivery device and was inspected. It was then passed through the sheath into the ventricle. The new valve was desheathed, placed across the old valve, and deployed in proper position. The delivery device was removed, followed by the sheath. The mini-sternotomy was closed in anatomic layers with Vicryl in the subcutaneous tissue and Dermabond on the skin. A Blake drain was inserted for intercostal drainage. The patient was returned to cardiothoracic ICU.

Code(s):

Ø2RF38H   **Replacement of Aortic Valve with Zooplastic Tissue, Transapical, Percutaneous Approach**

Rationale:

Aortic valve replacement is typically performed via open heart surgery. Transapical aortic valve replacement (TAVR) provides a minimally invasive alternative. A TAVR is performed through a small incision in the thorax, via access through the heart wall, without direct visualization of the heart. The native valve is not resected but is rendered nonfunctional with the new prosthetic valve deployed over the top of the native valve. This minimally invasive approach to replacing the aortic valve provides a means of treating diseased aortic valves in patients considered high risk for the traditional open replacement surgery and to which peripheral vascular access for transcatheter placement of the valve is contraindicated.

The procedure involves putting in biological material to take over the function of a body part, which meets the definition of root operation Replacement (R). The body part Aortic Valve (F) can be found in the Heart and Great Vessels (2) body system. There is no approach value for minimally invasive so the operative report documentation should be carefully reviewed to determine the best approach value. Although an incision was made in the thorax, the placement of the new heart valve was not directly visualized, making Percutaneous (3) the best option. The Sapien device is a bioprosthetic valve made from bovine tissue, correlating to the device value Zooplastic Tissue (8). The seventh-character Qualifier value, Transapical (H), completes the code signifying that the valve insertion was through the heart wall.

Definition
transapical. Through the wall of the heart.

Root Operation		
Replacement (R)	Definition:	Putting in or on biological or synthetic material that physically takes the place and/or function of all or a portion of a body part
	Explanation:	The body part may have been taken out or replaced, or may be taken out, physically eradicated, or rendered nonfunctional during the REPLACEMENT procedure. A REMOVAL procedure is coded for taking out the device used in a previous replacement procedure.

Spotlight
Although a small incision was made into the intercostal space for access (mini-sternotomy), the actual procedure of the valve replacement was performed using a Percutaneous approach through the catheter.

Robotic or Computer Assisted Surgery

AHA Coding Clinic

2015, 1Q, 33   Robotic-Assisted Laparoscopic Hysterectomy Converted to Open Procedure

2014, 4Q, 33   Radical Prostatectomy

Usually performed with minimally invasive surgery, robotic- or computer-assisted surgery allows complex procedures to be performed with more precision, control, and flexibility than conventional techniques. Through the use of a robotic system or computer, the surgeon guides the instrumentation from a console that also provides high definition, magnification, and 3D visualization. Two robotic systems that have received FDA approval include da Vinci and Zeus. Report a separate code from Other Procedures (8E0) for the robotic or computer assistance in addition to the code that captures the intent of the procedure.

Spotlight
The term Robotic Assisted Procedure as well as the term Computer Assisted Procedure in the ICD-10-PCS alphabetic index directs the user to table 8E0.

Case Study 6.18. Radical Prostatectomy, Robotic-assisted Laparoscopic

Preoperative diagnosis: Prostate malignancy.

Procedure description: A midline supraumbilical incision was made with a #15 blade, approximately 2 cm in length. This was deepened sharply to the rectus fascia. Stay sutures were placed on either side of the rectus fascia. A Veress needle was inserted into the peritoneal cavity. Pneumoperitoneum was created.

The Veress needle was replaced with a 12 mm trocar. The camera was introduced through this trocar and the peritoneal cavity was inspected. The left robotic trocar was inserted and laparoscopic scissors were used through this trocar in order to take down some adhesions in the right upper quadrant. The fourth arm trocar was inserted under direct vision followed by the right robotic trocar. A 12 mm trocar was placed in the right upper quadrant under direct vision and a 5 mm trocar was placed medial to this. All of these were inserted under direct laparoscopic vision. The da Vinci robot was docked to the robotic trocars.

The procedure started by reflecting the bladder off the anterior abdominal wall. The space of Retzius was dissected. The prostate was identified and cleaned off. Starting on the patient's right side, the endopelvic fascia was carefully dissected and opened in order to dissect the space between the prostate and the levator ani muscle. This was repeated on the patient's left side.

The anterior bladder neck was divided at the prostatovesical junction and dissection was continued posteriorly after the Foley was removed. The posterior bladder neck was divided carefully and the dissection was carried through the posterior layers of the bladder wall. The vas deferens and seminal vesicles were identified on either side and carefully dissected free and removed to an Endo Catch bag. Denonvilliers' fascia was divided at the plane between the posterior surface of the prostate so the rectum could be developed. The left prostatic pedicle was divided using a combination of blunt and sharp dissection and Hem-o-Lok clips.

Attention was turned to the right prostatic pedicle, which was taken down in a similar fashion. The apex of the prostate was approached. The dorsal vein complex and the apex of the prostate were divided carefully and the rectourethralis muscle was divided sharply. The prostate specimen was completely freed and placed in an Endo Catch bag. The anastomosis between the urethra and the bladder neck was completed using two continuous 2-0 Monocryl sutures tied to each other. Each of the sutures was 16 cm in length. The anastomosis was secured intermittently with laparoscopic tie absorbable clips. The JP drain was inserted through the exit of the fourth robotic trocar site. The drain was secured to the skin with a silk suture.

The robot was undocked from the patient. The patient was moved out of Trendelenburg position and the laparoscopic sites were closed under laparoscopic vision using a port closure device and 0 PDS interrupted suture. The midline incision was extended slightly in order to remove the specimen. The midline incision was closed with interrupted 0 PDS sutures. The skin was closed with 4-0 Vicryl sutures followed by Dermabond. The specimen was sent for pathologic analysis.

Code(s):

ØVT04ZZ	**Resection of Prostate, Percutaneous Endoscopic Approach**
ØVT34ZZ	**Resection of Bilateral Seminal Vesicles, Percutaneous Endoscopic Approach**
ØVTQ4ZZ	**Resection of Bilateral Vas Deferens, Percutaneous Endoscopic Approach**
8EØW4CZ	**Robotic Assisted Procedure of Trunk Region, Percutaneous Endoscopic Approach**

Rationale:

The ICD-10-PCS index for Prostatectomy lists *see* Excision, Prostate ØVBØ and *see* Resection, Prostate ØVTØ. In this example the entire Prostate (Ø) was removed, meeting the root operation definition of Resection (T). Additionally, the Seminal Vesicles, Bilateral (3) and Vas Deferens, Bilateral (Q) were removed in their entirety. According to the following multiple procedures guideline B3.2a, three codes are needed since three distinct body part values were removed.

PCS Guideline
Multiple procedures
B3.2a   During the same operative episode, multiple procedures are coded if:
a. The same root operation is performed on different body parts as defined by distinct values of the body part character.
Example: Diagnostic excision of liver and pancreas are coded separately.
Excision of lesion in the ascending colon and excision of lesion in the transverse colon are coded separately.

This laparoscopic procedure is reported with approach value Percutaneous Endoscopic (4). The robotic assistance is coded separately and can be found in the ICD-10-PCS index under Robotic Assisted Procedure, Trunk Region 8EØW.

Root Operation		
Resection (T)	Definition:	Cutting out or off, without replacement, all of a body part
	Explanation:	None

Via Natural or Artificial Opening with Percutaneous Endoscopic Assistance

Currently, the only tables that offer the approach option of Via Natural or Artificial Opening with Percutaneous Endoscopic Assistance (F) are the Excision root operation table of the Gastrointestinal System (ØDB), the Resection root operation table of the Gastrointestinal System (ØDT), and the Resection root operation table of the Female Reproductive System (ØUT). This approach is defined by the entry of instrumention through a natural or artificial external opening **and** entry by puncture or minor incision of instrumentation through the skin or mucous membrane and any other body layers necessary to aid in the performance of the procedure. Instrumentation is used for visualization.

Case Study 6.19. Hysterectomy, Laparoscopic-assisted Vaginal

Postoperative diagnoses: 1. Abnormal uterine bleeding. 2. Uterine fibroids.

Operation performed: Laparoscopic-assisted vaginal hysterectomy.

Procedure description: After adequate general endotracheal anesthesia, the patient was placed in the dorsal lithotomy position and prepped and draped in the usual manner for a laparoscopic procedure. A speculum was placed into the vagina. A single tooth tenaculum was utilized to grasp the anterior lip of the uterine cervix. A #10 RUMI cannula was utilized and attached for uterine manipulation. The single-tooth tenaculum and speculum were removed from the vagina. At this time, the infraumbilical area was injected with 0.25% Marcaine with epinephrine and an infraumbilical vertical skin incision was made through which a Veress needle was inserted into the abdominal cavity. The abdomen was insufflated with carbon dioxide. After adequate insufflation, the Veress needle was removed and an 11-mm separator trocar was introduced through the infraumbilical incision into the abdominal cavity. Through the trocar sheath, the laparoscope was inserted and adequate visualization of the pelvic structures was noted. A 5 mm skin incision was made and a 5 mm trocar was introduced into the abdominal cavity for instrumentation. At this time, the right cornu was grasped and the right fallopian tube, uteroovarian ligament, and round ligaments were doubly coagulated with bipolar electrocautery and transected without difficulty. The remainder of the uterine vessels and anterior and posterior leaves of the broad ligament, as well as the cardinal ligament, was coagulated and transected in a serial fashion down to level of the uterine artery. The uterine artery was identified. It was doubly coagulated with bipolar electrocautery and transected. The left fallopian tube, uteroovarian ligament, and round ligaments were doubly coagulated with bipolar electrocautery and transected. The remainder of the cardinal ligament, uterine vessels, and anterior and posterior sheaths of the broad ligament were coagulated and transected in a serial manner to the level of the uterine artery. The anterior leaf of the broad ligament was dissected to the midline bilaterally, establishing a bladder flap with a combination of blunt and sharp dissection. At this time, attention was made to the vaginal hysterectomy.

The laparoscope and RUMI cannula were removed and the anterior and posterior leafs of the cervix were grasped with Lahey tenaculum. A circumferential incision was made at the cervicovaginal portio. The anterior and posterior colpotomies were accomplished with a combination of blunt and sharp dissection without difficulty. The right and left uterosacral ligament was clamped, transected, and ligated with #0 Vicryl sutures. The parametrial tissue was clamped bilaterally, transected, and ligated with #0 Vicryl suture bilaterally. The uterus was removed and passed off the operative field. The uterosacral ligaments were suture fixated into the vaginal cuff angles with #0 Vicryl sutures. The vaginal cuff was closed in a running fashion with #0 Vicryl suture. At this time, the laparoscope was reinserted into the abdomen. The abdomen was reinsufflated. The suprapubic trocar sheath was removed under laparoscopic visualization. The laparoscope and the infraumbilical trocar sheath were removed. The skin incisions were closed with #4-0 Vicryl in subcuticular fashion.

Code(s):

ØUT9FZZ   **Resection of Uterus, Via Natural or Artificial Opening With Percutaneous Endoscopic Assistance**

Rationale:

Only one code is needed to capture the objective of this procedure, complete removal or Resection (T) of the body part Uterus (9), despite both the uterus and cervix being removed. The cervix removal, in PCS, is considered inherent in hysterectomy procedures and is not coded separately. This can be confirmed by consulting main term Hysterectomy, Total *see* Resection, Uterus 0UT9 in the alphabetic index. Total hysterectomy is the term most often used to describe removal of the cervix and uterus.

Spotlight
When the cervix is not removed during a hysterectomy procedure, it is considered a supracervical hysterectomy. The code assigned is built from the same Resection root operation table in the Female Reproductive body system with body part value Uterus (0UT9), but the qualifier Supracervical (L) is assigned to denote that only the uterus was removed.

Root Operation		
Resection (T)	Definition:	Cutting out or off, without replacement, all of a body part
	Explanation:	None

The body part Uterus (9), which captures both the uterus and the cervix removal, is found in the Female Reproductive (U) body system. The uterus and cervix were detached with laparoscopic assistance but removed through the natural opening, meeting the approach definition Via Natural or Artificial Opening with Percutaneous Endoscopic Assistance (F).

In a laparoscopic-assisted vaginal hysterectomy (LAVH), a laparoscope is used to visualize and detach the pelvic organs and ligaments to facilitate a vaginal removal of the resected organs. This LAVH approach can be beneficial for a woman with conditions that may complicate a normal vaginal hysterectomy, such as an enlarged uterus from fibroids, endometriosis, or adhesions from prior pelvic surgeries. The recovery is much shorter and easier than with a traditional abdominal hysterectomy.

Spotlight
If this procedure had been performed using robotic assistance, an additional code capturing the robotic assistance would be needed.

Lack of Approach Value

AHA Coding Clinic

2017, 1Q, 36	Approach Value for Mini Thoracotomy
2016, 3Q, 32	Transcatheter Tricuspid Valve Replacement
2016, 2Q, 20	Sialendoscopy with Stone Removal
2016, 1Q, 9	Anteversion of Retroverted Pregnant Uterus
2016, 1Q, 23	Transurethral Resection of Ejaculatory Ducts
2015, 3Q, 29	Approach Value for Esophageal Electrophysiology Study
2015, 2Q, 14	Intraoperative EMG Monitoring via Endotracheal Tube
2015, 2Q, 31	Thoracoscopic Talc Pleurodesis

There may be instances where a particular approach value is not available in an ICD-10-PCS table. *AHA Coding Clinic* advises that the closest equivalent approach value be used. For example, when percutaneous endoscopic is not available, the closest equivalent is percutaneous.

Approach Value for Devices

The approach used for Insertion (H) of a device may be different than the approach used with root operations Change (2), Removal (P), Replacement (R), Revision (W), and Supplement (U). Careful review of the documentation ensures appropriate approach character value selection.

Case Study 6.20. IUD Replacement

The patient was on the exam table with feet in stirrups. A speculum was inserted into the patient's vagina and IUD strings located. Pulling steadily on the strings, the IUD was removed. A new IUD was inserted and the speculum was removed.

Code(s):

ØU2DXHZ   Change Contraceptive Device in Uterus and Cervix, External Approach

Rationale:

In this example, a device was removed and immediately replaced with the same type of device, which meets the root operation definition of Change (2). An IUD is a Contraceptive Device (H) inserted in the uterus. The uterus is captured as body part Uterus and Cervix (D) found in the Female Reproductive (U) body system.

The Change (2) root operation only has External (X) as an approach option. There is no approach choice for via natural opening since all Change (2) procedures are coded as External (X). However, the initial Insertion (H) of the IUD would have used approach Via Natural or Artificial Opening (7) or Via Natural or Artificial Opening Endoscopic (8).

Root Operation		
Change (2)	Definition:	Taking out or off a device from a body part and putting back an identical or similar device in or on the same body part without cutting or puncturing the skin or a mucous membrane
	Explanation:	All CHANGE procedures are coded using the approach EXTERNAL
Insertion (H)	Definition:	Putting in a nonbiological appliance that monitors, assists, performs, or prevents a physiological function but does not physically take the place of a body part
	Explanation:	None

Chapter 7. Device Guidelines

Device Overview

Device: Character 6

Character 1	Character 2	Character 3	Character 4	Character 5	Character 6	Character 7
Section	Body System	Root Operation	Body Part	Approach	Device	Qualifier

Character six, Device, is one of the most quickly evolving PCS characters. New innovations and advances in devices are introduced more often than can be incorporated into PCS codes. Commonly used devices are represented by the descriptive terms contained in the device tables; newer devices may be located in the New Technology tables until they are more commonly put into practice. For more information regarding the New Technology (X) section, see chapter 9.

Spotlight
Many of the codes in the New Technology section are defined by the use of a newly developed device. It is advisable to check the New Technology section for a new device prior to building a code from the Medical and Surgical tables. The New Technology tables are all inclusive with all of the characters necessary to represent a potential new procedure, including the root operation, body part, and device values.

A variety of devices are reported with the sixth character of a PCS code. If the objective of a procedure is accomplished by means of a device, and the device remains in or on the procedure site at the conclusion of the procedure, then a specific device value is assigned in the sixth character. If no device is used to accomplish the objective with the exception of small devices that are considered integral to the performance of the procedure, then the sixth-character value No Device (Z) is assigned.

There are four major types of devices:

- Biological or synthetic material that takes the place of all or a portion of a body part (e.g., skin graft, joint prosthesis)
- Biological or synthetic material that assists or prevents a physiological function (e.g., IUD)
- Therapeutic material not absorbed by, eliminated by, or incorporated into a body part (e.g., radioactive implant)
- Mechanical or electronic appliances used to assist, monitor, take the place of, or prevent a physiological function (e.g., cardiac pacemaker, orthopedic pin)

The size, shape, complexity, or composition of a device does not influence whether a specific device value is coded. Devices can be too small to be seen by the naked eye (e.g., microcoils used to occlude vessels) or very large fixation devices. The following factors help determine whether a material is coded as a device:

- The device is used to achieve the objective of the procedure, not only to support the performance of the procedure.

  Example: Radiological markers used to achieve or support another objective, such as tumor excision, are not coded as a device. In contrast, insertion of radioactive brachytherapy seeds into a body site is coded as a device since the objective of the procedure is to treat the malignancy.

- An apparatus such as Drainage Device (Ø) used to accomplish an objective may be coded with a specific device value in one procedure; however, the same apparatus may be coded as No Device (Z) in a different procedure if it is an inherent part of the root operation.

  Example: A catheter such as a chest tube placed specifically for therapeutic or diagnostic purposes is coded to root operation Drainage (9) with a device value of Drainage Device (Ø). However, when a wound drain is placed at the surgical incision site at the conclusion of the procedure it is considered inherent in the procedure and not coded separately.

- Materials used to close procedure sites such as sutures, fibrin glue, Dermabond, special vessel closure devices, etc. are not coded as devices. In most cases, closure occurs in support of or as a necessary part of the procedure rather than the objective. If wound closure is the main objective of the procedure, such as for trauma or other reasons, root operation Repair (Q) with No Device (Z) value is used.

- Instruments used to visualize the procedure site are specified in the approach, not the device value.

- Equipment used to perform the procedure is not a device. Even though it may interface with the body, it is generally on the outside of the body and is only used temporarily to assist with the procedure. An example of this is mechanical ventilation or EEG electrodes. If reported, use codes from Extracorporeal or Systemic Assistance and Performance (5AØ-5A2) and Measurement and Monitoring (4AØ-4A1) respectively.

- Biologic or synthetic skin grafts are considered devices. Although often referred to as artificial or synthetic, Integra and Dermagraft skin substitutes are considered biologically derived and should be coded as nonautologous tissue substitutes according to *AHA Coding Clinic,* 2014, 2Q, 5.

Device vs. Substance

It may be difficult to ascertain whether a material is considered a device or a substance. Devices are represented by the sixth character in the Medical and Surgical (Ø) section whereas substances are represented by the sixth character in the Administration (3) section only.

One determining factor of whether a material is considered a device or a substance is its removability. After a device is placed, even if not logical, it is physically possible to remove.

Devices are also deliberately placed in a specific location where they remain unless intentionally or unintentionally removed or repositioned. A substance is meant to be disseminated or absorbed into the body.

Spotlight
If a device moves from its intended location, it may need to be "revised" in a subsequent procedure to move it back to its intended location.

Root Operations Involving Devices

Root operations Alteration, Bypass, Creation, Dilation, Drainage, Fusion, Occlusion, Reposition, and Restriction, depending upon the procedure performed, may require the use of a device value. However, the six root operations listed below **always** involve a device:

- Change (2)
- Insertion (H)
- Removal (P)
- Replacement (R)
- Supplement (U)
- Revision (W)

Correct code assignment depends on the objective of the procedure. If the objective of the procedure is to put in the device, the root operation is Insertion. If the device placed is to meet an objective other than insertion, the root operation defining the underlying objective of the procedure is used, with the device specified with the device value. For example, if a procedure to replace the hip joint is performed, the root operation Replacement is coded, and the prosthetic device is specified with the device value.

Root Operation		
Change (2)	Definition:	Taking out or off a device from a body part and putting back an identical or similar device in or on the same body part without cutting or puncturing the skin or a mucous membrane
	Explanation:	All CHANGE procedures are coded using the approach EXTERNAL
Insertion (H)	Definition:	Putting in a nonbiological appliance that monitors, assists, performs, or prevents a physiological function but does not physically take the place of a body part
	Explanation:	None
Removal (P)	Definition:	Taking out or off a device from a body part
	Explanation:	If a device is taken out and a similar device put in without cutting or puncturing the skin or mucous membrane, the procedure is coded to the root operation CHANGE. Otherwise, the procedure for taking out a device is coded to the root operation REMOVAL.
Replacement (R)	Definition:	Putting in or on a biological or synthetic material that physically takes the place and/or function of all or a portion of a body part
	Explanation:	The body part may have been taken out or replaced, or may be taken out, physically eradicated, or rendered nonfunctional during the REPLACEMENT procedure. A REMOVAL procedure is coded for taking out the device used in a previous replacement procedure.
Supplement (U)	Definition:	Putting in or on biological or synthetic material that physically reinforces and/or augments the function of a portion of a body part
	Explanation:	The biological material is non-living, or is living and from the same individual. The body part may have been previously replaced, and the SUPPLEMENT procedure is performed to physically reinforce and/or augment the function of the replaced body part.
Revision (W)	Definition:	Correcting, to the extent possible, a portion of a malfunctioning device or the position of a displaced device
	Explanation:	Revision can include correcting a malfunctioning or displaced device by taking out or putting in components of the device such as a screw or pin

Device Key, Aggregation Table, and Device Definitions

The tables described in the following section can be found in their entirety in the back of this book as Appendix F. Device Key and Aggregation Table, and Appendix G. Device Definitions.

The Device Key, Aggregation Table, and Device Definition table are published by CMS and updated annually. Since devices continue to evolve, it is important to consult the most recent tables. It is helpful to review these device tables to become familiar with the way that devices are defined in ICD-10-PCS. Several different types of devices may be classified to one PCS device value. For example, the PCS device value Drainage Device includes the following specific devices:

- Cystostomy tube
- Foley catheter
- Percutaneous nephrostomy catheter
- Thoracostomy tube

Spotlight
In many PCS tables, a value for Other Device (Y) is available to provide for future device value expansion.

Device Key

The Device Key lists specific devices used in the medical profession, such as stents or bovine pericardial valves, in alphabetic order by specific name brand (on the left side), with the appropriate ICD-10-PCS device value (on the right side), as shown in the following table excerpt.

Term	ICD-10-PCS Value
3f (Aortic) Bioprosthesis valve	Zooplastic Tissue in Heart and Great Vessels
AbioCor® Total Replacement Heart	Synthetic Substitute
Absolute Pro Vascular (OTW) Self-Expanding Stent System	Intraluminal Device
Acculink (RX) Carotid Stent System	Intraluminal Device
Acellular Hydrated Dermis	Nonautologous Tissue Substitute
Acetabular cup	Liner in Lower Joints
Activa PC neurostimulator	Stimulator Generator, Multiple Array for Insertion in Subcutaneous Tissue and Fascia

Aggregation Table

The Aggregation Table crosswalks specific device value definitions for specific root operations in a specific body system to the more general device value to be used when the root operation covers a wide range of body parts and the device value represents an entire family of devices.

For example, in the following Aggregation table excerpt, root operation Insertion in the Upper or Lower Joints body system contains very specific choices for the various types of spinal stabilization devices. However, if one of these devices is involved in another root operation, such as Removal, Reposition, or Revision, the appropriate device value based on this chart is Internal Fixation Device as listed in the General Device column. Only the root operations listed in the "for Operation" column of this table contain device values for the specific device, such as Pacemaker or Single Chamber Rate Responsive, while any other root operation involving this device is coded with the "General Device" term listed, such as Cardiac Rhythm Related Device.

Example: Spinal Stabilization Device, Facet Replacement (D) is coded with its own individual device value for the root operation Insertion; however, if root operations Removal (P), Reposition (S), or Revision (W) is performed, the device value is the more general Internal Fixation Device (4).

Specific Device	for Operation	in Body System	General Device
Pacemaker, Dual Chamber (6)	Insertion	Subcutaneous Tissue and Fascia	Cardiac Rhythm Related Device (P)
Pacemaker, Single Chamber (4)	Insertion	Subcutaneous Tissue and Fascia	Cardiac Rhythm Related Device (P)
Pacemaker, Single Chamber Rate Responsive (5)	Insertion	Subcutaneous Tissue and Fascia	Cardiac Rhythm Related Device (P)
Spinal Stabilization Device, Facet Replacement (D)	Insertion	Lower Joints Upper Joints	Internal Fixation Device (4)
Spinal Stabilization Device, Interspinous Process (B)	Insertion	Lower Joints Upper Joints	Internal Fixation Device (4)

AHA Coding Clinic

2015, 4Q, 18   Use of the ICD-10-PCS Device Key and Device Aggregation Table

Spotlight
While all devices can be removed, some cannot be removed without putting in another nonbiological appliance or body-part substitute. When a specific device value is used to identify the device for a root operation, such as Insertion, and that same device value is not an option for a more broad range root operation, such as Removal, select the general device value as indicated in the Device Aggregation Table.
For example, in the body system Heart and Great Vessels, the more **specific** Cardiac Lead, Pacemaker (J) is the device value in root operation Insertion. For the root operation Removal, the **general** device value Cardiac Lead (M) would be selected for the pacemaker lead.

Device Definitions

This resource is a reverse look-up to the Device Key. The user may reference this resource to see the specific devices that may be grouped to a particular device value (character 6). In the example following, some of the various name brands of cardiac devices that may be found in an operative report are listed (on the right side) and grouped into the appropriate PCS device value description (on the left side).

ICD-10-PCS Value	Definition
Cardiac Lead, Pacemaker for Insertion in Heart and Great Vessels	Includes: ACUITY™ Steerable Lead Attain Ability® lead Attain StarFix® (OTW) lead Cardiac resynchronization therapy (CRT) lead Corox (OTW) Bipolar Lead
Cardiac Resynchronization Defibrillator Pulse Generator for Insertion in Subcutaneous Tissue and Fascia	Includes: COGNIS® CRT-D Concerto II CRT-D Consulta CRT-D CONTAK RENEWA® 3 RF (HE) CRT-D LIVIAN™ CRT-D Maximo II DR CRT-D Ovatio™ CRT-D Protecta XT CRT-D Viva (XT)(S)

General Guidelines

There are three general guidelines for procedures involving a device and an additional guideline that pertains only to Drainage Devices. There has been much advice published in the ICD-10-PCS coding clinics regarding the use of devices. Some of the *AHA Coding Clinic* titles from third quarter 2012 - second quarter 2018 that pertain to specific device guidelines are listed below each guideline.

Guideline B6.1a

> **B6.1a** **A device is coded only if a device remains after the procedure is completed. If no device remains, the device value No Device is coded. In limited root operations, the classification provides the qualifier values Temporary and Intraoperative, for specific procedures involving clinically significant devices, where the purpose of the device is to be utilized for a brief duration during the procedure or current inpatient stay. If a device that is intended to remain after the procedure is completed requires removal before the end of the operative episode in which it was inserted (for example, the device size is inadequate or a complication occurs), both the insertion and removal of the device should be coded.**

AHA Coding Clinic

2018, 2Q, 3-4	Intra-Aortic Balloon Pump	2015, 3Q, 16	Revision of Previous Truncus Arteriosus Surgery with Ventricle to Pulmonary Artery Conduit
2018, 2Q, 17	Arthroscopic Drainage of Knee and Nonexcisional Debridement		
2018, 2Q, 19	Pacing Lead Attached to Automatic Implantable Cardioverter Defibrillator	2015, 3Q, 18	Total Hip Replacement with Acetabular Reconstruction
2018, 1Q, 22	Spinal Fusion Procedures without Bone Graft	2015, 3Q, 25	Placement of Inflatable Penile Prosthesis
		2015, 3Q, 35	Swan Ganz Catheterization
2017, 4Q, 31	Resuscitative Endovascular Balloon Occlusion of the Aorta	2015, 2Q, 3	Coronary Artery Intervention Site
		2015, 2Q, 11	Cystourethroscopic Deflux® Injection
2017, 4Q, 43-44	Insertion of External Heart Assist Devices	2015, 2Q, 23	Annuloplasty Ring
		2015, 2Q, 27	Uterine Artery Embolization Using Gelfoam
2017, 4Q, 63	Added and Revised Device Values	2015, 2Q, 28	Release and Replacement of Celiac Artery
2017, 4Q, 104	Placement of Watchman™ Left Atrial Appendage Device	2015, 2Q, 31	Leadless Pacemaker Insertion
		2015, 2Q, 33-35	Totally Implantable Central Venous Access Device (Port-a-Cath)
2017, 3Q, 8	First Stage of Gastroschisis Repair with Silo Placement		
2017, 3Q, 11	Placement of Peripherally Inserted Central Catheter using 3CG ECG Technology	2015, 2Q, 36	Insertion of Infusion Device into Peritoneal Cavity
		2015, 1Q, 28	Repair of Bronchopleural Fistula Using Omental Pedicle Graft
2017, 2Q, 23	Decompression of Spinal Cord and Placement of Instrumentation	2014, 4Q, 19	Ultrasound Accelerated Thrombolysis
2017, 2Q, 24	Tunneled Catheter versus Totally Implantable Catheter	2014, 4Q, 37	Endovascular Embolization of Arteriovenous Malformation Using Onyx-18 Liquid
2017, 1Q, 10	External Heart Assist Device	2014, 4Q, 37	Bovine Patch Arterioplasty
2017, 1Q, 21	Staged Scoliosis Surgery with Iliac Fixation and Spinal Fusion	2014, 3Q, 3	Blalock-Taussig Shunt Procedure
		2014, 3Q, 5	Use of Imaging Report to Confirm Catheter Placement
2017, 1Q, 23	Reconstruction of Mandible Using Titanium and Bone	2014, 3Q, 8	Coronary Artery Bypass Graft Utilizing Internal Mammary as Pedicle Graft
2017, 1Q, 30	Insertion of Umbilical Artery Catheter		
2017, 1Q, 32	Total Knee Replacement and Patellar Component	2014, 3Q, 16	Repair of Tetralogy of Fallot
		2014, 3Q, 20	MAZE Procedure Performed with Coronary Artery Bypass Graft
2016, 3Q, 40	Omentoplasty		
2016, 2Q, 11	Carotid Endarterectomy with Patch Angioplasty	2014, 3Q, 26	Coil Embolization of Gastroduodenal Artery with Chemoembolization of Hepatic Artery
2016, 1Q, 19	Embolization of Superior Hypophyseal Aneurysm Using Stent-Assisted Coil	2014, 3Q, 31	Closure of Paravalvular Leak Using Amplatzer® Vascular Plug
2015, 4Q, 22	Congenital Heart Corrective Procedures	2014, 2Q, 5	Acellular Dermal Replacement Graft
		2014, 2Q, 5	Oasis Acellular Matrix Graft
2015, 4Q, 26-32	Vascular Access Devices	2014, 2Q, 6	Composite Grafting (Synthetic versus Nonautologous Tissue Substitute)
2015, 4Q, 33	Externalization of Peritoneal Dialysis Catheter		
		2014, 2Q, 7	Anterior Cervical Thoracic Fusion with Total Discectomy
2015, 3Q, 13	Nonexcisional Debridement of Cranial Wound with Removal and Replacement of Hardware	2014, 2Q, 12	Percutaneous Vertebroplasty Using Cement

AHA Coding Clinic (Continued)

2014, 1Q, 9	Endovascular Repair of Abdominal Aortic Aneurysm	2013, 3Q, 24	Distraction Osteogenesis
2014, 1Q, 24	Endovascular Embolization for Gastrointestinal Bleeding	2013, 3Q, 25	360-Degree Spinal Fusion
		2013, 2Q, 34	Placement of Intrauterine Device via Open Approach
2013, 4Q, 116	Device Character for Port-A-Cath Placement	2013, 2Q, 36	Intrauterine Pressure Monitor
2013, 4Q, 117	Percutaneous Endoscopic Placement of Gastrostomy Tube	2013, 2Q, 39	Ankle Fusion, Osteotomy, and Removal of Hardware
2013, 4Q, 123	Urolift® Procedure	2013, 1Q, 21-23	Spinal Fusion of Thoracic and Lumbar Vertebrae
2013, 3Q, 18	Placement of Peripherally Inserted Central Catheter (PICC)	2013, 1Q, 29	Cervical and Thoracic Spinal Fusion
2013, 3Q, 18	Heart Transplant Surgery	2012, 4Q, 104	Placement of Subcutaneous Implantable Cardioverter Defibrillator

The rule of thumb when choosing to code a device value for character 6 is whether the device remains in or on the patient at the conclusion of the procedure, with the exception of those devices considered integral to the performance of the procedure. Guideline B6.1a outlines some additional exceptions to this rule.

Intraoperative and Temporary Devices

There are certain devices that, although clinically significant for the success of a procedure, are used only for a short period of time during the performance of a procedure or a short time after the procedure. Because these devices and procedures are an exception to the rule, qualifiers Intraoperative (J) and Temporary (J) have been added to a limited number of tables to represent these devices.

Examples include:

Intraoperative (J). Insertion of a Short-term External Heart Assist System (R) into the heart solely for use during a surgical procedure but not remaining in the patient at the conclusion of the procedure. The removal is inherent in the intraoperative qualifier and not coded separately if removed during the same operative episode. If the external short-term heart assist system remains in the patient temporarily after the completion of the surgery, use No Qualifier (Z). A separate code for Removal (P) of this device is applicable in those instances.

Temporary (J). Although they both have the same qualifier character J, Temporary and Intraoperative have different meanings and are found in entirely different tables. The qualifier Temporary (J) is found in tables:

Ø2L Heart and Great Vessel (2), Occlusion (L)

Ø4L Lower Arteries (2), Occlusion (L)

Ø4V Lower Arteries (2), Restriction (V)

These tables are used when a resuscitative endovascular balloon (REBOA) is placed in the Thoracic Aorta, Descending (W) or the Abdominal Aorta (Ø). This procedure uses a balloon catheter to close off the blood flow in the aorta for a brief time. This can be done when treating traumatic injuries to stop hemorrhaging or during a surgical procedure to prevent bleeding.

Spotlight
The qualifier values Intraoperative (J) or Temporary (J) are not an option when coding an intra-aortic balloon pump (IABP) nor should root operations Insertion (H) and Removal (P) be assigned when IABP is utilized. An intra-aortic balloon pump (IABP) is not considered a device in PCS, viewed only as auxiliary instrumentation, similar to cardiopulmonary bypass. When utilized during or after a surgical procedure, assign code 5A02210 Assistance with cardiac output using balloon pump, continuous from the section Extracorporeal or Systemic Assistance and Performance (5). See *AHA Coding Clinic,* 2018, 2Q, 3-5.

Devices Intended to Remain at the Conclusion of a Procedure

There are instances when a device is inserted in order to facilitate the objective of a procedure but due to complications or contraindications is not left in or on the patient at the conclusion of the procedure. Although contrary to the standard advice that a device must remain at the end of a procedure to be coded, it is appropriate to assign a code for the Insertion and a code for the Removal of that device, in these limited instances.

Practical Application for Guideline B6.1a

Case Study 7.1. Transjugular Intrahepatic Portosystemic Shunt (TIPS)

The procedure was performed under general anesthesia. The patient was placed in a supine position on the angiography table. The right neck was prepped and draped utilizing maximal sterile barrier technique. Local anesthesia was achieved with lidocaine and a small stab incision was made.

Under ultrasound guidance, using an access needle and wire, a long sheath was eventually advanced through the right internal jugular vein into the central venous circulation. After confirming position within the right hepatic vein, a needle was advanced through the sheath. A needle was used to puncture through the right hepatic vein into the right portal vein. A wire was placed from the right hepatic vein into the right portal vein and a catheter was advanced over the wire. The sheath was advanced over the wire into the main portal vein and a 10 mm x 6 cm/2 cm Viatorr shunt was advanced. The shunt was deployed in appropriate position so that the 2 cm uncovered portion was within the right portal vein and the 6 cm long covered portion extended through the hepatic parenchyma into the right hepatic vein at its confluence with the IVC. The wires, catheters, and sheath were removed and hemostasis was achieved.

Code(s):

Ø6183J4   **Bypass Portal Vein to Hepatic Vein with Synthetic Substitute, Percutaneous Approach**

Rationale:

As shown in the following illustration, the objective of a TIPS procedure is to insert a shunt through a tunnel through the liver to connect the portal vein with a hepatic vein. It is done typically for portal hypertension and cirrhosis to allow for better blood flow and to decrease portal vein pressure. The appropriate root operation is Bypass (1) because the blood is bypassing a damaged liver and flowing from the portal vein directly to the hepatic vein.

Root Operation		
Bypass (1)	Definition:	Altering the route of passage of the contents of a tubular body part
	Explanation:	Rerouting contents of a body part to a downstream area of the normal route, to a similar route and body part, or to an abnormal route and dissimilar body part. Includes one or more anastomoses, with or without the use of a device.

The body system is the Lower Veins (6) with the Portal Vein (8) as the body part value as it is the body part that the blood is flowing from. A Percutaneous (3) approach was performed via catheters.

The device used to complete the procedure is a shunt and because it was left in the patient's body, it is reported with a device value based on guideline B6.1a. The shunt is classified as a Synthetic Substitute (J).

The qualifier in the seventh character supplies the information concerning where the blood was bypassed to, which in this case is the Hepatic Vein (4).

Figure 7.1. Transjugular Intrahepatic Portosystemic Shunt (TIPS)

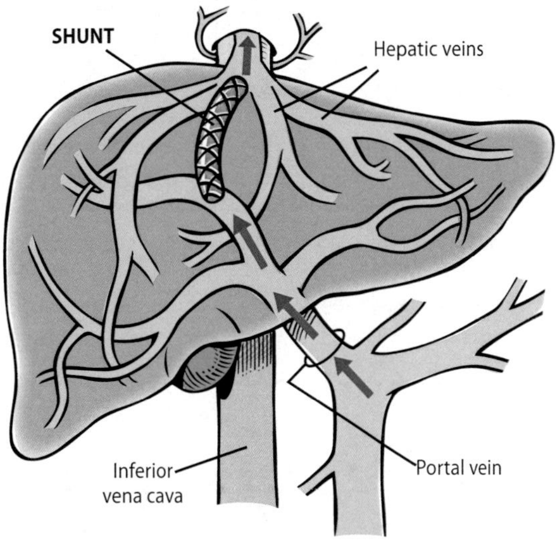

Case Study 7.2. Replacement, Unicondylar Knee, Bilateral

Preoperative diagnosis: Medial compartment osteoarthritis, bilateral knees.

Operation: Bilateral unicompartmental (medial compartment) knee replacements.

The patient was brought to the operating room and given a spinal anesthetic to augment the adductor canal block that was done in the holding room. A Foley catheter was placed. The bilateral lower extremities had tourniquets placed on the thighs and were sterilely prepped and draped in the usual fashion.

The left extremity was attended to first. After gravity exsanguination, the tourniquet was inflated to 300 mmHg pressure for a total of 54 minutes. A midline incision was made and carried down to the quads mechanism. Taking into account rotation and depth of slope, the tibial resection was made. The tibial size showed a three to be appropriate. With the knee in extension, the distal femoral cut was made. The finishing cuts and lug holes were made on the femur. The Keel punch and the lug holes were made for the tibial tray. The trial femur and the trial polyethylene were placed. Flexion, extension, and midflexion, showed good balance with the 8 mm polyethylene. The trials were removed. Bone ends were lavaged and dried. The tibia was first cemented on, followed by the femur. The extraneous cement was removed with the elevators. The polyethylene was snapped into position. The wound was irrigated and closed in the standard fashion and the tourniquet was let down.

The same procedure was taken with the right knee at this point. Once this was completed, the tourniquet was let down on the right side. Both knees were sterilely dressed.

Code(s):

ØSRCØL9   **Replacement of Right Knee Joint with Medial Unicondylar Synthetic Substitute, Cemented, Open Approach**

ØSRDØL9   **Replacement of Left Knee Joint with Medial Unicondylar Synthetic Substitute, Cemented, Open Approach**

Rationale:

A unicondylar (partial) knee only replaces the medial or lateral portion of the knee joint rather than the total joint. The components used are similar to those used in a total knee replacement with a femoral component and a tibial component with an insert that articulates against the femur. It is important to code these correctly as the data may be needed in the future if the joint needs to be converted to a total joint replacement. As defined in the following root operation table, Replacement (R) is the correct root operation, which requires no additional code for the removal of the body part.

Root Operation		
Replacement (R)	Definition:	Putting in or on a biological or synthetic material that physically takes the place and/or function of all or a portion of a body part
	Explanation:	The body part may have been taken out or replaced, or may be taken out, physically eradicated, or rendered nonfunctional during the REPLACEMENT procedure. A REMOVAL procedure is coded for taking out the device used in a previous replacement procedure.

Unicondylar knee replacements are procedures on the knee joints, not the bone (tibia, fibula, or femur); thus, the appropriate body system is Lower Joints (S). There is no body part value indicating bilateral so the Knee Joint, Right (C) and Knee Joint, Left (D) must be coded separately. This is consistent with the following advice given in Guideline B4.3.

PCS Guideline
Bilateral body part values
B4.3   Bilateral body part values are available for a limited number of body parts. If the identical procedure is performed on contralateral body parts, and a bilateral body part value exists for that body part, a single procedure is coded using the bilateral body part value. If no bilateral body part value exists, each procedure is coded separately using the appropriate body part value.
Example: The identical procedure performed on both fallopian tubes is coded once using the body part value Fallopian Tube, Bilateral.
The identical procedure performed on both knee joints is coded twice using the body part values Knee Joint, Right and Knee Joint, Left.

An Open (Ø) approach was used and since the device was left in the body, the device value is reported (Guideline B6.1a) as Synthetic Substitute, Unicondylar Medial (L). Other device options include Lateral and Patellofemoral devices, which emphasize the need for careful review of the operative report. Qualifier choices of Cemented, Uncemented, or No Qualifier are the same as in a total knee replacement. This example was Cemented (9).

Figure 7.2. Unicondylar Versus Total Knee Replacement

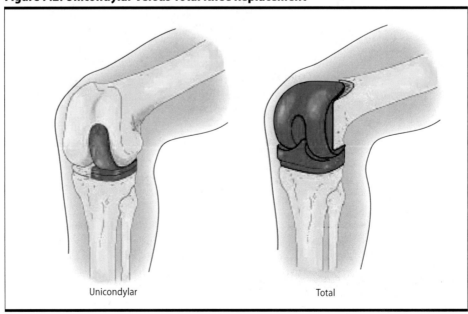

| Unicondylar | Total |

Case Study 7.3. Replacement, Hip

Operation Performed: Total Left Hip Arthroplasty.

With the patient in the left side up decubitus position and the operative site cleaned and prepped, an incision was made from the posterior third of the greater trochanter distally back approximately toward the posterior inferior iliac spine. It was taken down through the subcutaneous tissue, fascia, and the gluteus muscle split. Eventually access to the capsule was achieved. The hip was dislocated and appropriate resection was performed utilizing an oscillating saw. The acetabulum was visualized and careful reaming was performed in graduated fashion from small to large; trial components were tested and removed. The actual component was impacted in the acetabulum. A 10-degree lip **polyethylene** was also placed in the acetabular cap. This was impacted, placed, and checked to ensure that it was well seated with no loosening. Attention was then focused to the femur. A box osteotome was used to remove the cancellous portion of the femoral neck and the femoral canal was accessed. At this time, broaching was started beginning with size #10 and working up to #12. Range of motion testing did not demonstrate any instability. The trial broach was removed and an Alloclassic SL offset stem uncemented for taper component was impacted in place. Once seated, the 28 mm zero neck length **cobalt-chrome** femoral head was impacted in place. The hip was reduced within the acetabulum and again range of motion was checked, as well as ligamentous stability with gentle traction, external rotation, and hip flexion. Satisfaction was met for all of the components, as well as the alignment of the components. The wound was irrigated with normal saline and closed in layers.

Code(s):

ØSRBØ2A   **Replacement of Left Hip Joint with Metal on Polyethylene Synthetic Substitute, Uncemented, Open Approach**

Rationale:

Often surgeons refer to a total hip replacement as a total arthroplasty or a partial hip replacement as a hemiarthroplasty. The root operation for either of these procedures is Replacement (R).

Root Operation		
Replacement (R)	Definition:	Putting in or on biological or synthetic material that physically takes the place and/or function of all or a portion of a body part
	Explanation:	The body part may have been taken out or replaced, or may be taken out, physically eradicated, or rendered nonfunctional during the Replacement procedure. A Removal procedure is coded for taking out the device used in a previous replacement procedure.

The body part in this total hip arthroplasty is the Hip Joint, Left (B), located in the Lower Joints (S) body system. If the procedure is performed on the right and left hip joints, two separate codes are reported to indicate a bilateral procedure. The procedure was performed with an Open (Ø) approach. The operative report, plus the list of components that is often included, must be carefully reviewed to determine the correct bearing surface. The bearing surface identifies the material of the femoral head and the acetabular liner. This case indicated that a cobalt-chrome head and a polyethylene liner were used, which is reported with device value Synthetic Substitute, Metal on Polyethylene (2) as shown in the following illustration. A full list of device options with explanations follows. The qualifier choice of Uncemented (A) is appropriate in this case because the operative report specified that it was uncemented. The qualifier choices of Cemented (9), Uncemented (A), and No Qualifier (Z) can be difficult to discern or often times are not well documented. Meeting with the chief orthopedic surgeon is one way to find out which types of devices are used and whether cement is used at the facility.

Spotlight
A cemented joint replacement uses epoxy cement to attach the joint to the bone. An uncemented joint prosthesis contains holes on its surface that allows the growth of the patient's natural bone to hold the device in place. If documentation is insufficient to determine whether the synthetic joint prothesis is cemented or uncemented, use No Qualifier (Z) according to *AHA Coding Clinic,* 2016, 3Q, 35.

Table 7.1. Hip Bearing Surfaces

PCS Device Value	Bearing Surface	Explanation
Synthetic Substitute, Metal (1)	Metal on metal (MoM)	These are the oldest and first commonly used devices, but lost some popularity when poly was introduced. Better designs have increased demand as metal has resurfaced as stronger and longer lasting, especially in larger femoral heads. Usually made from cobalt chromium alloy, titanium alloy, or stainless steel.
Synthetic Substitute, Metal on Polyethylene (2)	Metal on plastic or polyethylene	These devices have been around since the 1950s. Older types of plastic had faster wear than other surfaces but the newer cross-linked poly has shown better durability and better long-term results. These are the most widely used and least expensive. Look for abbreviation(s): • UHMWPE-Ultra High Molecular Weight Poly • UHXLPE-Ultra Highly Cross-Linked Poly
Synthetic Substitute, Ceramic (3)	Ceramic on ceramic	Ceramic on ceramic offers numerous advantages over traditional bearing surfaces, including scratch resistance, superior wear resistance, and improved lubrication. There is no metal ion release, and the alumina particulate debris is less bio-reactive. Squeaking can sometimes occur. Earlier versions had fracturing issues but recent improvements in ceramic strength have reduced this. Used often in younger people. Most expensive of devices.
Synthetic Substitute, Ceramic on Polyethylene (4)	Ceramic on polyethylene	As with ceramic on ceramic, this is known for low wear, resulting in longevity and reliability. Better wear rate but more expensive than metal on poly but less expensive than ceramic on ceramic.
Synthetic Substitute, Oxidized Zirconium on Polyethylene (6)	Oxidized zirconium on polyethylene	Considered a ceramicised metal alloy, oxidized zirconium transforms the metal head into ceramic material resulting in increased durability and longer wear.
Synthetic Substitute (J)	Unspecified	

Figure 7.3. Hip Prosthetic Device

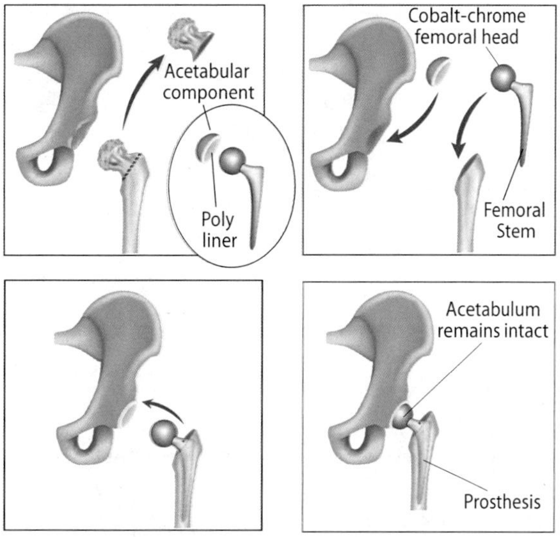

Case Study 7.4. Transvaginal Urethral Repair with Mesh

Indications: Stress urinary incontinence (SUI).

In the supine position and under satisfactory general anesthesia, the patient was placed in the dorsal lithotomy position in the Allen stirrups and prepped and draped in usual fashion for vaginal surgery.

A weighted speculum was placed in the posterior fornix of the vagina. The anterior vaginal wall was grasped with two Kocher clamps and the vaginal wall was opened in the midline with Metzenbaum scissors. That opening was continued up to the apex of the vagina. The vagina was carefully dissected off from the muscularis of the bladder back to the pubic rami bilaterally. The bladder wall and endopelvic fascia were then plicated with 2-0 Vicryl sutures, elevating the bladder and lengthening the urethra. A MiniArc Precise pubovaginal sling was passed on both sides until it was sitting nicely under the mid-urethra with no twisting, no tension, and allowed passage of a curved hemostat easily between it and the underlying tissue.

The bladder was left half full to perform a manual Valsalva maneuver that was negative. The Foley catheter was inserted, draining clear fluid. The patient was sent to the recovery room in stable condition.

Code(s):

ØTSDØZZ   Reposition Urethra, Open Approach

Rationale:

Although at initial review, it may seem logical to code the sling using root operation Supplement (U), the correct root operation assignment is Reposition (S). The urethra is not malfunctioning, but out of position. Correcting the urethra with the sling does not perform the function of the urethra, but moves it back into proper position (*AHA Coding Clinic,* 2016, 1Q, 15).

Body part Urethra (D) in the Urinary (T) body system is the focus of the procedure and was reached by cutting through the vaginal wall, which is coded as an Open (Ø) approach.

Although the sling was left in the body and according to guideline B6.1a a specific device value should be reported, at the current time, No Device (Z) is the only available option for the sixth character in the root operation Reposition (S) table.

Root Operation		
Reposition (S)	Definition:	Moving to its normal location, or other suitable location, all or a portion of a body part
	Explanation:	The body part is moved to a new location from an abnormal location, or from a normal location where it is not functioning correctly. The body part may or may not be cut out or off to be moved to the new location
Supplement (U)	Definition:	Putting in or on biological or synthetic material that physically reinforces and/or augments the function of a portion of a body part
	Explanation:	The biological material is non-living, or is living and from the same individual. The body part may have been previously replaced, and the Supplement procedure is performed to physically reinforce and/or augment the function of the replaced body part.

Figure 7.4. Urethral Sling

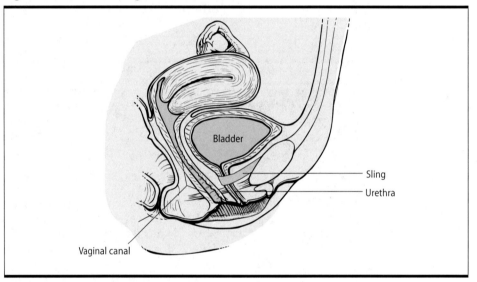

Case Study 7.5. Atherectomy with External Heart Assist

A patient with myocardial infarction was sent emergently to the cath lab with blockage of LAD due to chronic plaque and acute embolism. An Impella heart pump device was inserted for stabilization while transluminal atherectomy was performed with insertion of one DE stent. Blood flow was adequately restored and the Impella pump was removed at the conclusion of the procedure.

Code(s):

02C03ZZ	**Extirpation of Matter from Coronary Artery, One Artery, Percutaneous Approach**
027034Z	**Dilation of Coronary Artery, One Artery with Drug-eluting Intraluminal Device, Percutaneous Approach**
02HA3RJ	**Insertion of Short-term External Heart Assist System into Heart, Intraoperative, Percutaneous Approach**
5A0221D	**Assistance with Cardiac Output using Impeller Pump, Continuous**

Rationale:

A transluminal atherectomy of the left anterior descending artery is represented by the body part value Coronary Artery, One Artery (0) in the body system Heart and Great Vessels (2). This procedure employs a Percutaneous (3) approach to cut away the plaque, suctioning the plaque and emboli through a catheter. The root operation Extirpation (C) is appropriate, which is described as taking or cutting out solid matter from the body.

Since two different root operations with different objectives were performed on the same body part, Extirpation (C) and Dilation (7), multiple procedures guideline B3.2c applies and the root operation Dilation (7) is assigned for expanding the arterial lumen with a Intraluminal Device, Drug-eluting (4).

PCS Guideline	
B3.2	During the same operative episode, multiple procedures are coded if:
	c. Multiple root operations with distinct objectives are performed on the same body part.
	Example: Destruction of sigmoid lesion and bypass of sigmoid colon are coded separately.

An Impella® heart pump is an example of a Short-Term External Heart Assist System (R). Although the device is controlled externally by a console, the pump itself is inserted through a catheter and threaded into the heart. These devices can be used to mimic the heartbeat, keeping the blood flow stable during high-risk procedures. Insertion (H) is the root operation with a Percutaneous (3) approach of the device Short-term External Heart Assist Device (R). Since the device was removed at the conclusion of the procedure, it was only used during the surgery, which is identified with the qualifier Intraoperative (J). Because the Impella® device was only used during the operative episode, only the insertion of the device is required; removal of the device is not reported separately. (*AHA Coding Clinic* 2017, 4Q, 43)

Root Operation		
Medical and Surgical Section (0)		
Dilation (7)	Definition:	Expanding an orifice or the lumen of a tubular body part
	Explanation:	The orifice can be a natural orifice or an artificially created orifice. Accomplished by stretching a tubular body part using intraluminal pressure or by cutting part of the orifice or wall of the tubular body part.
Extirpation (C)	Definition:	Taking or cutting out solid matter from a body part
	Explanation:	The solid matter may be an abnormal byproduct of a biological function or a foreign body; it may be imbedded in a body part or in the lumen of a tubular body part. The solid matter may or may not have been previously broken into pieces.
Insertion (H)	Definition:	Putting in a nonbiological appliance that monitors, assists, performs, or prevents a physiological function but does not physically take the place of a body part
	Explanation:	None
Placement Section (2)		
Assistance (0)	Definition:	Taking over a portion of a physiological function by extracorporeal means

Figure 7.5. Impella Heart Assist Pump

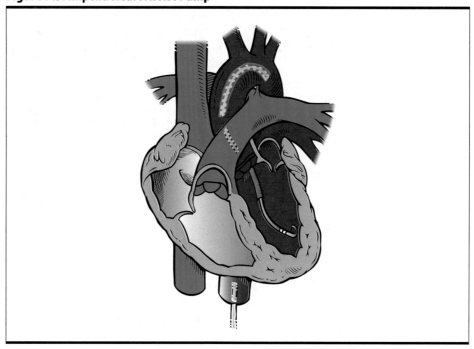

Case Study 7.6. Embolization

Indications: Patient with severe hormonal symptoms resulting from metastatic neuroendocrine tumor to the liver. The patient is not a surgical candidate and presents today for palliative embolization of the gastroduodenal artery (GDA) and right gastric artery to reduce blood flow into diseased liver.

Procedure description: The patient was prepped and draped in usual fashion. A catheter was inserted and advanced into the gastroduodenal artery. An MVP™ plug was attached to the pusher wire, advanced through the catheter, and rotated into position near the origin of the GDA. Following deployment of the plug, angiography was performed and although blood flow was reduced, the device appeared to have migrated from its desired position. Attempts made to reposition and stabilize the device were unsuccessful. The size of the device was determined to be inadequate and was removed. Due to the failed attempt at embolization in the GDA, embolization of the right gastric artery was not attempted.

Code(s):

Ø4H33DZ	**Insertion Intraluminal Device into Hepatic Artery, Percutaneous Approach**
Ø4PY3DZ	**Removal Intraluminal Device from Lower Artery, Percutaneous Approach**

Rationale:

A Micro Vascular Plug system (MVP™) is a device used to obstruct the flow of blood through a vessel. Successful insertion of this device meets the objective of root operation Occlusion (L), with the plug device left in the patient to completely close the lumen of a tubular body part.

Root Operation		
Occlusion (L)	Definition:	Completely closing an orifice or the lumen of a tubular body part
	Explanation:	The orifice can be a natural orifice or an artificially created orifice

In this case, the plug was not successfully inserted, requiring removal from the patient prior to the conclusion of the procedure. Although the device did not remain in the patient at the conclusion of this procedure, according to guideline B6.1a, if the original intent of a procedure was for a device to remain in the patient, codes can be reported to account for the work performed. Because the original objective was not accomplished, the root operation Occlusion (L) cannot be assigned; instead, root operations Insertion (H) and Removal (P) are reported.

Except for the root operation (character 3) value and the body part (character 4) value, all other characters needed to capture the procedures performed are identical. The two root operations performed were Insertion (H) and Removal (P), both found in the Lower Arteries (4) body system. The device that was placed inside the vessel is appropriately captured with device value Intraluminal Device (D) and was inserted and removed via a catheter for a Percutaneous (3) approach.

There is only one body part value, Lower Artery (Y), in the root operation table Removal (P). The Insertion (H) table has many body part values in addition to the Lower Artery (Y); however, none of the body part values are specific to gastroduodenal artery. Before defaulting to Lower Artery (Y), the Body Part Key should be consulted. According to the Body Part Key, gastroduodenal artery should be coded to body part value Hepatic Artery (3).

Root Operation		
Insertion (H)	Definition:	Putting in a nonbiological appliance that monitors, assists, performs, or prevents a physiological function but does not physically take the place of a body part
	Explanation:	None
Removal (P)	Definition:	Taking out or off a device from a body part
	Explanation:	If a device is taken out and a similar device put in without cutting or puncturing the skin or mucous membrane, the procedure is coded to the root operation CHANGE. Otherwise, the procedure for taking out a device is coded to the root operation REMOVAL.

Guideline B6.1b

B6.1b   Materials such as sutures, ligatures, radiological markers and temporary post-operative wound drains are considered integral to the performance of a procedure and are not coded as devices.

AHA Coding Clinic

2018, 1Q, 9	Craniectomy with DuraGuard Placement
2017, 4Q, 104	Intrauterine Brachytherapy & Placement of Tandems & Ovoids
2017, 3Q, 20	Creation of Indiana Pouch
2017, 3Q, 21	Augmentation Cystoplasty with Indiana Pouch and Continent Urinary Diversion
2015, 3Q, 30	Removal of Cervical Cerclage
2015, 2Q, 27	Uterine Artery Embolization Using Gelfoam
2014, 4Q, 31	Delayed Wound Closure Following Fracture Treatment
2014, 3Q, 9	Interspinous Ligamentoplasty
2014, 1Q, 9	Endovascular Repair of Endoleak
2014, 1Q, 20	Fiducial Marker Placement

Sutures, staples, glue, postoperative wound drains, operative site drains, wound vacs, and other similar medical supplies do not meet the definition of a device and are considered integral to the procedure. Some terms that indicate postoperative or wound drains are Jackson-Pratt (JP), Penrose, Blake Hemovac, Redivac™, Pigtail™ drain, or chest tube. Foley catheters (urinary) and nasogastric tubes are also not reported in PCS. Closure devices are also inherent to the definitive procedure and are not assigned a device value. No sixth-character device value is added for vascular closure devices such as Angio-Seal, Perclose, or StarClose as they are part of the closure and are inherent to the root operation that was performed.

For example, the StarClosure device is used to seal a percutaneously made access puncture into a vessel. The use of this device, similar to the use of a suture, is considered inherent to the closure of the procedure and based on the advice given in guideline B6.1b is not reported as a device.

Figure 7.6. StarClosure Vascular Closure Device

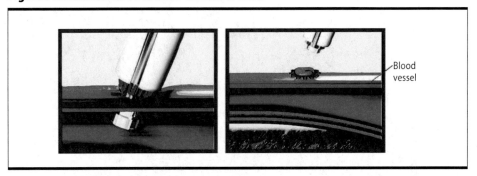

Practical Application for Guideline B6.1b

Case Study 7.7. Repair, Heart Laceration

Indication: Stab wound to chest with laceration to the left ventricle and hemothorax.

The midline of the sternum was identified externally and an incision was made over the midline of the sternum from the sternal notch down to the level of the xiphoid process. This incision was carried down through the skin and subcutaneous tissues to the level of the sternum with electrocautery. A sternal saw was used to cut the sternum and the chest cavity was entered. The pericardium was entered with Metzenbaum scissors. The heart was rotated slightly to the left and injury was noted to the left ventricle. A pledgeted 3-0 Prolene was used to place a U-stitch around the area of the injury to the heart. Care was taken not to compromise any coronary arteries in this process. After the stitch was tied down, there was noted to still be a small amount of bleeding so a second U-stitch was also placed. After this was tied, there was no further bleeding. A 40-French left-sided chest tube was placed to drain the wound and sewn into place with 0-Ethibond and was left in place.

Code(s):

Ø2QLØZZ   **Repair Left Ventricle, Open Approach**

Rationale:

The knife caused a laceration to the left ventricle of the heart, which was sewn closed with sutures. The appropriate root operation for this procedure is Repair (Q), which is used as a default when no other root operations are performed. There is a specific body part value in the Heart and Great Vessels (2) body system for Ventricle, Left (L). A sternal saw was used to cut open the sternum and enter the chest cavity, describing an Open (Ø) procedure. According to the preceding guideline B6.1b, sutures are not considered a device so No Device (Z) is reported, as well as No Qualifier (Z). Based on guideline B6.1b, no code is added for the chest tube as it was a postoperative wound drain and an inherent part of the procedure.

Root Operation		
Repair (Q)	Definition:	Restoring, to the extent possible, a body part to its normal anatomic structure and function
	Explanation:	Used only when the method to accomplish the repair is not one of the other root operations

Case Study 7.8. Brachytherapy

Indications: Prostate cancer.

Brachytherapy, permanent LDR Palladium 103 (Pd 103) seed implantation.

Total seeds placed 102.

The patient was brought to the OR and general anesthesia administered. He was placed in the dorsal lithotomy position and given preop antibiotics. Under ultrasound guidance, a total of 29 needles were placed in the periphery of the prostate, with a total of 102 seeds placed throughout the prostate. There were no seeds visualized in the bladder and all the seeds were very well distributed throughout the prostate under fluoroscopy. Please note that the Foley catheter was in place throughout the procedure. The plan was for the Foley to be left in place overnight since the patient has a history of urethral strictures. The patient is to follow up tomorrow to have the Foley removed.

Code(s):

ØVH31Z   **Insertion of Radioactive Element into Prostate, Percutaneous Approach**

DV1ØBBZ   **Low Dose Rate (LDR) Brachytherapy of Prostate using Palladium 1Ø3 (Pd-1Ø3)**

Rationale:

Brachytherapy is a type of radiation treatment that is well suited for the treatment of prostate cancer as it keeps the radiation localized to the prostate area and because the prostate is located close enough to the external skin for the brachytherapy needles to reach. Permanent seeds emit a low-dose rate over a period of time and remain in the prostate. High-dose temporary seeds remain for only a short period of time and are removed. Because treatment of the prostate cancer is the objective of this procedure, the brachytherapy seeds are considered a device that is coded.

Two codes are needed to fully capture this procedure: seed implantation is coded using root operation Insertion (H) in the Medical and Surgical (Ø) section and a second code from the Radiation Therapy (D) section is needed since the seeds are the radiation method.

Using root operation Insertion (H), the seeds are considered a Radioactive Element (6) device that was placed in the Prostate (Ø) found in the Male Reproductive System (V) using a Percutaneous (3) approach. No Qualifier (Z) is the only available option for the seventh character.

Root Operation		
Insertion (H)	Definition:	Putting in a nonbiological appliance that monitors, assists, performs, or prevents a physiological function but does not physically take the place of a body part
	Explanation:	None

The radiation component is captured in the Radiation Therapy (D) section. The body systems in this section are similar to the Medical and Surgical (Ø) section and the treatment site of Prostate (Ø) is found in the Male Reproductive System (V). The fifth character, called the modality qualifier, indicates whether a high or low dose is used, which if not specified may be determined by whether it is a permanent LDR (low dose) or a temporary HDR (high dose). This specific case used a Low Dose Rate (LDR) (B). The sixth character is determined by the type of isotope used, which can generally be identified by its initials; Palladium 103 or Pd-103 was used in this procedure and is represented by the PCS value B. The seventh character for brachytherapy is None (Z). Additionally, the ICD-10 PCS index listing for Brachytherapy Prostate directs the user to table DV10.

Although the Foley catheter remained in place at the conclusion of the procedure, it is considered inherent to the surgical procedure, not the objective of the procedure, and no code is assigned.

Figure 7.7. Prostate Brachytherapy Seeds

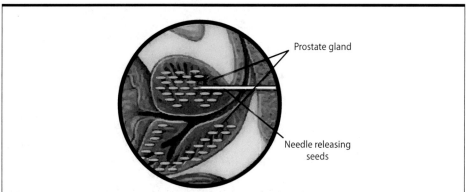

> ### Case Study 7.9. Fiducial Marker Placement
>
> **Indications:** Prostate cancer.
>
> The patient was brought to the OR for radiological marker placement for upcoming stereotactic radiotherapy. Local anesthesia was applied. A Foley catheter was placed. The patient was placed on his side in a fetal position. The patient had done bowel prep the day before. Rectal digital exam was performed. Using transrectal ultrasound guidance, three needles were inserted with three gold fiducial markers placed around the prostate. The Foley was removed. The patient was scheduled for external beam radiotherapy in two days.

Code(s):

ØDJD7ZZ   **Inspection of Lower Intestinal Tract, Via Natural or Artificial Opening**

Rationale:

In preparation for radiation therapy to the prostate, radiological markers are placed. However, based on guideline B6.1b no code is used for the insertion of radiological markers as they are merely placed to aid in the localization of radiation therapy. This example contrasts to the previous case where brachytherapy seeds are coded as a device because radiation therapy **was** the objective of the procedure.

The only code to report for this encounter is the root operation Inspection (J) for the rectal digital exam. Many of the body part values offered in the Inspection (J) table are nonspecific with Lower Intestinal Tract (D) being the correct body part value in the Gastrointestinal (D) body system. The exam was performed manually through the anus without a scope, which is described as Via Natural or Artificial Opening (7). The value for No Device (Z) and No Qualifier (Z) is reported.

Root Operation		
Inspection (J)	Definition:	Visually and/or manually exploring a body part
	Explanation:	Visual exploration may be performed with or without optical instrumentation. Manual exploration may be performed directly or through intervening body layers.

If the facility wishes to report the ultrasound guidance, code BV49ZZZ Ultrasonography of Prostate and Seminal Vesicles from the Imaging (B) section is appropriate.

The intraoperative Foley catheter is inherent to the procedure and is not reported separately. A Foley catheter is not reported in ICD-10-PCS unless it is the sole objective of the procedure and is left in at the conclusion, in which case root operation Drainage (9) with Drainage Device (0) is assigned.

Guideline B6.1c

B6.1c	**Procedures performed on a device only and not on a body part are specified in the root operations Change, Irrigation, Removal and Revision, and are coded to the procedure performed.** ***Example:*** **Irrigation of percutaneous nephrostomy tube is coded to the root operation Irrigation of indwelling device in the Administration section.**

AHA Coding Clinic

2018, 2Q, 16	Exchange of Tibial Polyethylene Component with Stabilizing Insert (Tibial Tray)
2018, 1Q, 8	Ventricular Peritoneal Shunt Ligation
2018, 1Q, 10	Revision of Transjugular Intrahepatic Portosystemic Shunt
2018, 1Q, 17	Repositioning of Impella Short-Term External Heart Assist Device
2018, 1Q, 20	Adjustment of Gastric Band
2017, 4Q, 111	Exchange of Ureteral Stent
2017, 3Q, 18	Intra-Aortic Balloon Pump Removal
2017, 2Q, 20	Exchange of Intramedullary Antibiotic Impregnated Spacer
2017, 2Q, 24	Tunneled Catheter versus Totally Implantable Catheter
2017, 2Q, 26	Exchange of Tunneled Catheter
2016, 4Q, 84	Coronary Artery, Number of Stents
2016, 4Q, 95	Intracardiac Pacemaker
2016, 4Q, 110	Removal and Revision of Hip and Knee Devices
2016, 3Q, 39	Revision of Arteriovenous Graft
2016, 2Q, 15	Removal and Replacement of Tunneled Internal Jugular Catheter
2016, 2Q, 27	Exchange of Ureteral Stents
2016, 2Q, 27	Removal of Nonviable Transverse Rectus Abdominis Myocutaneous (TRAM) Flaps
2015, 3Q, 13	Nonexcisional Debridement of Cranial Wound with Removal and Replacement of Hardware
2015, 2Q, 6	Planned Implant Break
2015, 2Q, 9	Revision of Ventriculoperitoneal (VP) Shunt
2015, 2Q, 18	Total Knee Revision
2015, 2Q, 19	Revision of Femoral Head and Acetabular Liner
2015, 1Q, 32	Deployment of Stent for Herniated/ Migrated Coil in Basilar Artery
2015, 1Q, 36	Revision of Femoropopliteal Bypass Graft
2014, 4Q, 26	Adjustment of VEPTR Lengthening Mechanism
2014, 4Q, 27	Bilateral Lengthening of Growing Rods
2014, 4Q, 28	Removal and Replacement of DisplacedGrowing Rods
2014, 3Q, 19	End of Life Replacement of Baclofen Pump
2014, 3Q, 25	Revision of Transjugular Intrahepatic Portosystemic Shunt (TIPS)
2014, 3Q, 30	Creation of Conduit from Right Ventricle to Pulmonary Artery
2014, 3Q, 31	Closure of Paravalvular Leak Using Amplatzer® Vascular Plug
2014, 1Q, 9	Endovascular Repair of Endoleak

Revision, Change, and Removal are ICD-10-PCS root operations used for procedures performed strictly on a device and not on a body part. Users should be vigilant when coding procedures involving previously placed devices to ensure the appropriate root operation assignment is selected, based on whether the procedure was performed on the patient's body part or only on the device. The root operation Irrigation (1) from the Administration (3) section can be used in the context of indwelling devices or body parts (physiological systems or anatomical regions).

Spotlight
Root operation Irrigation from the Administration section may apply to an indwelling device or a body part. When an indwelling device is irrigated, refer to table 3C1. Note that this table is comprised of a single code 3C1ZX8Z Irrigation of Indwelling Device using Irrigating Substance, External Approach and therefore is the only option available regardless of the type of indwelling device. When a body part is irrigated, refer to table 3E1. Various codes are available from table 3E1 in the Administration section that are specific to the body part or anatomical region, the approach technique, and whether an irrigating substance or dialysate was used. A qualifier value indicating whether the procedure was for diagnostic or therapeutic purposes is also available.

Root Operation		
Medical and Surgical Section (0)		
Change (2)	Definition:	Taking out or off a device from a body part and putting back an identical or similar device in or on the same body part without cutting or puncturing the skin or a mucous membrane
	Explanation:	All CHANGE procedures are coded using the approach EXTERNAL
Removal (P)	Definition:	Taking out or off a device from a body part
	Explanation:	If a device is taken out and a similar device put in without cutting or puncturing the skin or mucous membrane, the procedure is coded to the root operation CHANGE. Otherwise, the procedure for taking out a device is coded to the root operation REMOVAL.
Revision (W)	Definition:	Correcting, to the extent possible, a portion of a malfunctioning device or the position of a displaced device
	Explanation:	Revision can include correcting a malfunctioning or displaced device by taking out or putting in components of the device such as a screw or pin
Administration Section (3)		
Irrigation (1)	Definition:	Putting in or on a cleansing substance
	Explanation:	None

Selecting the appropriate root operation to use on procedures performed on a device can be confusing. The root operation Change is most often seen in an outpatient setting and rarely in an inpatient setting. This is due in part to the definition of Change that states that procedures with the root operation of Change are always done with an external approach. The root operation Change is generally used in tube or catheter changes, such as drainage tubes, chest tubes, tracheostomy tubes, or Foley catheters.

Revision is also not frequently used in an inpatient setting. Examples of revision surgery include re-cementing of a prosthetic joint or adjusting a pacemaker lead. If an entire device, rather than a minor component (such as screws or pins), is being removed and replaced rather than repositioned, then Removal and Replacement is more appropriate. If a device is removed and replaced with a different device, Removal and Insertion may be the better option.

Although documentation in many operative reports uses wording such as revision, exchange, or change, it is important to carefully review the intent of the procedure and the root operation definitions before choosing the root operations Revision or Change. Some of the following case studies include examples of this type of documentation.

Practical Application for Guideline B6.1c

> ### Case Study 7.10. Reposition, Interbody Fusion Device
>
> **Preoperative diagnosis:** L5-S1 interbody implant migration.
>
> **Procedure:** Repositioning of L5-S1 interbody implant.
>
> The patient was taken to the operating room and positioned in the lateral decubitus position, right side down, left side up on a bean bag covered with a gel pad. An axillary roll was placed. True AP and lateral confirmed with fluoroscopy. The patient was prepped and draped in sterile fashion. The left lower abdominal oblique incision was reopened. After the spine was identified, it was very clear the implant was not only loose but, as demonstrated on preoperative imaging, nearly one third out of the disk space. Using a tamp, it was impacted back into position. A loose screw was replaced with a screw and washer to act as a buttress plate. It nicely held the implant in position; implant was now wholly contained within the disk space. The lumbar wound was closed with inverted 2-0 Vicryl for the subcutaneous and a running 4-0 Monocryl suture was used for the skin edges.

Code(s):

ØSW3ØAZ   Revision of Interbody Fusion Device in Lumbosacral Joint, Open Approach

Rationale:

The interbody fusion device was moved back into its intended position without being removed or replaced. As noted in guideline B6.1c, root operation Revision (W) is used when the procedure is performed solely on the device and not the body part itself. No additional code is needed for the replacement of the screw and washer since Revision (W) can include correcting a malfunctioning or displaced device by taking out or putting in components of the device such as a screw or pin. The migrated device was in the Lumbosacral Joint (3) space of the body system Lower Joints (S). An Open (Ø) approach was used and the device was an Interbody Fusion Device (A). The seventh character is No Qualifier (Z).

Root Operation		
Revision (W)	Definition:	Correcting, to the extent possible, a portion of a malfunctioning device or the position of a displaced device
	Explanation:	Revision can include correcting a malfunctioning or displaced device by taking out or putting in components of the device such as a screw or pin

Case Study 7.11. AICD Upgrade with Revision to CRT-D

A 4 to 5 cm incision was made over the existing ICD pulse generator pocket and entered by cauterized dissection. The implantable defibrillator was removed from the pocket and disconnected from the defibrillator lead. The defibrillator leads at the right ventricular apex, as well as the right atrium, were found to have stable positioning with stable electrophysiologic parameters. Attention was turned to the left ventricular lead. Over the guidewire, a 9-French sheath was advanced in position. Through the sheath, a guided extended hook coronary sinus guiding sheath was advanced in position under fluoroscopic guidance in the right atrium. Through the sheath, a Cordis Webster deflectable quadripolar catheter was advanced and the coronary sinus was cannulated and the guiding sheath was advanced into the middle cardiac vein of the left ventricle. The deflectable catheter was removed. Through the coronary sinus guiding sheath, a Guidant left ventricular pacing lead, was advanced in position in the middle cardiac vein. The vascular introducing hardware was removed from the central circulation. The lead was secured in position using its lead stay. The new and the old leads were connected to the new implantable cardioverter defibrillator pulse generator device. The pocket was surgically revised to accommodate the new device. The hardware was tucked into the previously created pocket, which was flushed copiously with antibiotic solution and closed with three layers of Vicryl suture material. Final fluoroscopic confirmation of lead positioning was performed. Final programming of the device was performed.

Code(s):

ØJH6Ø9Z   **Insertion of Cardiac Resynchronization Defibrillator Pulse Generator into Chest Subcutaneous Tissue and Fascia, Open Approach**

02H43KZ   **Insertion of Defibrillator Lead into Coronary Vein, Percutaneous Approach**

ØJPTØPZ   **Removal of Cardiac Rhythm Related Device from Trunk Subcutaneous Tissue and Fascia, Open Approach**

Rationale:

Since the old defibrillator generator was replaced with a different type of device, Removal (P) of the old device and Insertion (H) of the new device are the appropriate root operations. Revision (W) is incorrect because the old device was not adjusted or repositioned but replaced with a different device. Change (2) is also not appropriate because it only pertains to External (X) approaches and the new Cardiac Resynchronization Defibrillator Pulse Generator (9) device was inserted using an Open (Ø) approach. The generator was inserted in a pocket in the subcutaneous tissue of the chest wall, which is reported as body part Subcutaneous Tissue and Fascia, Chest (6) of the Subcutaneous Tissue and Fascia (J) body system.

The CRT-D uses the leads in the right ventricle and right atrium, which were already intact from the previous ICD device, plus a third left ventricular lead that "synchronizes" the coordination of the heartbeat. An additional code must be reported for the Insertion (H) of the Cardiac Lead, Defibrillator (K). The coronary sinus is a collection of veins that form a large vein that runs through the heart. The lead was inserted through the coronary sinus to the middle coronary vein, which is one of the branches of the coronary sinus that goes through the left ventricle. Often the lead is placed in the lateral, posterior, anterior, or middle coronary vein. Body part Coronary Vein (4) may also be referred to as the posterior interventricular vein, and is located in the Heart and Great Vessels (2) body system. Percutaneous (3) approach is used for lead insertion.

Root Operation		
Insertion (H)	Definition:	Putting in a nonbiological appliance that monitors, assists, performs, or prevents a physiological function but does not physically take the place of a body part
	Explanation:	None
Removal (P)	Definition:	Taking out or off a device from a body part
	Explanation:	If a device is taken out and a similar device put in without cutting or puncturing the skin or mucous membrane, the procedure is coded to the root operation CHANGE. Otherwise, the procedure for taking out a device is coded to the root operation REMOVAL.

A third code is added for the Removal (P) of the previous device, which was extracted from a pocket formed in the Subcutaneous Tissue and Fascia, Trunk (T). This table (ØJP) in the Subcutaneous Tissue and Fascia (J) body system offers less specific body parts than some of the other root operations so chest is not an option. The device options in the table are also less specific with all of the individual heart rhythm devices categorized into the device value Cardiac Rhythm Related Device (P). All three of these codes use No Qualifier (Z) as a seventh character.

Definitions
cardiac contractility modulation device (CCM). Rather than regulating the heartbeats, this device is designed to provide low electrical signals to stimulate the heart muscle and over time strengthen the natural contraction of the left ventricle. At this time there is not a FDA approved product in wide use in the USA, although CCM devices are in use in Europe and other countries.   **cardiac resynchronization pacemaker pulse generator (CRT-P) and cardiac resynchronization defibrillator pulse generator (CRT-D).** These devices have three leads: one in the right atrium, one in the right ventricle, and a third lead in the left ventricle, which allows for smoother coordination or resynchronization of heart pumping. The CRT-P is only a pacemaker while the CRT-D acts as a pacemaker and defibrillator (ICD).   **pacemaker and defibrillator.** Pacemakers use low energy electrical impulses to regulate heart arrhythmias prompting it into a normal beat. An implantable cardioverter defibrillator (ICD) not only detects and regulates abnormal heart rate with low energy, but also sends a high energy shock when it senses a dangerously irregular heartbeat or cardiac arrest. Single chamber devices have a lead that goes into the right ventricle or right atrium, while dual chamber devices have a lead in both the right atrium and right ventricle.

Case Study 7.12. Change Ureteral Stent

Indications: Hydronephrosis.

Procedure performed: Exchange left ureteral stent.

Using a cystoscope, a guidewire was advanced to the preexisting left ureteral stent, which was found to be occluded distally. The ureteral stent and cystoscope were removed. A catheter was passed. Over a wire, a new ureteral stent was placed and confirmed with fluoroscopy, resulting in the spontaneous drainage of contrast and urine into the bladder.

Code(s):

ØT777DZ   **Dilation of Left Ureter with Intraluminal Device, Via Natural or Artificial Opening**

ØTP98DZ   **Removal of Intraluminal Device from Ureter, Via Natural or Artificial Opening Endoscopic**

Rationale:

The objective of this procedure was to expand the ureter with the insertion of a stent, which is reported with root operation Dilation (7). The dilation was performed on the body part Ureter, Left

(7) in the Urinary System (T). The approach for the insertion of the stent was performed Via Natural or Artificial Opening (7) with visualization using fluoroscopy. The stent is an Intraluminal Device (D). Although it may seem logical to use the root operation Change (2), the advice given by *AHA Coding Clinic,* 2016, 2Q, 27, states that because the definitive objective was to dilate the ureter, Change (2) is not appropriate. Additionally, the approach was not done externally, which is the only approach that can be used with Change (2) according to the root operation definition and explanation.

A second code describes the Removal (P) of the original, occluded stent. This table in the Urinary System (T) does not offer choices for Ureter (9) laterality. The procedure was performed with the aid of a cystoscope, which is best reported with Via Natural or Artificial Opening Endoscopic (8). The device removed was an Intraluminal Device (D).

Root Operation		
Change (2)	Definition:	Taking out or off a device from a body part and putting back an identical or similar device in or on the same body part without cutting or puncturing the skin or a mucous membrane
	Explanation:	All CHANGE procedures are coded using the approach EXTERNAL
Dilation (7)	Definition:	Expanding an orifice or the lumen of a tubular body part
	Explanation:	The orifice can be a natural orifice or an artificially created orifice. Accomplished by stretching a tubular body part using intraluminal pressure or by cutting part of the orifice or wall of the tubular body part.
Removal (P)	Definition:	Taking out or off a device from a body art
	Explanation:	If a device is taken out and a similar device put in without cutting or puncturing the skin or mucous membrane, the procedure is coded to the root operation CHANGE. Otherwise, the procedure for taking out a device is coded to the root operation REMOVAL.

Case Study 7.13. Knee Liner Revision

Procedure performed: Polyethylene liner exchange, right knee, with placement of STIMULAN antibiotic impregnated beads.

The patient's right lower extremity was prepped and draped in the usual sterile fashion. The leg was exsanguinated and the tourniquet inflated. The patient's previous midline skin incision was utilized. Dissection was carried down to the extensor. The superior aspect of the extensor repair had been disrupted and did communicate with the joint. The previously placed polyethylene insert was removed. The knee was thoroughly irrigated. At this point, all tissues were healthy-appearing. A new polyethylene liner was impacted into place. As a precaution, 25 mL of STIMULAN beads, which had been impregnated with vancomycin and tobramycin, were placed in the gutters. The wound was closed in layered fashion with #2 STRATAFIX for the extensor followed by 2-0 PDS in the deep subcutaneous tissue. Then 3-0 nylon mattress sutures were used to close the skin.

Code(s):
ØSUCØ9Z	**Supplement Right Knee Joint with Liner, Open**
ØSPCØ9Z	**Removal of Liner from Right Knee Joint, Open Approach**
3EØUØ29	**Introduction of Other Anti-infective into Joints, Open Approach**

Rationale:
The previous liner was completely taken out and replaced with another. The root operation Revision (W) is not used when a device is removed and replaced. Because a device was taken out, report root operation Removal (P) from Knee Joint, Right (C) in the Lower Joints (S) body systems. Table ØSP also contains a device value for Liner (9) and it was performed with an Open (Ø) approach.

The correct root operation for the new liner is Supplement (U) because the liner physically reinforces the replaced knee joint; Replacement (R) is not correct because it is defined as taking the place of, or functioning as, a body part. *AHA Coding Clinic,* 2015, 2Q, 19, gives another example of this with guidance supporting this rationale. The body part is Knee Joint, Right (C) from the Lower Joints (S) body system. An Open (Ø) approach was used to insert the polyethylene liner, which is reported with the device value Liner (9) and No Qualifier (Z).

If facility guidelines dictate, a code can also be reported for the insertion of the antibiotic beads, found in the Administration (3) section and Physiological Systems and Anatomical Regions (E). The root operation is Introduction (Ø) into the Joints (U) body system/region with Open (Ø) approach, since the beads are laid into the open joint. PCS refers to antibiotic substances, including beads as Anti-infectives (2). The qualifier is Other Anti-Infective (9).

Root Operation		
Medical and Surgical Section (0)		
Supplement (U)	Definition:	Putting in or on biological or synthetic material that physically reinforces and/or augments the function of a portion of a body part
	Explanation:	The biological material is non-living, or is living and from the same individual. The body part may have been previously replaced, and the Supplement procedure is performed to physically reinforce and/or augment the function of the replaced body part.
Removal (P)	Definition:	Taking out or off a device from a body part
	Explanation:	If a device is taken out and a similar device put in without cutting or puncturing the skin or mucous membrane, the procedure is coded to the root operation CHANGE. Otherwise, the procedure for taking out a device is coded to the root operation REMOVAL.
Administration Section (3)		
Introduction (Ø)	Definition:	Putting in or on a therapeutic, diagnostic, nutritional, physiological or prophylactic substance except blood or blood products.
	Explanation:	None

Case Study 7.14. Change Gastrostomy Tube (G-Tube)

Using a syringe from the side port, old water was removed, deflating the balloon. Once all of the water was removed, the old tube was gently pulled out. After lubricating the new tube and gently pushing it down into the stoma, the balloon was inflated using a small amount of water and the syringe.

Code(s):

ØD2ØXUZ   Change Feeding Device in Upper Intestinal Tract, External Approach

Rationale:
This is an instance where the root operation Change (2) is appropriate because the old gastrostomy tube is exchanged for a new Feeding Device (U) and the procedure is performed using an External (X) approach.

Root Operation		
Change (2)	Definition:	Taking out or off a device from a body part and putting back an identical or similar device in or on the same body part without cutting or puncturing the skin or a mucous membrane.
	Explanation:	All CHANGE procedures are coded using the approach EXTERNAL

The only body part choices in the Change (2) table in the Gastrointestinal System (D) for a feeding tube are the Upper and Lower Intestinal Tract. A gastrostomy tube inserts into the stomach and according to the following Guideline B4.8, the stomach is located in the Upper Intestinal Tract (Ø).

PCS Guideline
Upper and lower intestinal tract
B4.8   In the Gastrointestinal body system, the general body part values Upper Intestinal Tract and Lower Intestinal Tract are provided as an option for the root operations Change, Inspection, Removal and Revision. Upper Intestinal Tract includes the portion of the gastrointestinal tract from the esophagus down to and including the duodenum, and Lower Intestinal Tract includes the portion of the gastrointestinal tract from the jejunum down to and including the rectum and anus. *Example:* In the root operation Change table, change of a device in the jejunum is coded using the body part Lower Intestinal Tract.

Case Study 7.15. Wittmann Patch Removal

Operation: Removal of Wittmann patch.

After a previous hernia repair, getting the patient's fascia back together has been unsuccessful. He has been returned to the OR every two to three days for tightening of the Wittmann patch that is pulling his abdominal fascia together. It is now almost closed and he has developed Staph on the Wittmann patch, therefore it was felt to be removed and sewn completely together.

He was placed in a supine position and under general anesthesia the subcutaneous tissue was entered down into the fascial where the Wittmann patch suture was cut and the patch was removed from both edges of the fascia. The abdominal cavity was irrigated with sterile saline. A complex wound closure was then carried out in layers with 2-0 Vicryl suture. The skin was closed with staples and an abdominal binder placed.

Code(s):

ØJPTØJZ   **Removal of Synthetic Substitute from Trunk Subcutaneous Tissue and Fascia, Open Approach**

Rationale:

The Wittmann Patch is a device that assists with gradual pulling of abdominal wall fascia that is too far apart to close due to abdominal wall swelling or tissue loss. It is similar to Velcro® and is often used in conjunction with negative pressure dressings (wound vac). The patient returns to the OR every two or three days for tightening, inspection, and reapproximation of the fascia. When the fascial edges are pulled close enough together, the final abdominal layered closure is performed. In this example the patch was taken off, which is described by the root operation Removal (P). The procedure was performed on the abdominal wall fascia, reported with Subcutaneous Tissue and Fascia, Trunk (T) in the Subcutaneous Tissue and Fascia (J) body system. The skin and subcutaneous layers were entered to reach the fascia so the approach is Open (Ø). The correct device value for the Wittmann Patch is Synthetic Substitute (J) with No Qualifier (Z) as the seventh character.

Root Operation		
Removal (P)	Definition:	Taking out or off a device from a body part
	Explanation:	If a device is taken out and a similar device put in without cutting or puncturing the skin or mucous membrane, the procedure is coded to the root operation CHANGE. Otherwise, the procedure for taking out a device is coded to the root operation REMOVAL.

Case Study 7.16. Skin Grafts

Indication: The patient suffered a significant flame burn while trying to start a fire with gasoline. He underwent a previous burn excision and grafting with Integra. He was doing well and his burns were healing as expected with need for autografting.

Procedure: Removal of Integra allograft with placement of split thickness skin graft to the bilateral lower extremities and abdomen. Surface area grafted included the left anterior thigh, left posterior thigh, left knee and left lower anterior leg, left calf and another smaller burn on the left calf, right anterior thigh burns, right posterior thigh, right lower leg medial burn, right lower leg lateral burn, and abdominal burn.

Procedure Description: After consent was obtained, the patient was taken to the operating suite and placed in the supine position. Preoperative antibiotics were given per anesthesia. General anesthesia was induced by the anesthesia team. The abdomen and bilateral lower extremities were circumferentially prepped and draped in the usual sterile fashion. The allograft was clean and adherent at all sites without evidence of infection. This was easily excised down to healthy bleeding tissue using a #8 Weck blade. All superficial granulation tissue was debrided. Hemostasis was obtained using epinephrine soaks as well as meticulous electrocautery.

A standard pneumatic dermatome set at 0.012 of an inch depth was used to harvest skin for autografting. The skin was harvested from the skin on the upper back and the skin was meshed in a 2:1 ratio. The meshed autograft was applied in the standard fashion with the dermal side facing the wound to all excised regions. The skin was trimmed to accommodate the wound edges and was secured with skin staples. Sites grafted are as listed above. Final assessment of all sites revealed excellent graft adherence with excellent wound apposition and no evidence of hematoma, seroma, or other concern. The wounds were dressed with Xeroform, dry burn dressing followed by Kerlix, and Ace dressings. The donor sites were dressed with Mepitel Ag.

Code(s):

ØHR7X74	**Replacement of Abdomen Skin with Autologous Tissue Substitute, Partial Thickness, External Approach**
ØHRHX74	**Replacement of Right Upper Leg Skin with Autologous Tissue Substitute, Partial Thickness, External Approach**
ØHRKX74	**Replacement of Right Lower Leg Skin with Autologous Tissue Substitute, Partial Thickness, External Approach**
ØHRJX74	**Replacement of Left Upper Leg Skin with Autologous Tissue Substitute, Partial Thickness, External Approach**
ØHRLX74	**Replacement of Left Lower Leg Skin with Autologous Tissue Substitute, Partial Thickness, External Approach**
ØHB6XZZ	**Excision of Back Skin, External Approach**
ØHPPXKZ	**Removal of Nonautologous Tissue Substitute from Skin, External Approach**

Rationale:

The first five codes represent Replacement (R) of the previous allograft tissue with newly harvested autograft skin tissue. Each body part with an individual PCS body part value must be coded separately based on multiple procedure Guideline B3.2a. The separate sites, which are all located in the Skin and Breast (H) body system, include:

- Skin, Abdomen (7)
- Skin, Right Upper Leg (H)
- Skin, Right Lower Leg (K)
- Skin, Left Upper Leg (J)
- Skin, Left Lower Leg (L)

These codes include the skin of the anterior and posterior thighs, knees, and calves.

PCS Guideline
Multiple procedures
B3.2   During the same operative episode, multiple procedures are coded if: a. The same root operation is performed on different body parts as defined by distinct values of the body part character. *Example:* Diagnostic excision of liver and pancreas are coded separately. Excision of lesion in the ascending colon and excision of lesion in the transverse colon are coded separately.

The only approach value on all skin body parts is External (X). Skin grafts are considered a device and since this skin graft is made from the patient's own skin, Autologous Tissue Substitute (7) is the device value. The skin was harvested with 0.012 of an inch depth and meshed in a 2:1 ratio, reported with qualifier Partial Thickness (4). This is also often documented as a "split-thickness" or STSG.

According to Guideline B3.9, the harvest of the skin autograft must be coded separately. The root operation Excision (B) of the back is reported with Skin, Back (6) of the Skin and Breast (H) body system. An External (X) approach was used with No Device (Z) and No Qualifier (Z).

PCS Guideline
Excision for Graft
B3.9   If an autograft is obtained from a different procedure site in order to complete the objective of the procedure, a separate procedure is coded. *Example:* Coronary bypass with excision of saphenous vein graft, excision of saphenous vein is coded separately.

According to the root operation definition for Replacement (R), when a device is being replaced rather than a body part, the root operation Removal (P) must also be reported. The actual skin had been temporarily replaced with the allograft Integra in a previous episode and was now ready for its permanent autologous replacement. Since allograft Integra is considered a device, based on guideline B6.1c, Removal (P) of the Nonautologous Tissue Substitute (K) is reported from body part Skin (P) found in the Skin and Breast (H) body system, performed with an External (X) approach. If no allograft had been previously placed but rather the patient's own skin removed in this operative episode and directly replaced with the autologous grafts, no additional code would be required for the removal of the skin body part.

Spotlight
Biologic or synthetic skin grafts are considered devices. Although often referred to as artificial or synthetic, Integra and Dermagraft skin substitutes are considered biologically derived and should be coded as Nonautologous Tissue Substitute (K) according to *AHA Coding Clinic,* 2014, 2Q, 5.

Root Operation		
Replacement (R)	Definition:	Putting in or on biological or synthetic material that physically takes the place and/or function of all or a portion of a body part
	Explanation:	The body part may have been taken out or replaced, or may be taken out, physically eradicated, or rendered nonfunctional during the Replacement procedure. A Removal procedure is coded for taking out the device used in a previous replacement procedure.
Excision (B)	Definition:	Cutting out or off, without replacement, a portion of a body part
	Explanation:	The qualifier DIAGNOSTIC is used to identify excision procedures that are biopsies
Removal (P)	Definition:	Taking out or off a device from a body part
	Explanation:	If a device is taken out and a similar device put in without cutting or puncturing the skin or mucous membrane, the procedure is coded to the root operation CHANGE. Otherwise, the procedure for taking out a device is coded to the root operation REMOVAL.

Drainage Device

Guideline B6.2

Drainage device

B6.2   **A separate procedure to put in a drainage device is coded to the root operation Drainage with the device value Drainage Device.**

AHA Coding Clinic

2018, 2Q, 17   Arthroscopic Drainage of Knee and Nonexcisional Debridement
2017, 3Q, 19   Ureteral Stent Placement for Urinary Leakage
2015, 3Q, 11   Percutaneous Drainage of Subdural Hematoma
2015, 3Q, 12   Placement of Ventriculostomy Catheter via Burr Hole
2015, 3Q, 12   Subdural Evacuation Portal System (SEPS) Placement
2015, 3Q, 23   Incision and Drainage of Multiple Abscess Cavities Using Vessel Loop
2015, 2Q, 29   Insertion of Nasogastric Tube for Drainage and Feeding
2015, 2Q, 30   Drainage of Syrinx
2015, 1Q, 32   Percutaneous Transhepatic Biliary Drainage Catheter Placement
2014, 3Q, 15   Drainage of Pancreatic Pseudocyst

Placement of a drainage device is a commonly performed procedure on various sites throughout the body. The objective of the procedure is to drain the body part, which means root operation Drainage should be assigned. It should not be automatically assumed that initial placement of any device is assigned to the root operation Insertion. Appropriate root operation assignment requires a thorough understanding of the intent of a procedure.

Spotlight
A code for Drainage Device is only assigned when it is used to perform the objective of the procedure and remains in the body after the conclusion of the procedure.

Practical Application for Guideline B6.2

Case Study 7.17. Myringotomy with Tubes

Indications: Chronic otitis media with effusion.

Procedure performed: Right myringotomy with tympanostomy tube placement.

The patient was placed in supine position and the patient's head was turned to the left exposing the right ear. The operative microscope and small-sized ear speculum were placed and the cerumen from the external auditory canal was removed with a cerumen loop to suction. The tympanic membrane was brought into direct visualization with no signs of any gross retracted pockets or cholesteatoma. A myringotomy incision was made within the posterior inferior quadrant and the middle ear was suctioned until demonstrating dry contents. A short-term tube was placed in the myringotomy incision utilizing forceps. Cortisporin otic drops were placed followed by cotton balls.

Code(s):

Ø99500Z   **Drainage of Right Middle Ear with Drainage Device, Open Approach**

Rationale:

During a myringotomy, a small incision is made into the tympanic membrane (eardrum) to suction out fluid buildup and relieve pressure from the middle ear. A small tube, referred to as a tympanostomy or myringotomy tube, is placed in the middle ear incision to keep it aerated and to keep the fluid from accumulating. Since the purpose of the procedure is to drain the fluid and keep it from returning it is reported with root operation Drainage (9). Root operation Insertion (H) is not appropriate; Drainage (9) more accurately describes the procedure performed. The alphabetic index, under Myringotomy and Myringostomy, directs the user to *see* Drainage, Ear, Nose, Sinus Ø99.

The body part Middle Ear, Right (5) is reported since that was the part of the ear treated, found in the Ear, Nose and Sinus (9) body system. The correct approach is Open (Ø) because the eardrum was incised to access the middle ear. Review tables Ø995 carefully as one row offers only No Device (Z) but the correct option is found in the row that offers Drainage Device (Ø). When a drainage device is placed, and remains in situ at the completion of the procedure, assign the device value Drainage Device (Ø).

Root Operation		
Drainage (9)	Definition:	Taking or letting out fluids and/or gases from a body part
	Explanation:	The qualifier DIAGNOSTIC is used to identify drainage procedures that are biopsies
Insertion (H)	Definition:	Putting in a nonbiological appliance that monitors, assists, performs, or prevents a physiological function but does not physically take the place of a body part
	Explanation:	None

Figure 7.8. Myringotomy

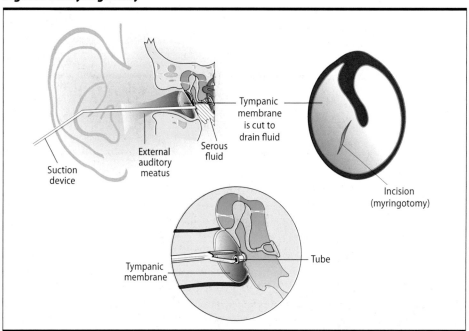

Case Study 7.18. Chest Tube for Pneumothorax

Operative procedure: The patient is a 67-year-old male who recently had port placement in his right chest. He was noted to have a postprocedural pneumothorax on the right with O_2 saturations of 30 to 40 percent. Therefore, the patient was sterilely prepped and draped in his bed. Xylocaine 1% was infiltrated along the right chest wall. A 24 French trocar chest tube was placed in the right chest and positioned high in the apex. The tube was secured with a silk suture. Tape was applied. The patient tolerated the procedure well with immediate response with O_2 saturations jumping from 80 percent to 97 percent. The chest tube was left in.

Code(s):

ØW993ØZ   Drainage of Right Pleural Cavity with Drainage Device, Percutaneous Approach

Rationale:

A pneumothorax is caused by air escaping from a lung into the chest cavity. This causes compression to the lung creating breathing difficulty and possibly a collapsed lung. The objective of this procedure was to let the air out of the chest cavity allowing the lung to expand normally. The definition of the root operation Drainage (9) not only includes removing fluids but also letting out gases or air. Guideline B2.1a states that when a procedure is performed on an anatomical region such as Drainage (9) of a body cavity, a code from Anatomical Region, General (W) is appropriate. The air was let out from the right chest cavity, which coincides with PCS body part value Pleural Cavity, Right (9). The chest tube was placed using a Percutaneous (3) approach and was left in at the conclusion of the procedure. According to guideline B6.2, the chest tube is reported with device value Drainage Device (Ø). The qualifier is No Qualifier (Z). If the chest tube is immediately removed, No Device (Z) value is reported.

PCS Guideline
General Guidelines
B2.1a   The procedure codes in the general anatomical regions body systems can be used when the procedure is performed on an anatomical region rather than a specific body part (e.g., root operations Control and Detachment, Drainage of a body cavity) or on the rare occasion when no information is available to support assignment of a code to a specific body part.
Example: Control of postoperative hemorrhage is coded to the root operation Control found in the general anatomical regions body systems.
Chest tube drainage of the pleural cavity is coded to the root operation Drainage found in the general anatomical regions body systems. Suture repair of the abdominal wall is coded to the root operation Repair in the general anatomical regions body system.

Figure 7.9. Chest Tube Placement for Pneumothorax

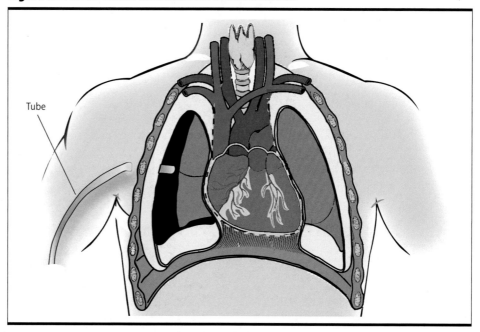

Tube

Chapter 8. Obstetrics Section Guidelines

Obstetrics Section Overview

Obstetrics Section: Character 1

The Obstetrics (1) section is one of nine sections found in the Medical and Surgical-Related section in ICD-10-PCS.

The seven characters that make up a PCS code in the Obstetrics (1) section are the same as those found in the Medical and Surgical (Ø) section.

Character 1	Character 2	Character 3	Character 4	Character 5	Character 6	Character 7
Section	Body System	Root Operation	Body Part	Approach	Device	Qualifier

Obstetrics Character Meanings

Character 1: Section (1)

The first character in an ICD-10-PCS obstetrics code is always Obstetrics (1).

Character 2: Body System (Ø)

There is only one valid body system value for character 2 in an obstetrics code: Pregnancy (Ø).

Character 3: Root Operation

There are 12 root operations in the Obstetrics section, two of which are unique to the section:

- **Abortion (A).** Artificially terminating a pregnancy.

  Abortion procedures are further differentiated based on whether a substance is used (e.g., abortifacient or laminaria) or whether the procedure is performed by mechanical (vacuum) means. If a substance or vacuum is used, the approach value is Via Natural or Artificial Opening (7) and is assigned the appropriate Qualifier (seventh character) value.

- **Delivery (E).** Assisting the passage of the products of conception from the genital canal.

  This root operation applies only to manually-assisted vaginal deliveries. Cesarean deliveries are coded to the root operation Extraction (D).

The following table provides a list of the 12 valid root operations with examples for the Obstetrics section.

Table 8.1. Obstetrics Root Operation

ICD-10-PCS Value		Definition
Change (2)	Definition:	Taking out or off a device from a body part and putting back an identical or similar device in or on the same body part without cutting or puncturing the skin or a mucous membrane
	Explanation:	None
	Example:	Replacement of fetal scalp electrode
Drainage (9)	Definition:	Taking or letting out fluids and/or gases from a body part
	Explanation:	None
	Example:	Biopsy of amniotic fluid
Abortion (A)	Definition:	Artificially terminating a pregnancy
	Explanation:	None
	Example:	Transvaginal abortion using vacuum aspiration technique
Extraction (D)	Definition:	Pulling or stripping out or off all or a portion of a body part by the use of force
	Explanation:	None
	Example:	Low-transverse C-section
Delivery (E)	Definition:	Assisting the passage of the products of conception from the genital canal
	Explanation:	None
	Example:	Manually-assisted delivery
Insertion (H)	Definition:	Putting in a nonbiological appliance that monitors, assists, performs, or prevents a physiological function but does not physically take the place of a body part
	Explanation:	None
	Example:	Placement of fetal scalp electrode
Inspection (J)	Definition:	Visually and/or manually exploring a body part
	Explanation:	Visual exploration may be performed with or without optical instrumentation. Manual exploration may be performed directly or through intervening body layers.
	Example:	Bimanual pregnancy exam
Removal (P)	Definition:	Taking out or off a device from a body part, region or orifice
	Explanation:	If a device is taken out and a similar device put in without cutting or puncturing the skin or mucous membrane, the procedure is coded to the root operation CHANGE. Otherwise, the procedure for taking out a device is coded to the root operation REMOVAL.
	Example:	Removal of fetal monitoring electrode
Repair (Q)	Definition:	Restoring, to the extent possible, a body part to its normal anatomic structure and function
	Explanation:	Used only when the method to accomplish the repair is not one of the other root operations
	Example:	In utero repair of congenital diaphragmatic hernia

ICD-10-PCS Value	Definition	
Reposition (S)	Definition:	Moving to its normal location, or other suitable location, all or a portion of a body part
	Explanation:	The body part is moved to a new location from an abnormal location, or from a normal location where it is not functioning correctly. The body part may or may not be cut out or off to be moved to the new location.
	Example:	External version of fetus
Resection (T)	Definition:	Cutting out or off, without replacement, all of a body part
	Explanation:	None
	Example:	Total excision of tubal pregnancy
Transplantation (Y)	Definition:	Putting in or on all or a portion of a living body part taken from another individual or animal to physically take the place and/or function of all or a portion of a similar body part
	Explanation:	The native body part may or may not be taken out, and the transplanted body part may take over all or a portion of its function
	Example:	In utero fetal kidney transplant

Character 4: Body Part

There are only three valid body part character values in the Obstetrics section, as follows:

- Products of Conception (Ø)
- Products of Conception, Retained (1)
- Products of Conception, Ectopic (2)

Character 5: Approach

The fifth character represents the approach, as defined in the Medical and Surgical section, with six approach values applicable to the Obstetrics (1) section. The following table provides an overview of the approaches used in the Obstetrics (1) section.

Table 8.2. Obstetrics Approach

Approach	Definition
Open (Ø)	Cutting through the skin or mucous membrane and any other body layers necessary to expose the site of the procedure.
Percutaneous (3)	Entry, by puncture or minor incision, of instrumentation through the skin or mucous membrane and any other body layers necessary to reach the site of the procedure.
Percutaneous Endoscopic (4)	Entry, by puncture or minor incision, of instrumentation through the skin or mucous membrane and any other body layers necessary to reach and visualize the site of the procedure.
Via Natural or Artificial Opening (7)	Entry of instrumentation through a natural or artificial external opening to reach the site of the procedure.
Via Natural or Artificial Opening Endoscopic (8)	Entry of instrumentation through a natural or artificial external opening to reach and visualize the site of the procedure.
External (X)	Procedures performed directly on the skin or mucous membrane and procedures performed indirectly by the application of external force through the skin or mucous membrane.

Character 6: Device

Sixth-character values for the Obstetrics section are limited to Monitoring Electrode (3), Other Device (Y), and No Device (Z). Monitoring Electrode (3) is most commonly assigned for procedures such as placement of a fetal pulse oximetry electrode.

Character 7: Qualifier

Seventh-character Qualifier provides detailed information for a variety of procedures. For example:

- Type of assisted delivery, such as Low Forceps (3), Mid Forceps (4), High Forceps (5), Vacuum (6), Internal Version (7), Other (8)
- Type of cesarean section, such as High (Ø), Low (1), Extraperitoneal (2)
- Type of fluid removed during a Drainage (9) procedure, such as Fetal Blood (9), Fetal Cerebrospinal Fluid (A), Fetal Fluid, Other (B), Amniotic Fluid, Therapeutic (C), Fluid, Other (D), or Amniotic Fluid, Diagnostic (U).
- Method used to terminate a pregnancy, such as Vacuum (6), Abortifacient (X), or Laminaria (W).
- Body system repaired during a fetal repair procedure, such as Nervous System (E), Cardiovascular System (F), Urinary System (S), etc.

Products of Conception

The most important guideline to keep in mind when coding procedures in the Obstetrics (1) section is that these procedures are **only** performed on products of conception. Procedures performed on the pregnant patient, other than on the embryo, fetus, or other product of conception, are coded elsewhere in PCS. Gestational age is not a part of the procedure code but can be addressed in the diagnosis code.

Definition
products of conception. Includes all physical components of a pregnancy, such as zygote, embryo, fetus, umbilical cord, amnion, and placenta.

Guideline C1

C1	Procedures performed on the products of conception are coded to the Obstetrics section. Procedures performed on the pregnant female other than the products of conception are coded to the appropriate root operation in the Medical and Surgical section.
	Example: **Amniocentesis is coded to the products of conception body part in the Obstetrics section. Repair of obstetric urethral laceration is coded to the urethra body part in the Medical and Surgical section.**

AHA Coding Clinic

2018, 2Q, 17	High Transverse Cesarean Section
2018, 1Q, 23	Tubal Ligation Procedure
2017, 4Q, 69	Manual Extraction of Retained Products of Conception
2017, 3Q, 5	Delivery of Placenta
2016, 2Q, 34	Assisted Vaginal Delivery
2016, 1Q, 9	Anteversion of Retroverted Pregnant Uterus
2016, 1Q, 9	Vaginal Delivery Assisted by Vacuum and Low Forceps Extraction
2015, 3Q, 31	Laparoscopic Partial Salpingectomy for Ectopic Pregnancy
2014, 4Q, 17	RH (D) Alloimmunization (Sensitization)
2014, 4Q, 43	Cesarean Delivery Assisted by Vacuum Extraction
2014, 4Q, 43	Vacuum Dilation and Curettage for Blighted Ovum
2014, 3Q, 12	Fetoscopic Laser Photocoagulation and Laser Microseptostomy for Twin-Twin Transfusion Syndrome
2014, 2Q, 9	Pitocin Administration to Augment Labor
2013, 2Q, 36	Intrauterine Pressure Monitor

Practical Application for Guideline C1

Products of Conception

Case Study 8.1. Abortion, Spontaneous Manually Assisted

Code(s):

10E0XZZ   Delivery of Products of Conception, External Approach

Rationale:

The pregnancy was not artificially terminated, so the manual assistance is coded to root operation Delivery (E). Information related to the abortion is found in the diagnosis code only. There is only one possible valid PCS code for table 10E.

Case Study 8.2. Abortion, Vacuum Aspiration

Code(s):

10A07Z6 Abortion of Products of Conception, Vacuum, Via Natural or Artificial Opening

Rationale:
Abortion refers to artificially terminating a pregnancy and is coded using Abortion (A). The method used to abort the products of conception was accomplished Via Natural or Artificial Opening (7) using a Vacuum (6). A vacuum is commonly used to facilitate an abortion procedure and is captured by the seventh-character (qualifier) assignment.

Case Study 8.3. Tubal Pregnancy, Laparoscopic Total Removal

Code(s):

10T24ZZ Resection of Products of Conception, Ectopic, Percutaneous Endoscopic Approach

Rationale:
Body part Products of Conception, Ectopic (2) should be assigned since the procedural statement indicated a tubal pregnancy. All of the products of conception were removed; Resection (T) is the most appropriate root operation.

Definition
ectopic pregnancy. Pregnancy in which a fertilized egg implants outside of the uterus. The most common site of an ectopic pregnancy is within a fallopian tube.

Case Study 8.4. Delivery, Breech with Vacuum

Code(s):

10D07Z6 Extraction of Products of Conception, Vacuum, Via Natural or Artificial Opening

Rationale:
Vacuum delivery is classified in PCS as an Extraction (D) root operation, with seventh-character Vacuum (6) designating the specific type of extraction.

Case Study 8.5. Delivery, Routine Vaginal Following Internal (or Transcervical) Fetal Rotation Due to Face-brow Presentation

Code(s):

10E0XZZ Delivery of Products of Conception, External Approach

10S07ZZ Reposition Products of Conception, Via Natural or Artificial Opening

Rationale:
Rotating the fetus prior to delivery is classified as a Reposition (S) root operation. Since the rotation was stated to be done internally, the approach is Via Natural or Artificial Opening (7). Code additionally the routine Delivery (E) via External (X) approach.

Case Study 8.6. Amniocentesis for Genetic Testing

Code(s):

10903ZU   **Drainage of Amniotic Fluid, Diagnostic from Products of Conception, Percutaneous Approach**

Rationale:

Fluid was removed from the amniotic cavity for diagnostic purposes, which meets the root operation definition of Drainage (9). Amniotic Fluid, Diagnostic (U) is used as the qualifier. An amniotic needle was inserted into the abdomen to aspirate the fluid and is reported as a Percutaneous (3) approach.

Case Study 8.7. Artificial Rupture of Membranes for Induction of Labor

Code(s):

10907ZC   **Drainage of Amniotic Fluid, Therapeutic from Products of Conception, Via Natural or Artificial Opening**

Rationale:

Artificial rupture of membranes is sometimes performed to induce labor or because membranes failed to rupture spontaneously during the course of labor. The objective of this procedure is to drain amniotic fluid from around the fetus. This objective meets the root operation definition for Drainage (9). Because the procedure is performed to assist in labor and delivery, the rupture of membranes is considered Therapeutic (C) (*AHA Coding Clinic*, 2014, 2Q, 9). Drainage is performed through the vagina so the approach value is via Natural or Artificial Opening (7).

Case Study 8.8. Transvaginal Placement of Fetal Pulse Oximetry Electrode

Code(s):

10H073Z   **Insertion of Monitoring Electrode into Products of Conception, Via Natural or Artificial Opening**

Rationale:

Insertion (H) is the correct root operation to use when an electrode is inserted to measure fetal oxygenation during labor.

Case Study 8.9. Cesarean Section, Low Cervical

Code(s):

10D00Z1   **Extraction of Products of Conception, Low, Open Approach**

Rationale:

By definition, a cesarean section (C-section) is removal of the fetus through an incision in the uterus. The fetus does not pass through the vagina in a C-section, ruling out the use of Delivery (E) as the root operation. Extraction (D) is the appropriate root operation using an Open (0) approach with the seventh character (qualifier) identifying the type of C-section.

Case Study 8.10. Amnioscopy

Code(s):

10J08ZZ   **Inspection of Products of Conception, Via Natural or Artificial Opening Endoscopic**

Rationale:

Amnioscopy is prenatal examination of the fetus and amniotic fluid by insertion of an endoscope through the cervix. Inspection (J) is the appropriate root operation with Via Natural or Artificial Opening Endoscopic (8) as the approach.

Case Study 8.11. Delivery, Vaginal with Perineal Laceration Repair

A patient was admitted at 40-weeks gestation in active labor, which progressed without incident. A single, liveborn infant was delivered spontaneously with manual assistance. A second-degree perineal tear was repaired with layered sutures.

Code(s):

10E0XZZ	Delivery of Products of Conception, External Approach
0KQM0ZZ	Repair Perineum Muscle, Open Approach

Rationale:

Manually assisted vaginal deliveries are coded using root operation Delivery (E) found in the Obstetrics (1) section. In ICD-10-PCS, infants are included in the body part Products of Conception (0). The only approach available is External (X).

Repair of the perineal tear is coded using Repair (Q) in the Medical and Surgical section (0) since this repair is being done on the pregnant female, not on the products of conception. A second-degree tear is coded using body part Perineum Muscle (M) in the Muscles (K) body system and an Open (0) approach.

Root Operation		
Obstetrics Section (1)		
Delivery (E)	Definition:	Assisting the passage of the products of conception from the genital canal
	Explanation:	None
Medical and Surgical Section (0)		
Repair (Q)	Definition:	Restoring, to the extent possible, a body part to its normal anatomic structure and function
	Explanation:	Used only when the method to accomplish the repair is not one of the other root operations

---

Case Study 8.12. Cesarean Section, Emergency

A 28-year-old female presented for medical induction of labor due to pre-eclampsia. Three trials of Cervidil failed to produce contractions of adequate strength and duration. On the third day of admission, Pitocin induction was attempted. Due to maternal exhaustion at the trials of labor, the decision was made to rupture membranes. Mid forceps and vacuum assistance were tried to no avail. Despite favorable prenatal cephalopelvic measurements, the patient was determined to be in obstructed labor due to disproportion. After three hours of pushing efforts with assistance and resultant maternal exhaustion, the decision was made to deliver by emergency cesarean section. The patient delivered a term liveborn female infant by low transverse cesarean section (LTCS).

Code(s):

10D00Z1	Extraction of Products of Conception, Low, Open Approach
10907ZC	Drainage of Amniotic Fluid, Therapeutic from Products of Conception, Via Natural or Artificial Opening
3E0P7VZ	Introduction of Hormone into Female Reproductive, Via Natural or Artificial Opening
3E033VJ	Introduction of Other Hormone into Peripheral Vein, Percutaneous Approach

Rationale:

Although delivery was attempted with the assistance of forceps and vacuum, neither of these techniques resulted in extraction; only the C-section is coded. The low cervical cesarean is coded using root operation Extraction (D), Open (0) approach, and qualifier Low (1).

Additional codes for the artificial rupture of membranes (AROM), Cervidil, and Pitocin should be reported. The rupture of membranes is considered a Drainage (9) procedure and the qualifier is Amniotic Fluid, Therapeutic (C) when used to induce and/or augment labor.

Spotlight
When vacuum assistance is used with a cesarean delivery, only the cesarean delivery is coded (*AHA Coding Clinic,* 2014, 4Q, 43).

Cervidil is coded using root operation Introduction (Ø) found in the Administration (3) section with substance Hormone (V). Cervidil is a vaginal insert that is reported with body system Female Reproductive (P) and not Products of Conception (E); approach is Via Natural or Artificial Opening (7).

Pitocin is a natural hormone administered intravenously. It is coded using root operation Introduction (Ø) found in the Administration (3) section, substance Hormone (V), and qualifier Other Hormone (J). Since it is administered intravenously, the body system is Peripheral Vein (3) and approach is Percutaneous (3).

Root Operation		
Obstetrics Section (1)		
Extraction (D)	Definition:	Pulling or stripping out or off all or a portion of a body part by the use of force
	Explanation:	None
Drainage (9)	Definition:	Taking or letting out fluids and/or gases from a body part
	Explanation:	None
Administration Section (3)		
Introduction (Ø)	Definition:	Putting in or on a therapeutic, diagnostic, nutritional, physiological, or prophylactic substance except blood or blood products
	Explanation:	None

Case Study 8.13. Delivery, Vaginal with Episiotomy and Repair

The patient was complete on cervical examination and was encouraged to push. When the fetal head was crowning, a right mediolateral episiotomy was made, and after that, a live female infant delivered in the occiput anterior position with tight nuchal cord x1 with Apgar of 8, 9, and 9. Weight was 3,350 grams and anterior shoulder and posterior shoulder delivered without any difficulties with the rest of the body. The cord was clamped and cut. The baby was handed to the awaiting pediatrician. The placenta was delivered spontaneously intact with three-vessel cord. Inspection of the perineum showed a second-degree left vaginal wall laceration, which was repaired with 2-0 Vicryl, and a right mediolateral episiotomy, which was repaired with 2-0 and 3-0 Vicryl. The patient tolerated the procedure very well.

Code(s):

1ØEØXZZ	**Delivery of Products of Conception, External Approach**
ØW8NXZZ	**Division of Female Perineum, External Approach**
ØKQMØZZ	**Repair Perineum Muscle, Open Approach**

Rationale:

Manually assisted vaginal deliveries are coded using root operation Delivery (E) in the Obstetrics (1) section, body part Products of Conception (Ø), and an External (X) approach.

Since the episiotomy was done on the pregnant female, and not the products of conception, it is coded in the Medical and Surgical (Ø) section using Anatomical Regions, General (W) body system. Root operation Division (8) captures the initial perineal incision done for the episiotomy.

Additionally, main term "Episiotomy" in the ICD-10-PCS alphabetical index directs the user to *see* Division, Perineum, Female ØW8N.

No repair code is needed for the episiotomy.

Repair (Q) is the appropriate root operation to use for suturing the vaginal wall laceration. Perineum Muscle (M), found in the Muscles (K) body system, is the correct body part as per *AHA Coding Clinic*, 2016, 1Q, 6. The approach is Open (Ø) and No Device (Z) and No Qualifier (Z) apply.

Root Operation		
Obstetrics Section (1)		
Delivery (E)	Definition:	Assisting the passage of the products of conception from the genital canal
	Explanation:	None
Medical and Surgical Section (Ø)		
Division (8)	Definition:	Cutting into a body part, without draining fluids and/or gases from the body part, in order to separate or transect a body part
	Explanation:	All or a portion of the body part is separated into two or more portions
Repair (Q)	Definition:	Restoring, to the extent possible, a body part to its normal anatomic structure and function
	Explanation:	Used only when the method to accomplish the repair is not one of the other root operations

---

Case Study 8.14. Delivery, Preterm Induced Vaginal of an Intrauterine Fetal Demise

The patient was admitted with a diagnosis of intrauterine fetal demise at 36 weeks gestation and was 3 cm dilated on admission. IV Pitocin was started for induction of labor, with an epidural placed for labor pain. The patient pushed for three contractions and delivered the fetal vertex in the right occiput anterior position followed by the remainder of the infant. There was a tight nuchal cord x 1 that was reduced after delivery. The cord was doubly clamped. The placenta delivered spontaneously and was carefully examined and found to be intact, without signs of abruption or abnormal cord insertion. The cord was examined and a three-vessel cord was confirmed. The vagina and perineum were carefully inspected. A small, first-degree midline laceration was repaired in normal running fashion with a 3-0 Vicryl suture.

Code(s):

10EØXZZ	**Delivery of Products of Conception, External Approach**
ØHQ9XZZ	**Repair Perineum Skin, External Approach**
3E033VJ	**Introduction of Other Hormone into Peripheral Vein, Percutaneous Approach**

Rationale:

The patient delivered via vaginal delivery. Main term "Delivery" and subterm "manually assisted" in the ICD-10-PCS alphabetic index leads to complete code 10EØXZZ. The fact that the fetus was preterm and stillborn has no bearing on the PCS code. That information is conveyed with ICD-10-CM codes.

During delivery, the patient sustained a small, first-degree perineal laceration that was repaired. Procedures performed on the pregnant female other than the products of conception are coded to the Medical and Surgical (Ø) section in ICD-10-PCS. Root operation Repair (Q) is appropriate, along with body part Skin, Perineum (9) for the first-degree laceration. The approach is External (X) since the suturing is done directly on the skin.

For the induction of labor with IV Pitocin (Oxytocin), main term "Induction of labor" and subterm "Oxytocin" in the ICD-10-PCS alphabetic index direct the user to *see* Introduction of Hormone.

Introduction (Ø) is found in the Administration (3) section. Peripheral Vein (3) is the body system for an intravenous line, approach is Percutaneous (3), the sixth character is Hormone (V), and the seventh character Other Hormone (J) completes the code for the Pitocin.

Root Operation		
Obstetrics Section (1)		
Delivery (E)	Definition:	Assisting the passage of the products of conception from the genital canal
	Explanation:	None
Medical and Surgical Section (Ø)		
Repair (Q)	Definition:	Restoring, to the extent possible, a body part to its normal anatomic structure and function
	Explanation:	Used only when the method to accomplish the repair is not one of the other root operations
Administration Section (3)		
Introduction (Ø)	Definition:	Putting in or on a therapeutic, diagnostic, nutritional, physiological, or prophylactic substance except blood or blood products
	Explanation:	None

Case Study 8.15. Fetal Surgical Repair

The patient at 25 1/2 weeks gestation carrying a male fetus with a left-sided diaphragmatic hernia elected to have fetal surgical repair. Preoperative testing revealed that most of the abdominal viscera of the fetus, including a dilated stomach, were herniated into the left chest, displacing the mediastinum to the right. There was little visible lung. There were no other detectable fetal abnormalities on ultrasonography, and prior amniocentesis revealed no additional defects.

After proper anesthesia was administered, the maternal abdomen was opened using a low transverse incision. Intraoperative ultrasonography confirmed that the placenta was on the anterior uterine wall, so the uterus was tilted forward and incised posteriorly after the amniotic fluid had been drained and preserved. The left arm of the fetus was brought outside the uterus, and the left chest and flank were positioned under the hysterotomy. The fetal heart rate and oxygen saturation were monitored.

Through a left subcostal incision in the fetus, the left lobe of the liver was carefully retracted, the herniated viscera (stomach, large and small intestine, and spleen) were removed from the chest, and the large diaphragmatic defect was closed with a Gore-Tex patch. The air in the emptied left chest cavity was replaced with warm Ringer's lactate, and the abdominal cavity was enlarged to accommodate the reduced viscera with a second Gore-Tex patch.

The uterus was closed in three layers. The amniotic-fluid volume was replenished with preserved amniotic fluid plus saline containing oxacillin. The fetus remained stable throughout the procedure.

Code(s):

1ØQ00YK   **Repair Respiratory System in Products of Conception with Other Device, Open Approach**

Rationale:

In this example, the diaphragm of the fetus was repaired in utero. Repair (Q) in the Obstetrics (1) section is the appropriate root operation since the fetus is part of the Products of Conception (Ø) body part. An Open (Ø) approach was used since the fetus was accessed through an abdominal incision. Other Device (Y) was reported to represent the Gore-Tex patch. The seventh-character qualifier identifies the organ system being repaired, which is the Respiratory System (K) since the diaphragm is classified in the Medical and Surgical (Ø) section in the Respiratory system (B).

Root Operation		
Repair (Q)	Definition:	Restoring, to the extent possible, a body part to its normal anatomic structure and function
	Explanation:	Used only when the method to accomplish the repair is not one of the other root operations

Case Study 8.16. Delivery, Vaginal Following McRoberts Rotation

The patient pushed through four contractions and the baby's head was delivered. Shoulder dystocia was encountered. Gentle downward traction was applied and McRoberts rotation was utilized. Suprapubic pressure was applied from the patient's left side on the baby's right shoulder. Rubin and woodscrew maneuvers were utilized and the shoulders delivered.

Code(s):

1ØEØXZZ   Delivery of Products of Conception, External Approach

Rationale:

In a McRoberts maneuver, which is used for shoulder dystocia, the mother's legs are sharply flexed to her abdomen while she is lying on her back. Although the objective of the McRoberts rotation is to maneuver the fetus to the proper position in the genital canal to allow for delivery, it is considered integral to the delivery as long as the procedure resulted in a delivery. The full definition of Delivery (E) reads "assisting the passage of the products of conception from the genital canal." There is only one code for a manually assisted delivery, found in the ICD-10-PCS alphabetic index under main term "Delivery" and subterm "Manually assisted," which leads to code 1ØEØXZZ.

If an external version had been performed before the fetus was in the genital canal, root operation Reposition (S) would be applicable.

Root Operation		
Delivery (E)	Definition:	Assisting the passage of the products of conception from the genital canal
	Explanation:	None

Procedures Following Delivery or Abortion

Guideline C2

C2	Procedures performed following a delivery or abortion for curettage of the endometrium or evacuation of retained products of conception are all coded in the Obstetrics section, to the root operation Extraction and the body part Products of Conception, Retained.
	Diagnostic or therapeutic dilation and curettage performed during times other than the postpartum or post-abortion period are all coded in the Medical and Surgical section, to the root operation Extraction and the body part Endometrium.

This guideline explains how to code the removal of residual products of conception after delivery or abortion. There is only one body part value that applies to this guideline: Products of Conception, Retained (1). Extraction (D) is the only root operation to use. One of the main distinctions with this guideline is when to use the Obstetrics (1) section and when the Medical and Surgical (Ø) section applies.

Root Operation		
Extraction (D)	Definition:	Pulling or stripping out or off all or a portion of a body part by the use of force
	Explanation:	None

Practical Application for Guideline C2

Case Study 8.17. Dilation and Curettage (D&C) Following Incomplete Spontaneous Abortion

Code(s):
10D17ZZ **Extraction of Products of Conception, Retained, Via Natural or Artificial Opening**

Rationale:
The spontaneous abortion was described as incomplete, which translates to body part Products of Conception, Retained (1). D&C, also called Dilation and Curettage, refers to the cervix being widened (dilated) and the removal of part of the lining of the uterus and/or contents of the uterus by scraping (curettage). This is represented by the root operation Extraction (D), which was performed through the vagina or Via Natural or Artificial Opening (7) approach. If a hysteroscope is used, Via Natural or Artificial Opening Endoscopic (8) is the correct approach.

Case Study 8.18. Dilation and Curettage, Nonobstetrical

Code(s):
ØUDB7ZZ **Extraction of Endometrium, Via Natural or Artificial Opening**

Rationale:
Since this is a nonobstetrical procedure, it must be coded using the Medical and Surgical (Ø) section and body part Endometrium (B), found in the Female Reproductive (U) system. Since there is no mention of the use of an endoscope, the correct approach is Via Natural or Artificial Opening (7).

Case Study 8.19. Manual Extraction of Retained Placenta

Code(s):

10D17Z9 **Manual Extraction of Products of Conception, Retained, Via Natural or Artificial Opening**

Rationale:

A retained placenta is generally defined as lack of expulsion of the placenta within 30 minutes to one hour following delivery of an infant. If complete expulsion requires the physician to sweep the uterus with a gloved hand, removing any remaining placenta, it is reported with body part value Products of Conception, Retained (1) and root operation Extraction (D). The approach is Via Natural or Artificial Opening (7) with qualifier value Manual (9).

Beyond the Guidelines

This section provides additional information about common Obstetrical terminology and procedures. Current guidelines may not specifically address these topics; however, *AHA Coding Clinic,* provide references for many of the topics.

Perineal Lacerations

AHA Coding Clinic

2018, 2Q, 25   Third and Fourth Degree Obstetric Lacerations

2016, 2Q, 34   Assisted Vaginal Delivery

2016, 1Q, 6   Obstetrical Perineal Laceration Repair

2014, 4Q, 18   Obstetrical Periurethral Laceration

2014, 4Q, 43   Second Degree Obstetric Perineal Laceration

2013, 4Q, 120   Repair of Second Degree Perineum Obstetric Laceration

2013, 4Q, 120   Repair of Clitoral Obstetric Laceration

During a vaginal delivery, the perineum may be strained and a perineal tear may result. Perineal lacerations are classified according to the depth of the tear. Careful review of the operative note assists in assigning the appropriate ICD-10-PCS code.

Degree	Injury Extends to:	PCS Code for Repair	PCS Description
1st degree	Outermost layer of perineum and vaginal mucosa	0HQ9XZZ	Repair Perineum Skin, External Approach
2nd degree	Vaginal wall and perineal muscle	0KQM0ZZ	Repair Perineum Muscle, Open Approach
3rd degree	Anal sphincter	0DQR0ZZ	Repair Anal Sphincter, Open Approach
4th degree	Rectal mucosa	0DQP0ZZ	Repair Rectum, Open Approach

Induction of Labor

AHA Coding Clinic

2014, 4Q, 17   RH (D) Alloimmunization (Sensitization)

2014, 2Q, 8   Medical Induction of Labor with Cervidil Tampon Insertion

2014, 2Q, 9   Pitocin Administration to Augment Labor

Induction of labor refers to the use of a procedure or medication to stimulate labor that has not started naturally. Augmentation refers to the assistance or acceleration of labor that has already begun.

Case Study 8.20. Ripening of the Cervix Cervidil (Dinoprostone/Prostaglandin Gel Insert)

Code(s):

3E0P7VZ   Introduction of Hormone into Female Reproductive, Via Natural or Artificial Opening

Case Study 8.21. Artificial Rupture of Membranes (AROM)

Code(s):

10907ZC   Drainage of Amniotic Fluid, Therapeutic from Products of Conception, Via Natural or Artificial Opening

Spotlight
AROM is reported when it is performed to induce as well as augment labor.

Case Study 8.22. Labor Induction with Intravenous Medications

Code(s):

3E033VJ   Introduction of Other Hormone into Peripheral Vein, Percutaneous Approach

Spotlight
The administration of Pitocin to **augment** labor is not coded separately.

Episiotomy

An episiotomy is a perineal surgical incision made just prior to delivery to enlarge the vaginal opening and ease delivery. The incision may be midline (median or midline episiotomy) or lateral, beginning at the vaginal orifice and continued to the right or left, away from the rectum (mediolateral). The PCS code for the episiotomy is derived from table 0W8 in the Medical and Surgical Section; Division (8) is the appropriate root operation as an episiotomy involves cutting into and separating the perineum.

Root Operation		
Division (8)	Definition:	Cutting into a body part, without draining fluids and/or gases from the body part, in order to separate or transect a body part
	Explanation:	All or a portion of the body part is separated into two or more portions

Following delivery, the episiotomy incision is repaired.

In the event that an episiotomy tears beyond the original incision, it is considered a laceration and the repair is coded to the extent (layer) documented.

Spotlight
Episiotomy repair following delivery is **not** reported separately unless it tears **beyond** the original incision.

Figure 8.1. Episiotomy

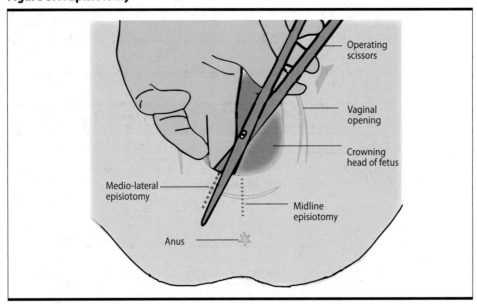

Assisted Delivery

AHA Coding Clinic

2016, 2Q, 34   Assisted Vaginal Delivery

2016, 1Q, 9   Vaginal Delivery Assisted by Vacuum and Low Forceps Extraction

2014, 4Q, 43   Vacuum Dilation and Curettage for Blighted Ovum

The use of forceps or a vacuum extractor to help deliver a baby when childbirth is not progressing in the pushing stage of labor is considered assisted delivery. Since both techniques require force, Extraction (D) is the appropriate root operation.

Figure 8.2. Assisted Delivery

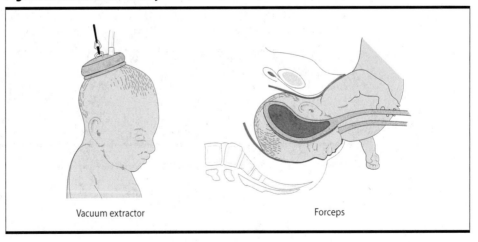

Vacuum extractor   Forceps

Vacuum Extractor Delivery

A vacuum (soft or rigid cup with a handle and vacuum pump) is applied to the baby's head and holds the baby in place. This prevents the baby's head from moving back up the birth canal between contractions and helps to guide the baby out of the birth canal.

10D07Z6   Extraction of Products of Conception, Vacuum, Via Natural or Artificial Opening

Spotlight
Vacuum assistance performed during a cesarean delivery is not coded separately. Only the cesarean delivery is coded (*AHA Coding Clinic,* 2014, 4Q, 43).

Forceps Delivery

With the use of forceps (device that resembles a long pair of spoons or tongs) gently pushed up on either side of the infant's head, the infant is pulled out. The American College of Obstetricians and Gynecologists (ACOG) classification system for forceps deliveries is based on station and amount of rotation and is reflected in the seventh character (qualifier). Shown below are the three forceps delivery codes in ICD-10-PCS, with the most often performed and safest being the outlet or Low where the head is less than +2 station, followed by Mid, which is not often performed, where the head is +2 and engaged. Although a code is available in PCS, High forceps is not included in the ACOG classification and is not recommended in modern medicine.

Low: 10D07Z3   Extraction of Products of Conception, Low Forceps, Via Natural or Artificial Opening

Mid: 10D07Z4   Extraction of Products of Conception, Mid Forceps, Via Natural or Artificial Opening

High: 10D07Z5   Extraction of Products of Conception, High Forceps, Via Natural or Artificial Opening

Monitoring During Labor

AHA Coding Clinic

2013, 2Q, 36   Intrauterine Pressure Monitor

Figure 8.3. Fetal Scalp Electrode (FSE) and Intrauterine Pressure Catheter (IUPC)

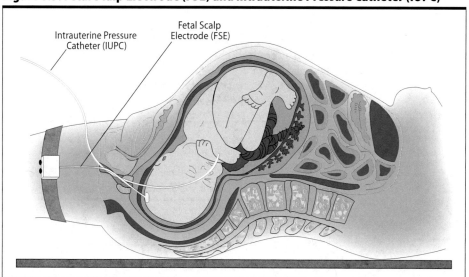

Case Study 8.23. Intrauterine Pressure Monitor

Code(s):

10H07YZ   Insertion of Other Device into Products of Conception, Via Natural or
Artificial Opening

Rationale:

An intrauterine pressure catheter (IUPC) is a pressure gauge that is inserted into the uterus to obtain accurate contraction measurements. The correct body part value is Products of Conception (0) in the Obstetrics (1) section. Currently, there is no separate device character for IUPC, so Other Device (Y) is the appropriate choice.

Case Study 8.24. Fetal Scalp Electrode

Code(s):

10H073Z   Insertion of Monitoring Electrode into Products of Conception, Via Natural or
Artificial Opening

Rationale:

Internal fetal monitoring may be done by placing an electrode on the fetal scalp through the cervix. This allows for monitoring of fetal heart rate during labor.

Spotlight
In addition to an insertion code, a code for the monitoring (found in the Measuring and Monitoring section) needs to be added: **4A1H7CZ Monitoring of Products of Conception, Cardiac Rate, Via Natural or Artificial Opening**

Cervical Cerclage

AHA Coding Clinic

2015, 3Q, 30   Insertion of Cervical Cerclage

2015, 3Q, 30   Removal of Cervical Cerclage

Obstetric cerclage is a surgical procedure that encircles an incompetent cervix with heavy suture material or wire for support in an attempt to retain a pregnancy and prevent preterm delivery. Cerclage is usually performed between 12 and 16 weeks gestation and is often employed in patients with a history of spontaneous abortion in otherwise normal pregnancies. The ligature is generally removed at 36 to 38 weeks.

Spotlight
Although performed on a pregnant female, the procedure takes place on the cervix, not on the products of conception. Therefore, codes for cervical cerclage are found in the Medical and Surgical (0) section, not Obstetrics (1).

Figure 8.4. Cervical Cerclage

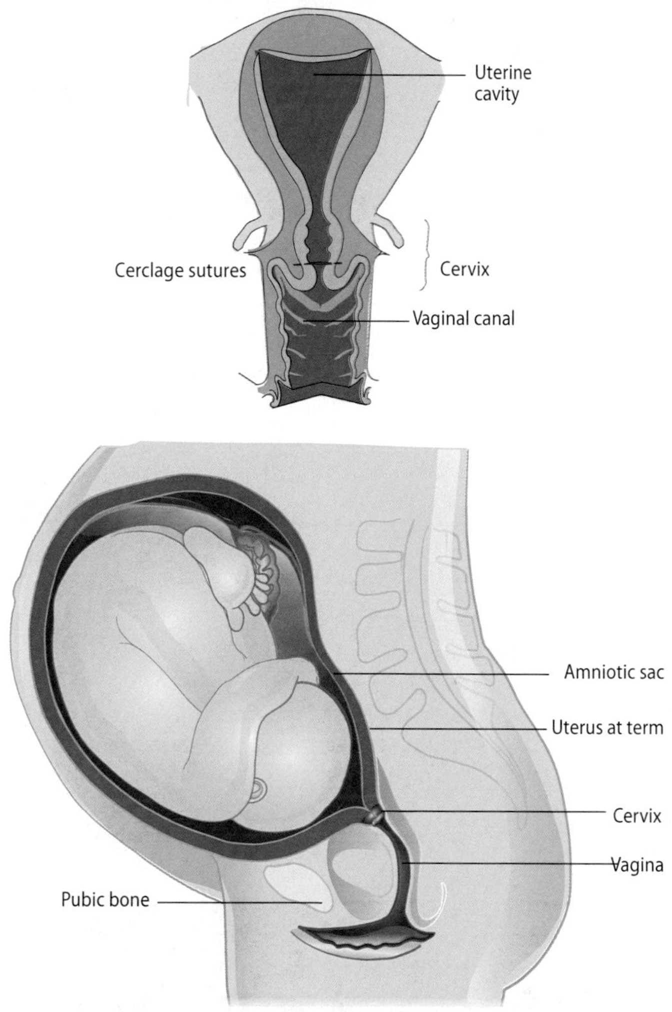

Case Study 8.25. Cervical Cerclage, Insertion

Code(s):

ØUVC7ZZ   **Restriction of Cervix, Via Natural or Artificial Opening**

Rationale:

The objective of the cerclage is to decrease the size of the cervical opening, which is reported with the root operation Restriction (V). Suture material, which is considered a surgical supply and not a device in ICD-10-PCS, is used to restrict the opening of the cervix.

Root Operation		
Restriction (V)	Definition:	Partially closing an orifice or the lumen of a tubular body part
	Explanation:	The orifice can be a natural orifice or an artificially created orifice

---

Case Study 8.26. Cervical Cerclage, Transvaginal Removal

Code(s):

ØUCC7ZZ   **Extirpation of Matter from Cervix, Via Natural or Artificial Opening**

Rationale:

A cerclage is a suture, which is considered a foreign body not a device. Therefore, the appropriate root operation for removal of the cerclage is Extirpation (C) rather than Removal (P) since Removal is only used for devices. Transvaginal refers to "through or via the vagina," which means the approach is Via Natural or Artificial Opening (7).

Root Operation		
Extirpation (C)	Definition:	Taking or cutting out solid matter from a body part
	Explanation:	The solid matter may be an abnormal byproduct of a biological function or a foreign body; it may be imbedded in a body part or in the lumen of a tubular body part. The solid matter may or may not have been previously broken into pieces.

Postpartum Contraception and Sterilization

AHA Coding Clinic

2015, 3Q, 31   Tubal Ligation for Sterilization

2013, 2Q, 34   Placement of Intrauterine Device via Open Approach

Contraception and sterilization procedures are commonly performed while a patient is still in the hospital following delivery. These procedures do not take place on the products of conception, however, and should not be coded using the Obstetrics (1) section. Instead, the appropriate root operation from the Medical and Surgical (Ø) section should be used.

Case Study 8.27. Tubal Sterilization Postpartum

Following delivery of a viable infant, the patient was taken to the OR and placed in the dorsal supine position. General endotracheal anesthesia was administered and the patient was prepped and draped in the usual manner. A transverse subumbilical incision was made and carried down through the subcutaneous tissue, fascia, and peritoneum. The right fallopian tube was identified, grasped, and pulled within the operative site. The proximal and distal tube was clamped, mid-section removed, and tied with 2-0 plain gut. No bleeding was noted. The ligated tube was allowed to return to the abdomen. A similar procedure was carried out on the left side.

Code(s):

ØUB7ØZZ   **Excision of Bilateral Fallopian Tubes, Open Approach**

Rationale:

Since the operative summary indicates that the segment of each tube between the sutures was removed, commonly referred to as Pomeroy technique, Excision (B) is the appropriate root operation. The correct body part is Fallopian Tubes, Bilateral (7), found in the Female Reproductive (U) body system within the Medical and Surgical (Ø) section. An incision was made, which meets the approach definition of Open (Ø). No Device (Z) was used and there was no indication that the fallopian tubes were being further evaluated so No Qualifier (Z) is the applicable seventh character.

Review the operative report carefully as there are many techniques or root operations used to perform tubal sterilization. Another method is Occlusion (L) of the tubes using rings, bands, or clips, which are classified as Extraluminal Device (C) as well as fulguration or Destruction (5) of the fallopian tubes.

Root Operation		
Excision (B)	Definition:	Cutting out or off, without replacement, a portion of a body part
	Explanation:	The qualifier DIAGNOSTIC is used to identify excision procedures that are biopsies
Occlusion (L)	Definition:	Completely closing an orifice or lumen of a tubular body part
	Explanation:	The orifice can be a natural orifice or an artificially created orifice
Destruction (5)	Definition:	Physical eradication of all or a portion of a body part by the direct use of energy, force, or a destructive agent
	Explanation:	None of the body part is physically taken out

Chapter 9. New Technology Guidelines

New Technology Overview

New Technology (X) is a section added to ICD-10-PCS beginning October 1, 2015. This section provides a place for codes that uniquely identify procedures requested via the New Technology Application Process or that capture other new technologies not currently classified in ICD-10-PCS.

Section X does not introduce any new coding concepts or unusual guidelines for correct coding. Although there are a few different body part values, most section X codes maintain continuity with the other sections in ICD-10-PCS by using the same root operation and body part values as their closest counterparts in other sections of ICD-10-PCS. One notable character value change is Character 7, which instead of Qualifier, indicates the New Technology Group year number.

Character 1	Character 2	Character 3	Character 4	Character 5	Character 6	Character 7
Section	Body System	Root Operation	Body Part	Approach	Device/ Substance/ Technology	New Technology Group #

New Technology (X) section codes are found by looking in the ICD-10-PCS index or by going directly to the New Technology (X) tables. In the index, the name of the new technology device, substance, or technology is included as a main term. In addition, all codes in New Technology (X) section are listed under the main term New Technology. The index entries for ceftazidime-avibactam are as follows:

Ceftazidime-Avibactam Anti-infective XWØ
New Technology
    Ceftazidime-Avibactam Anti-infective XWØ

New Technology Character Meaning
Section X codes are seven characters long like all ICD-10-PCS codes. Organized in tables containing valid combinations of values for each of the seven characters, the same type of information remains the same within a section. The seven characters are as follows:

Character 1: Section
The first character in an ICD-10-PCS New Technology code is always New Technology (X).

Character 2: Body System

The New Technology section does not use the same body system titles and values found in the other sections. They tend to be more general than the Medical and Surgical (Ø) section and vary depending on the procedures represented. Currently there are eight body system values:

Cardiovascular System (2)

Skin, Subcutaneous Tissue, Fascia and Breast (H)

Muscles, Tendons, Bursae and Ligaments (K)

Bones (N)

Joints (R)

Male Reproductive (V)

Anatomical Regions (W)

Extracorporeal (Y)

Spotlight
The body systems included in the New Technology (X) section may change from year to year with body systems added and/or deleted depending on the new technology being introduced and whether previous new technology codes were incorporated into the other sections of ICD-10-PCS.

Character 3: Root Operation

There are eight root operations currently applicable to the New Technology (X) section. These root operations are Assistance (A), Destruction (5), Extirpation (C), Fusion (G), Replacement (R), Reposition (S), Introduction (Ø), and Monitoring (2), all of which have the same definitions as their counterpart sections of ICD-10-PCS.

Table 9.1. New Technology Root Operation

ICD-10-PCS Value		Definition
Assistance (A)	Definition:	Taking over a portion of a physiological function by extracorporeal means
	Explanation:	None
Extirpation (C)	Definition:	Taking or cutting out solid matter from a body part
	Explanation:	The solid matter may be an abnormal byproduct of a biological function or a foreign body; it may be imbedded in a body part or in the lumen of a tubular body part. The solid matter may or may not have been previously broken into pieces.
Destruction (5)	Definition:	Physical eradication of all or a portion of a body part by the direct use of energy, force, or a destructive agent
	Explanation:	None of the body part is physically taken out
Fusion (G)	Definition:	Joining together portions of an articular body part rendering the articular body part immobile
	Explanation:	The body part is joined together by fixation device, bone graft, or other means

ICD-10-PCS Value	Definition	
Replacement (R)	Definition:	Putting in or on biological or synthetic material that physically takes the place and/or function of all or a portion of a body part
	Explanation:	The body part may have been taken out or replaced, or may be taken out, physically eradicated, or rendered nonfunctional during the Replacement procedure. A Removal procedure is coded for taking out the device used in a previous replacement procedure.
Reposition (S)	Definition:	Moving to its normal location, or other suitable location, all or a portion of a body part
	Explanation:	The body part is moved to a new location from an abnormal location, or from a normal location where it is not functioning correctly. The body part may or may not be cut out or off to be moved to the new location.
Introduction (Ø)	Definition:	Putting in or on a therapeutic, diagnostic, nutritional, physiological, or prophylactic substance except blood or blood products
	Explanation:	None
Monitoring (2)	Definition:	Determining the level of a physiological or physical function repetitively over a period of time
	Explanation:	None

Spotlight
The root operations included in the New Technology (X) section may change from year to year with root operations added and/or deleted depending on new technology being introduced and whether previous new technology codes were incorporated into the other sections of ICD-10-PCS.

Character 4: Body Part

The fourth-character body part values have a specific and direct relationship to the body system (character 2) value. In most cases this relationship holds the same meaning in this section as it does in its closest counterpart section of ICD-10-PCS; however, some new body parts have been added that are specific only to a particular new technology. Some of the body parts are very general while others are more specific.

Spotlight
The body part values included in the New Technology section may change from year to year with body part values added and/or deleted depending on new technology being introduced and whether previous new technology codes were incorporated into the other sections of ICD-10-PCS.

Character 5: Approach

Currently there are five valid fifth-character approach values within the New Technology (X) tables: Open (Ø), Percutaneous (3), Percutaneous Endoscopic (4), Via Natural or Artificial Opening Endoscopic (8), and External (X). Their definitions remain the same as in the Medical and Surgical (Ø) section.

Spotlight
The approach values included in the New Technology section may change from year to year with approach values added and/or deleted depending on new technology being introduced and whether previous new technology codes were incorporated into the other sections of ICD-10-PCS.

Character 6: Device/Substance/Technology

The sixth-character specifies the key feature of the new technology procedure. It may be specified as a new device, a new substance, or other new technology.

Some examples of sixth-character values are:

Sixth Character	Device, Substance, or Technology
L Skin Substitute, Porcine Liver Derived	Device
A Bezlotoxumab Monoclonal Antibody	Substance
6 Orbital Atherectomy Technology	Technology
F Interbody Fusion Device, Radiolucent Porous	Device
9 Defibrotide Sodium Anticoagulant	Substance
A Robotic Waterjet Ablation	Technology

Character 7: Qualifier

The seventh-character qualifier is used exclusively to specify the new technology group, a number that changes each year that new technology codes are added to the system. For example, New Technology (X) section, codes added for the first year have the seventh-character value New Technology Group 1 (1), new codes added for FY2017 have the seventh-character value New Technology Group 2 (2), and new codes added for FY2018 have the seventh-character value New Technology Group 3 (3) and so on. Changing the seventh-character value to a unique number every year that there are new codes added in the new technology section allows ICD-10-PCS to "recycle" the values in the third, fourth, and sixth characters as needed.

General Guidelines

Guideline D1

D1	**Section X codes are standalone codes. They are not supplemental codes. Section X codes fully represent the specific procedure described in the code title, and do not require any additional codes from other sections of ICD-10-PCS. When section X contains a code title which describes a specific new technology procedure, only that X code is reported for the procedure. There is no need to report a broader, non-specific code in another section of ICD-10-PCS.**
	Example: **XW04321 Introduction of Ceftazidime-Avibactam Anti-infective into Central Vein, Percutaneous Approach, New Technology Group 1, can be coded to indicate that Ceftazidime-Avibactam Anti-infective was administered via a central vein. A separate code from table 3E0 in the Administration section of ICD-10-PCS is not coded in addition to this code.**

AHA Coding Clinic

2017, 4Q, 74	Intramuscular autologous bone marrow cell therapy
2017, 4Q, 74-75	Magnetic Growth Rods
2017, 4Q, 76	Radiolucent Porous Interbody Fusion Device
2017, 4Q, 77	New Therapeutic Substances
2017, 4Q, 78	Intraoperative Treatment of Vascular Grafts
2016, 4Q, 117	Placement of Magnetic Growth Rods
2016, 4Q, 116	Aortic Valve Rapid Deployment
2016, 4Q, 116	Application of Wound Matrix
2016, 4Q, 115	Cerebral Embolic Filtration
2015, 4Q, 16	Changes to the ICD-10-PCS Official Guidelines for Coding and Reporting
2015, 4Q, 8-15	New Section X Codes—New Technology Procedures

New Technology (X) codes are standalone codes that can be coded as a single code if only one procedure is performed. However, if more than one procedure is performed during the same operative episode, multiple procedures (a New Technology code and code(s) from other sections of ICD-10-PCS) may be coded.

New Technology (X) Procedure Descriptions

The following are descriptions of some of the procedures in the New Technology Section (X) and may assist in discerning these procedures from procedures reported in another section, such as Medical and Surgical (0) or Administration (3).

Table X2A—Assistance, Cardiovascular System

During transcatheter aortic valve replacements (TAVR), embolic debris can be dislodged during endovascular procedures. This causes increased risk of stroke, dementia, and cognitive impairment postprocedure.

The Claret Medical™ Sentinel™ Cerebral Protection System protects the brain from this debris. The device includes two conically-shaped polyurethane filters that are delivered through a sheath placed in the right radial artery. The proximal filter is deployed in the brachiocephalic artery, and the distal filter is delivered to the left common carotid artery at the beginning of the TAVR procedure. At the completion of the TAVR procedure, the filters and captured debris are withdrawn into the catheter and removed from the patient. The filtration code (X2A5312) and a code for the TAVR should be reported.

Cerebral Embolic Filtration, Dual Filter (1) is reported as the Device/Substance/Technology value placed via Percutaneous (3) approach in the body part Innominate Artery and Left Common Carotid Artery (5), along with New Technology Group 2 (2) qualifier.

Table X2R—Replacement, Cardiovascular System
Current aortic valve replacement can involve a full sternotomy, excising the diseased aortic valve, and placing between 12 and 15 sutures through the aortic annulus and sewing ring of the valve to keep it in place.

The Edwards Intuity Elite™ Valve system utilizes a minimally invasive technique with a balloon expandable stent that allows precise positioning of the new valve with only three sutures, rather than the normal 12 to 15. The system uses a flexible deployment arm that allows the surgeon optimal access to anatomy for valve deployment and suturing. This technique allows rapid deployment of the valve for patients normally not suited for full sternotomy due to comorbid conditions.

The appropriate root operation is Replacement (R) of the Aortic Valve (F) body part with Zooplastic Tissue, Rapid Deployment Technique (3). The approach can be Open (0), Percutaneous (3), or Percutaneous Endoscopic (4), and the final character indicates the New Technology Group 2 (2).

Table XHR—Replacement, Skin, Subcutaneous Tissue, Fascia, and Breast
This table reflects a new acellular wound matrix that is derived from porcine (pig) liver. Other acellular biologic wound substitute products are derived from dermis, urinary bladder, or small intestine submucosa, all of which are thin, dense, and relatively avascular tissue compared to the open and highly-vascularized substrate present in the liver.

MIRODERM™ may be used in the management of wounds such as partial- and full-thickness wounds, pressure ulcers, venous ulcers, chronic vascular ulcers, diabetic ulcers, trauma wounds, drainage wounds, and surgical wounds (donor sites/grafts, post-Mohs' surgery, post-laser surgery, podiatric, wound dehiscence). MIRODERM™ is applied to contact the entire surface of the wound bed and extend slightly beyond all wound margins. After anchoring, a non-adherent wound dressing is applied over the MIRODERM matrix. A secondary dressing to manage the wound exudate should be applied in order to keep the MIRODERM™ matrix moist and keep all layers securely in place. Additional applications of MIRODERM™ are applied as needed until the wound closes.

Skin Substitute, Porcine Liver Derived (L) is reported as the Device/Substance/Technology value placed via External (X) approach on body part Skin (P), along with New Technology Group 2 (2) qualifier.

Table XNS—Reposition, Bones
The Ellipse Magec® System consists of one or two sterile, single use spinal rods implanted as fixation devices. The rods are used to brace the spine during growth to minimize the progression of scoliosis. The rods contain a small magnet that allows lengthening via an external remote controller. Periodic lengthening is performed by placing the external controller over the patient's spine. The implanted magnet is then activated, causing it to rotate and lengthen or shorten the rod. Once no longer needed, the rods are removed.

Magnetically Controlled Growth Rod(s) (3) is reported as the Device/Substance/Technology value placed into body part(s) Lumbar Vertebra (Ø), Cervical Vertebra (3), and/or Thoracic Vertebra (4), along with New Technology Group 2 (2) qualifier. Reposition (S) is used as the root operation since the intent of the procedure is to move the vertebrae into its normal location.

Table XRG—Fusion, Joints
Vertera Spine's COHERE® (Cervical) and COALESCE® (Lumbar) Interbody Fusion Devices are porous fusion devices developed from radiolucent plastic polyether ether ketone (PEEK). These devices combine the advantages of strength and optimal bone integration of porous metal with the ability afforded by plastics of unobscured visualization in X-ray, CT, or MRI imaging. Interbody Fusion

Device, Radiolucent Porous (F) is reported with an Open (Ø) approach, along with New Technology Group 3 (3) qualifier.

Titan Spine nanoLOCK™ is an interbody fusion device that uses a special nano-textured surface for spinal fusions. This surface technology uses proprietary manufacturing to create a roughened topography generating a better host-bone response to promote optimal bone growth for a faster and stronger fusion at the cellular level. Interbody Fusion Device, Nanotextured Surface (9) is reported as the Device/Substance/Technology value placed via Open (Ø) approach, along with New Technology Group 2 (2) qualifier.

Table XKØ—Introduction, Muscles, Tendon, Bursae, and Ligaments

- **Concentrated Bone Marrow Aspirate (Ø):** Intramuscular autologous bone marrow cell therapy is a new technique that involves the collection, concentration, and direct application of mononuclear stem cells originating in the patient's own bone marrow to promote the formation of new blood vessels. The new blood vessels revascularize the limbs compromised by peripheral artery disease (PAD). The aspirate is injected at multiple locations along a muscle in the affected limb.

Spotlight
Harvesting of the bone marrow would, in this case, be a separately reportable procedure as it is a specific objective using a different root operation, Extraction (D), performed on a different body part, such as Bone Marrow, Iliac (R).

Table XWØ–Introduction, Anatomical Regions

- **Ceftazidime-Avibactam Anti-infective (2):** This substance approved under brand name AVYCAZ® is a combination antibacterial drug containing ceftazidime, a cephalosporin, and avibactam, a beta-lactamase inhibitor. It is used to fight drug resistant, gram-negative infections particularly intra-abdominal and urinary tract infections.

- **Idarucizumab, Dabigatran Reversal Agent (3):** This substance is used as an antidote against the anticoagulant effects of dabigatran, a thrombin inhibitor. Dabigatran is widely prescribed for the treatment of DVT, PE, and also for patients with atrial fibrillation to reduce the risk of stroke and systemic embolism. Idarucizumab was developed for patients that experience abnormal bleeding while taking dabigatran because treatments such as protamine sulfate and vitamin K, used to reverse effects of heparin and warfarin, are not effective.

- **Isavuconazole Anti-Infective (4):** An intravenous (IV) or oral med known by the brand name CRESEMBA® that is used to treat invasive fungal infections, specifically aspergillosis and mucormycosis. Mucormycosis is mainly found in immunocompromised patients with lack of other effective treatment options. This code reports the intravenous use of this drug.

- **Blinatumomab Antineoplastic Immunotherapy (5):** Used to treat some types of acute lymphocytic leukemia (ALL), this substance is made up of two types of monoclonal antibodies that simultaneously attach to the protein of the leukemia/lymphoma cells and the protein of the immune T cells. The objective is to bring the cancer cells and immune cells together and cause the immune system to attack the cancer cells.

- **Andexanet Alfa, Factor Xa Inhibitor Reversal Agent (7):** Substance used as a universal antidote to direct factor Xa inhibitors. Factor Xa is a new class of anticoagulants for stroke prevention and systemic embolism in atrial fibrillation patients, plus those at risk for deep vein thrombosis or pulmonary embolism. A need to rapidly reverse the effects of anticoagulation due to serious bleeding episodes in patients taking these drugs has led to its development.

- **Uridine Triacetate (8):** Substance used for the emergency treatment of fluorouracil (5-FU) or capecitabine overexposure in adult and pediatric patients. It is an emergency oral treatment for overdose of, or severe adverse reactions to, fluorouracil or capecitabine and should be taken within 96 hours following the end of the chemotherapy administration.

- **Defibrotide Sodium Anticoagulant (9):** Substance used for the treatment of hepatic venoocclusive disease (VOD), also known as sinusoidal obstruction syndrome with evidence of multiorgan dysfunction following hematopoietic stem cell transplantation (HSCT). VOD is an early complication after HSCT that may develop due to cell injury from high-dose conditioning regimens prior to the transplant.

- **Bezlotoxumab Monoclonal Antibody (A):** This substance is a nonantibiotic drug used to reduce recurrence of *Clostridium difficile* infection (CDI), a common antibiotic-associated gastrointestinal infection.

- **Cytarabine and Daunorubicin Liposome Antineoplastic (B):** VYXEOS™ is a liposomal formulation of a combination chemotherapy cytarabine and daunorubicin for treatment of acute myeloid leukemia (AML), a blood and bone marrow cancer.

- **Engineered Autologous Chimeric Antigen Receptor T-cell Immunotherapy (C):** Also known as axicabtagene ciloleucel, it is an immunotherapy consisting of chimeric antigen receptor (CAR) construct T lymphocytes (T-cells) that recognize tumor antigen CD19-expressing cancer cells and normal B-cells. It is used to treat patients with relapsed or refractory aggressive B-cell non-Hodgkin lymphoma who, for various reasons, are not eligible for autologous stem cell transplant. The patient's own T-cells are harvested and genetically engineered using a disarmed virus to produce receptors on their surfaces, turning them into chimeric antigen receptors, or CARs. After being infused back into the patient, the new CAR T-cells recognize, target, activate, and kill the target cancer cells throughout the body.

Table XY0—Introduction, Extracorporeal

- **Endothelial Damage Inhibitor (8):** The intent of this intraoperative treatment of vascular grafts is to prevent vein graft disease (VGD) and vein graft failure following coronary artery bypass surgery or peripheral artery bypass surgery. After the vein graft is harvested, it is flushed with a tissue preservation solution that contains an endothelial damage inhibitor designed to inhibit damage to the endothelial cells lining the graft lumen. The graft soaks in the solution until immediately before the final bypass anastomosis takes place.

Practical Application for Guideline D1

Case Study 9.1. Intraoperative Monitoring of Right Knee Joint with Knee Replacement Sensor

Code(s):

XR2G021   Monitoring of Right Knee Joint using Intraoperative Knee Replacement Sensor, Open Approach, New Technology Group 1

Rationale:

An intraoperative knee replacement sensor is a sterile, disposable tibial insert used to aid orthopaedic surgeons in placing prosthetic joint components during knee replacement surgery. According to Official Guideline D1, only the New Technology (X) code is reported for this procedure. Insertion of the device is included in this code. Open (0) approach is the only option available in this table and the only available body parts are Knee Joint, Right (G) and Knee Joint, Left (H).

Case Study 9.2. Infusion, Bezlotoxumab Monoclonal Antibody via Central Vein

Code(s):

XW043A3   Introduction of Bezlotoxumab Monoclonal Antibody into Central Vein, Percutaneous Approach, New Technology Group 3

Rationale:
According to Official Guideline D1, this New Technology (X) code is a standalone code and does not require the addition of a code from table 3E0 in the Administration section of ICD-10-PCS. Bezlotoxumab Monoclonal Antibody is a new substance added to New Technology Group 3 (3), effective October 1, 2017.

Case Study 9.3. Percutaneous Orbital Atherectomy of RCA Calcified Lesion, Using Diamondback 360

Code(s):

X2C0361	Extirpation of Matter from Coronary Artery, One Artery using Orbital Atherectomy Technology, Percutaneous Approach, New Technology Group 1

Rationale:
An atherectomy procedure involves the removal of atherosclerosis from an artery, typically via a sharp blade on the end of a catheter or using rotational atherectomy. Orbital atherectomy also removes severely calcified atherosclerosis via a new technology using a diamond-coated crown on a coil placed in the plaque-filled artery and spun at variable rpms to debride the plaque from the arterial walls.

Orbital atherectomy can be accessed in the ICD-10-PCS index under main term "Extirpation" and subterm "Orbital Atherectomy Technology," leading the user to table X2C (New Technology Section/Cardiovascular System/Extirpation).

Spotlight
Stents are often deployed into the treated artery during this procedure. This is considered a separate objective, with an additional code reported for the Dilation of the coronary artery with an appropriate device value indicating the number and type of stent (*AHA Coding Clinic, 2015, 4Q, 13*).

Case Study 9.4. Infusion, Defibrotide Sodium Anticoagulant via Central Vein

Code(s):

XW04392	Introduction of Defibrotide Sodium Anticoagulant into Central Vein, Percutaneous Approach, New Technology Group 2

Rationale:
Defibrotide Sodium Anticoagulant (9) was among the substances added in New Technology Group 2 (2). According to Official Guideline D1, this New Technology (X) code is a standalone code and does not require the addition of a code from table 3E0 in the Administration section of ICD-10-PCS.

Case Study 9.5. Open Insertion of Ellipse Magec® System into Lumbar Vertebra to Correct Scoliosis

Code(s):

XNS0032	Reposition of Lumbar Vertebra using Magnetically Controlled Growth Rod(s), Open Approach, New Technology Group 2

Rationale:
The intent of the procedure is to move the vertebrae back into its normal location; Reposition (S) is the appropriate root operation. In this case, an Open (0) procedure was used to place the rod into the lumbar vertebral bone. The body part value lumbar vertebral joint is not appropriate as joints

are not an available option on this New Technology table. Ellipse Magec® System is a Magnetically Controlled Growth Rod(s) (3) found in the New Technology (X) section.

Case Study 9.6. Prostatectomy, Partial with Aquablation

With the patient properly placed and anesthetized, the transrectal ultrasound was mounted. Using the cystoscope, the bladder was accessed and the robotic hand piece employed. The physician mapped the depth and angle of the desired resection of prostate tissue and input the information into the console software. The Aquablation was employed with the robotic hand and, using various flow rates, the hyperplastic tissue was removed. The area was cauterized and the device removed. A Foley catheter was placed.

Code(s):

XV5Ø8A4   **Destruction of Prostate using Robotic Waterjet Ablation, Via Natural or Artificial Opening Endoscopic, New Technology Group 4**

Rationale:

Aquablation therapy uses the AquaBeam system, an ultrasound image-guided waterjet system with a robotically controlled and targeted high-velocity saline stream, to ablate obstructive prostate tissue in males suffering from lower urinary tract symptoms (LUTS) due to benign prostatic hyperplasia (BPH).

The tissue ablation is described by the root operation Destruction (5) of the body part Prostate (Ø) of the Male Reproductive System (V). It is performed with cystoscopy, which is Via Natural or Artificial Opening Endoscopic (8) approach. The Robotic Waterjet Ablation (A) is the sixth character and the New Technology Group 4 (4) is the seventh character.

Spotlight

Although the procedure was performed robotically, a separate code for the robotic assistance is not required. The robotic assistance is included in the procedure, recognized in the description of the Device/Substance/Technology value of Robotic Waterjet Ablation (A). Because all components of the code relate to the procedure performed, it does not meet the multiple procedure guidelines, and based on guideline D1 can appropriately be reported on its own.

Appendix A. ICD-10-PCS Official Guidelines for Coding and Reporting 2019

Narrative changes appear in **bold** text.

The Centers for Medicare and Medicaid Services (CMS) and the National Center for Health Statistics (NCHS), two departments within the U.S. Federal Government's Department of Health and Human Services (DHHS) provide the following guidelines for coding and reporting using the International Classification of Diseases, 10th Revision, Procedure Coding System (ICD-10-PCS). These guidelines should be used as a companion document to the official version of the ICD-10-PCS as published on the CMS website. The ICD-10-PCS is a procedure classification published by the United States for classifying procedures performed in hospital inpatient health care settings.

These guidelines have been approved by the four organizations that make up the Cooperating Parties for the ICD-10-PCS: the American Hospital Association (AHA), the American Health Information Management Association (AHIMA), CMS, and NCHS.

These guidelines are a set of rules that have been developed to accompany and complement the official conventions and instructions provided within the ICD-10-PCS itself. The instructions and conventions of the classification take precedence over guidelines. These guidelines are based on the coding and sequencing instructions in the Tables, Index and Definitions of ICD-10-PCS, but provide additional instruction. Adherence to these guidelines when assigning ICD-10-PCS procedure codes is required under the Health Insurance Portability and Accountability Act (HIPAA). The procedure codes have been adopted under HIPAA for hospital inpatient healthcare settings. A joint effort between the healthcare provider and the coder is essential to achieve complete and accurate documentation, code assignment, and reporting of diagnoses and procedures. These guidelines have been developed to assist both the healthcare provider and the coder in identifying those procedures that are to be reported. The importance of consistent, complete documentation in the medical record cannot be overemphasized. Without such documentation accurate coding cannot be achieved.

Conventions

A1. ICD-10-PCS codes are composed of seven characters. Each character is an axis of classification that specifies information about the procedure performed. Within a defined code range, a character specifies the same type of information in that axis of classification.

Example: The fifth axis of classification specifies the approach in sections Ø through 4 and 7 through 9 of the system.

A2. One of 34 possible values can be assigned to each axis of classification in the seven-character code: they are the numbers Ø through 9 and the alphabet (except I and O because they are easily confused with the numbers 1 and Ø). The number of unique values used in an axis of classification differs as needed.

Example: Where the fifth axis of classification specifies the approach, seven different approach values are currently used to specify the approach.

A3. The valid values for an axis of classification can be added to as needed.

Example: If a significantly distinct type of device is used in a new procedure, a new device value can be added to the system.

A4. As with words in their context, the meaning of any single value is a combination of its axis of classification and any preceding values on which it may be dependent.

Example: The meaning of a body part value in the Medical and Surgical section is always dependent on the body system value. The body part value Ø in the Central Nervous body system specifies Brain and the body part value Ø in the Peripheral Nervous body system specifies Cervical Plexus.

A5. As the system is expanded to become increasingly detailed, over time more values will depend on preceding values for their meaning.

Example: In the Lower Joints body system, the device value 3 in the root operation Insertion specifies Infusion Device and the device value 3 in the root operation Replacement specifies Ceramic Synthetic Substitute.

A6. The purpose of the alphabetic index is to locate the appropriate table that contains all information necessary to construct a procedure code. The PCS Tables should always be consulted to find the most appropriate valid code.

A7. It is not required to consult the index first before proceeding to the tables to complete the code. A valid code may be chosen directly from the tables.

A8. All seven characters must be specified to be a valid code. If the documentation is incomplete for coding purposes, the physician should be queried for the necessary information.

A9. Within a PCS table, valid codes include all combinations of choices in characters 4 through 7 contained in the same row of the table. In the example below, ØJHT3VZ is a valid code, and ØJHW3VZ is *not* a valid code.

Section:	Ø	**Medical and Surgical**
Body System:	J	**Subcutaneous Tissue and Fascia**
Operation:	H	**Insertion** Putting in a nonbiological appliance that monitors, assists, performs, or prevents a physiological function but does not physically take the place of a body part

Body Part	Approach	Device	Qualifier
S Subcutaneous Tissue and Fascia, Head and Neck **V** Subcutaneous Tissue and Fascia, Upper Extremity **W** Subcutaneous Tissue and Fascia, Lower Extremity	**Ø** Open **3** Percutaneous	**1** Radioactive Element **3** Infusion Device	**Z** No Qualifier
T Subcutaneous Tissue and Fascia, Trunk	**Ø** Open **3** Percutaneous	**1** Radioactive Element **3** Infusion Device **V** Infusion Pump	**Z** No Qualifier

A10. "And," when used in a code description, means "and/or," **except when used to describe a combination of multiple body parts for which separate values exist for each body part (e.g., Skin and Subcutaneous Tissue used as a qualifier, where there are separate body part values for "Skin" and "Subcutaneous Tissue").**

Example: Lower Arm and Wrist Muscle means lower arm and/or wrist muscle.

A11. Many of the terms used to construct PCS codes are defined within the system. It is the coder's responsibility to determine what the documentation in the medical record equates to in the PCS definitions. The physician is not expected to use the terms used in PCS code descriptions, nor is the coder required to query the physician when the correlation between the documentation and the defined PCS terms is clear.

Example: When the physician documents "partial resection" the coder can independently correlate "partial resection" to the root operation Excision without querying the physician for clarification.

Medical and Surgical Section Guidelines (section Ø)

B2. Body System

General guidelines

B2.1a. The procedure codes in the general anatomical regions body systems can be used when the procedure is performed on an anatomical region rather than a specific body part (e.g., root operations Control and Detachment, Drainage of a body cavity) or on the rare occasion when no information is available to support assignment of a code to a specific body part.

Examples: Control of postoperative hemorrhage is coded to the root operation Control found in the general anatomical regions body systems.

Chest tube drainage of the pleural cavity is coded to the root operation Drainage found in the general anatomical regions body systems. Suture repair of the abdominal wall is coded to the root operation Repair in the general anatomical regions body system.

B2.1b. Where the general body part values "upper" and "lower" are provided as an option in the Upper Arteries, Lower Arteries, Upper Veins, Lower Veins, Muscles and Tendons body systems, "upper" or "lower "specifies body parts located above or below the diaphragm respectively.

Example: Vein body parts above the diaphragm are found in the Upper Veins body system; vein body parts below the diaphragm are found in the Lower Veins body system.

B3. Root Operation

General guidelines

B3.1a. In order to determine the appropriate root operation, the full definition of the root operation as contained in the PCS Tables must be applied.

B3.1b. Components of a procedure specified in the root operation definition and explanation are not coded separately. Procedural steps necessary to reach the operative site and close the operative site, including anastomosis of a tubular body part, are also not coded separately.

Examples: Resection of a joint as part of a joint replacement procedure is included in the root operation definition of Replacement and is not coded separately.

Laparotomy performed to reach the site of an open liver biopsy is not coded separately. In a resection of sigmoid colon with anastomosis of descending colon to rectum, the anastomosis is not coded separately.

Multiple procedures

B3.2. During the same operative episode, multiple procedures are coded if:

    a.   The same root operation is performed on different body parts as defined by distinct values of the body part character.

        Examples: Diagnostic excision of liver and pancreas are coded separately.

        Excision of lesion in the ascending colon and excision of lesion in the transverse colon are coded separately.

    b.   The same root operation is repeated in multiple body parts, and those body parts are separate and distinct body parts classified to a single ICD-10-PCS body part value.

        Examples: Excision of the sartorius muscle and excision of the gracilis muscle are both included in the upper leg muscle body part value, and multiple procedures are coded.

        Extraction of multiple toenails are coded separately.

    c.   Multiple root operations with distinct objectives are performed on the same body part.

        Example: Destruction of sigmoid lesion and bypass of sigmoid colon are coded separately.

    d.   The intended root operation is attempted using one approach, but is converted to a different approach.

        Example: Laparoscopic cholecystectomy converted to an open cholecystectomy is coded as percutaneous endoscopic Inspection and open Resection.

Discontinued or incomplete procedures

B3.3. If the intended procedure is discontinued or otherwise not completed, code the procedure to the root operation performed. If a procedure is discontinued before any other root operation is performed, code the root operation Inspection of the body part or anatomical region inspected.

Example: A planned aortic valve replacement procedure is discontinued after the initial thoracotomy and before any incision is made in the heart muscle, when the patient becomes hemodynamically unstable. This procedure is coded as an open Inspection of the mediastinum.

Biopsy procedures

B3.4a. Biopsy procedures are coded using the root operations Excision, Extraction, or Drainage and the qualifier Diagnostic.

Examples: Fine needle aspiration biopsy of fluid in the lung is coded to the root operation Drainage with the qualifier Diagnostic.

Biopsy of bone marrow is coded to the root operation Extraction with the qualifier Diagnostic.

Lymph node sampling for biopsy is coded to the root operation Excision with the qualifier Diagnostic.

Biopsy followed by more definitive treatment

B3.4b. If a diagnostic Excision, Extraction, or Drainage procedure (biopsy) is followed by a more definitive procedure, such as Destruction, Excision or Resection at the same procedure site, both the biopsy and the more definitive treatment are coded.

Example: Biopsy of breast followed by partial mastectomy at the same procedure site, both the biopsy and the partial mastectomy procedure are coded.

Overlapping body layers

B3.5. If the root operations Excision, Repair or Inspection are performed on overlapping layers of the musculoskeletal system, the body part specifying the deepest layer is coded.

Example: Excisional debridement that includes skin and subcutaneous tissue and muscle is coded to the muscle body part.

Bypass procedures

B3.6a. Bypass procedures are coded by identifying the body part bypassed "from" and the body part bypassed "to." The fourth character body part specifies the body part bypassed from, and the qualifier specifies the body part bypassed to.

Example: Bypass from stomach to jejunum, stomach is the body part and jejunum is the qualifier.

B3.6b. Coronary artery bypass procedures are coded differently than other bypass procedures as described in the previous guideline. Rather than identifying the body part bypassed from, the body part identifies the number of coronary arteries bypassed to, and the qualifier specifies the vessel bypassed from.

Example: Aortocoronary artery bypass of the left anterior descending coronary artery and the obtuse marginal coronary artery is classified in the body part axis of classification as two coronary arteries, and the qualifier specifies the aorta as the body part bypassed from.

B3.6c. If multiple coronary arteries are bypassed, a separate procedure is coded for each coronary artery that uses a different device and/or qualifier.

Example: Aortocoronary artery bypass and internal mammary coronary artery bypass are coded separately.

Control vs. more definitive root operations

B3.7. The root operation Control is defined as, "Stopping, or attempting to stop, postprocedural or other acute bleeding." If an attempt to stop postprocedural or other acute bleeding is ~~initially~~ unsuccessful, and to stop the bleeding requires performing a more definitive root operation, such as Bypass, Detachment, Excision, Extraction, Reposition, Replacement, or Resection, then the more definitive root operation is coded instead of Control.

Example: Resection of spleen to stop bleeding is coded to Resection instead of Control.

Excision vs. Resection

B3.8. PCS contains specific body parts for anatomical subdivisions of a body part, such as lobes of the lungs or liver and regions of the intestine. Resection of the specific body part is coded whenever all of the body part is cut out or off, rather than coding Excision of a less specific body part.

Example: Left upper lung lobectomy is coded to Resection of Upper Lung Lobe, Left rather than Excision of Lung, Left.

Excision for graft

B3.9. If an autograft is obtained from a different procedure site in order to complete the objective of the procedure, a separate procedure is coded.

Example: Coronary bypass with excision of saphenous vein graft, excision of saphenous vein is coded separately.

Fusion procedures of the spine

B3.10a. The body part coded for a spinal vertebral joint(s) rendered immobile by a spinal fusion procedure is classified by the level of the spine (e.g. thoracic). There are distinct body part values for a single vertebral joint and for multiple vertebral joints at each spinal level.

Example: Body part values specify Lumbar Vertebral Joint, Lumbar Vertebral Joints, 2 or More and Lumbosacral Vertebral Joint.

B3.10b. If multiple vertebral joints are fused, a separate procedure is coded for each vertebral joint that uses a different device and/or qualifier.

Example: Fusion of lumbar vertebral joint, posterior approach, anterior column and fusion of lumbar vertebral joint, posterior approach, posterior column are coded separately.

B3.10c. Combinations of devices and materials are often used on a vertebral joint to render the joint immobile. When combinations of devices are used on the same vertebral joint, the device value coded for the procedure is as follows:

- If an interbody fusion device is used to render the joint immobile (alone or containing other material like bone graft), the procedure is coded with the device value Interbody Fusion Device

- If bone graft is the *only* device used to render the joint immobile, the procedure is coded with the device value Nonautologous Tissue Substitute or Autologous Tissue Substitute

- If a mixture of autologous and nonautologous bone graft (with or without biological or synthetic extenders or binders) is used to render the joint immobile, code the procedure with the device value Autologous Tissue Substitute

Examples: Fusion of a vertebral joint using a cage style interbody fusion device containing morsellized bone graft is coded to the device Interbody Fusion Device.

Fusion of a vertebral joint using a bone dowel interbody fusion device made of cadaver bone and packed with a mixture of local morsellized bone and demineralized bone matrix is coded to the device Interbody Fusion Device.

Fusion of a vertebral joint using both autologous bone graft and bone bank bone graft is coded to the device Autologous Tissue Substitute.

Inspection procedures

B3.11a. Inspection of a body part(s) performed in order to achieve the objective of a procedure is not coded separately.

Example: Fiberoptic bronchoscopy performed for irrigation of bronchus, only the irrigation procedure is coded.

B3.11b. If multiple tubular body parts are inspected, the most distal body part (the body part furthest from the starting point of the inspection) is coded. If multiple non-tubular body parts in a region are inspected, the body part that specifies the entire area inspected is coded.

Examples: Cystoureteroscopy with inspection of bladder and ureters is coded to the ureter body part value.

Exploratory laparotomy with general inspection of abdominal contents is coded to the peritoneal cavity body part value.

B3.11c. When both an Inspection procedure and another procedure are performed on the same body part during the same episode, if the Inspection procedure is performed using a different approach than the other procedure, the Inspection procedure is coded separately.

Example: Endoscopic Inspection of the duodenum is coded separately when open Excision of the duodenum is performed during the same procedural episode.

Occlusion vs. Restriction for vessel embolization procedures

B3.12. If the objective of an embolization procedure is to completely close a vessel, the root operation Occlusion is coded. If the objective of an embolization procedure is to narrow the lumen of a vessel, the root operation Restriction is coded.

Examples: Tumor embolization is coded to the root operation Occlusion, because the objective of the procedure is to cut off the blood supply to the vessel.

Embolization of a cerebral aneurysm is coded to the root operation Restriction, because the objective of the procedure is not to close off the vessel entirely, but to narrow the lumen of the vessel at the site of the aneurysm where it is abnormally wide.

Release procedures

B3.13. In the root operation Release, the body part value coded is the body part being freed and not the tissue being manipulated or cut to free the body part.

Example: Lysis of intestinal adhesions is coded to the specific intestine body part value.

Release vs. Division

B3.14. If the sole objective of the procedure is freeing a body part without cutting the body part, the root operation is Release. If the sole objective of the procedure is separating or transecting a body part, the root operation is Division.

Examples: Freeing a nerve root from surrounding scar tissue to relieve pain is coded to the root operation Release.

Severing a nerve root to relieve pain is coded to the root operation Division.

Reposition for fracture treatment

B3.15. Reduction of a displaced fracture is coded to the root operation Reposition and the application of a cast or splint in conjunction with the Reposition procedure is not coded separately. Treatment of a nondisplaced fracture is coded to the procedure performed.

Examples: Casting of a nondisplaced fracture is coded to the root operation Immobilization in the Placement section.

Putting a pin in a nondisplaced fracture is coded to the root operation Insertion.

Transplantation vs. Administration

B3.16. Putting in a mature and functioning living body part taken from another individual or animal is coded to the root operation Transplantation. Putting in autologous or nonautologous cells is coded to the Administration section.

Example: Putting in autologous or nonautologous bone marrow, pancreatic islet cells or stem cells is coded to the Administration section.

Transfer procedures using multiple tissue layers

B3.17. The root operation Transfer contains qualifiers that can be used to specify when a transfer flap is composed of more than one tissue layer, such as a musculocutaneous flap. For procedures involving transfer of multiple tissue layers including skin, subcutaneous tissue, fascia or muscle, the procedure is coded to the body part value that describes the deepest tissue layer in the flap, and the qualifier can be used to describe the other tissue layer(s) in the transfer flap.

***Example: A* musculocutaneous flap transfer is coded to the appropriate body part value in the body system Muscles, and the qualifier is used to describe the additional tissue layer(s) in the transfer flap.**

B4. Body Part

General guidelines

B4.1a. If a procedure is performed on a portion of a body part that does not have a separate body part value, code the body part value corresponding to the whole body part.

Example: A procedure performed on the alveolar process of the mandible is coded to the mandible body part.

B4.1b. If the prefix "peri" is combined with a body part to identify the site of the procedure, and the site of the procedure is not further specified, then the procedure is coded to the body part named. This guideline applies only when a more specific body part value is not available.

Examples: A procedure site identified as perirenal is coded to the kidney body part when the site of the procedure is not further specified.

A procedure site described in the documentation as peri-urethral, and the documentation also indicates that it is the vulvar tissue and not the urethral tissue that is the site of the procedure, then the procedure is coded to the vulva body part.

B4.1c. If a procedure is performed on a continuous section of a tubular body part, code the body part value corresponding to the furthest anatomical site from the point of entry.

Example: A procedure performed on a continuous section of artery from the femoral artery to the external iliac artery with the point of entry at the femoral artery is coded to the external iliac body part.

Branches of body parts

B4.2. Where a specific branch of a body part does not have its own body part value in PCS, the body part is typically coded to the closest proximal branch that has a specific body part value. In the cardiovascular body systems, if a general body part is available in the correct root operation table, and coding to a proximal branch would require assigning a code in a different body system, the procedure is coded using the general body part value.

Examples: A procedure performed on the mandibular branch of the trigeminal nerve is coded to the trigeminal nerve body part value.

Occlusion of the bronchial artery is coded to the body part value Upper Artery in the body system Upper Arteries, and not to the body part value Thoracic Aorta, Descending in the body system Heart and Great Vessels.

Bilateral body part values

B4.3. Bilateral body part values are available for a limited number of body parts. If the identical procedure is performed on contralateral body parts, and a bilateral body part value exists for that body part, a single procedure is coded using the bilateral body part value. If no bilateral body part value exists, each procedure is coded separately using the appropriate body part value.

Examples: The identical procedure performed on both fallopian tubes is coded once using the body part value Fallopian Tube, Bilateral.

The identical procedure performed on both knee joints is coded twice using the body part values Knee Joint, Right and Knee Joint, Left.

Coronary arteries

B4.4. The coronary arteries are classified as a single body part that is further specified by number of arteries treated. One procedure code specifying multiple arteries is used when the same procedure is performed, including the same device and qualifier values.

Examples: Angioplasty of two distinct coronary arteries with placement of two stents is coded as Dilation of Coronary Artery, Two Arteries with Two Intraluminal Devices.

Angioplasty of two distinct coronary arteries, one with stent placed and one without, is coded separately as Dilation of Coronary Artery, One Artery with Intraluminal Device, and Dilation of Coronary Artery, One Artery with no device.

Tendons, ligaments, bursae and fascia near a joint

B4.5. Procedures performed on tendons, ligaments, bursae and fascia supporting a joint are coded to the body part in the respective body system that is the focus of the procedure. Procedures performed on joint structures themselves are coded to the body part in the joint body systems.

Examples: Repair of the anterior cruciate ligament of the knee is coded to the knee bursa and ligament body part in the bursae and ligaments body system.

Knee arthroscopy with shaving of articular cartilage is coded to the knee joint body part in the Lower Joints body system.

Skin, subcutaneous tissue and fascia overlying a joint

B4.6. If a procedure is performed on the skin, subcutaneous tissue or fascia overlying a joint, the procedure is coded to the following body part:

- Shoulder is coded to Upper Arm
- Elbow is coded to Lower Arm
- Wrist is coded to Lower Arm
- Hip is coded to Upper Leg
- Knee is coded to Lower Leg
- Ankle is coded to Foot

Fingers and toes

B4.7. If a body system does not contain a separate body part value for fingers, procedures performed on the fingers are coded to the body part value for the hand. If a body system does not contain a separate body part value for toes, procedures performed on the toes are coded to the body part value for the foot.

Example: Excision of finger muscle is coded to one of the hand muscle body part values in the Muscles body system.

Upper and lower intestinal tract

B4.8. In the Gastrointestinal body system, the general body part values Upper Intestinal Tract and Lower Intestinal Tract are provided as an option for the root operations Change, Inspection, Removal and Revision. Upper Intestinal Tract includes the portion of the gastrointestinal tract from the esophagus down to and including the duodenum, and Lower Intestinal Tract includes the portion of the gastrointestinal tract from the jejunum down to and including the rectum and anus.

Example: In the root operation Change table, change of a device in the jejunum is coded using the body part Lower Intestinal Tract.

B5. Approach

Open approach with percutaneous endoscopic assistance

B5.2. Procedures performed using the open approach with percutaneous endoscopic assistance are coded to the approach Open.

Example: Laparoscopic-assisted sigmoidectomy is coded to the approach Open.

External approach

B5.3a. Procedures performed within an orifice on structures that are visible without the aid of any instrumentation are coded to the approach External.

Example: Resection of tonsils is coded to the approach External.

B5.3b. Procedures performed indirectly by the application of external force through the intervening body layers are coded to the approach External.

Example: Closed reduction of fracture is coded to the approach External.

Percutaneous procedure via device

B5.4. Procedures performed percutaneously via a device placed for the procedure are coded to the approach Percutaneous.

Example: Fragmentation of kidney stone performed via percutaneous nephrostomy is coded to the approach Percutaneous.

B6. Device

General guidelines

B6.1a. A device is coded only if a device remains after the procedure is completed. If no device remains, the device value No Device is coded. In limited root operations, the classification provides the qualifier values Temporary and Intraoperative, for specific procedures involving clinically significant devices, where the purpose of the device is to be utilized for a brief duration during the procedure or current inpatient stay. **If a device that is intended to remain after the procedure is completed requires removal before the end of the operative episode in which it was inserted (for example, the device size is inadequate or a complication occurs), both the insertion and removal of the device should be coded.**

B6.1b. Materials such as sutures, ligatures, radiological markers and temporary post-operative wound drains are considered integral to the performance of a procedure and are not coded as devices.

B6.1c. Procedures performed on a device only and not on a body part are specified in the root operations Change, Irrigation, Removal and Revision, and are coded to the procedure performed.

Example: Irrigation of percutaneous nephrostomy tube is coded to the root operation Irrigation of indwelling device in the Administration section.

Drainage device

B6.2. A separate procedure to put in a drainage device is coded to the root operation Drainage with the device value Drainage Device.

Obstetric Section Guidelines (section 1)

C. Obstetrics Section

Products of conception

C1. Procedures performed on the products of conception are coded to the Obstetrics section. Procedures performed on the pregnant female other than the products of conception are coded to the appropriate root operation in the Medical and Surgical section.

Example: Amniocentesis is coded to the products of conception body part in the Obstetrics section. Repair of obstetric urethral laceration is coded to the urethra body part in the Medical and Surgical section.

Procedures following delivery or abortion

C2. Procedures performed following a delivery or abortion for curettage of the endometrium or evacuation of retained products of conception are all coded in the Obstetrics section, to the root operation Extraction and the body part Products of Conception, Retained.

Diagnostic or therapeutic dilation and curettage performed during times other than the postpartum or post-abortion period are all coded in the Medical and Surgical section, to the root operation Extraction and the body part Endometrium.

New Technology Section Guidelines (section X)

D. New Technology Section

General guidelines

D1. Section X codes are standalone codes. They are not supplemental codes. Section X codes fully represent the specific procedure described in the code title, and do not require any additional codes from other sections of ICD-10-PCS. When section X contains a code title which describes a specific new technology procedure, only that X code is reported for the procedure. There is no need to report a broader, non-specific code in another section of ICD-10-PCS.

Example: XW04321 Introduction of Ceftazidime-Avibactam Anti-infective into Central Vein, Percutaneous Approach, New Technology Group 1, can be coded to indicate that Ceftazidime-Avibactam Anti-infective was administered via a central vein. A separate code from table 3E0 in the Administration section of ICD-10-PCS is not coded in addition to this code.

Selection of Principal Procedure

The following instructions should be applied in the selection of principal procedure and clarification on the importance of the relation to the principal diagnosis when more than one procedure is performed:

1. Procedure performed for definitive treatment of both principal diagnosis and secondary diagnosis

    a. Sequence procedure performed for definitive treatment most related to principal diagnosis as principal procedure.

2. Procedure performed for definitive treatment and diagnostic procedures performed for both principal diagnosis and secondary diagnosis.

    a. Sequence procedure performed for definitive treatment most related to principal diagnosis as principal procedure

3. A diagnostic procedure was performed for the principal diagnosis and a procedure is performed for definitive treatment of a secondary diagnosis.

    a. Sequence diagnostic procedure as principal procedure, since the procedure most related to the principal diagnosis takes precedence.

4. No procedures performed that are related to principal diagnosis; procedures performed for definitive treatment and diagnostic procedures were performed for secondary diagnosis

    a. Sequence procedure performed for definitive treatment of secondary diagnosis as principal procedure, since there are no procedures (definitive or nondefinitive treatment) related to principal diagnosis.

Appendix B. Components of the Medical and Surgical Approach Definitions

ICD-10-PCS Value	Definition	Access Location	Method	Type of Instrumentation	Example
Open (Ø)	Cutting through the skin or mucous membrane and any other body layers necessary to expose the site of the procedure	Skin or mucous membrane, any other body layers	Cutting	None	Abdominal hysterectomy
Percutaneous (3)	Entry, by puncture or minor incision, of instrumentation through the skin or mucous membrane and any other body layers necessary to reach the site of the procedure	Skin or mucous membrane, any other body layers	Puncture or minor incision	Without visualization	Needle biopsy of liver, Liposuction
Percutaneous endoscopic (4)	Entry, by puncture or minor incision, of instrumentation through the skin or mucous membrane and any other body layers necessary to reach and visualize the site of the procedure	Skin or mucous membrane, any other body layers	Puncture or minor incision	With visualization	Arthroscopy, Laparoscopic cholecystectomy
Via natural or artificial opening (7)	Entry of instrumentation through a natural or artificial external opening to reach the site of the procedure	Natural or artificial external opening	Direct entry	Without visualization	Endotracheal tube insertion, Foley catheter placement
Via natural or artificial opening endoscopic (8)	Entry of instrumentation through a natural or artificial external opening to reach and visualize the site of the procedure	Natural or artificial external opening	Direct entry	With visualization	Sigmoidoscopy, EGD, ERCP
Via natural or artificial opening with percutaneous endoscopic assistance (F)	Entry of instrumentation through a natural or artificial external opening and entry, by puncture or minor incision, of instrumentation through the skin or mucous membrane and any other body layers necessary to aid in the performance of the procedure	Skin or mucous membrane, any other body layers	Direct entry with puncture or minor incision for instrumentation only	With visualization	Laparoscopic-assisted vaginal hysterectomy
External (X)	Procedures performed directly on the skin or mucous membrane and procedures performed indirectly by the application of external force through the skin or mucous membrane	Skin or mucous membrane	Direct or indirect application	None	Closed fracture reduction, Resection of tonsils

Appendix C. Root Operation Definitions

Ø Medical and Surgical

	ICD-10-PCS Value		Definition
Ø	Alteration	Definition:	Modifying the anatomic structure of a body part without affecting the function of the body part
		Explanation:	Principal purpose is to improve appearance
		Examples:	Face lift, breast augmentation
1	Bypass	Definition:	Altering the route of passage of the contents of a tubular body part
		Explanation:	Rerouting contents of a body part to a downstream area of the normal route, to a similar route and body part, or to an abnormal route and dissimilar body part. Includes one or more anastomoses, with or without the use of a device.
		Examples:	Coronary artery bypass, colostomy formation
2	Change	Definition:	Taking out or off a device from a body part and putting back an identical or similar device in or on the same body part without cutting or puncturing the skin or a mucous membrane
		Explanation:	All CHANGE procedures are coded using the approach EXTERNAL
		Example:	Urinary catheter change, gastrostomy tube change
3	Control	Definition:	Stopping, or attempting to stop, postprocedural or other acute bleeding
		Explanation:	The site of the bleeding is coded as an anatomical region and not to a specific body part
		Examples:	Control of post-prostatectomy hemorrhage, control of intracranial subdural hemorrhage, control of bleeding duodenal ulcer, control of retroperitoneal hemorrhage
4	Creation	Definition:	Putting in or on biological or synthetic material to form a new body part that to the extent possible replicates the anatomic structure or function of an absent body part
		Explanation:	Used for gender reassignment surgery and corrective procedures in individuals with congenital anomalies
		Examples:	Creation of vagina in a male, creation of right and left atrioventricular valve from common atrioventricular valve
5	Destruction	Definition:	Physical eradication of all or a portion of a body part by the direct use of energy, force, or a destructive agent
		Explanation:	None of the body part is physically taken out
		Examples:	Fulguration of rectal polyp, cautery of skin lesion
6	Detachment	Definition:	Cutting off all or a portion of the upper or lower extremities
		Explanation:	The body part value is the site of the detachment, with a qualifier if applicable to further specify the level where the extremity was detached
		Examples:	Below knee amputation, disarticulation of shoulder
7	Dilation	Definition:	Expanding an orifice or the lumen of a tubular body part
		Explanation:	The orifice can be a natural orifice or an artificially created orifice. Accomplished by stretching a tubular body part using intraluminal pressure or by cutting part of the orifice or wall of the tubular body part.
		Examples:	Percutaneous transluminal angioplasty, internal urethrotomy
8	Division	Definition:	Cutting into a body part, without draining fluids and/or gases from the body part, in order to separate or transect a body part
		Explanation:	All or a portion of the body part is separated into two or more portions
		Examples:	Spinal cordotomy, osteotomy
9	Drainage	Definition:	Taking or letting out fluids and/or gases from a body part
		Explanation:	The qualifier DIAGNOSTIC is used to identify drainage procedures that are biopsies
		Examples:	Thoracentesis, incision and drainage

Continued on next page

Ø Medical and Surgical (continued)

ICD-10-PCS Value		Definition	
B	Excision	Definition:	Cutting out or off, without replacement, a portion of a body part
		Explanation:	The qualifier DIAGNOSTIC is used to identify excision procedures that are biopsies
		Examples:	Partial nephrectomy, liver biopsy
C	Extirpation	Definition:	Taking or cutting out solid matter from a body part
		Explanation:	The solid matter may be an abnormal byproduct of a biological function or a foreign body; it may be imbedded in a body part or in the lumen of a tubular body part. The solid matter may or may not have been previously broken into pieces.
		Examples:	Thrombectomy, choledocholithotomy
D	Extraction	Definition:	Pulling or stripping out or off all or a portion of a body part by the use of force
		Explanation:	The qualifier DIAGNOSTIC is used to identify extractions that are biopsies
		Examples:	Dilation and curettage, vein stripping
F	Fragmentation	Definition:	Breaking solid matter in a body part into pieces
		Explanation:	Physical force (e.g., manual, ultrasonic) applied directly or indirectly is used to break the solid matter into pieces. The solid matter may be an abnormal byproduct of a biological function or a foreign body. The pieces of solid matter are not taken out.
		Examples:	Extracorporeal shockwave lithotripsy, transurethral lithotripsy
G	Fusion	Definition:	Joining together portions of an articular body part rendering the articular body part immobile
		Explanation:	The body part is joined together by fixation device, bone graft, or other means
		Examples:	Spinal fusion, ankle arthrodesis
H	Insertion	Definition:	Putting in a nonbiological appliance that monitors, assists, performs, or prevents a physiological function but does not physically take the place of a body part
		Explanation:	None
		Examples:	Insertion of radioactive implant, insertion of central venous catheter
J	Inspection	Definition:	Visually and/or manually exploring a body part
		Explanation:	Visual exploration may be performed with or without optical instrumentation. Manual exploration may be performed directly or through intervening body layers.
		Examples:	Diagnostic arthroscopy, exploratory laparotomy
K	Map	Definition:	Locating the route of passage of electrical impulses and/or locating functional areas in a body part
		Explanation:	Applicable only to the cardiac conduction mechanism and the central nervous system
		Examples:	Cardiac mapping, cortical mapping
L	Occlusion	Definition:	Completely closing an orifice or lumen of a tubular body part
		Explanation:	The orifice can be a natural orifice or an artificially created orifice
		Examples:	Fallopian tube ligation, ligation of inferior vena cava
M	Reattachment	Definition:	Putting back in or on all or a portion of a separated body part to its normal location or other suitable location
		Explanation:	Vascular circulation and nervous pathways may or may not be reestablished
		Examples:	Reattachment of hand, reattachment of avulsed kidney
N	Release	Definition:	Freeing a body part from an abnormal physical constraint by cutting or by use of force
		Explanation:	Some of the restraining tissue may be taken out but none of the body part is taken out
		Examples:	Adhesiolysis, carpal tunnel release
P	Removal	Definition:	Taking out or off a device from a body part
		Explanation:	If a device is taken out and a similar device put in without cutting or puncturing the skin or mucous membrane, the procedure is coded to the root operation CHANGE. Otherwise, the procedure for taking out a device is coded to the root operation REMOVAL.
		Examples:	Drainage tube removal, cardiac pacemaker removal

Continued on next page

Ø Medical and Surgical (continued)

ICD-10-PCS Value			Definition
Q	Repair	Definition:	Restoring, to the extent possible, a body part to its normal anatomic structure and function
		Explanation:	Used only when the method to accomplish the repair is not one of the other root operations
		Examples:	Colostomy takedown, suture of laceration
R	Replacement	Definition:	Putting in or on biological or synthetic material that physically takes the place and/or function of all or a portion of a body part
		Explanation:	The body part may have been taken out or replaced, or may be taken out, physically eradicated, or rendered nonfunctional during the REPLACEMENT procedure. A REMOVAL procedure is coded for taking out the device used in a previous replacement procedure.
		Examples:	Total hip replacement, bone graft, free skin graft
S	Reposition	Definition:	Moving to its normal location, or other suitable location, all or a portion of a body part
		Explanation:	The body part is moved to a new location from an abnormal location, or from a normal location where it is not functioning correctly. The body part may or may not be cut out or off to be moved to the new location.
		Examples:	Reposition of undescended testicle, fracture reduction
T	Resection	Definition:	Cutting out or off, without replacement, all of a body part
		Explanation:	None
		Examples:	Total nephrectomy, total lobectomy of lung
V	Restriction	Definition:	Partially closing an orifice or the lumen of a tubular body part
		Explanation:	The orifice can be a natural orifice or an artificially created orifice
		Examples:	Esophagogastric fundoplication, cervical cerclage
W	Revision	Definition:	Correcting, to the extent possible, a portion of a malfunctioning device or the position of a displaced device
		Explanation:	Revision can include correcting a malfunctioning or displaced device by taking out or putting in components of the device such as a screw or pin
		Examples:	Adjustment of position of pacemaker lead, recementing of hip prosthesis
U	Supplement	Definition:	Putting in or on biological or synthetic material that physically reinforces and/or augments the function of a portion of a body part
		Explanation:	The biological material is non-living, or is living and from the same individual. The body part may have been previously replaced, and the SUPPLEMENT procedure is performed to physically reinforce and/or augment the function of the replaced body part.
		Examples:	Herniorrhaphy using mesh, free nerve graft, mitral valve ring annuloplasty, put a new acetabular liner in a previous hip replacement
X	Transfer	Definition:	Moving, without taking out, all or a portion of a body part to another location to take over the function of all or a portion of a body part
		Explanation:	The body part transferred remains connected to its vascular and nervous supply
		Examples:	Tendon transfer, skin pedicle flap transfer
Y	Transplantation	Definition:	Putting in or on all or a portion of a living body part taken from another individual or animal to physically take the place and/or function of all or a portion of a similar body part
		Explanation:	The native body part may or may not be taken out, and the transplanted body part may take over all or a portion of its function
		Examples:	Kidney transplant, heart transplant

Root Operation Definitions for Other Sections

1 Obstetrics

ICD-10-PCS Value			Definition
2	Change	Definition:	Taking out or off a device from a body part and putting back an identical or similar device in or on the same body part without cutting or puncturing the skin or a mucous membrane
		Explanation:	None
		Examples:	Replacement of fetal scalp electrode
9	Drainage	Definition:	Taking or letting out fluids and/or gases from a body part
		Explanation:	None
		Examples:	Biopsy of amniotic fluid
A	Abortion	Definition:	Artificially terminating a pregnancy
		Explanation:	None
		Examples:	Transvaginal abortion using vacuum aspiration technique
D	Extraction	Definition:	Pulling or stripping out or off all or a portion of a body part by the use of force
		Explanation:	None
		Examples:	Low-transverse C-section
E	Delivery	Definition:	Assisting the passage of the products of conception from the genital canal
		Explanation:	None
		Examples:	Manually-assisted delivery
H	Insertion	Definition:	Putting in a nonbiological appliance that monitors, assists, performs, or prevents a physiological function but does not physically take the place of a body part
		Explanation:	None
		Examples:	Placement of fetal scalp electrode
J	Inspection	Definition:	Visually and/or manually exploring a body part
		Explanation:	Visual exploration may be performed with or without optical instrumentation. Manual exploration may be performed directly or through intervening body layers.
		Examples:	Bimanual pregnancy exam
P	Removal	Definition:	Taking out or off a device from a body part, region or orifice
		Explanation:	If a device is taken out and a similar device put in without cutting or puncturing the skin or mucous membrane, the procedure is coded to the root operation CHANGE. Otherwise, the procedure for taking out a device is coded to the root operation REMOVAL.
		Examples:	Removal of fetal monitoring electrode
Q	Repair	Definition:	Restoring, to the extent possible, a body part to its normal anatomic structure and function
		Explanation:	Used only when the method to accomplish the repair is not one of the other root operations
		Examples:	In utero repair of congenital diaphragmatic hernia
S	Reposition	Definition:	Moving to its normal location, or other suitable location, all or a portion of a body part
		Explanation:	The body part is moved to a new location from an abnormal location, or from a normal location where it is not functioning correctly. The body part may or may not be cut out or off to be moved to the new location.
		Examples:	External version of fetus
T	Resection	Definition:	Cutting out or off, without replacement, all of a body part
		Explanation:	None
		Examples:	Total excision of tubal pregnancy
Y	Transplantation	Definition:	Putting in or on all or a portion of a living body part taken from another individual or animal to physically take the place and/or function of all or a portion of a similar body part
		Explanation:	The native body part may or may not be taken out, and the transplanted body part may take over all or a portion of its function
		Examples:	In utero fetal kidney transplant

2 Placement

ICD-10-PCS Value			Definition
Ø	Change	Definition:	Taking out or off a device from a body part and putting back an identical or similar device in or on the same body part without cutting or puncturing the skin or a mucous membrane
		Examples:	Change of vaginal packing
1	Compression	Definition:	Putting pressure on a body region
		Examples:	Placement of pressure dressing on abdominal wall
2	Dressing	Definition:	Putting material on a body region for protection
		Examples:	Application of sterile dressing to head wound
3	Immobilization	Definition:	Limiting or preventing motion of a body region
		Examples:	Placement of splint on left finger
4	Packing	Definition:	Putting material in a body region or orifice
		Examples:	Placement of nasal packing
5	Removal	Definition:	Taking out or off a device from a body part
		Examples:	Removal of stereotactic head frame
6	Traction	Definition:	Exerting a pulling force on a body region in a distal direction
		Examples:	Lumbar traction using motorized split-traction table

3 Administration

ICD-10-PCS Value			Definition
Ø	Introduction	Definition:	Putting in or on a therapeutic, diagnostic, nutritional, physiological, or prophylactic substance except blood or blood products
		Examples:	Nerve block injection to median nerve
1	Irrigation	Definition:	Putting in or on a cleansing substance
		Examples:	Flushing of eye
2	Transfusion	Definition:	Putting in blood or blood products
		Examples:	Transfusion of cell saver red cells into central venous line

4 Measurement and Monitoring

ICD-10-PCS Value			Definition
Ø	Measurement	Definition:	Determining the level of a physiological or physical function at a point in time
		Examples:	External electrocardiogram(EKG), single reading
1	Monitoring	Definition:	Determining the level of a physiological or physical function repetitively over a period of time
		Examples:	Urinary pressure monitoring

5 Extracorporeal or Systemic Assistance and Performance

ICD-10-PCS Value			Definition
Ø	Assistance	Definition:	Taking over a portion of a physiological function by extracorporeal means
		Examples:	Hyperbaric oxygenation of wound
1	Performance	Definition:	Completely taking over a physiological function by extracorporeal means
		Examples:	Cardiopulmonary bypass in conjunction with CABG
2	Restoration	Definition:	Returning, or attempting to return, a physiological function to its original state by extracorporeal means
		Examples:	Attempted cardiac defibrillation, unsuccessful

6 Extracorporeal or Systemic Therapies

ICD-10-PCS Value		Definition	
Ø	Atmospheric Control	Definition:	Extracorporeal control of atmospheric pressure and composition
		Examples:	Antigen-free air conditioning, series treatment
1	Decompression	Definition:	Extracorporeal elimination of undissolved gas from body fluids
		Examples:	Hyperbaric decompression treatment, single
2	Electromagnetic Therapy	Definition:	Extracorporeal treatment by electromagnetic rays
		Examples:	TMS (transcranial magnetic stimulation), series treatment
3	Hyperthermia	Definition:	Extracorporeal raising of body temperature
		Examples:	None
4	Hypothermia	Definition:	Extracorporeal lowering of body temperature
		Examples:	Whole body hypothermia treatment for temperature imbalances, series
5	Pheresis	Definition:	Extracorporeal separation of blood products
		Examples:	Therapeutic leukopheresis, single treatment
6	Phototherapy	Definition:	Extracorporeal treatment by light rays
		Examples:	Phototherapy of circulatory system, series treatment
7	Ultrasound Therapy	Definition:	Extracorporeal treatment by ultrasound
		Examples:	Therapeutic ultrasound of peripheral vessels, single treatment
8	Ultraviolet Light Therapy	Definition:	Extracorporeal treatment by ultraviolet light
		Examples:	Ultraviolet light phototherapy, series treatment
9	Shock Wave Therapy	Definition:	Extracorporeal treatment by shock waves
		Examples:	Shockwave therapy of plantar fascia, single treatment
B	Perfusion	Definition:	Extracorporeal treatment by diffusion of therapeutic fluid
		Examples:	Perfusion of donor liver while preparing transplant patient

7 Osteopathic

ICD-10-PCS Value		Definition	
Ø	Treatment	Definition:	Manual treatment to eliminate or alleviate somatic dysfunction and related disorders
		Examples:	Fascial release of abdomen, osteopathic treatment

8 Other Procedures

ICD-10-PCS Value		Definition	
Ø	Other Procedures	Definition:	Methodologies which attempt to remediate or cure a disorder or disease
		Examples:	Acupuncture, yoga therapy

9 Chiropractic

ICD-10-PCS Value		Definition	
B	Manipulation	Definition:	Manual procedure that involves a directed thrust to move a joint past the physiological range of motion, without exceeding the anatomical limit
		Examples:	Chiropractic treatment of cervical spine, short lever specific contact

Appendix D. Body Part Key

Term	ICD-10-PCS Value
Abdominal aortic plexus	Abdominal Sympathetic Nerve
Abdominal esophagus	Esophagus, Lower
Abductor hallucis muscle	Foot Muscle, Right
	Foot Muscle, Left
Accessory cephalic vein	Cephalic Vein, Right
	Cephalic Vein, Left
Accessory obturator nerve	Lumbar Plexus
Accessory phrenic nerve	Phrenic nerve
Accessory spleen	Spleen
Acetabulofemoral joint	Hip Joint, Right
	Hip Joint, Left
Achilles tendon	Lower Leg Tendon, Right
	Lower Leg Tendon, Left
Acromioclavicular ligament	Shoulder Bursa and Ligament, Right
	Shoulder Bursa and Ligament, Left
Acromion (process)	Scapula, Right
	Scapula, Left
Adductor brevis muscle	Upper Leg Muscle, Right
	Upper Leg Muscle, Left
Adductor hallucis muscle	Foot Muscle, Right
	Foot Muscle, Left
Adductor longus muscle	Upper Leg Muscle, Right
	Upper Leg Muscle, Left
Adductor magnus muscle	Upper Leg Muscle, Right
	Upper Leg Muscle, Left
Adenohypophysis	Pituitary Gland
Alar ligament of axis	Head and Neck Bursa and Ligament
Alveolar process of mandible	Mandible, Right
	Mandible, Left
Alveolar process of maxilla	Maxilla
Anal orifice	Anus
Anatomical snuffbox	Lower Arm and Wrist Muscle, Right
	Lower Arm and Wrist Muscle, Left
Angular artery	Face Artery
Angular vein	Face Vein, Right
	Face Vein, Left
Annular ligament	Elbow Bursa and Ligament, Right
	Elbow Bursa and Ligament, Left
Anorectal junction	Rectum
Ansa cervicalis	Cervical Plexus
Antebrachial fascia	Subcutaneous Tissue and Fascia, Right Lower Arm
	Subcutaneous Tissue and Fascia, Left Lower Arm

Term	ICD-10-PCS Value
Anterior (pectoral) lymph node	Lymphatic, Right Axillary
	Lymphatic, Left Axillary
Anterior cerebral artery	Intracranial Artery
Anterior cerebral vein	Intracranial Vein
Anterior choroidal artery	Intracranial Artery
Anterior circumflex humeral artery	Axillary Artery, Right
	Axillary Artery, Left
Anterior communicating artery	Intracranial Artery
Anterior cruciate ligament (ACL)	Knee Bursa and Ligament, Right
	Knee Bursa and Ligament, Left
Anterior crural nerve	Femoral Nerve
Anterior facial vein	Face Vein, Right
	Face Vein, Left
Anterior intercostal artery	Internal Mammary Artery, Right
	Internal Mammary Artery, Left
Anterior interosseous nerve	Median Nerve
Anterior lateral malleolar artery	Anterior Tibial Artery, Right
	Anterior Tibial Artery, Left
Anterior lingual gland	Minor Salivary Gland
Anterior medial malleolar artery	Anterior Tibial Artery, Right
	Anterior Tibial Artery, Left
Anterior spinal artery	Vertebral Artery, Right
	Vertebral Artery, Left
Anterior tibial recurrent artery	Anterior Tibial Artery, Right
	Anterior Tibial Artery, Left
Anterior ulnar recurrent artery	Ulnar Artery, Right
	Ulnar Artery, Left
Anterior vagal trunk	Vagus Nerve
Anterior vertebral muscle	Neck Muscle, Right
	Neck Muscle, Left
Antihelix	External Ear, Right
	External Ear, Left
	External Ear, Bilateral
Antitragus	External Ear, Right
	External Ear, Left
	External Ear, Bilateral
Antrum of Highmore	Maxillary Sinus, Right
	Maxillary Sinus, Left
Aortic annulus	Aortic Valve
Aortic arch	Thoracic Aorta, Ascending/Arch
Aortic intercostal artery	Upper Artery
Apical (subclavicular) lymph node	Lymphatic, Right Axillary
	Lymphatic, Left Axillary
Apneustic center	Pons
Aqueduct of Sylvius	Cerebral Ventricle

Term	ICD-10-PCS Value
Aqueous humour	Anterior Chamber, Right
	Anterior Chamber, Left
Arachnoid mater, intracranial	Cerebral Meninges
Arachnoid mater, spinal	Spinal Meninges
Arcuate artery	Foot Artery, Right
	Foot Artery, Left
Areola	Nipple, Right
	Nipple, Left
Arterial canal (duct)	Pulmonary Artery, Left
Aryepiglottic fold	Larynx
Arytenoid cartilage	Larynx
Arytenoid muscle	Neck Muscle, Right
	Neck Muscle, Left
Ascending aorta	Thoracic Aorta, Ascending/Arch
Ascending palatine artery	Face Artery
Ascending pharyngeal artery	External Carotid Artery, Right
	External Carotid Artery, Left
Atlantoaxial joint	Cervical Vertebral Joint
Atrioventricular node	Conduction Mechanism
Atrium dextrum cordis	Atrium, Right
Atrium pulmonale	Atrium, Left
Auditory tube	Eustachian Tube, Right
	Eustachian Tube, Left
Auerbach's (myenteric)plexus	Abdominal Sympathetic Nerve
Auricle	External Ear, Right
	External Ear, Left
	External Ear, Bilateral
Auricularis muscle	Head Muscle
Axillary fascia	Subcutaneous Tissue and Fascia, Right Upper Arm
	Subcutaneous Tissue and Fascia, Left Upper Arm
Axillary nerve	Brachial Plexus
Bartholin's (greater vestibular) gland	Vestibular Gland
Basal (internal) cerebral vein	Intracranial Vein
Basal nuclei	Basal Ganglia
Base of tongue	Pharynx
Basilar artery	Intracranial Artery
Basis pontis	Pons
Biceps brachii muscle	Upper Arm Muscle, Right
	Upper Arm Muscle, Left
Biceps femoris muscle	Upper Leg Muscle, Right
	Upper Leg Muscle, Left
Bicipital aponeurosis	Subcutaneous Tissue and Fascia, Right Lower Arm
	Subcutaneous Tissue and Fascia, Left Lower Arm
Bicuspid valve	Mitral Valve
Body of femur	Femoral Shaft, Right
	Femoral Shaft, Left

Term	ICD-10-PCS Value
Body of fibula	Fibula, Right
	Fibula, Left
Bony labyrinth	Inner Ear, Right
	Inner Ear, Left
Bony orbit	Orbit, Right
	Orbit, Left
Bony vestibule	Inner Ear, Right
	Inner Ear, Left
Botallo's duct	Pulmonary Artery, Left
Brachial (lateral) lymph node	Lymphatic, Right Axillary
	Lymphatic, Left Axillary
Brachialis muscle	Upper Arm Muscle, Right
	Upper Arm Muscle, Left
Brachiocephalic artery	Innominate Artery
Brachiocephalic trunk	Innominate Artery
Brachiocephalic vein	Innominate Vein, Right
	Innominate Vein, Left
Brachioradialis muscle	Lower Arm and Wrist Muscle, Right
	Lower Arm and Wrist Muscle, Left
Broad ligament	Uterine Supporting Structure
Bronchial artery	Upper Artery
Bronchus intermedius	Main Bronchus, Right
Buccal gland	Buccal Mucosa
Buccinator lymph node	Lymphatic, Head
Buccinator muscle	Facial Muscle
Bulbospongiosus muscle	Perineum Muscle
Bulbourethral (Cowper's) gland	Urethra
Bundle of His	Conduction Mechanism
Bundle of Kent	Conduction Mechanism
Calcaneocuboid joint	Tarsal Joint, Right
	Tarsal Joint, Left
Calcaneocuboid ligament	Foot Bursa and Ligament, Right
	Foot Bursa and Ligament, Left
Calcaneofibular ligament	Ankle Bursa and Ligament, Right
	Ankle Bursa and Ligament, Left
Calcaneus	Tarsal, Right
	Tarsal, Left
Capitate bone	Carpal, Right
	Carpal, Left
Cardia	Esophagogastric Junction
Cardiac plexus	Thoracic Sympathetic Nerve
Cardioesophageal junction	Esophagogastric Junction
Caroticotympanic artery	Internal Carotid Artery, Right
	Internal Carotid Artery, Left
Carotid glomus	Carotid Body, Right
	Carotid Body, Left
	Carotid Bodies, Bilateral
Carotid sinus	Internal Carotid Artery, Right
	Internal Carotid Artery, Left
Carotid sinus nerve	Glossopharyngeal Nerve

Term	ICD-10-PCS Value
Carpometacarpal ligament	Hand Bursa and Ligament, Right
	Hand Bursa and Ligament, Left
Cauda equina	Lumbar Spinal Cord
Cavernous plexus	Head and Neck Sympathetic Nerve
Celiac ganglion	Abdominal Sympathetic Nerve
Celiac (solar) plexus	Abdominal Sympathetic Nerve
Celiac lymph node	Lymphatic, Aortic
Celiac trunk	Celiac Artery
Central axillary lymph node	Lymphatic, Right Axillary
	Lymphatic, Left Axillary
Cerebral aqueduct (Sylvius)	Cerebral Ventricle
Cerebrum	Brain
Cervical esophagus	Esophagus, Upper
Cervical facet joint	Cervical Vertebral Joint
	Cervical Vertebral Joints, 2 or more
Cervical ganglion	Head and Neck Sympathetic Nerve
Cervical interspinous ligament	Head and Neck Bursa and Ligament
Cervical intertransverse ligament	Head and Neck Bursa and Ligament
Cervical ligamentum flavum	Head and Neck Bursa and Ligament
Cervical lymph node	Lymphatic, Right Neck
	Lymphatic, Left Neck
Cervicothoracic facet joint	Cervicothoracic Vertebral Joint
Choana	Nasopharynx
Chondroglossus muscle	Tongue, Palate, Pharynx Muscle
Chorda tympani	Facial Nerve
Choroid plexus	Cerebral Ventricle
Ciliary body	Eye, Right
	Eye, Left
Ciliary ganglion	Head and Neck Sympathetic Nerve
Circle of Willis	Intracranial Artery
Circumflex illiac artery	Femoral Artery, Right
	Femoral Artery, Left
Claustrum	Basal Ganglia
Coccygeal body	Coccygeal Glomus
Coccygeus muscle	Trunk Muscle, Right
	Trunk Muscle, Left
Cochlea	Inner Ear, Right
	Inner Ear, Left
Cochlear nerve	Acoustic Nerve
Columella	Nasal Mucosa and Soft Tissue
Common digital vein	Foot Vein, Right
	Foot Vein, Left
Common facial vein	Face Vein, Right
	Face Vein, Left
Common fibular nerve	Peroneal Nerve
Common hepatic artery	Hepatic Artery
Common iliac (subaortic) lymph node	Lymphatic, Pelvis

Term	ICD-10-PCS Value
Common interosseous artery	Ulnar Artery, Right
	Ulnar Artery, Left
Common peroneal nerve	Peroneal Nerve
Condyloid process	Mandible, Right
	Mandible, Left
Conus arteriosus	Ventricle, Right
Conus medullaris	Lumbar Spinal Cord
Coracoacromial ligament	Shoulder Bursa and Ligament, Right
	Shoulder Bursa and Ligament, Left
Coracobrachialis muscle	Upper Arm Muscle, Right
	Upper Arm Muscle, Left
Coracoclavicular ligament	Shoulder Bursa and Ligament, Right
	Shoulder Bursa and Ligament, Left
Coracohumeral ligament	Shoulder Bursa and Ligament, Right
	Shoulder Bursa and Ligament, Left
Coracoid process	Scapula, Right
	Scapula, Left
Corniculate cartilage	Larynx
Corpus callosum	Brain
Corpus cavernosum	Penis
Corpus spongiosum	Penis
Corpus striatum	Basal Ganglia
Corrugator supercilii muscle	Facial Muscle
Costocervical trunk	Subclavian Artery, Right
	Subclavian Artery, Left
Costoclavicular ligament	Shoulder Bursa and Ligament, Right
	Shoulder Bursa and Ligament, Left
Costotransverse joint	Thoracic Vertebral Joint
Costotransverse ligament	Rib(s) Bursa and Ligament
Costovertebral joint	Thoracic Vertebral Joint
Costoxiphoid ligament	Sternum Bursa and Ligament
Cowper's (bulbourethral) gland	Urethra
Cremaster muscle	Perineum Muscle
Cribriform plate	Ethmoid Bone, Right
	Ethmoid Bone, Left
Cricoid cartilage	Trachea
Cricothyroid artery	Thyroid Artery, Right
	Thyroid Artery, Left
Cricothyroid muscle	Neck Muscle, Right
	Neck Muscle, Left
Crural fascia	Subcutaneous Tissue and Fascia, Right Upper Leg
	Subcutaneous Tissue and Fascia, Left Upper Leg
Cubital lymph node	Lymphatic, Right Upper Extremity
	Lymphatic, Left Upper Extremity
Cubital nerve	Ulnar Nerve
Cuboid bone	Tarsal, Right
	Tarsal, Left

Term	ICD-10-PCS Value
Cuboideonavicular joint	Tarsal Joint, Right
	Tarsal Joint, Left
Culmen	Cerebellum
Cuneiform cartilage	Larynx
Cuneonavicular joint	Tarsal Joint, Right
	Tarsal Joint, Left
Cuneonavicular ligament	Foot Bursa and Ligament, Right
	Foot Bursa and Ligament, Left
Cutaneous (transverse) cervical nerve	Cervical Plexus
Deep cervical fascia	Subcutaneous Tissue and Fascia, Right Neck
	Subcutaneous Tissue and Fascia, Left Neck
Deep cervical vein	Vertebral Vein, Right
	Vertebral Vein, Left
Deep circumflex iliac artery	External Iliac Artery, Right
	External Iliac Artery, Left
Deep facial vein	Face Vein, Right
	Face Vein, Left
Deep femoral artery	Femoral Artery, Right
	Femoral Artery, Left
Deep femoral (profunda femoris) vein	Femoral Vein, Right
	Femoral Vein, Left
Deep palmar arch	Hand Artery, Right
	Hand Artery, Left
Deep transverse perineal muscle	Perineum Muscle
Deferential artery	Internal Iliac Artery, Right
	Internal Iliac Artery, Left
Deltoid fascia	Subcutaneous Tissue and Fascia, Right Upper Arm
	Subcutaneous Tissue and Fascia, Left Upper Arm
Deltoid ligament	Ankle Bursa and Ligament, Right
	Ankle Bursa and Ligament, Left
Deltoid muscle	Shoulder Muscle, Right
	Shoulder Muscle, Left
Deltopectoral (infraclavicular) lymph node	Lymphatic, Right Upper Extremity
	Lymphatic, Left Upper Extremity
Dens	Cervical Vertebra
Denticulate (dentate) ligament	Spinal Meninges
Depressor anguli oris muscle	Facial Muscle
Depressor labii inferioris muscle	Facial Muscle
Depressor septi nasi muscle	Facial Muscle
Depressor supercilii muscle	Facial Muscle
Dermis	Skin
Descending genicular artery	Femoral Artery, Right
	Femoral Artery, Left
Diaphragma sellae	Dura Mater

Term	ICD-10-PCS Value
Distal humerus	Humeral Shaft, Right
	Humeral Shaft, Left
Distal humerus, involving joint	Elbow Joint, Right
	Elbow Joint, Left
Distal radioulnar joint	Wrist Joint, Right
	Wrist Joint, Left
Dorsal digital nerve	Radial Nerve
Dorsal metacarpal vein	Hand Vein, Right
	Hand Vein, Left
Dorsal metatarsal artery	Foot Artery, Right
	Foot Artery, Left
Dorsal metatarsal vein	Foot Vein, Right
	Foot Vein, Left
Dorsal scapular artery	Subclavian Artery, Right
	Subclavian Artery, Left
Dorsal scapular nerve	Brachial Plexus
Dorsal venous arch	Foot Vein, Right
	Foot Vein, Left
Dorsalis pedis artery	Anterior Tibial Artery, Right
	Anterior Tibial Artery, Left
Duct of Santorini	Pancreatic Duct, Accessory
Duct of Wirsung	Pancreatic Duct
Ductus deferens	Vas Deferens, Right
	Vas Deferens, Left
	Vas Deferens, Bilateral
	Vas Deferens
Duodenal ampulla	Ampulla of Vater
Duodenojejunal flexure	Jejunum
Dura mater, intracranial	Dura Mater
Dura mater, spinal	Spinal Meninges
Dural venous sinus	Intracranial Vein
Earlobe	External Ear, Right
	External Ear, Left
	External Ear, Bilateral
Eighth cranial nerve	Acoustic Nerve
Ejaculatory duct	Vas Deferens, Right
	Vas Deferens, Left
	Vas Deferens, Bilateral
	Vas Deferens
Eleventh cranial nerve	Accessory Nerve
Encephalon	Brain
Ependyma	Cerebral Ventricle
Epidermis	Skin
Epidural space, spinal	Spinal Canal
Epiploic foramen	Peritoneum
Epithalamus	Thalamus
Epitroclear lymph node	Lymphatic, Right Upper Extremity
	Lymphatic, Left Upper Extremity
Erector spinae muscle	Trunk Muscle, Right
	Trunk Muscle, Left
Esophageal artery	Upper Artery
Esophageal plexus	Thoracic Sympathetic Nerve

Term	ICD-10-PCS Value
Ethmoidal air cell	Ethmoid Sinus, Right
	Ethmoid Sinus, Left
Extensor carpi radialis muscle	Lower Arm and Wrist Muscle, Right
Extensor carpi ulnaris muscle	Lower Arm and Wrist Muscle, Left
Extensor digitorum brevis muscle	Foot Muscle, Right
	Foot Muscle, Left
Extensor digitorum longus muscle	Lower Leg Muscle, Right
	Lower Leg Muscle, Left
Extensor hallucis brevis muscle	Foot Muscle, Right
	Foot Muscle, Left
Extensor hallucis longus muscle	Lower Leg Muscle, Right
	Lower Leg Muscle, Left
External anal sphincter	Anal Sphincter
External auditory meatus	External Auditory Canal, Right
	External Auditory Canal, Left
External maxillary artery	Face Artery
External naris	Nasal Mucosa and Soft Tissue
External oblique aponeurosis	Subcutaneous Tissue and Fascia, Trunk
External oblique muscle	Abdomen Muscle, Right
	Abdomen Muscle, Left
External popliteal nerve	Peroneal Nerve
External pudendal artery	Femoral Artery, Right
	Femoral Artery, Left
External pudenal vein	Saphenous Vein, Right
	Saphenous Vein, Left
External urethral sphincter	Urethra
Extradural space, intracranial	Epidural Space, Intracranial
Extradural space, spinal	Spinal Canal
Facial artery	Face Artery
False vocal cord	Larynx
Falx cerebri	Dura Mater
Fascia lata	Subcutaneous Tissue and Fascia, Right Upper Leg
	Subcutaneous Tissue and Fascia, Left Upper Leg
Femoral head	Upper Femur, Right
	Upper Femur, Left
Femoral lymph node	Lymphatic, Right Lower Extremity
	Lymphatic, Left Lower Extremity
Femoropatellar joint	Knee Joint, Right
	Knee Joint, Left
	Knee Joint, Femoral Surface, Right
	Knee Joint, Femoral Surface, Left
Femorotibial joint	Knee Joint, Right
	Knee Joint, Left
	Knee Joint, Tibial Surface, Right
	Knee Joint, Tibial Surface, Left
Fibular artery	Peroneal Artery, Right
	Peroneal Artery, Left

Term	ICD-10-PCS Value
Fibularis brevis muscle	Lower Leg Muscle, Right
	Lower Leg Muscle, Left
Fibularis longus muscle	Lower Leg Muscle, Right
	Lower Leg Muscle, Left
Fifth cranial nerve	Trigeminal Nerve
Filum terminale	Spinal Meninges
First cranial nerve	Olfactory Nerve
First intercostal nerve	Brachial Plexus
Flexor carpi radialis muscle	Lower Arm and Wrist Muscle, Right
	Lower Arm and Wrist Muscle, Left
Flexor carpi ulnaris muscle	Lower Arm and Wrist Muscle, Right
	Lower Arm and Wrist Muscle, Left
Flexor digitorum brevis muscle	Foot Muscle, Right
	Foot Muscle, Left
Flexor digitorum longus muscle	Lower Leg Muscle, Right
	Lower Leg Muscle, Left
Flexor hallucis brevis muscle	Foot Muscle, Right
	Foot Muscle, Left
Flexor hallucis longus muscle	Lower Leg Muscle, Right
	Lower Leg Muscle, Left
Flexor pollicis longus muscle	Lower Arm and Wrist Muscle, Right
	Lower Arm and Wrist Muscle, Left
Foramen magnum	Occipital Bone
Foramen of Monro (intraventricular)	Cerebral Ventricle
Foreskin	Prepuce
Fossa of Rosenmuller	Nasopharynx
Fourth cranial nerve	Trochlear Nerve
Fourth ventricle	Cerebral Ventricle
Fovea	Retina, Right
	Retina, Left
Frenulum labii inferioris	Lower Lip
Frenulum labii superioris	Upper Lip
Frenulum linguae	Tongue
Frontal lobe	Cerebral Hemisphere
Frontal vein	Face Vein, Right
	Face Vein, Left
Fundus uteri	Uterus
Galea aponeurotica	Subcutaneous Tissue and Fascia, Scalp
Ganglion impar (ganglion of Walther)	Sacral Sympathetic Nerve
Gasserian ganglion	Trigeminal Nerve
Gastric lymph node	Lymphatic, Aortic
Gastric plexus	Abdominal Sympathetic Nerve
Gastrocnemius muscle	Lower Leg Muscle, Right
	Lower Leg Muscle, Left
Gastrocolic ligament	Omentum
Gastrocolic omentum	Omentum
Gastroduodenal artery	Hepatic Artery
Gastroesophageal (GE) junction	Esophagogastric Junction
Gastrohepatic omentum	Omentum

Term	ICD-10-PCS Value
Gastrophrenic ligament	Omentum
Gastrosplenic ligament	Omentum
Gemellus muscle	Hip Muscle, Right
	Hip Muscle, Left
Geniculate ganglion	Facial Nerve
Geniculate nucleus	Thalamus
Genioglossus muscle	Tongue, Palate, Pharynx Muscle
Genitofemoral nerve	Lumbar Plexus
Glans penis	Prepuce
Glenohumeral joint	Shoulder Joint, Right
	Shoulder Joint, Left
Glenohumeral ligament	Shoulder Bursa and Ligament, Right
	Shoulder Bursa and Ligament, Left
Glenoid fossa (of scapula)	Glenoid Cavity, Right
	Glenoid Cavity, Left
Glenoid ligament (labrum)	Shoulder Joint, Right
	Shoulder Joint, Left
Globus pallidus	Basal Ganglia
Glossoepiglottic fold	Epiglottis
Glottis	Larynx
Gluteal lymph node	Lymphatic, Pelvis
Gluteal vein	Hypogastric Vein, Right
	Hypogastric Vein, Left
Gluteus maximus muscle	Hip Muscle, Right
	Hip Muscle, Left
Gluteus medius muscle	Hip Muscle, Right
	Hip Muscle, Left
Gluteus minimus muscle	Hip Muscle, Right
	Hip Muscle, Left
Gracilis muscle	Upper Leg Muscle, Right
	Upper Leg Muscle, Left
Great auricular nerve	Cervical Plexus
Great cerebral vein	Intracranial Vein
Great(er) saphenous vein	Saphenous Vein, Right
	Saphenous Vein, Left
Greater alar cartilage	Nasal Mucosa and Soft Tissue
Greater occipital nerve	Cervical Nerve
Greater omentum	Omentum
Greater splanchnic nerve	Thoracic Sympathetic Nerve
Greater superficial petrosal nerve	Facial Nerve
Greater trochanter	Upper Femur, Right
	Upper Femur, Left
Greater tuberosity	Humeral Head, Right
	Humeral Head, Left
Greater vestibular (Bartholin's) gland	Vestibular Gland
Greater wing	Sphenoid Bone
Hallux	1st Toe, Right
	1st Toe, Left
Hamate bone	Carpal, Right
	Carpal, Left

Term	ICD-10-PCS Value
Head of fibula	Fibula, Right
	Fibula, Left
Helix	External Ear, Right
	External Ear, Left
	External Ear, Bilateral
Hepatic artery proper	Hepatic Artery
Hepatic flexure	Transverse Colon
Hepatic lymph node	Lymphatic, Aortic
Hepatic plexus	Abdominal Sympathetic Nerve
Hepatic portal vein	Portal Vein
Hepatogastric ligament	Omentum
Hepatopancreatic ampulla	Ampulla of Vater
Humeroradial joint	Elbow Joint, Right
	Elbow Joint, Left
Humeroulnar joint	Elbow Joint, Right
	Elbow Joint, Left
Humerus, distal	Humeral Shaft, Right
	Humeral Shaft, Left
Hyoglossus muscle	Tongue, Palate, Pharynx Muscle
Hyoid artery	Thyroid Artery, Right
	Thyroid Artery, Left
Hypogastric artery	Internal Iliac Artery, Right
	Internal Iliac Artery, Left
Hypopharynx	Pharynx
Hypophysis	Pituitary Gland
Hypothenar muscle	Hand Muscle, Right
	Hand Muscle, Left
Ileal artery	Superior Mesenteric Artery
Ileocolic artery	Superior Mesenteric Artery
Ileocolic vein	Colic Vein
Iliac crest	Pelvic Bone, Right
	Pelvic Bone, Left
Iliac fascia	Subcutaneous Tissue and Fascia, Right Upper Leg
	Subcutaneous Tissue and Fascia, Left Upper Leg
Iliac lymph node	Lymphatic, Pelvis
Iliacus muscle	Hip Muscle, Right
	Hip Muscle, Left
Iliofemoral ligament	Hip Bursa and Ligament, Right
	Hip Bursa and Ligament, Left
Iliohypogastric nerve	Lumbar Plexus
Ilioinguinal nerve	Lumbar Plexus
Iliolumbar artery	Internal Iliac Artery, Right
	Internal Iliac Artery, Left
Iliolumbar ligament	Lower Spine Bursa and Ligament
Iliotibial tract (band)	Subcutaneous Tissue and Fascia, Right Upper Leg
	Subcutaneous Tissue and Fascia, Left Upper Leg
Ilium	Pelvic Bone, Right
	Pelvic Bone, Left

Term	ICD-10-PCS Value
Incus	Auditory Ossicle, Right
	Auditory Ossicle, Left
Inferior cardiac nerve	Thoracic Sympathetic Nerve
Inferior cerebellar vein	Intracranial Vein
Inferior cerebral vein	Intracranial Vein
Inferior epigastric artery	External Iliac Artery, Right
	External Iliac Artery, Left
Inferior epigastric lymph node	Lymphatic, Pelvis
Inferior genicular artery	Popliteal Artery, Right
	Popliteal Artery, Left
Inferior gluteal artery	Internal Iliac Artery, Right
	Internal Iliac Artery, Left
Inferior gluteal nerve	Sacral Plexus
Inferior hypogastric plexus	Abdominal Sympathetic Nerve
Inferior labial artery	Face Artery
Inferior longitudinal muscle	Tongue, Palate, Pharynx Muscle
Inferior mesenteric ganglion	Abdominal Sympathetic Nerve
Inferior mesenteric lymph node	Lymphatic, Mesenteric
Inferior mesenteric plexus	Abdominal Sympathetic Nerve
Inferior oblique muscle	Extraocular Muscle, Right
	Extraocular Muscle, Left
Inferior pancreaticoduo-denal artery	Superior Mesenteric Artery
Inferior phrenic artery	Abdominal Aorta
Inferior rectus muscle	Extraocular Muscle, Right
	Extraocular Muscle, Left
Inferior suprarenal artery	Renal Artery, Right
	Renal Artery, Left
Inferior tarsal plate	Lower Eyelid, Right
	Lower Eyelid, Left
Inferior thyroid vein	Innominate Vein, Right
	Innominate Vein, Left
Inferior tibiofibular joint	Ankle Joint, Right
	Ankle Joint, Left
Inferior turbinate	Nasal Turbinate
Inferior ulnar collateral artery	Brachial Artery, Right
	Brachial Artery, Left
Inferior vesical artery	Internal Iliac Artery, Right
	Internal Iliac Artery, Left
Infraauricular lymph node	Lymphatic, Head
Infraclavicular (deltopectoral) lymph node	Lymphatic, Right Upper Extremity
	Lymphatic, Left Upper Extremity
Infrahyoid muscle	Neck Muscle, Right
	Neck Muscle, Left
Infraparotid lymph node	Lymphatic, Head

Term	ICD-10-PCS Value
Infraspinatus fascia	Subcutaneous Tissue and Fascia, Right Upper Arm
	Subcutaneous Tissue and Fascia, Left Upper Arm
Infraspinatus muscle	Shoulder Muscle, Right
	Shoulder Muscle, Left
Infundibulopelvic ligament	Uterine Supporting Structure
Inguinal canal	Inguinal Region, Right
	Inguinal Region, Left
	Inguinal Region, Bilateral
Inguinal triangle	Inguinal Region, Right
	Inguinal Region, Left
	Inguinal Region, Bilateral
Interatrial septum	Atrial Septum
Intercarpal joint	Carpal Joint, Right
	Carpal Joint, Left
Intercarpal ligament	Hand Bursa and Ligament, Right
	Hand Bursa and Ligament, Left
Interclavicular ligament	Shoulder Bursa and Ligament, Right
	Shoulder Bursa and Ligament, Left
Intercostal lymph node	Lymphatic, Thorax
Intercostal muscle	Thorax Muscle, Right
	Thorax Muscle, Left
Intercostal nerve	Thoracic Nerve
Intercostobrachial nerve	Thoracic Nerve
Intercuneiform joint	Tarsal Joint, Right
	Tarsal Joint, Left
Intercuneiform ligament	Foot Bursa and Ligament, Right
	Foot Bursa and Ligament, Left
Intermediate bronchus	Main Bronchus, Right
Intermediate cuneiform bone	Tarsal, Right
	Tarsal, Left
Internal anal sphincter	Anal Sphincter
Internal (basal) cerebral vein	Intracranial Vein
Internal carotid artery, intracranial portion	Intracranial Artery
Internal carotid plexus	Head and Neck Sympathetic Nerve
Internal iliac vein	Hypogastric Vein, Right
	Hypogastric Vein, Left
Internal maxillary artery	External Carotid Artery, Right
	External Carotid Artery, Left
Internal naris	Nasal Mucosa and Soft Tissue
Internal oblique muscle	Abdomen Muscle, Right
	Abdomen Muscle, Left
Internal pudendal artery	Internal Iliac Artery, Right
	Internal Iliac Artery, Left
Internal pudendal vein	Hypogastric Vein, Right
	Hypogastric Vein, Left

Term	ICD-10-PCS Value
Internal thoracic artery	Internal Mammary Artery, Right
	Internal Mammary Artery, Left
	Subclavian Artery, Right
	Subclavian Artery, Left
Internal urethral sphincter	Urethra
Interphalangeal (IP) joint	Finger Phalangeal Joint, Right
	Finger Phalangeal Joint, Left
	Toe Phalangeal Joint, Right
	Toe Phalangeal Joint, Left
Interphalangeal ligament	Foot Bursa and Ligament, Right
	Foot Bursa and Ligament, Left
	Hand Bursa and Ligament, Right
	Hand Bursa and Ligament, Left
Interspinalis muscle	Trunk Muscle, Right
	Trunk Muscle, Left
Interspinous ligament, cervical	Head and Neck Bursa and Ligament
Interspinous ligament, lumbar	Lower Spine Bursa and Ligament
Interspinous ligament, thoracic	Upper Spine Bursa and Ligament
Intertransversarius muscle	Trunk Muscle, Right
	Trunk Muscle, Left
Intertransverse ligament, cervical	Head and Neck Bursa and Ligament
Intertransverse ligament, lumbar	Lower Spine Bursa and Ligament
Intertransverse ligament, thoracic	Upper Spine Bursa and Ligament
Interventricular foramen (Monro)	Cerebral Ventricle
Interventricular septum	Ventricular Septum
Intestinal lymphatic trunk	Cisterna Chyli
Ischiatic nerve	Sciatic Nerve
Ischiocavernosus muscle	Perineum Muscle
Ischiofemoral ligament	Hip Bursa and Ligament, Right
	Hip Bursa and Ligament, Left
Ischium	Pelvic Bone, Right
	Pelvic Bone, Left
Jejunal artery	Superior Mesenteric Artery
Jugular body	Glomus Jugulare
Jugular lymph node	Lymphatic, Right Neck
	Lymphatic, Left Neck
Labia majora	Vulva
Labia minora	Vulva
Labial gland	Upper Lip
	Lower Lip
Lacrimal canaliculus	Lacrimal Duct, Right
	Lacrimal Duct, Left
Lacrimal punctum	Lacrimal Duct, Right
	Lacrimal Duct, Left

Term	ICD-10-PCS Value
Lacrimal sac	Lacrimal Duct, Right
	Lacrimal Duct, Left
Laryngopharynx	Pharynx
Lateral (brachial) lymph node	Lymphatic, Right Axillary
	Lymphatic, Left Axillary
Lateral canthus	Upper Eyelid, Right
	Upper Eyelid, Left
Lateral collateral ligament (LCL)	Knee Bursa and Ligament, Right
	Knee Bursa and Ligament, Left
Lateral condyle of femur	Lower Femur, Right
	Lower Femur, Left
Lateral condyle of tibia	Tibia, Right
	Tibia, Left
Lateral cuneiform bone	Tarsal, Right
	Tarsal, Left
Lateral epicondyle of femur	Lower Femur, Right
	Lower Femur, Left
Lateral epicondyle of humerus	Humeral Shaft, Right
	Humeral Shaft, Left
Lateral femoral cutaneous nerve	Lumbar Plexus
Lateral malleolus	Fibula, Right
	Fibula, Left
Lateral meniscus	Knee Joint, Right
	Knee Joint, Left
Lateral nasal cartilage	Nasal Mucosa and Soft Tissue
Lateral plantar artery	Foot Artery, Right
	Foot Artery, Left
Lateral plantar nerve	Tibial Nerve
Lateral rectus muscle	Extraocular Muscle, Right
	Extraocular Muscle, Left
Lateral sacral artery	Internal Iliac Artery, Right
	Internal Iliac Artery, Left
Lateral sacral vein	Hypogastric Vein, Right
	Hypogastric Vein, Left
Lateral sural cutaneous nerve	Peroneal Nerve
Lateral tarsal artery	Foot Artery, Right
	Foot Artery, Left
Lateral temporo-mandibular ligament	Head and Neck Bursa and Ligament
Lateral thoracic artery	Axillary Artery, Right
	Axillary Artery, Left
Latissimus dorsi muscle	Trunk Muscle, Right
	Trunk Muscle, Left
Least splanchnic nerve	Thoracic Sympathetic Nerve
Left ascending lumbar vein	Hemiazygos Vein
Left atrioventricular valve	Mitral Valve
Left auricular appendix	Atrium, Left
Left colic vein	Colic Vein
Left coronary sulcus	Heart, Left
Left gastric artery	Gastric Artery

Term	ICD-10-PCS Value
Left gastroepiploic artery	Splenic Artery
Left gastroepiploic vein	Splenic Vein
Left inferior phrenic vein	Renal Vein, Left
Left inferior pulmonary vein	Pulmonary Vein, Left
Left jugular trunk	Thoracic Duct
Left lateral ventricle	Cerebral Ventricle
Left ovarian vein	Renal Vein, Left
Left second lumbar vein	Renal Vein, Left
Left subclavian trunk	Thoracic Duct
Left subcostal vein	Hemiazygos Vein
Left superior pulmonary vein	Pulmonary Vein, Left
Left suprarenal vein	Renal Vein, Left
Left testicular vein	Renal Vein, Left
Leptomeninges, intracranial	Cerebral Meninges
Leptomeninges, spinal	Spinal Meninges
Lesser alar cartilage	Nasal Mucosa and Soft Tissue
Lesser occipital nerve	Cervical Plexus
Lesser omentum	Omentum
Lesser saphenous vein	Saphenous Vein, Right
	Saphenous Vein, Left
Lesser splanchnic nerve	Thoracic Sympathetic Nerve
Lesser trochanter	Upper Femur, Right
	Upper Femur, Left
Lesser tuberosity	Humeral Head, Right
	Humeral Head, Left
Lesser wing	Sphenoid Bone
Levator anguli oris muscle	Facial Muscle
Levator ani muscle	Perineum Muscle
Levator labii superioris alaeque nasi muscle	Facial Muscle
Levator labii superioris muscle	Facial Muscle
Levator palpebrae superioris muscle	Upper Eyelid, Right
	Upper Eyelid, Left
Levator scapulae muscle	Neck Muscle, Right
	Neck Muscle, Left
Levator veli palatini muscle	Tongue, Palate, Pharynx Muscle
Levatores costarum muscle	Thorax Muscle, Right
	Thorax Muscle, Left
Ligament of head of fibula	Knee Bursa and Ligament, Right
	Knee Bursa and Ligament, Left
Ligament of the lateral malleolus	Ankle Bursa and Ligament, Right
	Ankle Bursa and Ligament, Left
Ligamentum flavum, cervical	Head and Neck Bursa and Ligament
Ligamentum flavum, lumbar	Lower Spine Bursa and Ligament
Ligamentum flavum, thoracic	Upper Spine Bursa and Ligament

Term	ICD-10-PCS Value
Lingual artery	External Carotid Artery, Right
	External Carotid Artery, Left
Lingual tonsil	Pharynx
Locus ceruleus	Pons
Long thoracic nerve	Brachial Plexus
Lumbar artery	Abdominal Aorta
Lumbar facet joint	Lumbar Vertebral Joint
Lumbar ganglion	Lumbar Sympathetic Nerve
Lumbar lymph node	Lymphatic, Aortic
Lumbar lymphatic trunk	Cisterna Chyli
Lumbar splanchnic nerve	Lumbar Sympathetic Nerve
Lumbosacral facet joint	Lumbosacral Joint
Lumbosacral trunk	Lumbar Nerve
Lunate bone	Carpal, Right
	Carpal, Left
Lunotriquetral ligament	Hand Bursa and Ligament, Right
	Hand Bursa and Ligament, Left
Macula	Retina, Right
	Retina, Left
Malleus	Auditory Ossicle, Right
	Auditory Ossicle, Left
Mammary duct	Breast, Right
	Breast, Left
	Breast, Bilateral
Mammary gland	Breast, Right
	Breast, Left
	Breast, Bilateral
Mammillary body	Hypothalamus
Mandibular nerve	Trigeminal Nerve
Mandibular notch	Mandible, Right
	Mandible, Left
Manubrium	Sternum
Masseter muscle	Head Muscle
Masseteric fascia	Subcutaneous Tissue and Fascia, Face
Mastoid (postauricular) lymph node	Lymphatic, Right Neck
	Lymphatic, Left Neck
Mastoid air cells	Mastoid Sinus, Right
	Mastoid Sinus, Left
Mastoid process	Temporal Bone, Right
	Temporal Bone, Left
Maxillary artery	External Carotid Artery, Right
	External Carotid Artery, Left
Maxillary nerve	Trigeminal Nerve
Medial canthus	Lower Eyelid, Right
	Lower Eyelid, Left
Medial collateral ligament (MCL)	Knee Bursa and Ligament, Right
	Knee Bursa and Ligament, Left
Medial condyle of femur	Lower Femur, Right
	Lower Femur, Left
Medial condyle of tibia	Tibia, Right
	Tibia, Left

Term	ICD-10-PCS Value
Medial cuneiform bone	Tarsal, Right
	Tarsal, Left
Medial epicondyle of femur	Lower Femur, Right
	Lower Femur, Left
Medial epicondyle of humerus	Humeral Shaft, Right
	Humeral Shaft, Left
Medial malleolus	Tibia, Right
	Tibia, Left
Medial meniscus	Knee Joint, Right
	Knee Joint, Left
Medial plantar artery	Foot Artery, Right
	Foot Artery, Left
Medial plantar nerve	Tibial Nerve
Medial popliteal nerve	Tibial Nerve
Medial rectus muscle	Extraocular Muscle, Right
	Extraocular Muscle, Left
Medial sural cutaneous nerve	Tibial Nerve
Median antebrachial vein	Basilic Vein, Right
	Basilic Vein, Left
Median cubital vein	Basilic Vein, Right
	Basilic Vein, Left
Median sacral artery	Abdominal Aorta
Mediastinal cavity	Mediastinum
Mediastinal lymph node	Lymphatic, Thorax
Mediastinal space	Mediastinum
Meissner's (submucous) plexus	Abdominal Sympathetic Nerve
Membranous urethra	Urethra
Mental foramen	Mandible, Right
	Mandible, Left
Mentalis muscle	Facial Muscle
Mesoappendix	Mesentery
Mesocolon	Mesentery
Metacarpal ligament	Hand Bursa and Ligament, Right
	Hand Bursa and Ligament, Left
Metacarpophalangeal ligament	Hand Bursa and Ligament, Right
	Hand Bursa and Ligament, Left
Metatarsal ligament	Foot Bursa and Ligament, Right
	Foot Bursa and Ligament, Left
Metatarsophalangeal ligament	Foot Bursa and Ligament, Right
	Foot Bursa and Ligament, Left
Metatarsophalangeal (MTP) joint	Metatarsal-Phalangeal Joint, Right
	Metatarsal-Phalangeal Joint, Left
Metathalamus	Thalamus
Midcarpal joint	Carpal Joint, Right
	Carpal Joint, Left
Middle cardiac nerve	Thoracic Sympathetic Nerve
Middle cerebral artery	Intracranial Artery
Middle cerebral vein	Intracranial Vein
Middle colic vein	Colic Vein

Term	ICD-10-PCS Value
Middle genicular artery	Popliteal Artery, Right
	Popliteal Artery, Left
Middle hemorrhoidal vein	Hypogastric Vein, Right
	Hypogastric Vein, Left
Middle rectal artery	Internal Iliac Artery, Right
	Internal Iliac Artery, Left
Middle suprarenal artery	Abdominal Aorta
Middle temporal artery	Temporal Artery, Right
	Temporal Artery, Left
Middle turbinate	Nasal Turbinate
Mitral annulus	Mitral Valve
Molar gland	Buccal Mucosa
Musculocutaneous nerve	Brachial Plexus
Musculophrenic artery	Internal Mammary Artery, Right
	Internal Mammary Artery, Left
Musculospiral nerve	Radial Nerve
Myelencephalon	Medulla Oblongata
Myenteric (Auerbach's) plexus	Abdominal Sympathetic Nerve
Myometrium	Uterus
Nail bed	Finger Nail
	Toe Nail
Nail plate	Finger Nail
	Toe Nail
Nasal cavity	Nasal Mucosa and Soft Tissue
Nasal concha	Nasal Turbinate
Nasalis muscle	Facial Muscle
Nasolacrimal duct	Lacrimal Duct, Right
	Lacrimal Duct, Left
Navicular bone	Tarsal, Right
	Tarsal, Left
Neck of femur	Upper Femur, Right
	Upper Femur, Left
Neck of humerus (anatomical) (surgical)	Humeral Head, Right
	Humeral Head, Left
Nerve to the stapedius	Facial Nerve
Neurohypophysis	Pituitary Gland
Ninth cranial nerve	Glossopharyngeal Nerve
Nostril	Nasal Mucosa and Soft Tissue
Obturator artery	Internal Iliac Artery, Right
	Internal Iliac Artery, Left
Obturator lymph node	Lymphatic, Pelvis
Obturator muscle	Hip Muscle, Right
	Hip Muscle, Left
Obturator nerve	Lumbar Plexus
Obturator vein	Hypogastric Vein, Right
	Hypogastric Vein, Left
Obtuse margin	Heart, Left
Occipital artery	External Carotid Artery, Right
	External Carotid Artery, Left
Occipital lobe	Cerebral Hemisphere

Term	ICD-10-PCS Value
Occipital lymph node	Lymphatic, Right Neck
	Lymphatic, Left Neck
Occipitofrontalis muscle	Facial Muscle
Odontoid process	Cervical Vertebra
Olecranon bursa	Elbow Bursa and Ligament, Right
	Elbow Bursa and Ligament, Left
Olecranon process	Ulna, Right
	Ulna, Left
Olfactory bulb	Olfactory Nerve
Ophthalmic artery	Intracranial Artery
Ophthalmic nerve	Trigeminal Nerve
Ophthalmic vein	Intracranial Vein
Optic chiasma	Optic Nerve
Optic disc	Retina, Right
	Retina, Left
Optic foramen	Sphenoid Bone
Orbicularis oculi muscle	Upper Eyelid, Right
	Upper Eyelid, Left
Orbicularis oris muscle	Facial Muscle
Orbital fascia	Subcutaneous Tissue and Fascia, Face
Orbital portion of ethmoid bone	Orbit, Right
	Orbit, Left
Orbital portion of frontal bone	Orbit, Right
	Orbit, Left
Orbital portion of lacrimal bone	Orbit, Right
	Orbit, Left
Orbital portion of maxilla	Orbit, Right
	Orbit, Left
Orbital portion of palatine bone	Orbit, Right
	Orbit, Left
Orbital portion of sphenoid bone	Orbit, Right
	Orbit, Left
Orbital portion of zygomatic bone	Orbit, Right
	Orbit, Left
Oropharynx	Pharynx
Otic ganglion	Head and Neck Sympathetic Nerve
Oval window	Middle Ear, Right
	Middle Ear, Left
Ovarian artery	Abdominal Aorta
Ovarian ligament	Uterine Supporting Structure
Oviduct	Fallopian Tube, Right
	Fallopian Tube, Left
Palatine gland	Buccal Mucosa
Palatine tonsil	Tonsils
Palatine uvula	Uvula
Palatoglossal muscle	Tongue, Palate, Pharynx Muscle
Palatopharyngeal muscle	Tongue, Palate, Pharynx Muscle
Palmar (volar) digital vein	Hand Vein, Right
	Hand Vein, Left
Palmar (volar) metacarpal vein	Hand Vein, Right
	Hand Vein, Left

Term	ICD-10-PCS Value
Palmar cutaneous nerve	Median Nerve
	Radial Nerve
Palmar fascia (aponeurosis)	Subcutaneous Tissue and Fascia, Right Hand
	Subcutaneous Tissue and Fascia, Left Hand
Palmar interosseous muscle	Hand Muscle, Right
	Hand Muscle, Left
Palmar ulnocarpal ligament	Wrist Bursa and Ligament, Right
	Wrist Bursa and Ligament, Left
Palmaris longus muscle	Lower Arm and Wrist Muscle, Right
	Lower Arm and Wrist Muscle, Left
Pancreatic artery	Splenic Artery
Pancreatic plexus	Abdominal Sympathetic Nerve
Pancreatic vein	Splenic Vein
Pancreaticosplenic lymph node	Lymphatic, Aortic
Paraaortic lymph node	Lymphatic, Aortic
Pararectal lymph node	Lymphatic, Mesenteric
Parasternal lymph node	Lymphatic, Thorax
Paratracheal lymph node	Lymphatic, Thorax
Paraurethral (Skene's) gland	Vestibular Gland
Parietal lobe	Cerebral Hemisphere
Parotid lymph node	Lymphatic, Head
Parotid plexus	Facial Nerve
Pars flaccida	Tympanic Membrane, Right
	Tympanic Membrane, Left
Patellar ligament	Knee Bursa and Ligament, Right
	Knee Bursa and Ligament, Left
Patellar tendon	Knee Tendon, Right
	Knee Tendon, Left
Patellofemoral joint	Knee Joint, Right
	Knee Joint, Left
	Knee Joint, Femoral Surface, Right
	Knee Joint, Femoral Surface, Left
Pectineus muscle	Upper Leg Muscle, Right
	Upper Leg Muscle, Left
Pectoral (anterior) lymph node	Lymphatic, Right Axillary
	Lymphatic, Left Axillary
Pectoral fascia	Subcutaneous Tissue and Fascia, Chest
Pectoralis major muscle	Thorax Muscle, Right
	Thorax Muscle, Left
Pectoralis minor muscle	Thorax Muscle, Right
	Thorax Muscle, Left
Pelvic splanchnic nerve	Abdominal Sympathetic Nerve
	Sacral Sympathetic Nerve
Penile urethra	Urethra
Pericardiophrenic artery	Internal Mammary Artery, Right
	Internal Mammary Artery, Left
Perimetrium	Uterus

Term	ICD-10-PCS Value
Peroneus brevis muscle	Lower Leg Muscle, Right
	Lower Leg Muscle, Left
Peroneus longus muscle	Lower Leg Muscle, Right
	Lower Leg Muscle, Left
Petrous part of temporal bone	Temporal Bone, Right
	Temporal Bone, Left
Pharyngeal constrictor muscle	Tongue, Palate, Pharynx Muscle
Pharyngeal plexus	Vagus Nerve
Pharyngeal recess	Nasopharynx
Pharyngeal tonsil	Adenoids
Pharyngotympanic tube	Eustachian Tube, Right
	Eustachian Tube, Left
Pia mater, intracranial	Cerebral Meninges
Pia mater, spinal	Spinal Meninges
Pinna	External Ear, Right
	External Ear, Left
	External Ear, Bilateral
Piriform recess (sinus)	Pharynx
Piriformis muscle	Hip Muscle, Right
	Hip Muscle, Left
Pisiform bone	Carpal, Right
	Carpal, Left
Pisohamate ligament	Hand Bursa and Ligament, Right
	Hand Bursa and Ligament, Left
Pisometacarpal ligament	Hand Bursa and Ligament, Right
	Hand Bursa and Ligament, Left
Plantar digital vein	Foot Vein, Right
	Foot Vein, Left
Plantar fascia (aponeurosis)	Subcutaneous Tissue and Fascia, Right Foot
	Subcutaneous Tissue and Fascia, Left Foot
Plantar metatarsal vein	Foot Vein, Right
	Foot Vein, Left
Plantar venous arch	Foot Vein, Right
	Foot Vein, Left
Platysma muscle	Neck Muscle, Right
	Neck Muscle, Left
Plica semilunaris	Conjunctiva, Right
	Conjunctiva, Left
Pneumogastric nerve	Vagus Nerve
Pneumotaxic center	Pons
Pontine tegmentum	Pons
Popliteal ligament	Knee Bursa and Ligament, Right
	Knee Bursa and Ligament, Left
Popliteal lymph node	Lymphatic, Left Lower Extremity
	Lymphatic, Right Lower Extremity
Popliteal vein	Femoral Vein, Right
	Femoral Vein, Left
Popliteus muscle	Lower Leg Muscle, Right
	Lower Leg Muscle, Left

Term	ICD-10-PCS Value
Postauricular (mastoid) lymph node	Lymphatic, Right Neck
	Lymphatic, Left Neck
Postcava	Inferior Vena Cava
Posterior (subscapular) lymph node	Lymphatic, Right Axillary
	Lymphatic, Left Axillary
Posterior auricular artery	External Carotid Artery, Right
	External Carotid Artery, Left
Posterior auricular nerve	Facial Nerve
Posterior auricular vein	External Jugular Vein, Right
	External Jugular Vein, Left
Posterior cerebral artery	Intracranial Artery
Posterior chamber	Eye, Right
	Eye, Left
Posterior circumflex humeral artery	Axillary Artery, Right
	Axillary Artery, Left
Posterior communicating artery	Intracranial Artery
Posterior cruciate ligament (PCL)	Knee Bursa and Ligament, Right
	Knee Bursa and Ligament, Left
Posterior facial (retromandibular) vein	Face Vein, Right
	Face Vein, Left
Posterior femoral cutaneous nerve	Sacral Plexus
Posterior inferior cerebellar artery (PICA)	Intracranial Artery
Posterior interosseous nerve	Radial Nerve
Posterior labial nerve	Pudendal Nerve
Posterior scrotal nerve	Pudendal Nerve
Posterior spinal artery	Vertebral Artery, Right
	Vertebral Artery, Left
Posterior tibial recurrent artery	Anterior Tibial Artery, Right
	Anterior Tibial Artery, Left
Posterior ulnar recurrent artery	Ulnar Artery, Right
	Ulnar Artery, Left
Posterior vagal trunk	Vagus Nerve
Preauricular lymph node	Lymphatic, Head
Precava	Superior Vena Cava
Prepatellar bursa	Knee Bursa and Ligament, Right
	Knee Bursa and Ligament, Left
Pretracheal fascia	Subcutaneous Tissue and Fascia, Right Neck
	Subcutaneous Tissue and Fascia, Left Neck
Prevertebral fascia	Subcutaneous Tissue and Fascia, Right Neck
	Subcutaneous Tissue and Fascia, Left Neck
Princeps pollicis artery	Hand Artery, Right
	Hand Artery, Left
Procerus muscle	Facial Muscle

Term	ICD-10-PCS Value
Profunda brachii	Brachial Artery, Right
	Brachial Artery, Left
Profunda femoris (deep femoral) vein	Femoral Vein, Right
	Femoral Vein, Left
Pronator quadratus muscle	Lower Arm and Wrist Muscle, Right
	Lower Arm and Wrist Muscle, Left
Pronator teres muscle	Lower Arm and Wrist Muscle, Right
	Lower Arm and Wrist Muscle, Left
Prostatic urethra	Urethra
Proximal radioulnar joint	Elbow Joint, Right
	Elbow Joint, Left
Psoas muscle	Hip Muscle, Right
	Hip Muscle, Left
Pterygoid muscle	Head Muscle
Pterygoid process	Sphenoid Bone
Pterygopalatine (sphenopalatine) ganglion	Head and Neck Sympathetic Nerve
Pubis	Pelvic Bone, Right
	Pelvic Bone, Left
Pubofemoral ligament	Hip Bursa and Ligament, Right
	Hip Bursa and Ligament, Left
Pudendal nerve	Sacral Plexus
Pulmoaortic canal	Pulmonary Artery, Left
Pulmonary annulus	Pulmonary Valve
Pulmonary plexus	Thoracic Sympathetic Nerve
	Vagus Nerve
Pulmonic valve	Pulmonary Valve
Pulvinar	Thalamus
Pyloric antrum	Stomach, Pylorus
Pyloric canal	Stomach, Pylorus
Pyloric sphincter	Stomach, Pylorus
Pyramidalis muscle	Abdomen Muscle, Right
	Abdomen Muscle, Left
Quadrangular cartilage	Nasal Septum
Quadrate lobe	Liver
Quadratus femoris muscle	Hip Muscle, Right
	Hip Muscle, Left
Quadratus lumborum muscle	Trunk Muscle, Right
	Trunk Muscle, Left
Quadratus plantae muscle	Foot Muscle, Right
	Foot Muscle, Left
Quadriceps (femoris)	Upper Leg Muscle, Right
	Upper Leg Muscle, Left
Radial collateral carpal ligament	Wrist Bursa and Ligament, Right
	Wrist Bursa and Ligament, Left
Radial collateral ligament	Elbow Bursa and Ligament, Right
	Elbow Bursa and Ligament, Left
Radial notch	Ulna, Right
	Ulna, Left
Radial recurrent artery	Radial Artery, Right
	Radial Artery, Left

Term	ICD-10-PCS Value
Radial vein	Brachial Vein, Right
	Brachial Vein, Left
Radialis indicis	Hand Artery, Right
	Hand Artery, Left
Radiocarpal joint	Wrist Joint, Right
	Wrist Joint, Left
Radiocarpal ligament	Wrist Bursa and Ligament, Right
	Wrist Bursa and Ligament, Left
Radioulnar ligament	Wrist Bursa and Ligament, Right
	Wrist Bursa and Ligament, Left
Rectosigmoid junction	Sigmoid Colon
Rectus abdominis muscle	Abdomen Muscle, Right
	Abdomen Muscle, Left
Rectus femoris muscle	Upper Leg Muscle, Right
	Upper Leg Muscle, Left
Recurrent laryngeal nerve	Vagus Nerve
Renal calyx	Kidney, Right
	Kidney, Left
	Kidneys, Bilateral
	Kidney
Renal capsule	Kidney, Right
	Kidney, Left
	Kidneys, Bilateral
	Kidney
Renal cortex	Kidney, Right
	Kidney, Left
	Kidneys, Bilateral
	Kidney
Renal plexus	Abdominal Sympathetic Nerve
Renal segment	Kidney, Right
	Kidney, Left
	Kidneys, Bilateral
	Kidney
Renal segmental artery	Renal Artery, Right
	Renal Artery, Left
Retroperitoneal cavity	Retroperitoneum
Retroperitoneal lymph node	Lymphatic, Aortic
Retroperitoneal space	Retroperitoneum
Retropharyngeal lymph node	Lymphatic, Right Neck
	Lymphatic, Left Neck
Retropubic space	Pelvic Cavity
Rhinopharynx	Nasopharynx
Rhomboid major muscle	Trunk Muscle, Right
	Trunk Muscle, Left
Rhomboid minor muscle	Trunk Muscle, Right
	Trunk Muscle, Left
Right ascending lumbar vein	Azygos Vein
Right atrioventricular valve	Tricuspid Valve
Right auricular appendix	Atrium, Right

Term	ICD-10-PCS Value
Right colic vein	Colic Vein
Right coronary sulcus	Heart, Right
Right gastric artery	Gastric Artery
Right gastroepiploic vein	Superior Mesenteric Vein
Right inferior phrenic vein	Inferior Vena Cava
Right inferior pulmonary vein	Pulmonary Vein, Right
Right jugular trunk	Lymphatic, Right Neck
Right lateral ventricle	Cerebral Ventricle
Right lymphatic duct	Lymphatic, Right Neck
Right ovarian vein	Inferior Vena Cava
Right second lumbar vein	Inferior Vena Cava
Right subclavian trunk	Lymphatic, Right Neck
Right subcostal vein	Azygos Vein
Right superior pulmonary vein	Pulmonary Vein, Right
Right suprarenal vein	Inferior Vena Cava
Right testicular vein	Inferior Vena Cava
Rima glottidis	Larynx
Risorius muscle	Facial Muscle
Round ligament of uterus	Uterine Supporting Structure
Round window	Inner Ear, Right
	Inner Ear, Left
Sacral ganglion	Sacral Sympathetic Nerve
Sacral lymph node	Lymphatic, Pelvis
Sacral splanchnic nerve	Sacral Sympathetic Nerve
Sacrococcygeal ligament	Lower Spine Bursa and Ligament
Sacrococcygeal symphysis	Sacrococcygeal Joint
Sacroiliac ligament	Lower Spine Bursa and Ligament
Sacrospinous ligament	Lower Spine Bursa and Ligament
Sacrotuberous ligament	Lower Spine Bursa and Ligament
Salpingopharyngeus muscle	Tongue, Palate, Pharynx Muscle
Salpinx	Fallopian Tube, Right
	Fallopian Tube, Left
Saphenous nerve	Femoral Nerve
Sartorius muscle	Upper Leg Muscle, Right
	Upper Leg Muscle, Left
Scalene muscle	Neck Muscle, Right
	Neck Muscle, Left
Scaphoid bone	Carpal, Right
	Carpal, Left
Scapholunate ligament	Hand Bursa and Ligament, Right
	Hand Bursa and Ligament, Left
Scaphotrapezium ligament	Hand Bursa and Ligament, Right
	Hand Bursa and Ligament, Left
Scarpa's (vestibular) ganglion	Acoustic Nerve
Sebaceous gland	Skin

Term	ICD-10-PCS Value
Second cranial nerve	Optic Nerve
Sella turcica	Sphenoid Bone
Semicircular canal	Inner Ear, Right
	Inner Ear, Left
Semimembranosus muscle	Upper Leg Muscle, Right
	Upper Leg Muscle, Left
Semitendinosus muscle	Upper Leg Muscle, Right
	Upper Leg Muscle, Left
Septal cartilage	Nasal Septum
Serratus anterior muscle	Thorax Muscle, Right
	Thorax Muscle, Left
Serratus posterior muscle	Trunk Muscle, Right
	Trunk Muscle, Left
Seventh cranial nerve	Facial Nerve
Short gastric artery	Splenic Artery
Sigmoid artery	Inferior Mesenteric Artery
Sigmoid flexure	Sigmoid Colon
Sigmoid vein	Inferior Mesenteric Vein
Sinoatrial node	Conduction Mechanism
Sinus venosus	Atrium, Right
Sixth cranial nerve	Abducens Nerve
Skene's (paraurethral) gland	Vestibular Gland
Small saphenous vein	Saphenous Vein, Right
	Saphenous Vein, Left
Solar (celiac) plexus	Abdominal Sympathetic Nerve
Soleus muscle	Lower Leg Muscle, Right
	Lower Leg Muscle, Left
Sphenomandibular ligament	Head and Neck Bursa and Ligament
Sphenopalatine (pterygopalatine) ganglion	Head and Neck Sympathetic Nerve
Spinal nerve, cervical	Cervical Nerve
Spinal nerve, lumbar	Lumbar Nerve
Spinal nerve, sacral	Sacral Nerve
Spinal nerve, thoracic	Thoracic Nerve
Spinous process	Cervical Vertebra
	Lumbar Vertebra
	Thoracic Vertebra
Spiral ganglion	Acoustic Nerve
Splenic flexure	Transverse Colon
Splenic plexus	Abdominal Sympathetic Nerve
Splenius capitis muscle	Head Muscle
Splenius cervicis muscle	Neck Muscle, Right
	Neck Muscle, Left
Stapes	Auditory Ossicle, Right
	Auditory Ossicle, Left
Stellate ganglion	Head and Neck Sympathetic Nerve
Stensen's duct	Parotid Duct, Right
	Parotid Duct, Left
Sternoclavicular ligament	Shoulder Bursa and Ligament, Right
	Shoulder Bursa and Ligament, Left

Term	ICD-10-PCS Value
Sternocleidomastoid artery	Thyroid Artery, Right
	Thyroid Artery, Left
Sternocleidomastoid muscle	Neck Muscle, Right
	Neck Muscle, Left
Sternocostal ligament	Sternum Bursa and Ligament
Styloglossus muscle	Tongue, Palate, Pharynx Muscle
Stylomandibular ligament	Head and Neck Bursa and Ligament
Stylopharyngeus muscle	Tongue, Palate, Pharynx Muscle
Subacromial bursa	Shoulder Bursa and Ligament, Right
	Shoulder Bursa and Ligament, Left
Subaortic (common iliac) lymph node	Lymphatic, Pelvis
Subarachnoid space, spinal	Spinal Canal
Subclavicular (apical) lymph node	Lymphatic, Right Axillary
	Lymphatic, Left Axillary
Subclavius muscle	Thorax Muscle, Right
	Thorax Muscle, Left
Subclavius nerve	Brachial Plexus
Subcostal artery	Upper Artery
Subcostal muscle	Thorax Muscle, Right
	Thorax Muscle, Left
Subcostal nerve	Thoracic Nerve
Subdural space, spinal	Spinal Canal
Submandibular ganglion	Facial Nerve
	Head and Neck Sympathetic Nerve
Submandibular gland	Submaxillary Gland, Right
	Submaxillary Gland, Left
Submandibular lymph node	Lymphatic, Head
Submaxillary ganglion	Head and Neck Sympathetic Nerve
Submaxillary lymph node	Lymphatic, Head
Submental artery	Face Artery
Submental lymph node	Lymphatic, Head
Submucous (Meissner's) plexus	Abdominal Sympathetic Nerve
Suboccipital nerve	Cervical Nerve
Suboccipital venous plexus	Vertebral Vein, Right
	Vertebral Vein, Left
Subparotid lymph node	Lymphatic, Head
Subscapular aponeurosis	Subcutaneous Tissue and Fascia, Right Upper Arm
	Subcutaneous Tissue and Fascia, Left Upper Arm
Subscapular artery	Axillary Artery, Right
	Axillary Artery, Left
Subscapular (posterior) lymph node	Lymphatic, Right Axillary
	Lymphatic, Left Axillary
Subscapularis muscle	Shoulder Muscle, Right
	Shoulder Muscle, Left
Substantia nigra	Basal Ganglia

Term	ICD-10-PCS Value
Subtalar (talocalcaneal) joint	Tarsal Joint, Right
	Tarsal Joint, Left
Subtalar ligament	Foot Bursa and Ligament, Right
	Foot Bursa and Ligament, Left
Subthalamic nucleus	Basal Ganglia
Superficial circumflex iliac vein	Saphenous Vein, Right
	Saphenous Vein, Left
Superficial epigastric artery	Femoral Artery, Right
	Femoral Artery, Left
Superficial epigastric vein	Saphenous Vein, Right
	Saphenous Vein, Left
Superficial palmar arch	Hand Artery, Right
	Hand Artery, Left
Superficial palmar venous arch	Hand Vein, Right
	Hand Vein, Left
Superficial temporal artery	Temporal Artery, Right
	Temporal Artery, Left
Superficial transverse perineal muscle	Perineum Muscle
Superior cardiac nerve	Thoracic Sympathetic Nerve
Superior cerebellar vein	Intracranial Vein
Superior cerebral vein	Intracranial Vein
Superior clunic (cluneal) nerve	Lumbar Nerve
Superior epigastric artery	Internal Mammary Artery, Right
	Internal Mammary Artery, Left
Superior genicular artery	Popliteal Artery, Right
	Popliteal Artery, Left
Superior gluteal artery	Internal Iliac Artery, Right
	Internal Iliac Artery, Left
Superior gluteal nerve	Lumbar Plexus
Superior hypogastric plexus	Abdominal Sympathetic Nerve
Superior labial artery	Face Artery
Superior laryngeal artery	Thyroid Artery, Right
	Thyroid Artery, Left
Superior laryngeal nerve	Vagus Nerve
Superior longitudinal muscle	Tongue, Palate, Pharynx Muscle
Superior mesenteric ganglion	Abdominal Sympathetic Nerve
Superior mesenteric lymph node	Lymphatic, Mesenteric
Superior mesenteric plexus	Abdominal Sympathetic Nerve
Superior oblique muscle	Extraocular Muscle, Right
	Extraocular Muscle, Left
Superior olivary nucleus	Pons
Superior rectal artery	Inferior Mesenteric Artery
Superior rectal vein	Inferior Mesenteric Vein
Superior rectus muscle	Extraocular Muscle, Right
	Extraocular Muscle, Left

Term	ICD-10-PCS Value
Superior tarsal plate	Upper Eyelid, Right
	Upper Eyelid, Left
Superior thoracic artery	Axillary Artery, Right
	Axillary Artery, Left
Superior thyroid artery	External Carotid Artery, Right
	External Carotid Artery, Left
	Thyroid Artery, Right
	Thyroid Artery, Left
Superior turbinate	Nasal Turbinate
Superior ulnar collateral artery	Brachial Artery, Right
	Brachial Artery, Left
Supraclavicular nerve	Cervical Plexus
Supraclavicular (Virchow's) lymph node	Lymphatic, Right Neck
	Lymphatic, Left Neck
Suprahyoid lymph node	Lymphatic, Head
Suprahyoid muscle	Neck Muscle, Right
	Neck Muscle, Left
Suprainguinal lymph node	Lymphatic, Pelvis
Supraorbital vein	Face Vein, Right
	Face Vein, Left
Suprarenal gland	Adrenal Gland, Right
	Adrenal Gland, Left
	Adrenal Glands, Bilateral
	Adrenal Gland
Suprarenal plexus	Abdominal Sympathetic Nerve
Suprascapular nerve	Brachial Plexus
Supraspinatus fascia	Subcutaneous Tissue and Fascia, Right Upper Arm
	Subcutaneous Tissue and Fascia, Left Upper Arm
Supraspinatus muscle	Shoulder Muscle, Right
	Shoulder Muscle, Left
Supraspinous ligament	Upper Spine Bursa and Ligament
	Lower Spine Bursa and Ligament
Suprasternal notch	Sternum
Supratrochlear lymph node	Lymphatic, Right Upper Extremity
	Lymphatic, Left Upper Extremity
Sural artery	Popliteal Artery, Right
	Popliteal Artery, Left
Sweat gland	Skin
Talocalcaneal ligament	Foot Bursa and Ligament, Right
	Foot Bursa and Ligament, Left
Talocalcaneal (subtalar) joint	Tarsal Joint, Right
	Tarsal Joint, Left
Talocalcaneonavicular joint	Tarsal Joint, Right
	Tarsal Joint, Left
Talocalcaneonavicular ligament	Foot Bursa and Ligament, Right
	Foot Bursa and Ligament, Left
Talocrural joint	Ankle Joint, Right
	Ankle Joint, Left
Talofibular ligament	Ankle Bursa and Ligament, Right
	Ankle Bursa and Ligament, Left

Term	ICD-10-PCS Value
Talus bone	Tarsal, Right
	Tarsal, Left
Tarsometatarsal ligament	Foot Bursa and Ligament, Right
	Foot Bursa and Ligament, Left
Temporal lobe	Cerebral Hemisphere
Temporalis muscle	Head Muscle
Temporoparietalis muscle	Head Muscle
Tensor fasciae latae muscle	Hip Muscle, Right
	Hip Muscle, Left
Tensor veli palatini muscle	Tongue, Palate, Pharynx Muscle
Tenth cranial nerve	Vagus Nerve
Tentorium cerebelli	Dura Mater
Teres major muscle	Shoulder Muscle, Right
	Shoulder Muscle, Left
Teres minor muscle	Shoulder Muscle, Right
	Shoulder Muscle, Left
Testicular artery	Abdominal Aorta
Thenar muscle	Hand Muscle, Right
	Hand Muscle, Left
Third cranial nerve	Oculomotor Nerve
Third occipital nerve	Cervical Nerve
Third ventricle	Cerebral Ventricle
Thoracic aortic plexus	Thoracic Sympathetic Nerve
Thoracic esophagus	Esophagus, Middle
Thoracic facet joint	Thoracic Vertebral Joint
Thoracic ganglion	Thoracic Sympathetic Nerve
Thoracoacromial artery	Axillary Artery, Right
	Axillary Artery, Left
Thoracolumbar facet joint	Thoracolumbar Vertebral Joint
Thymus gland	Thymus
Thyroarytenoid muscle	Neck Muscle, Right
	Neck Muscle, Left
Thyrocervical trunk	Thyroid Artery, Right
	Thyroid Artery, Left
Thyroid cartilage	Larynx
Tibialis anterior muscle	Lower Leg Muscle, Right
	Lower Leg Muscle, Left
Tibialis posterior muscle	Lower Leg Muscle, Right
	Lower Leg Muscle, Left
Tibiofemoral joint	Knee Joint, Right
	Knee Joint, Left
	Knee Joint, Tibial Surface, Right
	Knee Joint, Tibial Surface, Left
Tongue, base of	Pharynx
Tracheobronchial lymph node	Lymphatic, Thorax
Tragus	External Ear, Right
	External Ear, Left
	External Ear, Bilateral
Transversalis fascia	Subcutaneous Tissue and Fascia, Trunk

Term	ICD-10-PCS Value
Transverse acetabular ligament	Hip Bursa and Ligament, Right
	Hip Bursa and Ligament, Left
Transverse (cutaneous) cervical nerve	Cervical Plexus
Transverse facial artery	Temporal Artery, Right
	Temporal Artery, Left
Transverse foramen	Cervical Vertebra
Transverse humeral ligament	Shoulder Bursa and Ligament, Right
	Shoulder Bursa and Ligament, Left
Transverse ligament of atlas	Head and Neck Bursa and Ligament
Transverse process	Cervical Vertebra
	Thoracic Vertebra
	Lumbar Vertebra
Transverse scapular ligament	Shoulder Bursa and Ligament, Right
	Shoulder Bursa and Ligament, Left
Transverse thoracis muscle	Thorax Muscle, Right
	Thorax Muscle, Left
Transversospinalis muscle	Trunk Muscle, Right
	Trunk Muscle, Left
Transversus abdominis muscle	Abdomen Muscle, Right
	Abdomen Muscle, Left
Trapezium bone	Carpal, Right
	Carpal, Left
Trapezius muscle	Trunk Muscle, Right
	Trunk Muscle, Left
Trapezoid bone	Carpal, Right
	Carpal, Left
Triceps brachii muscle	Upper Arm Muscle, Right
	Upper Arm Muscle, Left
Tricuspid annulus	Tricuspid Valve
Trifacial nerve	Trigeminal Nerve
Trigone of bladder	Bladder
Triquetral bone	Carpal, Right
	Carpal, Left
Trochantericbursa	Hip Bursa and Ligament, Right
	Hip Bursa and Ligament, Left
Twelfth cranial nerve	Hypoglossal Nerve
Tympanic cavity	Middle Ear, Right
	Middle Ear, Left
Tympanic nerve	Glossopharyngeal Nerve
Tympanic part of temoporal bone	Temporal Bone, Right
	Temporal Bone, Left
Ulnar collateral carpal ligament	Wrist Bursa and Ligament, Right
	Wrist Bursa and Ligament, Left
Ulnar collateral ligament	Elbow Bursa and Ligament, Right
	Elbow Bursa and Ligament, Left
Ulnar notch	Radius, Right
	Radius, Left
Ulnar vein	Brachial Vein, Right
	Brachial Vein, Left

Term	ICD-10-PCS Value
Umbilical artery	Internal Iliac Artery, Right
	Internal Iliac Artery, Left
	Lower Artery
Ureteral orifice	Ureter, Right
	Ureter, Left
	Ureters, Bilateral
	Ureter
Ureteropelvic junction (UPJ)	Kidney Pelvis, Right
	Kidney Pelvis, Left
Ureterovesical orifice	Ureter, Right
	Ureter, Left
	Ureters, Bilateral
	Ureter
Uterine artery	Internal Iliac Artery, Right
	Internal Iliac Artery, Left
Uterine cornu	Uterus
Uterine tube	Fallopian Tube, Right
	Fallopian Tube, Left
Uterine vein	Hypogastric Vein, Right
	Hypogastric Vein, Left
Vaginal artery	Internal Iliac Artery, Right
	Internal Iliac Artery, Left
Vaginal vein	Hypogastric Vein, Right
	Hypogastric Vein, Left
Vastus intermedius muscle	Upper Leg Muscle, Right
	Upper Leg Muscle, Left
Vastus lateralis muscle	Upper Leg Muscle, Right
	Upper Leg Muscle, Left
Vastus medialis muscle	Upper Leg Muscle, Right
	Upper Leg Muscle, Left
Ventricular fold	Larynx
Vermiform appendix	Appendix
Vermilion border	Upper Lip
	Lower Lip
Vertebral arch	Cervical Vertebra
	Lumbar Vertebra
	Thoracic Vertebra
Vertebral body	Cervical Vertebra
	Lumbar Vertebra
	Thoracic Vertebra
Vertebral canal	Spinal Canal
Vertebral foramen	Cervical Vertebra
	Lumbar Vertebra
	Thoracic Vertebra
Vertebral lamina	Cervical Vertebra
	Lumbar Vertebra
	Thoracic Vertebra
Vertebral pedicle	Cervical Vertebra
	Lumbar Vertebra
	Thoracic Vertebra
Vesical vein	Hypogastric Vein, Right
	Hypogastric Vein, Left

Term	ICD-10-PCS Value
Vestibular (Scarpa's) ganglion	Acoustic Nerve
Vestibular nerve	Acoustic Nerve
Vestibulocochlear nerve	Acoustic Nerve
Virchow's (supraclavicular) lymph node	Lymphatic, Right Neck
	Lymphatic, Left Neck
Vitreous body	Vitreous, Right
	Vitreous, Left
Vocal fold	Vocal Cord, Right
	Vocal Cord, Left
Volar (palmar) digital vein	Hand Vein, Right
	Hand Vein, Left
Volar (palmar) metacarpal vein	Hand Vein, Right
	Hand Vein, Left
Vomer bone	Nasal Septum

Term	ICD-10-PCS Value
Vomer of nasal septum	Nasal Bone
Xiphoid process	Sternum
Zonule of Zinn	Lens, Right
	Lens, Left
Zygomatic process of frontal bone	Frontal Bone
Zygomatic process of temporal bone	Temporal Bone, Right
	Temporal Bone, Left
Zygomaticus muscle	Facial Muscle

Appendix E. Body Part Definitions

ICD-10-PCS Value	Definition
1st Toe, Left **1st Toe, Right**	**Includes:** Hallux
Abdomen Muscle, Left **Abdomen Muscle, Right**	**Includes:** External oblique muscle Internal oblique muscle Pyramidalis muscle Rectus abdominis muscle Transversus abdominis muscle
Abdominal Aorta	**Includes:** Inferior phrenic artery Lumbar artery Median sacral artery Middle suprarenal artery Ovarian artery Testicular artery
Abdominal Sympathetic Nerve	**Includes:** Abdominal aortic plexus Auerbach's (myenteric) plexus Celiac (solar) plexus Celiac ganglion Gastric plexus Hepatic plexus Inferior hypogastric plexus Inferior mesenteric ganglion Inferior mesenteric plexus Meissner's (submucous) plexus Myenteric (Auerbach's) plexus Pancreatic plexus Pelvic splanchnic nerve Renal plexus Solar (celiac) plexus Splenic plexus Submucous (Meissner's) plexus Superior hypogastric plexus Superior mesenteric ganglion Superior mesenteric plexus Suprarenal plexus
Abducens Nerve	**Includes:** Sixth cranial nerve
Accessory Nerve	**Includes:** Eleventh cranial nerve
Acoustic Nerve	**Includes:** Cochlear nerve Eighth cranial nerve Scarpa's (vestibular) ganglion Spiral ganglion Vestibular (Scarpa's) ganglion Vestibular nerve Vestibulocochlear nerve
Adenoids	**Includes:** Pharyngeal tonsil
Adrenal Gland **Adrenal Gland, Left** **Adrenal Gland, Right** **Adrenal Glands, Bilateral**	**Includes:** Suprarenal gland
Ampulla of Vater	**Includes:** Duodenal ampulla Hepatopancreatic ampulla

ICD-10-PCS Value	Definition
Anal Sphincter	**Includes:** External anal sphincter Internal anal sphincter
Ankle Bursa and Ligament, Left **Ankle Bursa and Ligament, Right**	**Includes:** Calcaneofibular ligament Deltoid ligament Ligament of the lateral malleolus Talofibular ligament
Ankle Joint, Left **Ankle Joint, Right**	**Includes:** Inferior tibiofibular joint Talocrural joint
Anterior Chamber, Left **Anterior Chamber, Right**	**Includes:** Aqueous humour
Anterior Tibial Artery, Left **Anterior Tibial Artery, Right**	**Includes:** Anterior lateral malleolar artery Anterior medial malleolar artery Anterior tibial recurrent artery Dorsalis pedis artery Posterior tibial recurrent artery
Anus	**Includes:** Anal orifice
Aortic Valve	**Includes:** Aortic annulus
Appendix	**Includes:** Vermiform appendix
Atrial Septum	**Includes:** Interatrial septum
Atrium, Left	**Includes:** Atrium pulmonale Left auricular appendix
Atrium, Right	**Includes:** Atrium dextrum cordis Right auricular appendix Sinus venosus
Auditory Ossicle, Left **Auditory Ossicle, Right**	**Includes:** Incus Malleus Stapes
Axillary Artery, Left **Axillary Artery, Right**	**Includes:** Anterior circumflex humeral artery Lateral thoracic artery Posterior circumflex humeral artery Subscapular artery Superior thoracic artery Thoracoacromial artery
Azygos Vein	**Includes:** Right ascending lumbar vein Right subcostal vein
Basal Ganglia	**Includes:** Basal nuclei Claustrum Corpus striatum Globus pallidus Substantia nigra Subthalamic nucleus

ICD-10-PCS Value	Definition
Basilic Vein, Left Basilic Vein, Right	**Includes:** Median antebrachial vein Median cubital vein
Bladder	**Includes:** Trigone of bladder
Brachial Artery, Left Brachial Artery, Right	**Includes:** Inferior ulnar collateral artery Profunda brachii Superior ulnar collateral artery
Brachial Plexus	**Includes:** Axillary nerve Dorsal scapular nerve First intercostal nerve Long thoracic nerve Musculocutaneous nerve Subclavius nerve Suprascapular nerve
Brachial Vein, Left Brachial Vein, Right	**Includes:** Radial vein Ulnar vein
Brain	**Includes:** Cerebrum Corpus callosum Encephalon
Breast, Bilateral Breast, Left Breast, Right	**Includes:** Mammary duct Mammary gland
Buccal Mucosa	**Includes:** Buccal gland Molar gland Palatine gland
Carotid Bodies, Bilateral Carotid Body, Left Carotid Body, Right	**Includes:** Carotid glomus
Carpal Joint, Left Carpal Joint, Right	**Includes:** Intercarpal joint Midcarpal joint
Carpal, Left Carpal, Right	**Includes:** Capitate bone Hamate bone Lunate bone Pisiform bone Scaphoid bone Trapezium bone Trapezoid bone Triquetral bone
Celiac Artery	**Includes:** Celiac trunk
Cephalic Vein, Left Cephalic Vein, Right	**Includes:** Accessory cephalic vein
Cerebellum	**Includes:** Culmen
Cerebral Hemisphere	**Includes:** Frontal lobe Occipital lobe Parietal lobe Temporal lobe
Cerebral Meninges	**Includes:** Arachnoid mater, intracranial Leptomeninges, intracranial Pia mater, intracranial

ICD-10-PCS Value	Definition
Cerebral Ventricle	**Includes:** Aqueduct of Sylvius Cerebral aqueduct (Sylvius) Choroid plexus Ependyma Foramen of Monro (intraventricular) Fourth ventricle Interventricular foramen (Monro) Left lateral ventricle Right lateral ventricle Third ventricle
Cervical Nerve	**Includes:** Greater occipital nerve Spinal nerve, cervical Suboccipital nerve Third occipital nerve
Cervical Plexus	**Includes:** Ansa cervicalis Cutaneous (transverse) cervical nerve Great auricular nerve Lesser occipital nerve Supraclavicular nerve Transverse (cutaneous) cervical nerve
Cervical Vertebra	**Includes:** Dens Odontoid process Spinous process Transverse foramen Transverse process Vertebral arch Vertebral body Vertebral foramen Vertebral lamina Vertebral pedicle
Cervical Vertebral Joint	**Includes:** Atlantoaxial joint Cervical facet joint
Cervical Vertebral Joints, 2 or more	**Includes:** Cervical facet joint
Cervicothoracic Vertebral Joint	**Includes:** Cervicothoracic facet joint
Cisterna Chyli	**Includes:** Intestinal lymphatic trunk Lumbar lymphatic trunk
Coccygeal Glomus	**Includes:** Coccygeal body
Colic Vein	**Includes:** Ileocolic vein Left colic vein Middle colic vein Right colic vein
Conduction Mechanism	**Includes:** Atrioventricular node Bundle of His Bundle of Kent Sinoatrial node
Conjunctiva, Left Conjunctiva, Right	**Includes:** Plica semilunaris

ICD-10-PCS Value	Definition
Dura Mater	**Includes:** Diaphragma sellae Dura mater, intracranial Falx cerebri Tentorium cerebelli
Elbow Bursa and Ligament, Left Elbow Bursa and Ligament, Right	**Includes:** Annular ligament Olecranon bursa Radial collateral ligament Ulnar collateral ligament
Elbow Joint, Left Elbow Joint, Right	**Includes:** Distal humerus, involving joint Humeroradial joint Humeroulnar joint Proximal radioulnar joint
Epidural Space, Intracranial	**Includes:** Extradural space, intracranial
Epiglottis	**Includes:** Glossoepiglottic fold
Esophagogastric Junction	**Includes:** Cardia Cardioesophageal junction Gastroesophageal (GE) junction
Esophagus, Lower	**Includes:** Abdominal esophagus
Esophagus, Middle	**Includes:** Thoracic esophagus
Esophagus, Upper	**Includes:** Cervical esophagus
Ethmoid Bone, Left Ethmoid Bone, Right	**Includes:** Cribriform plate
Ethmoid Sinus, Left Ethmoid Sinus, Right	**Includes:** Ethmoidal air cell
Eustachian Tube, Left Eustachian Tube, Right	**Includes:** Auditory tube Pharyngotympanic tube
External Auditory Canal, Left External Auditory Canal, Right	**Includes:** External auditory meatus
External Carotid Artery, Left External Carotid Artery, Right	**Includes:** Ascending pharyngeal artery Internal maxillary artery Lingual artery Maxillary artery Occipital artery Posterior auricular artery Superior thyroid artery
External Ear, Bilateral External Ear, Left External Ear, Right	**Includes:** Antihelix Antitragus Auricle Earlobe Helix Pinna Tragus
External Iliac Artery, Left External Iliac Artery, Right	**Includes:** Deep circumflex iliac artery Inferior epigastric artery

ICD-10-PCS Value	Definition
External Jugular Vein, Left External Jugular Vein, Right	**Includes:** Posterior auricular vein
Extraocular Muscle, Left Extraocular Muscle, Right	**Includes:** Inferior oblique muscle Inferior rectus muscle Lateral rectus muscle Medial rectus muscle Superior oblique muscle Superior rectus muscle
Eye, Left Eye, Right	**Includes:** Ciliary body Posterior chamber
Face Artery	**Includes:** Angular artery Ascending palatine artery External maxillary artery Facial artery Inferior labial artery Submental artery Superior labial artery
Face Vein, Left Face Vein, Right	**Includes:** Angular vein Anterior facial vein Common facial vein Deep facial vein Frontal vein Posterior facial (retromandibular) vein Supraorbital vein
Facial Muscle	**Includes:** Buccinator muscle Corrugator supercilii muscle Depressor anguli oris muscle Depressor labii inferioris muscle Depressor septi nasi muscle Depressor supercilii muscle Levator anguli oris muscle Levator labii superioris alaeque nasi muscle Levator labii superioris muscle Mentalis muscle Nasalis muscle Occipitofrontalis muscle Orbicularis oris muscle Procerus muscle Risorius muscle Zygomaticus muscle
Facial Nerve	**Includes:** Chorda tympani Geniculate ganglion Greater superficial petrosal nerve Nerve to the stapedius Parotid plexus Posterior auricular nerve Seventh cranial nerve Submandibular ganglion
Fallopian Tube, Left Fallopian Tube, Right	**Includes:** Oviduct Salpinx Uterine tube

ICD-10-PCS Value	Definition
Femoral Artery, Left Femoral Artery, Right	**Includes:** Circumflex iliac artery Deep femoral artery Descending genicular artery External pudendal artery Superficial epigastric artery
Femoral Nerve	**Includes:** Anterior crural nerve Saphenous nerve
Femoral Shaft, Left Femoral Shaft, Right	**Includes:** Body of femur
Femoral Vein, Left Femoral Vein, Right	**Includes:** Deep femoral (profunda femoris) vein Popliteal vein Profunda femoris (deep femoral) vein
Fibula, Left Fibula, Right	**Includes:** Body of fibula Head of fibula Lateral malleolus
Finger Nail	**Includes:** Nail bed Nail plate
Finger Phalangeal Joint, Left Finger Phalangeal Joint, Right	**Includes:** Interphalangeal (IP) joint
Foot Artery, Left Foot Artery, Right	**Includes:** Arcuate artery Dorsal metatarsal artery Lateral plantar artery Lateral tarsal artery Medial plantar artery
Foot Bursa and Ligament, Left Foot Bursa and Ligament, Right	**Includes:** Calcaneocuboid ligament Cuneonavicular ligament Intercuneiform ligament Interphalangeal ligament Metatarsal ligament Metatarsophalangeal ligament Subtalar ligament Talocalcaneal ligament Talocalcaneonavicular ligament Tarsometatarsal ligament
Foot Muscle, Left Foot Muscle, Right	**Includes:** Abductor hallucis muscle Adductor hallucis muscle Extensor digitorum brevis muscle Extensor hallucis brevis muscle Flexor digitorum brevis muscle Flexor hallucis brevis muscle Quadratus plantae muscle
Foot Vein, Left Foot Vein, Right	**Includes:** Common digital vein Dorsal metatarsal vein Dorsal venous arch Plantar digital vein Plantar metatarsal vein Plantar venous arch
Frontal Bone	**Includes:** Zygomatic process of frontal bone

ICD-10-PCS Value	Definition
Gastric Artery	**Includes:** Left gastric artery Right gastric artery
Glenoid Cavity, Left Glenoid Cavity, Right	**Includes:** Glenoid fossa (of scapula)
Glomus Jugulare	**Includes:** Jugular body
Glossopharyngeal Nerve	**Includes:** Carotid sinus nerve Ninth cranial nerve Tympanic nerve
Hand Artery, Left Hand Artery, Right	**Includes:** Deep palmar arch Princeps pollicis artery Radialis indicis Superficial palmar arch
Hand Bursa and Ligament, Left Hand Bursa and Ligament, Right	**Includes:** Carpometacarpal ligament Intercarpal ligament Interphalangeal ligament Lunotriquetral ligament Metacarpal ligament Metacarpophalangeal ligament Pisohamate ligament Pisometacarpal ligament Scapholunate ligament Scaphotrapezium ligament
Hand Muscle, Left Hand Muscle, Right	**Includes:** Hypothenar muscle Palmar interosseous muscle Thenar muscle
Hand Vein, Left Hand Vein, Right	**Includes:** Dorsal metacarpal vein Palmar (volar) digital vein Palmar (volar) metacarpal vein Superficial palmar venous arch Volar (palmar) digital vein Volar (palmar) metacarpal vein
Head and Neck Bursa and Ligament	**Includes:** Alar ligament of axis Cervical interspinous ligament Cervical intertransverse ligament Cervical ligamentum flavum Interspinous ligament, cervical Intertransverse ligament, cervical Lateral temporomandibular ligament Ligamentum flavum, cervical Sphenomandibular ligament Stylomandibular ligament Transverse ligament of atlas
Head and Neck Sympathetic Nerve	**Includes:** Cavernous plexus Cervical ganglion Ciliary ganglion Internal carotid plexus Otic ganglion Pterygopalatine (sphenopalatine) ganglion Sphenopalatine (pterygopalatine) ganglion Stellate ganglion Submandibular ganglion Submaxillary ganglion

ICD-10-PCS Value	Definition
Head Muscle	**Includes:** Auricularis muscle Masseter muscle Pterygoid muscle Splenius capitis muscle Temporalis muscle Temporoparietalis muscle
Heart, Left	**Includes:** Left coronary sulcus Obtuse margin
Heart, Right	**Includes:** Right coronary sulcus
Hemiazygos Vein	**Includes:** Left ascending lumbar vein Left subcostal vein
Hepatic Artery	**Includes:** Common hepatic artery Gastroduodenal artery Hepatic artery proper
Hip Bursa and Ligament, Left Hip Bursa and Ligament, Right	**Includes:** Iliofemoral ligament Ischiofemoral ligament Pubofemoral ligament Transverse acetabular ligament Trochanteric bursa
Hip Joint, Left Hip Joint, Right	**Includes:** Acetabulofemoral joint
Hip Muscle, Left Hip Muscle, Right	**Includes:** Gemellus muscle Gluteus maximus muscle Gluteus medius muscle Gluteus minimus muscle Iliacus muscle Obturator muscle Piriformis muscle Psoas muscle Quadratus femoris muscle Tensor fasciae latae muscle
Humeral Head, Left Humeral Head, Right	**Includes:** Greater tuberosity Lesser tuberosity Neck of humerus (anatomical)(surgical)
Humeral Shaft, Left Humeral Shaft, Right	**Includes:** Distal humerus Humerus, distal Lateral epicondyle of humerus Medial epicondyle of humerus
Hypogastric Vein, Left Hypogastric Vein, Right	**Includes:** Gluteal vein Internal iliac vein Internal pudendal vein Lateral sacral vein Middle hemorrhoidal vein Obturator vein Uterine vein Vaginal vein Vesical vein
Hypoglossal Nerve	**Includes:** Twelfth cranial nerve
Hypothalamus	**Includes:** Mammillary body

ICD-10-PCS Value	Definition
Inferior Mesenteric Artery	**Includes:** Sigmoid artery Superior rectal artery
Inferior Mesenteric Vein	**Includes:** Sigmoid vein Superior rectal vein
Inferior Vena Cava	**Includes:** Postcava Right inferior phrenic vein Right ovarian vein Right second lumbar vein Right suprarenal vein Right testicular vein
Inguinal Region, Bilateral Inguinal Region, Left Inguinal Region, Right	**Includes:** Inguinal canal Inguinal triangle
Inner Ear, Left Inner Ear, Right	**Includes:** Bony labyrinth Bony vestibule Cochlea Round window Semicircular canal
Innominate Artery	**Includes:** Brachiocephalic artery Brachiocephalic trunk
Innominate Vein, Left Innominate Vein, Right	**Includes:** Brachiocephalic vein Inferior thyroid vein
Internal Carotid Artery, Left Internal Carotid Artery, Right	**Includes:** Caroticotympanic artery Carotid sinus
Internal Iliac Artery, Left Internal Iliac Artery, Right	**Includes:** Deferential artery Hypogastric artery Iliolumbar artery Inferior gluteal artery Inferior vesical artery Internal pudendal artery Lateral sacral artery Middle rectal artery Obturator artery Superior gluteal artery Umbilical artery Uterine artery Vaginal artery
Internal Mammary Artery, Left Internal Mammary Artery, Right	**Includes:** Anterior intercostal artery Internal thoracic artery Musculophrenic artery Pericardiophrenic artery Superior epigastric artery

ICD-10-PCS Value	Definition
Intracranial Artery	**Includes:** Anterior cerebral artery Anterior choroidal artery Anterior communicating artery Basilar artery Circle of Willis Internal carotid artery, intracranial portion Middle cerebral artery Ophthalmic artery Posterior cerebral artery Posterior communicating artery Posterior inferior cerebellar artery (PICA)
Intracranial Vein	**Includes:** Anterior cerebral vein Basal (internal) cerebral vein Dural venous sinus Great cerebral vein Inferior cerebellar vein Inferior cerebral vein Internal (basal) cerebral vein Middle cerebral vein Ophthalmic vein Superior cerebellar vein Superior cerebral vein
Jejunum	**Includes:** Duodenojejunal flexure
Kidney	**Includes:** Renal calyx Renal capsule Renal cortex Renal segment
Kidney Pelvis, Left Kidney Pelvis, Right	**Includes:** Ureteropelvic junction (UPJ)
Kidney, Left Kidney, Right Kidneys, Bilateral	**Includes:** Renal calyx Renal capsule Renal cortex Renal segment
Knee Bursa and Ligament, Left Knee Bursa and Ligament, Right	**Includes:** Anterior cruciate ligament (ACL) Lateral collateral ligament (LCL) Ligament of head of fibula Medial collateral ligament (MCL) Patellar ligament Popliteal ligament Posterior cruciate ligament (PCL) Prepatellar bursa
Knee Joint, Femoral Surface, Left Knee Joint, Femoral Surface, Right	**Includes:** Femoropatellar joint Patellofemoral joint
Knee Joint, Left Knee Joint, Right	**Includes:** Femoropatellar joint Femorotibial joint Lateral meniscus Medial meniscus Patellofemoral joint Tibiofemoral joint
Knee Joint, Tibial Surface, Left Knee Joint, Tibial Surface, Right	**Includes:** Femorotibial joint Tibiofemoral joint

ICD-10-PCS Value	Definition
Knee Tendon, Left Knee Tendon, Right	**Includes:** Patellar tendon
Lacrimal Duct, Left Lacrimal Duct, Right	**Includes:** Lacrimal canaliculus Lacrimal punctum Lacrimal sac Nasolacrimal duct
Larynx	**Includes:** Aryepiglottic fold Arytenoid cartilage Corniculate cartilage Cuneiform cartilage False vocal cord Glottis Rima glottidis Thyroid cartilage Ventricular fold
Lens, Left Lens, Right	**Includes:** Zonule of Zinn
Liver	**Includes:** Quadrate lobe
Lower Arm and Wrist Muscle, Left Lower Arm and Wrist Muscle, Right	**Includes:** Anatomical snuffbox Brachioradialis muscle Extensor carpi radialis muscle Extensor carpi ulnaris muscle Flexor carpi radialis muscle Flexor carpi ulnaris muscle Flexor pollicis longus muscle Palmaris longus muscle Pronator quadratus muscle Pronator teres muscle
Lower Artery	**Includes:** Umbilical artery
Lower Eyelid, Left Lower Eyelid, Right	**Includes:** Inferior tarsal plate Medial canthus
Lower Femur, Left Lower Femur, Right	**Includes:** Lateral condyle of femur Lateral epicondyle of femur Medial condyle of femur Medial epicondyle of femur
Lower Leg Muscle, Left Lower Leg Muscle, Right	**Includes:** Extensor digitorum longus muscle Extensor hallucis longus muscle Fibularis brevis muscle Fibularis longus muscle Flexor digitorum longus muscle Flexor hallucis longus muscle Gastrocnemius muscle Peroneus brevis muscle Peroneus longus muscle Popliteus muscle Soleus muscle Tibialis anterior muscle Tibialis posterior muscle
Lower Leg Tendon, Left Lower Leg Tendon, Right	**Includes:** Achilles tendon
Lower Lip	**Includes:** Frenulum labii inferioris Labial gland Vermilion border

ICD-10-PCS Value	Definition
Lower Spine Bursa and Ligament	**Includes:** Iliolumbar ligament Interspinous ligament, lumbar Intertransverse ligament, lumbar Ligamentum flavum, lumbar Sacrococcygeal ligament Sacroiliac ligament Sacrospinous ligament Sacrotuberous ligament Supraspinous ligament
Lumbar Nerve	**Includes:** Lumbosacral trunk Spinal nerve, lumbar Superior clunic (cluneal) nerve
Lumbar Plexus	**Includes:** Accessory obturator nerve Genitofemoral nerve Iliohypogastric nerve Ilioinguinal nerve Lateral femoral cutaneous nerve Obturator nerve Superior gluteal nerve
Lumbar Spinal Cord	**Includes:** Cauda equina Conus medullaris
Lumbar Sympathetic Nerve	**Includes:** Lumbar ganglion Lumbar splanchnic nerve
Lumbar Vertebra	**Includes:** Spinous process Transverse process Vertebral arch Vertebral body Vertebral foramen Vertebral lamina Vertebral pedicle
Lumbar Vertebral Joint	**Includes:** Lumbar facet joint
Lumbosacral Joint	**Includes:** Lumbosacral facet joint
Lymphatic, Aortic	**Includes:** Celiac lymph node Gastric lymph node Hepatic lymph node Lumbar lymph node Pancreaticosplenic lymph node Paraaortic lymph node Retroperitoneal lymph node
Lymphatic, Head	**Includes:** Buccinator lymph node Infraauricular lymph node Infraparotid lymph node Parotid lymph node Preauricular lymph node Submandibular lymph node Submaxillary lymph node Submental lymph node Subparotid lymph node Suprahyoid lymph node

ICD-10-PCS Value	Definition
Lymphatic, Left Axillary	**Includes:** Anterior (pectoral) lymph node Apical (subclavicular) lymph node Brachial (lateral) lymph node Central axillary lymph node Lateral (brachial) lymph node Pectoral (anterior) lymph node Posterior (subscapular) lymph node Subclavicular (apical) lymph node Subscapular (posterior) lymph node
Lymphatic, Left Lower Extremity	**Includes:** Femoral lymph node Popliteal lymph node
Lymphatic, Left Neck	**Includes:** Cervical lymph node Jugular lymph node Mastoid (postauricular) lymph node Occipital lymph node Postauricular (mastoid) lymph node Retropharyngeal lymph node Supraclavicular (Virchow's) lymph node Virchow's (supraclavicular) lymph node
Lymphatic, Left Upper Extremity	**Includes:** Cubital lymph node Deltopectoral (infraclavicular) lymph node Epitrochlear lymph node Infraclavicular (deltopectoral) lymph node Supratrochlear lymph node
Lymphatic, Mesenteric	**Includes:** Inferior mesenteric lymph node Pararectal lymph node Superior mesenteric lymph node
Lymphatic, Pelvis	**Includes:** Common iliac (subaortic) lymph node Gluteal lymph node Iliac lymph node Inferior epigastric lymph node Obturator lymph node Sacral lymph node Subaortic (common iliac) lymph node Suprainguinal lymph node
Lymphatic, Right Axillary	**Includes:** Anterior (pectoral) lymph node Apical (subclavicular) lymph node Brachial (lateral) lymph node Central axillary lymph node Lateral (brachial) lymph node Pectoral (anterior) lymph node Posterior (subscapular) lymph node Subclavicular (apical) lymph node Subscapular (posterior) lymph node

ICD-10-PCS Value	Definition
Lymphatic, Right Lower Extremity	Includes: Femoral lymph node Popliteal lymph node
Lymphatic, Right Neck	Includes: Cervical lymph node Jugular lymph node Mastoid (postauricular) lymph node Occipital lymph node Postauricular (mastoid) lymph node Retropharyngeal lymph node Right jugular trunk Right lymphatic duct Right subclavian trunk Supraclavicular (Virchow's) lymph node Virchow's (supraclavicular) lymph node
Lymphatic, Right Upper Extremity	Includes: Cubital lymph node Deltopectoral (infraclavicular) lymph node Epitrochlear lymph node Infraclavicular (deltopectoral) lymph node Supratrochlear lymph node
Lymphatic, Thorax	Includes: Intercostal lymph node Mediastinal lymph node Parasternal lymph node Paratracheal lymph node Tracheobronchial lymph node
Main Bronchus, Right	Includes: Bronchus intermedius Intermediate bronchus
Mandible, Left Mandible, Right	Includes: Alveolar process of mandible Condyloid process Mandibular notch Mental foramen
Mastoid Sinus, Left Mastoid Sinus, Right	Includes: Mastoid air cells
Maxilla	Includes: Alveolar process of maxilla
Maxillary Sinus, Left Maxillary Sinus, Right	Includes: Antrum of Highmore
Median Nerve	Includes: Anterior interosseous nerve Palmar cutaneous nerve
Mediastinum	Includes: Mediastinal cavity Mediastinal space
Medulla Oblongata	Includes: Myelencephalon
Mesentery	Includes: Mesoappendix Mesocolon
Metatarsal-Phalangeal Joint, Left Metatarsal-Phalangeal Joint, Right	Includes: Metatarsophalangeal (MTP) joint

ICD-10-PCS Value	Definition
Middle Ear, Left Middle Ear, Right	Includes: Oval window Tympanic cavity
Minor Salivary Gland	Includes: Anterior lingual gland
Mitral Valve	Includes: Bicuspid valve Left atrioventricular valve Mitral annulus
Nasal Bone	Includes: Vomer of nasal septum
Nasal Mucosa and Soft Tissue	Includes: Columella External naris Greater alar cartilage Internal naris Lateral nasal cartilage Lesser alar cartilage Nasal cavity Nostril
Nasal Septum	Includes: Quadrangular cartilage Septal cartilage Vomer bone
Nasal Turbinate	Includes: Inferior turbinate Middle turbinate Nasal concha Superior turbinate
Nasopharynx	Includes: Choana Fossa of Rosenmuller Pharyngeal recess Rhinopharynx
Neck Muscle, Left Neck Muscle, Right	Includes: Anterior vertebral muscle Arytenoid muscle Cricothyroid muscle Infrahyoid muscle Levator scapulae muscle Platysma muscle Scalene muscle Splenius cervicis muscle Sternocleidomastoid muscle Suprahyoid muscle Thyroarytenoid muscle
Nipple, Left Nipple, Right	Includes: Areola
Occipital Bone	Includes: Foramen magnum
Oculomotor Nerve	Includes: Third cranial nerve
Olfactory Nerve	Includes: First cranial nerve Olfactory bulb

ICD-10-PCS Value	Definition
Omentum	**Includes:** Gastrocolic ligament Gastrocolic omentum Gastrohepatic omentum Gastrophrenic ligament Gastrosplenic ligament Greater Omentum Hepatogastric ligament Lesser Omentum
Optic Nerve	**Includes:** Optic chiasma Second cranial nerve
Orbit, Left Orbit, Right	**Includes:** Bony orbit Orbital portion of ethmoid bone Orbital portion of frontal bone Orbital portion of lacrimal bone Orbital portion of maxilla Orbital portion of palatine bone Orbital portion of sphenoid bone Orbital portion of zygomatic bone
Pancreatic Duct	**Includes:** Duct of Wirsung
Pancreatic Duct, Accessory	**Includes:** Duct of Santorini
Parotid Duct, Left Parotid Duct, Right	**Includes:** Stensen's duct
Pelvic Bone, Left Pelvic Bone, Right	**Includes:** Iliac crest Ilium Ischium Pubis
Pelvic Cavity	**Includes:** Retropubic space
Penis	**Includes:** Corpus cavernosum Corpus spongiosum
Perineum Muscle	**Includes:** Bulbospongiosus muscle Cremaster muscle Deep transverse perineal muscle Ischiocavernosus muscle Levator ani muscle Superficial transverse perineal muscle
Peritoneum	**Includes:** Epiploic foramen
Peroneal Artery, Left Peroneal Artery, Right	**Includes:** Fibular artery
Peroneal Nerve	**Includes:** Common fibular nerve Common peroneal nerve External popliteal nerve Lateral sural cutaneous nerve
Pharynx	**Includes:** Base of Tongue Hypopharynx Laryngopharynx Lingual tonsil Oropharynx Piriform recess (sinus) Tongue, base of

ICD-10-PCS Value	Definition
Phrenic Nerve	**Includes:** Accessory phrenic nerve
Pituitary Gland	**Includes:** Adenohypophysis Hypophysis Neurohypophysis
Pons	**Includes:** Apneustic center Basis pontis Locus ceruleus Pneumotaxic center Pontine tegmentum Superior olivary nucleus
Popliteal Artery, Left Popliteal Artery, Right	**Includes:** Inferior genicular artery Middle genicular artery Superior genicular artery Sural artery
Portal Vein	**Includes:** Hepatic portal vein
Prepuce	**Includes:** Foreskin Glans penis
Pudendal Nerve	**Includes:** Posterior labial nerve Posterior scrotal nerve
Pulmonary Artery, Left	**Includes:** Arterial canal (duct) Botallo's duct Pulmoaortic canal
Pulmonary Valve	**Includes:** Pulmonary annulus Pulmonic valve
Pulmonary Vein, Left	**Includes:** Left inferior pulmonary vein Left superior pulmonary vein
Pulmonary Vein, Right	**Includes:** Right inferior pulmonary vein Right superior pulmonary vein
Radial Artery, Left Radial Artery, Right	**Includes:** Radial recurrent artery
Radial Nerve	**Includes:** Dorsal digital nerve Musculospiral nerve Palmar cutaneous nerve Posterior interosseous nerve
Radius, Left Radius, Right	**Includes:** Ulnar notch
Rectum	**Includes:** Anorectal junction
Renal Artery, Left Renal Artery, Right	**Includes:** Inferior suprarenal artery Renal segmental artery
Renal Vein, Left	**Includes:** Left inferior phrenic vein Left ovarian vein Left second lumbar vein Left suprarenal vein Left testicular vein

ICD-10-PCS Value	Definition
Retina, Left Retina, Right	Includes: Fovea Macula Optic disc
Retroperitoneum	Includes: Retroperitoneal cavity Retroperitoneal space
Rib(s) Bursa and Ligament	Includes: Costotransverse ligament
Sacral Nerve	Includes: Spinal nerve, sacral
Sacral Plexus	Includes: Inferior gluteal nerve Posterior femoral cutaneous nerve Pudendal nerve
Sacral Sympathetic Nerve	Includes: Ganglion impar (ganglion of Walther) Pelvic splanchnic nerve Sacral ganglion Sacral splanchnic nerve
Sacrococcygeal Joint	Includes: Sacrococcygeal symphysis
Saphenous Vein, Left Saphenous Vein, Right	Includes: External pudendal vein Great(er) saphenous vein Lesser saphenous vein Small saphenous vein Superficial circumflex iliac vein Superficial epigastric vein
Scapula, Left Scapula, Right	Includes: Acromion (process) Coracoid process
Sciatic Nerve	Includes: Ischiatic nerve
Shoulder Bursa and Ligament, Left Shoulder Bursa and Ligament, Right	Includes: Acromioclavicular ligament Coracoacromial ligament Coracoclavicular ligament Coracohumeral ligament Costoclavicular ligament Glenohumeral ligament Interclavicular ligament Sternoclavicular ligament Subacromial bursa Transverse humeral ligament Transverse scapular ligament
Shoulder Joint, Left Shoulder Joint, Right	Includes: Glenohumeral joint Glenoid ligament (labrum)
Shoulder Muscle, Left Shoulder Muscle, Right	Includes: Deltoid muscle Infraspinatus muscle Subscapularis muscle Supraspinatus muscle Teres major muscle Teres minor muscle
Sigmoid Colon	Includes: Rectosigmoid junction Sigmoid flexure

ICD-10-PCS Value	Definition
Skin	Includes: Dermis Epidermis Sebaceous gland Sweat gland
Sphenoid Bone	Includes: Greater wing Lesser wing Optic foramen Pterygoid process Sella turcica
Spinal Canal	Includes: Epidural space, spinal Extradural space, spinal Subarachnoid space, spinal Subdural space, spinal Vertebral canal
Spinal Meninges	Includes: Arachnoid mater, spinal Denticulate (dentate) ligament Dura mater, spinal Filum terminale Leptomeninges, spinal Pia mater, spinal
Spleen	Includes: Accessory spleen
Splenic Artery	Includes: Left gastroepiploic artery Pancreatic artery Short gastric artery
Splenic Vein	Includes: Left gastroepiploic vein Pancreatic vein
Sternum	Includes: Manubrium Suprasternal notch Xiphoid process
Sternum Bursa and Ligament	Includes: Costoxiphoid ligament Sternocostal ligament
Stomach, Pylorus	Includes: Pyloric antrum Pyloric canal Pyloric sphincter
Subclavian Artery, Left Subclavian Artery, Right	Includes: Costocervical trunk Dorsal scapular artery Internal thoracic artery
Subcutaneous Tissue and Fascia, Chest	Includes: Pectoral fascia
Subcutaneous Tissue and Fascia, Face	Includes: Masseteric fascia Orbital fascia
Subcutaneous Tissue and Fascia, Left Foot	Includes: Plantar fascia (aponeurosis)
Subcutaneous Tissue and Fascia, Left Hand	Includes: Palmar fascia (aponeurosis)
Subcutaneous Tissue and Fascia, Left Lower Arm	Includes: Antebrachial fascia Bicipital aponeurosis

ICD-10-PCS Value	Definition
Subcutaneous Tissue and Fascia, Left Neck	Includes: Deep cervical fascia Pretracheal fascia Prevertebral fascia
Subcutaneous Tissue and Fascia, Left Upper Arm	Includes: Axillary fascia Deltoid fascia Infraspinatus fascia Subscapular aponeurosis Supraspinatus fascia
Subcutaneous Tissue and Fascia, Left Upper Leg	Includes: Crural fascia Fascia lata Iliac fascia Iliotibial tract (band)
Subcutaneous Tissue and Fascia, Right Foot	Includes: Plantar fascia (aponeurosis)
Subcutaneous Tissue and Fascia, Right Hand	Includes: Palmar fascia (aponeurosis)
Subcutaneous Tissue and Fascia, Right Lower Arm	Includes: Antebrachial fascia Bicipital aponeurosis
Subcutaneous Tissue and Fascia, Right Neck	Includes: Deep cervical fascia Pretracheal fascia Prevertebral fascia
Subcutaneous Tissue and Fascia, Right Upper Arm	Includes: Axillary fascia Deltoid fascia Infraspinatus fascia Subscapular aponeurosis Supraspinatus fascia
Subcutaneous Tissue and Fascia, Right Upper Leg	Includes: Crural fascia Fascia lata Iliac fascia Iliotibial tract (band)
Subcutaneous Tissue and Fascia, Scalp	Includes: Galea aponeurotica
Subcutaneous Tissue and Fascia, Trunk	Includes: External oblique aponeurosis Transversalis fascia
Submaxillary Gland, Left Submaxillary Gland, Right	Includes: Submandibular gland
Superior Mesenteric Artery	Includes: Ileal artery Ileocolic artery Inferior pancreaticoduodenal artery Jejunal artery
Superior Mesenteric Vein	Includes: Right gastroepiploic vein
Superior Vena Cava	Includes: Precava

ICD-10-PCS Value	Definition
Tarsal Joint, Left Tarsal Joint, Right	Includes: Calcaneocuboid joint Cuboideonavicular joint Cuneonavicular joint Intercuneiform joint Subtalar (talocalcaneal) joint Talocalcaneal (subtalar) joint Talocalcaneonavicular joint
Tarsal, Left Tarsal, Right	Includes: Calcaneus Cuboid bone Intermediate cuneiform bone Lateral cuneiform bone Medial cuneiform bone Navicular bone Talus bone
Temporal Artery, Left Temporal Artery, Right	Includes: Middle temporal artery Superficial temporal artery Transverse facial artery
Temporal Bone, Left Temporal Bone, Right	Includes: Mastoid process Petrous part of temporal bone Tympanic part of temporal bone Zygomatic process of temporal bone
Thalamus	Includes: Epithalamus Geniculate nucleus Metathalamus Pulvinar
Thoracic Aorta, Ascending/Arch	Includes: Aortic arch Ascending aorta
Thoracic Duct	Includes: Left jugular trunk Left subclavian trunk
Thoracic Nerve	Includes: Intercostal nerve Intercostobrachial nerve Spinal nerve, thoracic Subcostal nerve
Thoracic Sympathetic Nerve	Includes: Cardiac plexus Esophageal plexus Greater splanchnic nerve Inferior cardiac nerve Least splanchnic nerve Lesser splanchnic nerve Middle cardiac nerve Pulmonary plexus Superior cardiac nerve Thoracic aortic plexus Thoracic ganglion
Thoracic Vertebra	Includes: Spinous process Transverse process Vertebral arch Vertebral body Vertebral foramen Vertebral lamina Vertebral pedicle

ICD-10-PCS Value	Definition
Thoracic Vertebral Joint	**Includes:** Costotransverse joint Costovertebral joint Thoracic facet joint
Thoracolumbar Vertebral Joint	**Includes:** Thoracolumbar facet joint
Thorax Muscle, Left **Thorax Muscle, Right**	**Includes:** Intercostal muscle Levatores costarum muscle Pectoralis major muscle Pectoralis minor muscle Serratus anterior muscle Subclavius muscle Subcostal muscle Transverse thoracis muscle
Thymus	**Includes:** Thymus gland
Thyroid Artery, Left **Thyroid Artery, Right**	**Includes:** Cricothyroid artery Hyoid artery Sternocleidomastoid artery Superior laryngeal artery Superior thyroid artery Thyrocervical trunk
Tibia, Left **Tibia, Right**	**Includes:** Lateral condyle of tibia Medial condyle of tibia Medial malleolus
Tibial Nerve	**Includes:** Lateral plantar nerve Medial plantar nerve Medial popliteal nerve Medial sural cutaneous nerve
Toe Nail	**Includes:** Nail bed Nail plate
Toe Phalangeal Joint, Left **Toe Phalangeal Joint, Right**	**Includes:** Interphalangeal (IP) joint
Tongue	**Includes:** Frenulum linguae
Tongue, Palate, Pharynx Muscle	**Includes:** Chondroglossus muscle Genioglossus muscle Hyoglossus muscle Inferior longitudinal muscle Levator veli palatini muscle Palatoglossal muscle Palatopharyngeal muscle Pharyngeal constrictor muscle Salpingopharyngeus muscle Styloglossus muscle Stylopharyngeus muscle Superior longitudinal muscle Tensor veli palatini muscle
Tonsils	**Includes:** Palatine tonsil
Trachea	**Includes:** Cricoid cartilage
Transverse Colon	**Includes:** Hepatic flexure Splenic flexure

ICD-10-PCS Value	Definition
Tricuspid Valve	**Includes:** Right atrioventricular valve Tricuspid annulus
Trigeminal Nerve	**Includes:** Fifth cranial nerve Gasserian ganglion Mandibular nerve Maxillary nerve Ophthalmic nerve Trifacial nerve
Trochlear Nerve	**Includes:** Fourth cranial nerve
Trunk Muscle, Left **Trunk Muscle, Right**	**Includes:** Coccygeus muscle Erector spinae muscle Interspinalis muscle Intertransversarius muscle Latissimus dorsi muscle Quadratus lumborum muscle Rhomboid major muscle Rhomboid minor muscle Serratus posterior muscle Transversospinalis muscle Trapezius muscle
Tympanic Membrane, Left **Tympanic Membrane, Right**	**Includes:** Pars flaccida
Ulna, Left **Ulna, Right**	**Includes:** Olecranon process Radial notch
Ulnar Artery, Left **Ulnar Artery, Right**	**Includes:** Anterior ulnar recurrent artery Common interosseous artery Posterior ulnar recurrent artery
Ulnar Nerve	**Includes:** Cubital nerve
Upper Arm Muscle, Left **Upper Arm Muscle, Right**	**Includes:** Biceps brachii muscle Brachialis muscle Coracobrachialis muscle Triceps brachii muscle
Upper Artery	**Includes:** Aortic intercostal artery Bronchial artery Esophageal artery Subcostal artery
Upper Eyelid, Left **Upper Eyelid, Right**	**Includes:** Lateral canthus Levator palpebrae superioris muscle Orbicularis oculi muscle Superior tarsal plate
Upper Femur, Left **Upper Femur, Right**	**Includes:** Femoral head Greater trochanter Lesser trochanter Neck of femur

ICD-10-PCS Value	Definition
Upper Leg Muscle, Left Upper Leg Muscle, Right	**Includes:** Adductor brevis muscle Adductor longus muscle Adductor magnus muscle Biceps femoris muscle Gracilis muscle Pectineus muscle Quadriceps (femoris) Rectus femoris muscle Sartorius muscle Semimembranosus muscle Semitendinosus muscle Vastus intermedius muscle Vastus lateralis muscle Vastus medialis muscle
Upper Lip	**Includes:** Frenulum labii superioris Labial gland Vermilion border
Upper Spine Bursa and Ligament	**Includes:** Interspinous ligament, thoracic Intertransverse ligament, thoracic Ligamentum flavum, thoracic Supraspinous ligament
Ureter Ureter, Left Ureter, Right Ureters, Bilateral	**Includes:** Ureteral orifice Ureterovesical orifice
Urethra	**Includes:** Bulbourethral (Cowper's) gland Cowper's (bulbourethral) gland External urethral sphincter Internal urethral sphincter Membranous urethra Penile urethra Prostatic urethra
Uterine Supporting Structure	**Includes:** Broad ligament Infundibulopelvic ligament Ovarian ligament Round ligament of uterus
Uterus	**Includes:** Fundus uteri Myometrium Perimetrium Uterine cornu
Uvula	**Includes:** Palatine uvula
Vagus Nerve	**Includes:** Anterior vagal trunk Pharyngeal plexus Pneumogastric nerve Posterior vagal trunk Pulmonary plexus Recurrent laryngeal nerve Superior laryngeal nerve Tenth cranial nerve

ICD-10-PCS Value	Definition
Vas Deferens Vas Deferens, Bilateral Vas Deferens, Left Vas Deferens, Right	**Includes:** Ductus deferens Ejaculatory duct
Ventricle, Right	**Includes:** Conus arteriosus
Ventricular Septum	**Includes:** Interventricular septum
Vertebral Artery, Left Vertebral Artery, Right	**Includes:** Anterior spinal artery Posterior spinal artery
Vertebral Vein, Left Vertebral Vein, Right	**Includes:** Deep cervical vein Suboccipital venous plexus
Vestibular Gland	**Includes:** Bartholin's (greater vestibular) gland Greater vestibular (Bartholin's) gland Paraurethral (Skene's) gland Skene's (paraurethral) gland
Vitreous, Left Vitreous, Right	**Includes:** Vitreous body
Vocal Cord, Left Vocal Cord, Right	**Includes:** Vocal fold
Vulva	**Includes:** Labia majora Labia minora
Wrist Bursa and Ligament, Left Wrist Bursa and Ligament, Right	**Includes:** Palmar ulnocarpal ligament Radial collateral carpal ligament Radiocarpal ligament Radioulnar ligament Ulnar collateral carpal ligament
Wrist Joint, Left Wrist Joint, Right	**Includes:** Distal radioulnar joint Radiocarpal joint

Appendix F. Device Key and Aggregation Table

Device Key

Term	ICD-10-PCS Value
3f (Aortic) Bioprosthesis valve	Zooplastic Tissue in Heart and Great Vessels
AbioCor® Total Replacement Heart	Synthetic Substitute
Absolute Pro Vascular (OTW) Self-Expanding Stent System	Intraluminal Device
Acculink (RX) Carotid Stent System	Intraluminal Device
Acellular Hydrated Dermis	Nonautologous Tissue Substitute
Acetabular cup	Liner in Lower Joints
Activa PC neurostimulator	Stimulator Generator, Multiple Array for Insertion in Subcutaneous Tissue and Fascia
Activa RC neurostimulator	Stimulator Generator, Multiple Array Rechargeable for Insertion in Subcutaneous Tissue and Fascia
Activa SC neurostimulator	Stimulator Generator, Single Array for Insertion in Subcutaneous Tissue and Fascia
ACUITY™ Steerable Lead	Cardiac Lead, Pacemaker for Insertion in Heart and Great Vessels Cardiac Lead, Defibrillator for Insertion in Heart and Great Vessels
Advisa (MRI)	Pacemaker, Dual Chamber for Insertion in Subcutaneous Tissue and Fascia
AFX® Endovascular AAA System	Intraluminal Device
AMPLATZER® Muscular VSD Occluder	Synthetic Substitute
AMS 8ØØ® Urinary Control System	Artificial Sphincter in Urinary System
AneuRx® AAA Advantage®	Intraluminal Device
Annuloplasty ring	Synthetic Substitute
Articulating Spacer (Antibiotic)	Articulating Spacer in Lower Joints
Artificial anal sphincter (AAS)	Artificial Sphincter in Gastrointestinal System
Artificial bowel sphincter (neosphincter)	Artificial Sphincter in Gastrointestinal System
Artificial urinary sphincter (AUS)	Artificial Sphincter in Urinary System
Ascenda Intrathecal Catheter	Infusion Device
Assurant (Cobalt) stent	Intraluminal Device
AtriClip LAA Exclusion System	Extraluminal Device

Term	ICD-10-PCS Value
Attain Ability® Lead	Cardiac Lead, Pacemaker for Insertion in Heart and Great Vessels Cardiac Lead, Defibrillator for Insertion in Heart and Great Vessels
Attain StarFix® (OTW) Lead	Cardiac Lead, Pacemaker for Insertion in Heart and Great Vessels Cardiac Lead, Defibrillator for Insertion in Heart and Great Vessels
Autograft	Autologous Tissue Substitute
Autologous artery graft	Autologous Arterial Tissue in Heart and Great Vessels Autologous Arterial Tissue in Upper Arteries Autologous Arterial Tissue in Lower Arteries Autologous Arterial Tissue in Upper Veins Autologous Arterial Tissue in Lower Veins
Autologous vein graft	Autologous Venous Tissue in Heart and Great Vessels Autologous Venous Tissue in Upper Arteries Autologous Venous Tissue in Lower Arteries Autologous Venous Tissue in Upper Veins Autologous Venous Tissue in Lower Veins
Axial Lumbar Interbody Fusion System	Interbody Fusion Device in Lower Joints
AxiaLIF® System	Interbody Fusion Device in Lower Joints
BAK/C® Interbody Cervical Fusion System	Interbody Fusion Device in Upper Joints
Bard® Composix® (E/X)(LP) mesh	Synthetic Substitute
Bard® Composix® Kugel® patch	Synthetic Substitute
Bard® Dulex™ mesh	Synthetic Substitute
Bard® Ventralex™ hernia patch	Synthetic Substitute
Baroreflex Activation Therapy® (BAT®)	Stimulator Lead in Upper Arteries Stimulator Generator in Subcutaneous Tissue and Fascia
Berlin Heart Ventricular Assist Device	Implantable Heart Assist System in Heart and Great Vessels

Term	ICD-10-PCS Value
Bioactive embolization coil(s)	Intraluminal Device, Bioactive in Upper Arteries
Biventricular external heart assist system	Short-term External Heart Assist System in Heart and Great Vessels
Blood glucose monitoring system	Monitoring Device
Bone anchored hearing device	Hearing Device, Bone Conduction for Insertion in Ear, Nose, Sinus Hearing Device, in Head and Facial Bones
Bone bank bone graft	Nonautologous Tissue Substitute
Bone screw (interlocking)(lag)(pedicle)(recessed)	Internal Fixation Device in Head and Facial Bones Internal Fixation Device in Upper Bones Internal Fixation Device in Lower Bones
Bovine pericardial valve	Zooplastic Tissue in Heart and Great Vessels
Bovine pericardium graft	Zooplastic Tissue in Heart and Great Vessels
Brachytherapy seeds	Radioactive Element
BRYAN® Cervical Disc System	Synthetic Substitute
BVS 5000 Ventricular Assist Device	Short-term External Heart Assist System in Heart and Great Vessels
Cardiac contractility modulation lead	Cardiac Lead in Heart and Great Vessels
Cardiac event recorder	Monitoring Device
Cardiac resynchronization therapy (CRT) lead	Cardiac Lead, Pacemaker for Insertion in Heart and Great Vessels Cardiac Lead, Defibrillator for Insertion in Heart and Great Vessels
CardioMEMS® pressure sensor	Monitoring Device, Pressure Sensor for Insertion in Heart and Great Vessels
Carotid (artery) sinus (baroreceptor) lead	Stimulator Lead in Upper Arteries
Carotid WALLSTENT® Monorail® Endoprosthesis	Intraluminal Device
Centrimag® Blood Pump	Short-term External Heart Assist System in Heart and Great Vessels
Ceramic on ceramic bearing surface	Synthetic Substitute, Ceramic for Replacement in Lower Joints
Cesium-131 Collagen Implant	Radioactive Element, Cesium-131 Collagen Implant for Insertion in Central Nervous System and Cranial Nerves
Clamp and rod internal fixation system (CRIF)	Internal Fixation Device in Upper Bones Internal Fixation Device in Lower Bones
COALESCE® radiolucent interbody fusion device	Interbody Fusion Device, Radiolucent Porous in New Technology
CoAxia NeuroFlo catheter	Intraluminal Device
Cobalt/chromium head and polyethylene socket	Synthetic Substitute, Metal on Polyethylene for Replacement in Lower Joints

Term	ICD-10-PCS Value
Cobalt/chromium head and socket	Synthetic Substitute, Metal for Replacement in Lower Joints
Cochlear implant (CI), multiple channel (electrode)	Hearing Device, Multiple Channel Cochlear Prosthesis for Insertion in Ear, Nose, Sinus
Cochlear implant (CI), single channel (electrode)	Hearing Device, Single Channel Cochlear Prosthesis for Insertion in Ear, Nose, Sinus
COGNIS® CRT-D	Cardiac Resynchronization Defibrillator Pulse Generator for Insertion in Subcutaneous Tissue and Fascia
COHERE® radiolucent interbody fusion device	Interbody Fusion Device, Radiolucent Porous in New Technology
Colonic Z-Stent®	Intraluminal Device
Complete (SE) stent	Intraluminal Device
Concerto II CRT-D	Cardiac Resynchronization Defibrillator Pulse Generator for Insertion in Subcutaneous Tissue and Fascia
CONSERVE® PLUS Total Resurfacing Hip System	Resurfacing Device in Lower Joints
Consulta CRT-D	Cardiac Resynchronization Defibrillator Pulse Generator for Insertion in Subcutaneous Tissue and Fascia
Consulta CRT-P	Cardiac Resynchronization Pacemaker Pulse Generator for Insertion in Subcutaneous Tissue and Fascia
CONTAK RENEWAL® 3 RF (HE) CRT-D	Cardiac Resynchronization Defibrillator Pulse Generator for Insertion in Subcutaneous Tissue and Fascia
Contegra Pulmonary Valved Conduit	Zooplastic Tissue in Heart and Great Vessels
Continuous Glucose Monitoring (CGM) device	Monitoring Device
Cook Biodesign® Fistula Plug(s)	Nonautologous Tissue Substitute
Cook Biodesign® Hernia Graft(s)	Nonautologous Tissue Substitute
Cook Biodesign® Layered Graft(s)	Nonautologous Tissue Substitute
Cook Zenapro™ Layered Graft(s)	Nonautologous Tissue Substitute
Cook Zenith AAA Endovascular Graft	Intraluminal Device Intraluminal Device, Branched or Fenestrated, One or Two Arteries for Restriction in Lower Arteries Intraluminal Device, Branched or Fenestrated, Three or More Arteries for Restriction in Lower Arteries
CoreValve transcatheter aortic valve	Zooplastic Tissue in Heart and Great Vessels
Cormet Hip Resurfacing System	Resurfacing Device in Lower Joints

Term	ICD-10-PCS Value
CoRoent® XL	Interbody Fusion Device in Lower Joints
Corox (OTW) Bipolar Lead	Cardiac Lead, Pacemaker for Insertion in Heart and Great Vessels Cardiac Lead, Defibrillator for Insertion in Heart and Great Vessels
Cortical strip neurostimulator lead	Neurostimulator Lead in Central Nervous System and Cranial Nerves
Cultured epidermal cell autograft	Autologous Tissue Substitute
CYPHER® Stent	Intraluminal Device, Drug-eluting in Heart and Great Vessels
Cystostomy tube	Drainage Device
DBS lead	Neurostimulator Lead in Central Nervous System and Cranial Nerves
DeBakey Left Ventricular Assist Device	Implantable Heart Assist System in Heart and Great Vessels
Deep brain neurostimulator lead	Neurostimulator Lead in Central Nervous System and Cranial Nerves
Delta frame external fixator	External Fixation Device, Hybrid for Insertion in Upper Bones External Fixation Device, Hybrid for Reposition in Upper Bones External Fixation Device, Hybrid for Insertion in Lower Bones External Fixation Device, Hybrid for Reposition in Lower Bones
Delta III Reverse shoulder prosthesis	Synthetic Substitute, Reverse Ball and Socket for Replacement in Upper Joints
Diaphragmatic pacemaker generator	Stimulator Generator in Subcutaneous Tissue and Fascia
Direct Lateral Interbody Fusion (DLIF) device	Interbody Fusion Device in Lower Joints
Driver stent (RX) (OTW)	Intraluminal Device
DuraHeart Left Ventricular Assist System	Implantable Heart Assist System in Heart and Great Vessels
Durata® Defibrillation Lead	Cardiac Lead, Defibrillator for Insertion in Heart and Great Vessels
Dynesys® Dynamic Stabilization System	Spinal Stabilization Device, Pedicle-Based for Insertion in Upper Joints Spinal Stabilization Device, Pedicle-Based for Insertion in Lower Joints
E-Luminexx™ (Biliary)(Vascular) Stent	Intraluminal Device
EDWARDS INTUITY Elite valve system	Zooplastic Tissue, Rapid Deployment Technique in New Technology

Term	ICD-10-PCS Value
Electrical bone growth stimulator (EBGS)	Bone Growth Stimulator in Head and Facial Bones Bone Growth Stimulator in Upper Bones Bone Growth Stimulator in Lower Bones
Electrical muscle stimulation (EMS) lead	Stimulator Lead in Muscles
Electronic muscle stimulator lead	Stimulator Lead in Muscles
Embolization coil(s)	Intraluminal Device
Endeavor® (III)(IV) (Sprint) Zotarolimus-eluting Coronary Stent System	Intraluminal Device, Drug-eluting in Heart and Great Vessels
Endologix AFX® Endovascular AAA System	Intraluminal Device
EndoSure® sensor	Monitoring Device, Pressure Sensor for Insertion in Heart and Great Vessels
ENDOTAK RELIANCE® (G) Defibrillation Lead	Cardiac Lead, Defibrillator for Insertion in Heart and Great Vessels
Endotracheal tube (cuffed)(double-lumen)	Intraluminal Device, Endotracheal Airway in Respiratory System
Endurant® Endovascular Stent Graft	Intraluminal Device
Endurant® II AAA stent graft system	Intraluminal Device
EnRhythm	Pacemaker, Dual Chamber for Insertion in Subcutaneous Tissue and Fascia
Enterra gastric neurostimulator	Stimulator Generator, Multiple Array for Insertion in Subcutaneous Tissue and Fascia
Epic™ Stented Tissue Valve (aortic)	Zooplastic Tissue in Heart and Great Vessels
Epicel® cultured epidermal autograft	Autologous Tissue Substitute
Esophageal obturator airway (EOA)	Intraluminal Device, Airway in Gastrointestinal System
Esteem® implantable hearing system	Hearing Device in Ear, Nose, Sinus
Evera (XT)(S)(DR/VR)	Defibrillator Generator for Insertion in Subcutaneous Tissue and Fascia
Everolimus-eluting coronary stent	Intraluminal Device, Drug-eluting in Heart and Great Vessels
Ex-PRESS™ mini glaucoma shunt	Synthetic Substitute
EXCLUDER® AAA Endoprosthesis	Intraluminal Device Intraluminal Device, Branched or Fenestrated, One or Two Arteries for Restriction in Lower Arteries Intraluminal Device, Branched or Fenestrated, Three or More Arteries for Restriction in Lower Arteries
EXCLUDER® IBE Endoprosthesis	Intraluminal Device, Branched or Fenestrated, One or Two Arteries for Restriction in Lower Arteries

Term	ICD-10-PCS Value
Express® (LD) Premounted Stent System	Intraluminal Device
Express® Biliary SD Monorail® Premounted Stent System	Intraluminal Device
Express® SD Renal Monorail® Premounted Stent System	Intraluminal Device
External fixator	External Fixation Device in Head and Facial Bones External Fixation Device in Upper Bones External Fixation Device in Lower Bones External Fixation Device in Upper Joints External Fixation Device in Lower Joints
EXtreme Lateral Interbody Fusion (XLIF) device	Interbody Fusion Device in Lower Joints
Facet replacement spinal stabilization device	Spinal Stabilization Device, Facet Replacement for Insertion in Upper Joints Spinal Stabilization Device, Facet Replacement for Insertion in Lower Joints
FLAIR® Endovascular Stent Graft	Intraluminal Device
Flexible Composite Mesh	Synthetic Substitute
Foley catheter	Drainage Device
Formula™ Balloon-Expandable Renal Stent System	Intraluminal Device
Freestyle (Stentless) Aortic Root Bioprosthesis	Zooplastic Tissue in Heart and Great Vessels
Fusion screw (compression)(lag)(locking)	Internal Fixation Device in Upper Joints Internal Fixation Device in Lower Joints
GammaTile™	Radioactive Element, Cesium-131 Collagen Implant for Insertion in Central Nervous System and Cranial Nerves
Gastric electrical stimulation (GES) lead	Stimulator Lead in Gastrointestinal System
Gastric pacemaker lead	Stimulator Lead in Gastrointestinal System
GORE EXCLUDER® AAA Endoprosthesis	Intraluminal Device Intraluminal Device, Branched or Fenestrated, One or Two Arteries for Restriction in Lower Arteries Intraluminal Device, Branched or Fenestrated, Three or More Arteries for Restriction in Lower Arteries
GORE EXCLUDER® IBE Endoprosthesis	Intraluminal Device, Branched or Fenestrated, One or Two Arteries for Restriction in Lower Arteries
GORE TAG® Thoracic Endoprosthesis	Intraluminal Device
GORE® DUALMESH®	Synthetic Substitute
Guedel airway	Intraluminal Device, Airway in Mouth and Throat

Term	ICD-10-PCS Value
Hancock Bioprosthesis (aortic)(mitral) valve	Zooplastic Tissue in Heart and Great Vessels
Hancock Bioprosthetic Valved Conduit	Zooplastic Tissue in Heart and Great Vessels
HeartMate 3™ LVAS	Implantable Heart Assist System in Heart and Great Vessels
HeartMate II® Left Ventricular Assist Device (LVAD)	Implantable Heart Assist System in Heart and Great Vessels
HeartMate XVE® Left Ventricular Assist Device (LVAD)	Implantable Heart Assist System in Heart and Great Vessels
Herculink (RX) Elite Renal Stent System	Intraluminal Device
Hip (joint) liner	Liner in Lower Joints
Holter valve ventricular shunt	Synthetic Substitute
Ilizarov external fixator	External Fixation Device, Ring for Insertion in Upper Bones External Fixation Device, Ring for Reposition in Upper Bones External Fixation Device, Ring for Insertion in Lower Bones External Fixation Device, Ring for Reposition in Lower Bones
Ilizarov-Vecklich device	External Fixation Device, Limb Lengthening for Insertion in Upper Bones External Fixation Device, Limb Lengthening for Insertion in Lower Bones
Impella® heart pump	Short-term External Heart Assist System in Heart and Great Vessels
Implantable cardioverter-defibrillator (ICD)	Defibrillator Generator for Insertion in Subcutaneous Tissue and Fascia
Implantable drug infusion pump (anti-spasmodic) (chemotherapy)(pain)	Infusion Device, Pump in Subcutaneous Tissue and Fascia
Implantable glucose monitoring device	Monitoring Device
Implantable hemodynamic monitor (IHM)	Monitoring Device, Hemodynamic for Insertion in Subcutaneous Tissue and Fascia
Implantable hemodynamic monitoring system (IHMS)	Monitoring Device, Hemodynamic for Insertion in Subcutaneous Tissue and Fascia
Implantable Miniature Telescope™ (IMT)	Synthetic Substitute, Intraocular Telescope for Replacement in Eye
Implanted (venous)(access) port	Vascular Access Device, Totally Implantable in Subcutaneous Tissue and Fascia
InDura, intrathecal catheter (1P) (spinal)	Infusion Device
Injection reservoir, port	Vascular Access Device, Totally Implantable in Subcutaneous Tissue and Fascia
Injection reservoir, pump	Infusion Device, Pump in Subcutaneous Tissue and Fascia

Term	ICD-10-PCS Value
Interbody fusion (spine) cage	Interbody Fusion Device in Upper Joints Interbody Fusion Device in Lower Joints
Interspinous process spinal stabilization device	Spinal Stabilization Device, Interspinous Process for Insertion in Upper Joints Spinal Stabilization Device, Interspinous Process for Insertion in Lower Joints
InterStim® Therapy lead	Neurostimulator Lead in Peripheral Nervous System
InterStim® Therapy neurostimulator	Stimulator Generator, Single Array for Insertion in Subcutaneous Tissue and Fascia
Intramedullary (IM) rod (nail)	Internal Fixation Device, Intramedullary in Upper Bones Internal Fixation Device, Intramedullary in Lower Bones
Intramedullary skeletal kinetic distractor (ISKD)	Internal Fixation Device, Intramedullary in Upper Bones Internal Fixation Device, Intramedullary in Lower Bones
Intrauterine Device (IUD)	Contraceptive Device in Female Reproductive System
INTUITY Elite valve system, EDWARDS	Zooplastic Tissue, Rapid Deployment Technique in New Technology
Itrel (3)(4) neurostimulator	Stimulator Generator, Single Array for Insertion in Subcutaneous Tissue and Fascia
Joint fixation plate	Internal Fixation Device in Upper Joints Internal Fixation Device in Lower Joints
Joint liner (insert)	Liner in Lower Joints
Joint spacer (antibiotic)	Spacer in Upper Joints Spacer in Lower Joints
Kappa	Pacemaker, Dual Chamber for Insertion in Subcutaneous Tissue and Fascia
Kirschner wire (K-wire)	Internal Fixation Device in Head and Facial Bones Internal Fixation Device in Upper Bones Internal Fixation Device in Lower Bones Internal Fixation Device in Upper Joints Internal Fixation Device in Lower Joints
Knee (implant) insert	Liner in Lower Joints
Kuntscher nail	Internal Fixation Device, Intramedullary in Upper Bones Internal Fixation Device, Intramedullary in Lower Bones
LAP-BAND® adjustable gastric banding system	Extraluminal Device
LifeStent® (Flexstar)(XL) Vascular Stent System	Intraluminal Device

Term	ICD-10-PCS Value
LIVIAN™ CRT-D	Cardiac Resynchronization Defibrillator Pulse Generator for Insertion in Subcutaneous Tissue and Fascia
Loop recorder, implantable	Monitoring Device
MAGEC® Spinal Bracing and Distraction System	Magnetically Controlled Growth Rod(s) in New Technology
Mark IV Breathing Pacemaker System	Stimulator Generator in Subcutaneous Tissue and Fascia
Maximo II DR (VR)	Defibrillator Generator for Insertion in Subcutaneous Tissue and Fascia
Maximo II DR CRT-D	Cardiac Resynchronization Defibrillator Pulse Generator for Insertion in Subcutaneous Tissue and Fascia
Medtronic Endurant® II AAA stent graft system	Intraluminal Device
Melody® transcatheter pulmonary valve	Zooplastic Tissue in Heart and Great Vessels
Metal on metal bearing surface	Synthetic Substitute, Metal for Replacement in Lower Joints
Micro-Driver stent (RX) (OTW)	Intraluminal Device
MicroMed HeartAssist	Implantable Heart Assist System in Heart and Great Vessels
Micrus CERECYTE microcoil	Intraluminal Device, Bioactive in Upper Arteries
MIRODERM™ Biologic Wound Matrix	Skin Substitute, Porcine Liver Derived in New Technology
MitraClip valve repair system	Synthetic Substitute
Mitroflow® Aortic Pericardial Heart Valve	Zooplastic Tissue in Heart and Great Vessels
Mosaic Bioprosthesis (aortic) (mitral) valve	Zooplastic Tissue in Heart and Great Vessels
MULTI-LINK (VISION)(MINI-VISION)(ULTRA) Coronary Stent System	Intraluminal Device
nanoLOCK™ interbody fusion device	Interbody Fusion Device, Nanotextured Surface in New Technology
Nasopharyngeal airway (NPA)	Intraluminal Device, Airway in Ear, Nose, Sinus
Neuromuscular electrical stimulation (NEMS) lead	Stimulator Lead in Muscles
Neurostimulator generator, multiple channel	Stimulator Generator, Multiple Array for Insertion in Subcutaneous Tissue and Fascia
Neurostimulator generator, multiple channel rechargeable	Stimulator Generator, Multiple Array Rechargeable for Insertion in Subcutaneous Tissue and Fascia
Neurostimulator generator, single channel	Stimulator Generator, Single Array for Insertion in Subcutaneous Tissue and Fascia
Neurostimulator generator, single channel rechargeable	Stimulator Generator, Single Array Rechargeable for Insertion in Subcutaneous Tissue and Fascia

Term	ICD-10-PCS Value
Neutralization plate	Internal Fixation Device in Head and Facial Bones Internal Fixation Device in Upper Bones Internal Fixation Device in Lower Bones
Nitinol framed polymer mesh	Synthetic Substitute
Non-tunneled central venous catheter	Infusion Device
Novacor Left Ventricular Assist Device	Implantable Heart Assist System in Heart and Great Vessels
Novation® Ceramic AHS® (Articulation Hip System)	Synthetic Substitute, Ceramic for Replacement in Lower Joints
Omnilink Elite Vascular Balloon Expandable Stent System	Intraluminal Device
Open Pivot Aortic Valve Graft (AVG)	Synthetic Substitute
Open Pivot (mechanical) Valve	Synthetic Substitute
Optimizer™ III implantable pulse generator	Contractility Modulation Device for Insertion in Subcutaneous Tissue and Fascia
Oropharyngeal airway (OPA)	Intraluminal Device, Airway in Mouth and Throat
Ovatio™ CRT-D	Cardiac Resynchronization Defibrillator Pulse Generator for Insertion in Subcutaneous Tissue and Fascia
OXINIUM	Synthetic Substitute, Oxidized Zirconium on Polyethylene for Replacement in Lower Joints
Paclitaxel-eluting coronary stent	Intraluminal Device, Drug-eluting in Heart and Great Vessels
Paclitaxel-eluting peripheral stent	Intraluminal Device, Drug-eluting in Upper Arteries Intraluminal Device, Drug-eluting in Lower Arteries
Partially absorbable mesh	Synthetic Substitute
Pedicle-based dynamic stabilization device	Spinal Stabilization Device, Pedicle-Based for Insertion in Upper Joints Spinal Stabilization Device, Pedicle-Based for Insertion in Lower Joints
Perceval sutureless valve	Zooplastic Tissue, Rapid Deployment Technique in New Technology
Percutaneous endoscopic gastrojejunostomy (PEG/J) tube	Feeding Device in Gastrointestinal System
Percutaneous endoscopic gastrostomy (PEG) tube	Feeding Device in Gastrointestinal System
Percutaneous nephrostomy catheter	Drainage Device
Peripherally inserted central catheter (PICC)	Infusion Device
Pessary ring	Intraluminal Device, Pessary in Female Reproductive System

Term	ICD-10-PCS Value
Phrenic nerve stimulator generator	Stimulator Generator in Subcutaneous Tissue and Fascia
Phrenic nerve stimulator lead	Diaphragmatic Pacemaker Lead in Respiratory System
PHYSIOMESH™ Flexible Composite Mesh	Synthetic Substitute
Pipeline™ Embolization device (PED)	Intraluminal Device
Polyethylene socket	Synthetic Substitute, Polyethylene for Replacement in Lower Joints
Polymethylmethacrylate (PMMA)	Synthetic Substitute
Polypropylene mesh	Synthetic Substitute
Porcine (bioprosthetic) valve	Zooplastic Tissue in Heart and Great Vessels
PRESTIGE® Cervical Disc	Synthetic Substitute
PrimeAdvanced neurostimulator (SureScan)(MRI Safe)	Stimulator Generator, Multiple Array for Insertion in Subcutaneous Tissue and Fascia
PROCEED™ Ventral Patch	Synthetic Substitute
Prodisc-C	Synthetic Substitute
Prodisc-L	Synthetic Substitute
PROLENE Polypropylene Hernia System (PHS)	Synthetic Substitute
Protecta XT CRT-D	Cardiac Resynchronization Defibrillator Pulse Generator for Insertion in Subcutaneous Tissue and Fascia
Protecta XT DR (XT VR)	Defibrillator Generator for Insertion in Subcutaneous Tissue and Fascia
Protégé® RX Carotid Stent System	Intraluminal Device
Pump reservoir	Infusion Device, Pump in Subcutaneous Tissue and Fascia
REALIZE® Adjustable Gastric Band	Extraluminal Device
Rebound HRD® (Hernia Repair Device)	Synthetic Substitute
RestoreAdvanced neurostimulator (SureScan)(MRI Safe)	Stimulator Generator, Multiple Array Rechargeable for Insertion in Subcutaneous Tissue and Fascia
RestoreSensor neurostimulator (SureScan)(MRI Safe)	Stimulator Generator, Multiple Array Rechargeable for Insertion in Subcutaneous Tissue and Fascia
RestoreUltra neurostimulator (SureScan)(MRI Safe)	Stimulator Generator, Multiple Array Rechargeable for Insertion in Subcutaneous Tissue and Fascia
Reveal (DX)(XT)	Monitoring Device
Reverse® Shoulder Prosthesis	Synthetic Substitute, Reverse Ball and Socket for Replacement in Upper Joints
Revo MRI™ SureScan® pacemaker	Pacemaker, Dual Chamber for Insertion in Subcutaneous Tissue and Fascia
Rheos® System device	Stimulator Generator in Subcutaneous Tissue and Fascia
Rheos® System lead	Stimulator Lead in Upper Arteries

Term	ICD-10-PCS Value
RNS System lead	Neurostimulator Lead in Central Nervous System and Cranial Nerves
RNS system neurostimulator generator	Neurostimulator Generator in Head and Facial Bones
Sacral nerve modulation (SNM) lead	Stimulator Lead in Urinary System
Sacral neuromodulation lead	Stimulator Lead in Urinary System
SAPIEN transcatheter aortic valve	Zooplastic Tissue in Heart and Great Vessels
Secura (DR) (VR)	Defibrillator Generator for Insertion in Subcutaneous Tissue and Fascia
Sheffield hybrid external fixator	External Fixation Device, Hybrid for Insertion in Upper Bones External Fixation Device, Hybrid for Reposition in Upper Bones External Fixation Device, Hybrid for Insertion in Lower Bones External Fixation Device, Hybrid for Reposition in Lower Bones
Sheffield ring external fixator	External Fixation Device, Ring for Insertion in Upper Bones External Fixation Device, Ring for Reposition in Upper Bones External Fixation Device, Ring for Insertion in Lower Bones External Fixation Device, Ring for Reposition in Lower Bones
Single lead pacemaker (atrium)(ventricle)	Pacemaker, Single Chamber for Insertion in Subcutaneous Tissue and Fascia
Single lead rate responsive pacemaker (atrium)(ventricle)	Pacemaker, Single Chamber Rate Responsive for Insertion in Subcutaneous Tissue and Fascia
Sirolimus-eluting coronary stent	Intraluminal Device, Drug-eluting in Heart and Great Vessels
SJM Biocor® Stented Valve System	Zooplastic Tissue in Heart and Great Vessels
Spacer, Articulating (Antibiotic)	Articulating Spacer in Lower Joints
Spacer, Static (Antibiotic)	Spacer in Lower Joints
Spinal cord neurostimulator lead	Neurostimulator Lead in Central Nervous System and Cranial Nerves
Spinal growth rods, magnetically controlled	Magnetically Controlled Growth Rod(s) in New Technology
Spiration IBV™ Valve System	Intraluminal Device, Endobronchial Valve in Respiratory System
Static Spacer (Antibiotic)	Spacer in Lower Joints
Stent, intraluminal (cardiovascular) (gastrointestinal) (hepatobiliary)(urinary)	Intraluminal Device
Stented tissue valve	Zooplastic Tissue in Heart and Great Vessels
Stratos LV	Cardiac Resynchronization Pacemaker Pulse Generator for Insertion in Subcutaneous Tissue and Fascia

Term	ICD-10-PCS Value
Subcutaneous injection reservoir, port	Vascular Access Device, Totally Implantable in Subcutaneous Tissue and Fascia
Subcutaneous injection reservoir, pump	Infusion Device, Pump in Subcutaneous Tissue and Fascia
Subdermal progesterone implant	Contraceptive Device in Subcutaneous Tissue and Fascia
Sutureless valve, Perceval	Zooplastic Tissue, Rapid Deployment Technique in New Technology
SynCardia Total Artificial Heart	Synthetic Substitute
Synchra CRT-P	Cardiac Resynchronization Pacemaker Pulse Generator for Insertion in Subcutaneous Tissue and Fascia
SyncroMed Pump	Infusion Device, Pump in Subcutaneous Tissue and Fascia
Talent® Converter	Intraluminal Device
Talent® Occluder	Intraluminal Device
Talent® Stent Graft (abdominal)(thoracic)	Intraluminal Device
TandemHeart® System	Short-term External Heart Assist System in Heart and Great Vessels
TAXUS® Liberté® Paclitaxel-eluting Coronary Stent System	Intraluminal Device, Drug-eluting in Heart and Great Vessels
Therapeutic occlusion coil(s)	Intraluminal Device
Thoracostomy tube	Drainage Device
Thoratec IVAD (Implantable Ventricular Assist Device)	Implantable Heart Assist System in Heart and Great Vessels
Thoratec Paracorporeal Ventricular Assist Device	Short-term External Heart Assist System in Heart and Great Vessels
Tibial insert	Liner in Lower Joints
Tissue bank graft	Nonautologous Tissue Substitute
Tissue expander (inflatable)(injectable)	Tissue Expander in Skin and Breast Tissue Expander in Subcutaneous Tissue and Fascia
Titanium Sternal Fixation System (TSFS)	Internal Fixation Device, Rigid Plate for Insertion in Upper Bones Internal Fixation Device, Rigid Plate for Reposition in Upper Bones
Total artificial (replacement) heart	Synthetic Substitute
Tracheostomy tube	Tracheostomy Device in Respiratory System
Trifecta™ Valve (aortic)	Zooplastic Tissue in Heart and Great Vessels
Tunneled central venous catheter	Vascular Access Device, Tunneled in Subcutaneous Tissue and Fascia
Tunneled spinal (intrathecal) catheter	Infusion Device
Two lead pacemaker	Pacemaker, Dual Chamber for Insertion in Subcutaneous Tissue and Fascia
Ultraflex™ Precision Colonic Stent System	Intraluminal Device

Term	ICD-10-PCS Value
ULTRAPRO Hernia System (UHS)	Synthetic Substitute
ULTRAPRO Partially Absorbable Lightweight Mesh	Synthetic Substitute
ULTRAPRO Plug	Synthetic Substitute
Ultrasonic osteogenic stimulator	Bone Growth Stimulator in Head and Facial Bones Bone Growth Stimulator in Upper Bones Bone Growth Stimulator in Lower Bones
Ultrasound bone healing system	Bone Growth Stimulator in Head and Facial Bones Bone Growth Stimulator in Upper Bones Bone Growth Stimulator in Lower Bones
Uniplanar external fixator	External Fixation Device, Monoplanar for Insertion in Upper Bones External Fixation Device, Monoplanar for Reposition in Upper Bones External Fixation Device, Monoplanar for Insertion in Lower Bones External Fixation Device, Monoplanar for Reposition in Lower Bones
Urinary incontinence stimulator lead	Stimulator Lead in Urinary System
Vaginal pessary	Intraluminal Device, Pessary in Female Reproductive System
Valiant Thoracic Stent Graft	Intraluminal Device
Vectra® Vascular Access Graft	Vascular Access Device, Tunneled in Subcutaneous Tissue and Fascia
Ventrio™ Hernia Patch	Synthetic Substitute
Versa	Pacemaker, Dual Chamber for Insertion in Subcutaneous Tissue and Fascia
Virtuoso (II) (DR) (VR)	Defibrillator Generator for Insertion in Subcutaneous Tissue and Fascia
Viva(XT)(S)	Cardiac Resynchronization Defibrillator Pulse Generator for Insertion in Subcutaneous Tissue and Fascia
WALLSTENT® Endoprosthesis	Intraluminal Device

Term	ICD-10-PCS Value
X-STOP® Spacer	Spinal Stabilization Device, Interspinous Process for Insertion in Upper Joints Spinal Stabilization Device, Interspinous Process for Insertion in Lower Joints
Xact Carotid Stent System	Intraluminal Device
Xenograft	Zooplastic Tissue in Heart and Great Vessels
XIENCE Everolimus Eluting Coronary Stent System	Intraluminal Device, Drug-eluting in Heart and Great Vessels
XLIF® System	Interbody Fusion Device in Lower Joints
Zenith AAA Endovascular Graft	Intraluminal Device, Branched or Fenestrated, One or Two Arteries for Restriction in Lower Arteries Intraluminal Device, Branched or Fenestrated, Three or More Arteries for Restriction in Lower Arteries Intraluminal Device
Zenith Flex® AAA Endovascular Graft	Intraluminal Device
Zenith TX2® TAA Endovascular Graft	Intraluminal Device
Zenith® Renu™ AAA Ancillary Graft	Intraluminal Device
Zilver® PTX® (paclitaxel) Drug-Eluting Peripheral Stent	Intraluminal Device, Drug-eluting in Upper Arteries Intraluminal Device, Drug-eluting in Lower Arteries
Zimmer® NexGen® LPS Mobile Bearing Knee	Synthetic Substitute
Zimmer® NexGen® LPS-Flex Mobile Knee	Synthetic Substitute
Zotarolimus-eluting coronary stent	Intraluminal Device, Drug-eluting in Heart and Great Vessels

Device Aggregation Table

This table crosswalks specific device character value definitions for specific root operations in a specific body system to the more general device character value to be used when the root operation covers a wide range of body parts and the device character represents an entire family of devices.

Specific Device	for Operation	in Body System	General Device	
Autologous Arterial Tissue (A)	All applicable	Heart and Great Vessels Lower Arteries Lower Veins Upper Arteries Upper Veins	7	Autologous Tissue Substitute
Autologous Venous Tissue (9)	All applicable	Heart and Great Vessels Lower Arteries Lower Veins Upper Arteries Upper Veins	7	Autologous Tissue Substitute
Cardiac Lead, Defibrillator (K)	Insertion	Heart and Great Vessels	M	Cardiac Lead
Cardiac Lead, Pacemaker (J)	Insertion	Heart and Great Vessels	M	Cardiac Lead
Cardiac Resynchronization Defibrillator Pulse Generator (9)	Insertion	Subcutaneous Tissue and Fascia	P	Cardiac Rhythm Related Device
Cardiac Resynchronization Pacemaker Pulse Generator (7)	Insertion	Subcutaneous Tissue and Fascia	P	Cardiac Rhythm Related Device
Contractility Modulation Device (A)	Insertion	Subcutaneous Tissue and Fascia	P	Cardiac Rhythm Related Device
Defibrillator Generator (8)	Insertion	Subcutaneous Tissue and Fascia	P	Cardiac Rhythm Related Device
Epiretinal Visual Prosthesis (5)	All applicable	Eye	J	Synthetic Substitute
External Fixation Device, Hybrid (D)	Insertion	Lower Bones Upper Bones	5	External Fixation Device
External Fixation Device, Hybrid (D)	Reposition	Lower Bones Upper Bones	5	External Fixation Device
External Fixation Device, Limb Lengthening (8)	Insertion	Lower Bones Upper Bones	5	External Fixation Device
External Fixation Device, Monoplanar (B)	Insertion	Lower Bones Upper Bones	5	External Fixation Device
External Fixation Device, Monoplanar (B)	Reposition	Lower Bones Upper Bones	5	External Fixation Device
External Fixation Device, Ring (C)	Insertion	Lower Bones Upper Bones	5	External Fixation Device
External Fixation Device, Ring (C)	Reposition	Lower Bones Upper Bones	5	External Fixation Device
Hearing Device, Bone Conduction (4)	Insertion	Ear, Nose, Sinus	S	Hearing Device
Hearing Device, Multiple Channel Cochlear Prosthesis (6)	Insertion	Ear, Nose, Sinus	S	Hearing Device
Hearing Device, Single Channel Cochlear Prosthesis (5)	Insertion	Ear, Nose, Sinus	S	Hearing Device
Internal Fixation Device, Intramedullary (6)	All applicable	Lower Bones Upper Bones	4	Internal Fixation Device
Internal Fixation Device, Rigid Plate (Ø)	Insertion	Upper Bones	4	Internal Fixation Device
Internal Fixation Device, Rigid Plate (Ø)	Reposition	Upper Bones	4	Internal Fixation Device
Intraluminal Device, Airway (B)	All applicable	Ear, Nose, Sinus Gastrointestinal System Mouth and Throat	D	Intraluminal Device
Intraluminal Device, Bioactive (B)	All applicable	Upper Arteries	D	Intraluminal Device
Intraluminal Device, Branched or Fenestrated, One or Two Arteries (E)	Restriction	Heart and Great Vessels Lower Arteries	D	Intraluminal Device
Intraluminal Device, Branched or Fenestrated, Three or More Arteries (F)	Restriction	Heart and Great Vessels Lower Arteries	D	Intraluminal Device

Specific Device	for Operation	in Body System	General Device
Intraluminal Device, Drug-eluting (4)	All applicable	Heart and Great Vessels Lower Arteries Upper Arteries	**D** Intraluminal Device
Intraluminal Device, Drug-eluting, Four or More (7)	All applicable	Heart and Great Vessels Lower Arteries Upper Arteries	**D** Intraluminal Device
Intraluminal Device, Drug-eluting, Three (6)	All applicable	Heart and Great Vessels Lower Arteries Upper Arteries	**D** Intraluminal Device
Intraluminal Device, Drug-eluting, Two (5)	All applicable	Heart and Great Vessels Lower Arteries Upper Arteries	**D** Intraluminal Device
Intraluminal Device, Endobronchial Valve (G)	All applicable	Respiratory System	**D** Intraluminal Device
Intraluminal Device, Endotracheal Airway (E)	All applicable	Respiratory System	**D** Intraluminal Device
Intraluminal Device, Four or More (G)	All applicable	Heart and Great Vessels Lower Arteries Upper Arteries	**D** Intraluminal Device
Intraluminal Device, Pessary (G)	All applicable	Female Reproductive System	**D** Intraluminal Device
Intraluminal Device, Radioactive (T)	All applicable	Heart and Great Vessels	**D** Intraluminal Device
Intraluminal Device, Three (F)	All applicable	Heart and Great Vessels Lower Arteries Upper Arteries	**D** Intraluminal Device
Intraluminal Device, Two (E)	All applicable	Heart and Great Vessels Lower Arteries Upper Arteries	**D** Intraluminal Device
Monitoring Device, Hemodynamic (Ø)	Insertion	Subcutaneous Tissue and Fascia	**2** Monitoring Device
Monitoring Device, Pressure Sensor (Ø)	Insertion	Heart and Great Vessels	**2** Monitoring Device
Pacemaker, Dual Chamber (6)	Insertion	Subcutaneous Tissue and Fascia	**P** Cardiac Rhythm Related Device
Pacemaker, Single Chamber (4)	Insertion	Subcutaneous Tissue and Fascia	**P** Cardiac Rhythm Related Device
Pacemaker, Single Chamber Rate Responsive (5)	Insertion	Subcutaneous Tissue and Fascia	**P** Cardiac Rhythm Related Device
Spinal Stabilization Device, Facet Replacement (D)	Insertion	Lower Joints Upper Joints	**4** Internal Fixation Device
Spinal Stabilization Device, Interspinous Process (B)	Insertion	Lower Joints Upper Joints	**4** Internal Fixation Device
Spinal Stabilization Device, Pedicle-Based (C)	Insertion	Lower Joints Upper Joints	**4** Internal Fixation Device
Stimulator Generator, Multiple Array (D)	Insertion	Subcutaneous Tissue and Fascia	**M** Stimulator Generator
Stimulator Generator, Multiple Array Rechargeable (E)	Insertion	Subcutaneous Tissue and Fascia	**M** Stimulator Generator
Stimulator Generator, Single Array (B)	Insertion	Subcutaneous Tissue and Fascia	**M** Stimulator Generator
Stimulator Generator, Single Array Rechargeable (C)	Insertion	Subcutaneous Tissue and Fascia	**M** Stimulator Generator
Synthetic Substitute, Ceramic (3)	Replacement	Lower Joints	**J** Synthetic Substitute
Synthetic Substitute, Ceramic on Polyethylene (4)	Replacement	Lower Joints	**J** Synthetic Substitute
Synthetic Substitute, Intraocular Telescope (Ø)	Replacement	Eye	**J** Synthetic Substitute
Synthetic Substitute, Metal (1)	Replacement	Lower Joints	**J** Synthetic Substitute
Synthetic Substitute, Metal on Polyethylene (2)	Replacement	Lower Joints	**J** Synthetic Substitute
Synthetic Substitute, Oxidized Zirconium on Polyethylene (6)	Replacement	Lower Joints	**J** Synthetic Substitute
Synthetic Substitute, Polyethylene (Ø)	Replacement	Lower Joints	**J** Synthetic Substitute
Synthetic Substitute, Reverse Ball and Socket (Ø)	Replacement	Upper Joints	**J** Synthetic Substitute

Appendix G. Device Definitions

ICD-10-PCS Value	Definition
Articulating Spacer in Lower Joints	**Includes:** Articulating Spacer (Antibiotic) Spacer, Articulating (Antibiotic)
Artificial Sphincter in Gastrointestinal System	**Includes:** Artificial anal sphincter (AAS) Artificial bowel sphincter (neosphincter)
Artificial Sphincter in Urinary System	**Includes:** AMS 800® Urinary Control System Artificial urinary sphincter (AUS)
Autologous Arterial Tissue in Heart and Great Vessels	**Includes:** Autologous artery graft
Autologous Arterial Tissue in Lower Arteries	**Includes:** Autologous artery graft
Autologous Arterial Tissue in Lower Veins	**Includes:** Autologous artery graft
Autologous Arterial Tissue in Upper Arteries	**Includes:** Autologous artery graft
Autologous Arterial Tissue in Upper Veins	**Includes:** Autologous artery graft
Autologous Tissue Substitute	**Includes:** Autograft Cultured epidermal cell autograft Epicel® cultured epidermal autograft
Autologous Venous Tissue in Heart and Great Vessels	**Includes:** Autologous vein graft
Autologous Venous Tissue in Lower Arteries	**Includes:** Autologous vein graft
Autologous Venous Tissue in Lower Veins	**Includes:** Autologous vein graft
Autologous Venous Tissue in Upper Arteries	**Includes:** Autologous vein graft
Autologous Venous Tissue in Upper Veins	**Includes:** Autologous vein graft
Bone Growth Stimulator in Head and Facial Bones	**Includes:** Electrical bone growth stimulator (EBGS) Ultrasonic osteogenic stimulator Ultrasound bone healing system
Bone Growth Stimulator in Lower Bones	**Includes:** Electrical bone growth stimulator (EBGS) Ultrasonic osteogenic stimulator Ultrasound bone healing system
Bone Growth Stimulator in Upper Bones	**Includes:** Electrical bone growth stimulator (EBGS) Ultrasonic osteogenic stimulator Ultrasound bone healing system

ICD-10-PCS Value	Definition
Cardiac Lead in Heart and Great Vessels	**Includes:** Cardiac contractility modulation lead
Cardiac Lead, Defibrillator for Insertion in Heart and Great Vessels	**Includes:** ACUITY™ Steerable Lead Attain Ability® lead Attain StarFix® (OTW) lead Cardiac resynchronization therapy (CRT) lead Corox (OTW) Bipolar Lead Durata® Defibrillation Lead ENDOTAK RELIANCE® (G) Defibrillation Lead
Cardiac Lead, Pacemaker for Insertion in Heart and Great Vessels	**Includes:** ACUITY™ Steerable Lead Attain Ability® lead Attain StarFix® (OTW) lead Cardiac resynchronization therapy (CRT) lead Corox (OTW) Bipolar Lead
Cardiac Resynchronization Defibrillator Pulse Generator for Insertion in Subcutaneous Tissue and Fascia	**Includes:** COGNIS® CRT-D Concerto II CRT-D Consulta CRT-D CONTAK RENEWA® 3 RF (HE) CRT-D LIVIAN™ CRT-D Maximo II DR CRT-D Ovatio™ CRT-D Protecta XT CRT-D Viva (XT)(S)
Cardiac Resynchronization Pacemaker Pulse Generator for Insertion in Subcutaneous Tissue and Fascia	**Includes:** Consulta CRT-P Stratos LV Synchra CRT-P
Contraceptive Device in Female Reproductive System	**Includes:** Intrauterine device (IUD)
Contraceptive Device in Subcutaneous Tissue and Fascia	**Includes:** Subdermal progesterone implant
Contractility Modulation Device for Insertion in Subcutaneous Tissue and Fascia	**Includes:** Optimizer™ III implantable pulse generator
Defibrillator Generator for Insertion in Subcutaneous Tissue and Fascia	**Includes:** Evera (XT)(S)(DR/VR) Implantable cardioverter-defibrillator (ICD) Maximo II DR (VR) Protecta XT DR (XT VR) Secura (DR) (VR) Virtuoso (II) (DR) (VR)
Diaphragmatic Pacemaker Lead in Respiratory System	**Includes:** Phrenic nerve stimulator lead

ICD-10-PCS Value	Definition
Drainage Device	**Includes:** Cystostomy tube Foley catheter Percutaneous nephrostomy catheter Thoracostomy tube
External Fixation Device in Head and Facial Bones	**Includes:** External fixator
External Fixation Device in Lower Bones	**Includes:** External fixator
External Fixation Device in Lower Joints	**Includes:** External fixator
External Fixation Device in Upper Bones	**Includes:** External fixator
External Fixation Device in Upper Joints	**Includes:** External fixator
External Fixation Device, Hybrid for Insertion in Lower Bones	**Includes:** Delta frame external fixator Sheffield hybrid external fixator
External Fixation Device, Hybrid for Insertion in Upper Bones	**Includes:** Delta frame external fixator Sheffield hybrid external fixator
External Fixation Device, Hybrid for Reposition in Lower Bones	**Includes:** Delta frame external fixator Sheffield hybrid external fixator
External Fixation Device, Hybrid for Reposition in Upper Bones	**Includes:** Delta frame external fixator Sheffield hybrid external fixator
External Fixation Device, Limb Lengthening for Insertion in Lower Bones	**Includes:** Ilizarov-Vecklich device
External Fixation Device, Limb Lengthening for Insertion in Upper Bones	**Includes:** Ilizarov-Vecklich device
External Fixation Device, Monoplanar for Insertion in Lower Bones	**Includes:** Uniplanar external fixator
External Fixation Device, Monoplanar for Insertion in Upper Bones	**Includes:** Uniplanar external fixator
External Fixation Device, Monoplanar for Reposition in Lower Bones	**Includes:** Uniplanar external fixator
External Fixation Device, Monoplanar for Reposition in Upper Bones	**Includes:** Uniplanar external fixator
External Fixation Device, Ring for Insertion in Lower Bones	**Includes:** Ilizarov external fixator Sheffield ring external fixator
External Fixation Device, Ring for Insertion in Upper Bones	**Includes:** Ilizarov external fixator Sheffield ring external fixator
External Fixation Device, Ring for Reposition in Lower Bones	**Includes:** Ilizarov external fixator Sheffield ring external fixator

ICD-10-PCS Value	Definition
External Fixation Device, Ring for Reposition in Upper Bones	**Includes:** Ilizarov external fixator Sheffield ring external fixator
Extraluminal Device	**Includes:** AtriClip LAA Exclusion System LAP-BAND® adjustable gastric banding system REALIZE® Adjustable Gastric Band

Feeding Device in Gastrointestinal System	**Includes:**
	Percutaneous endoscopic
	  gastrojejunostomy (PEG/J) tube
	Percutaneous endoscopic
	  gastrostomy (PEG) tube

Hearing Device in Ear, Nose, Sinus	**Includes:** Esteem® implantable hearing system
Hearing Device in Head and Facial Bones	**Includes:** Bone anchored hearing device
Hearing Device, Bone Conduction for Insertion in Ear, Nose, Sinus	**Includes:** Bone anchored hearing device
Hearing Device, Multiple Channel Cochlear Prosthesis for Insertion in Ear, Nose, Sinus	**Includes:** Cochlear implant (CI), multiple channel (electrode)
Hearing Device, Single Channel Cochlear Prosthesis for Insertion in Ear, Nose, Sinus	**Includes:** Cochlear implant (CI), single channel (electrode)

Implantable Heart Assist System in Heart and Great Vessels	**Includes:**
	Berlin Heart Ventricular Assist
	  Device
	DeBakey Left Ventricular Assist
	  Device
	DuraHeart Left Ventricular Assist
	  System
	HeartMate 3™ LVAS
	HeartMate II® Left Ventricular
	  Assist Device (LVAD)
	HeartMate XVE® Left Ventricular
	  Assist Device (LVAD)
	MicroMed HeartAssist
	Novacor Left Ventricular Assist
	  Device
	Thoratec IVAD (Implantable
	  Ventricular Assist Device)

Infusion Device	**Includes:**
	Ascenda Intrathecal Catheter
	InDura, intrathecal catheter (1P)
	  (spinal)
	Non-tunneled central venous
	  catheter
	Peripherally inserted central
	  catheter (PICC)
	Tunneled spinal (intrathecal)
	  catheter

ICD-10-PCS Value	Definition
Infusion Device, Pump in Subcutaneous Tissue and Fascia	**Includes:** Implantable drug infusion pump (anti-spasmodic)(chemotherapy)(pain) Injection reservoir, pump Pump reservoir Subcutaneous injection reservoir, pump SynchroMed pump
Interbody Fusion Device in Lower Joints	**Includes:** Axial Lumbar Interbody Fusion System AxiaLIF® System CoRoent® XL Direct Lateral Interbody Fusion (DLIF) device EXtreme Lateral Interbody Fusion (XLIF) device Interbody fusion (spine) cage XLIF® System
Interbody Fusion Device in Upper Joints	**Includes:** BAK/C® Interbody Cervical Fusion System Interbody fusion (spine) cage
Interbody Fusion Device, Nanotextured Surface in New Technology	**Includes:** nanoLOCK™ interbody fusion device
Interbody Fusion Device, Radiolucent Porous in New Technology	**Includes:** COALESCE® radiolucent interbody fusion device COHERE® radiolucent interbody fusion device
Internal Fixation Device in Head and Facial Bones	**Includes:** Bone screw (interlocking)(lag)(pedicle)(recessed) Kirschner wire (K-wire) Neutralization plate
Internal Fixation Device in Lower Bones	**Includes:** Bone screw (interlocking)(lag)(pedicle)(recessed) Clamp and rod internal fixation system (CRIF) Kirschner wire (K-wire) Neutralization plate
Internal Fixation Device in Lower Joints	**Includes:** Fusion screw (compression)(lag)(locking) Joint fixation plate Kirschner wire (K-wire)
Internal Fixation Device in Upper Bones	**Includes:** Bone screw (interlocking)(lag)(pedicle)(recessed) Clamp and rod internal fixation system (CRIF) Kirschner wire (K-wire) Neutralization plate

ICD-10-PCS Value	Definition
Internal Fixation Device in Upper Joints	**Includes:** Fusion screw (compression)(lag)(locking) Joint fixation plate Kirschner wire (K-wire)
Internal Fixation Device, Intramedullary in Lower Bones	**Includes:** Intramedullary (IM) rod (nail) Intramedullary skeletal kinetic distractor (ISKD) Kuntscher nail
Internal Fixation Device, Intramedullary in Upper Bones	**Includes:** Intramedullary (IM) rod (nail) Intramedullary skeletal kinetic distractor (ISKD) Kuntscher nail
Internal Fixation Device, Rigid Plate for Insertion in Upper Bones	**Includes:** Titanium Sternal Fixation System (TSFS)
Internal Fixation Device, Rigid Plate for Reposition in Upper Bones	**Includes:** Titanium Sternal Fixation System (TSFS)
Intraluminal Device	**Includes:** Absolute Pro Vascular (OTW) Self-Expanding Stent System Acculink (RX) Carotid Stent System AFX® Endovascular AAA System AneuRx® AAA Advantage® Assurant (Cobalt) stent Carotid WALLSTENT® Monorail® Endoprosthesis CoAxia NeuroFlo catheter Colonic Z-Stent® Complete (SE) stent Cook Zenith AAA Endovascular Graft Driver stent (RX) (OTW) E-Luminexx™ (Biliary)(Vascular) Stent Embolization coil(s) Endologix AFX® Endovascular AAA System Endurant® Endovascular Stent Graft Endurant® II AAA stent graft system EXCLUDER® AAA Endoprosthesis Express® (LD) Premounted Stent System Express® Biliary SD Monorail® Premounted Stent System Express® SD Renal Monorail® Premounted Stent System FLAIR® Endovascular Stent Graft Formula™ Balloon-Expandable Renal Stent System GORE EXCLUDER® AAA Endoprosthesis GORE TAG® Thoracic Endoprosthesis Herculink (RX) Elite Renal Stent System LifeStent® (Flexstar)(XL) Vascular Stent System

Continued on next page

ICD-10-PCS Value	Definition
Intraluminal Device (continued)	**Includes:** Medtronic Endurant® II AAA stent graft system Micro-Driver stent (RX) (OTW) MULTI-LINK (VISION)(MINI-VISION)(ULTRA) Coronary Stent System Omnilink Elite Vascular Balloon Expandable Stent System Pipeline™ Embolization device (PED) Protege® RX Carotid Stent System Stent, intraluminal (cardiovascular) (gastrointestinal)(hepatobiliary) (urinary) Talent® Converter Talent® Occluder Talent® Stent Graft (abdominal)(thoracic) Therapeutic occlusion coil(s) Ultraflex™ Precision Colonic Stent System Valiant Thoracic Stent Graft WALLSTENT® Endoprosthesis Xact Carotid Stent System Zenith AAA Endovascular Graft Zenith Flex® AAA Endovascular Graft Zenith TX2® TAA Endovascular Graft Zenith® Renu™ AAA Ancillary Graft
Intraluminal Device, Airway in Ear, Nose, Sinus	**Includes:** Nasopharyngeal airway (NPA)
Intraluminal Device, Airway in Gastrointestinal System	**Includes:** Esophageal obturator airway (EOA)
Intraluminal Device, Airway in Mouth and Throat	**Includes:** Guedel airway Oropharyngeal airway (OPA)
Intraluminal Device, Bioactive in Upper Arteries	**Includes:** Bioactive embolization coil(s) Micrus CERECYTE microcoil
Intraluminal Device, Branched or Fenestrated, One or Two Arteries for Restriction in Lower Arteries	**Includes:** Cook Zenith AAA Endovascular Graft EXCLUDER® AAA Endoprosthesis EXCLUDER® IBE Endoprosthesis GORE EXCLUDER® AAA Endoprosthesis GORE EXCLUDER®IBE Endoprosthesis Zenith AAA Endovascular Graft
Intraluminal Device, Branched or Fenestrated, Three or More Arteries for Restriction in Lower Arteries	**Includes:** Cook Zenith AAA Endovascular Graft EXCLUDER® AAA Endoprosthesis GORE EXCLUDER® AAA Endoprosthesis Zenith AAA Endovascular Graft

ICD-10-PCS Value	Definition
Intraluminal Device, Drug-eluting in Heart and Great Vessels	**Includes:** CYPHER® Stent Endeavor® (III)(IV) (Sprint) Zotarolimus-eluting Coronary Stent System Everolimus-eluting coronary stent Paclitaxel-eluting coronary stent Sirolimus-eluting coronary stent TAXUS® Liberte® Paclitaxel-eluting Coronary Stent System XIENCE Everolimus Eluting Coronary Stent System Zotarolimus-eluting coronary stent
Intraluminal Device, Drug-eluting in Lower Arteries	**Includes:** Paclitaxel-eluting peripheral stent Zilver® PTX® (paclitaxel) Drug-Eluting Peripheral Stent
Intraluminal Device, Drug-eluting in Upper Arteries	**Includes:** Paclitaxel-eluting peripheral stent Zilver® PTX® (paclitaxel) Drug-Eluting Peripheral Stent
Intraluminal Device, Endobronchial Valve in Respiratory System	**Includes:** Spiration IBV™ Valve System
Intraluminal Device, Endotracheal Airway in Respiratory System	**Includes:** Endotracheal tube (cuffed)(double-lumen)
Intraluminal Device, Pessary in Female Reproductive System	**Includes:** Pessary ring Vaginal pessary
Liner in Lower Joints	**Includes:** Acetabular cup Hip (joint) liner Joint liner (insert) Knee (implant) insert Tibial insert
Magnetically Controlled Growth Rod(s) in New Technology	**Includes:** MAGEC® Spinal Bracing and Distraction System Spinal growth rods, magnetically controlled
Monitoring Device	**Includes:** Blood glucose monitoring system Cardiac event recorder Continuous Glucose Monitoring (CGM) device Implantable glucose monitoring device Loop recorder, implantable Reveal (DX)(XT)
Monitoring Device, Hemodynamic for Insertion in Subcutaneous Tissue and Fascia	**Includes:** Implantable hemodynamic monitor (IHM) Implantable hemodynamic monitoring system (IHMS)
Monitoring Device, Pressure Sensor for Insertion in Heart and Great Vessels	**Includes:** CardioMEMS® pressure sensor EndoSure® sensor
Neurostimulator Generator in Head and Facial Bones	**Includes:** RNS system neurostimulator generator

ICD-10-PCS Value	Definition
Neurostimulator Lead in Central Nervous System and Cranial Nerves	**Includes:** Cortical strip neurostimulator lead DBS lead Deep brain neurostimulator lead RNS System lead Spinal cord neurostimulator lead
Neurostimulator Lead in Peripheral Nervous System	**Includes:** InterStim® Therapy lead
Nonautologous Tissue Substitute	**Includes:** Acellular Hydrated Dermis Bone bank bone graft Cook Biodesign® Fistula Plug(s) Cook Biodesign® Hernia Graft(s) Cook Biodesign® Layered Graft(s) Cook Zenapro™ Layered Graft(s) Tissue bank graft
Pacemaker, Dual Chamber for Insertion in Subcutaneous Tissue and Fascia	**Includes:** Advisa (MRI) EnRhythm Kappa Revo MRI™ SureScan® pacemaker Two lead pacemaker Versa
Pacemaker, Single Chamber for Insertion in Subcutaneous Tissue and Fascia	**Includes:** Single lead pacemaker (atrium)(ventricle)
Pacemaker, Single Chamber Rate Responsive for Insertion in Subcutaneous Tissue and Fascia	**Includes:** Single lead rate responsive pacemaker (atrium)(ventricle)
Radioactive Element	**Includes:** Brachytherapy seeds
Radioactive Element, Cesium-131 Collagen Implant for Insertion in Central Nervous System and Cranial Nerves	**Includes:** Cesium-131 Collagen Implant GammaTile™
Resurfacing Device in Lower Joints	**Includes:** CONSERVE® PLUS Total Resurfacing Hip System Cormet Hip Resurfacing System
Short-term External Heart Assist System in Heart and Great Vessels	**Includes:** Biventricular external heart assist system BVS 5000 Ventricular Assist Device Centrimag® Blood Pump Impella® heart pump TandemHeart® System Thoratec Paracorporeal Ventricular Assist Device
Skin Substitute, Porcine Liver Derived in New Technology	**Includes:** MIRODERM™ Biologic Wound Matrix
Spacer in Lower Joints	**Includes:** Joint spacer (antibiotic) Spacer, Static (antibiotic) Static Spacer (antibiotic)
Spacer in Upper Joints	**Includes:** Joint spacer (antibiotic)

ICD-10-PCS Value	Definition
Spinal Stabilization Device, Facet Replacement for Insertion in Lower Joints	**Includes:** Facet replacement spinal stabilization device
Spinal Stabilization Device, Facet Replacement for Insertion in Upper Joints	**Includes:** Facet replacement spinal stabilization device
Spinal Stabilization Device, Interspinous Process for Insertion in Lower Joints	**Includes:** Interspinous process spinal stabilization device X-STOP® Spacer
Spinal Stabilization Device, Interspinous Process for Insertion in Upper Joints	**Includes:** Interspinous process spinal stabilization device X-STOP® Spacer
Spinal Stabilization Device, Pedicle- Based for Insertion in Lower Joints	**Includes:** Dynesys® Dynamic Stabilization System Pedicle-based dynamic stabilization device
Spinal Stabilization Device, Pedicle-Based for Insertion in Upper Joints	**Includes:** Dynesys® Dynamic Stabilization System Pedicle-based dynamic stabilization device
Stimulator Generator in Subcutaneous Tissue and Fascia	**Includes:** Baroreflex Activation Therapy® (BAT®) Diaphragmatic pacemaker generator Mark IV Breathing Pacemaker System Phrenic nerve stimulator generator Rheos® System device
Stimulator Generator, Multiple Array for Insertion in Subcutaneous Tissue and Fascia	**Includes:** Activa PC neurostimulator Enterra gastric neurostimulator Neurostimulator generator, multiple channel PrimeAdvanced neurostimulator (SureScan)(MRI Safe)
Stimulator Generator, Multiple Array Rechargeable for Insertion in Subcutaneous Tissue and Fascia	**Includes:** Activa RC neurostimulator Neurostimulator generator, multiple channel rechargeable RestoreAdvanced neurostimulator (SureScan)(MRI Safe) RestoreSensor neurostimulator (SureScan)(MRI Safe) RestoreUltra neurostimulator (SureScan)(MRI Safe)
Stimulator Generator, Single Array for Insertion in Subcutaneous Tissue and Fascia	**Includes:** Activa SC neurostimulator InterStim® Therapy neurostimulator Itrel (3)(4) neurostimulator Neurostimulator generator, single channel

ICD-10-PCS Value	Definition
Stimulator Generator, Single Array Rechargeable for Insertion in Subcutaneous Tissue and Fascia	**Includes:** Neurostimulator generator, single channel rechargeable
Stimulator Lead in Gastrointestinal System	**Includes:** Gastric electrical stimulation (GES) lead Gastric pacemaker lead
Stimulator Lead in Muscles	**Includes:** Electrical muscle stimulation (EMS) lead Electronic muscle stimulator lead Neuromuscular electrical stimulation (NEMS) lead
Stimulator Lead in Upper Arteries	**Includes:** Baroreflex Activation Therapy® (BAT®) Carotid (artery) sinus (baroreceptor) lead Rheos® System lead
Stimulator Lead in Urinary System	**Includes:** Sacral nerve modulation (SNM) lead Sacral neuromodulation lead Urinary incontinence stimulator lead
Synthetic Substitute	**Includes:** AbioCor® Total Replacement Heart AMPLATZER® Muscular VSD Occluder Annuloplasty ring Bard® Composix® (E/X) (LP) mesh Bard® Composix® Kugel® patch Bard® Dulex™ mesh Bard® Ventralex™ hernia patch BRYAN® Cervical Disc System Ex-PRESS™ mini glaucoma shunt Flexible Composite Mesh GORE® DUALMESH® Holter valve ventricular shunt MitraClip valve repair system Nitinol framed polymer mesh Open Pivot (mechanical) valve Open Pivot Aortic Valve Graft (AVG) Partially absorbable mesh PHYSIOMESH™ Flexible Composite Mesh Polymethylmethacrylate (PMMA) Polypropylene mesh PRESTIGE® Cervical Disc PROCEED™ Ventral Patch Prodisc-C Prodisc-L PROLENE Polypropylene Hernia System (PHS) Rebound HRD® (Hernia Repair Device) SynCardia Total Artificial Heart Total artificial (replacement) heart ULTRAPRO Hernia System (UHS)

ICD-10-PCS Value	Definition
Synthetic Substitute (continued)	**Includes:** ULTRAPRO Partially Absorbable Lightweight Mesh ULTRAPRO Plug Ventrio™ Hernia Patch Zimmer® NexGen® LPS Mobile Bearing Knee Zimmer® NexGen® LPS-Flex Mobile Knee
Synthetic Substitute, Ceramic for Replacement in Lower Joints	**Includes:** Ceramic on ceramic bearing surface Novation® Ceramic AHS® (Articulation Hip System)
Synthetic Substitute, Intraocular Telescope for Replacement in Eye	**Includes:** Implantable Miniature Telescope™ (IMT)
Synthetic Substitute, Metal for Replacement in Lower Joints	**Includes:** Cobalt/chromium head and socket Metal on metal bearing surface
Synthetic Substitute, Metal on Polyethylene for Replacement in Lower Joints	**Includes:** Cobalt/chromium head and polyethylene socket
Synthetic Substitute, Oxidized Zirconium on Polyethylene for Replacement in Lower Joints	**Includes:** OXINIUM
Synthetic Substitute, Polyethylene for Replacement in Lower Joints	**Includes:** Polyethylene socket
Synthetic Substitute, Reverse Ball and Socket for Replacement in Upper Joints	**Includes:** Delta III Reverse shoulder prosthesis Reverse® Shoulder Prosthesis
Tissue Expander in Skin and Breast	**Includes:** Tissue expander (inflatable) (injectable)
Tissue Expander in Subcutaneous Tissue and Fascia	**Includes:** Tissue expander (inflatable) (injectable)
Tracheostomy Device in Respiratory System	**Includes:** Tracheostomy tube
Vascular Access Device, Totally Implantable in Subcutaneous Tissue and Fascia	**Includes:** Implanted (venous)(access) port Injection reservoir, port Subcutaneous injection reservoir, port
Vascular Access Device, Tunneled in Subcutaneous Tissue and Fascia	**Includes:** Tunneled central venous catheter Vectra® Vascular Access Graft

ICD-10-PCS Value	Definition
Zooplastic Tissue in Heart and Great Vessels	**Includes:** 3f (Aortic) Bioprosthesis valve Bovine pericardial valve Bovine pericardium graft Contegra Pulmonary Valved Conduit CoreValve transcatheter aortic valve Epic™ Stented Tissue Valve (aortic) Freestyle (Stentless) Aortic Root Bioprosthesis Hancock Bioprosthesis (aortic) (mitral) valve Hancock Bioprosthetic Valved Conduit Melody® transcatheter pulmonary valve Mitroflow® Aortic Pericardial Heart Valve Mosaic Bioprosthesis (aortic) (mitral) valve Porcine (bioprosthetic) valve SAPIEN transcatheter aortic valve SJM Biocor® Stented Valve System Stented tissue valve Trifecta™ Valve (aortic) Xenograft
Zooplastic Tissue, Rapid Deployment Technique in New Technology	**Includes:** EDWARDS INTUITY Elite valve system INTUITY Elite valve system, EDWARDS Perceval sutureless valve Sutureless valve, Perceval

Appendix H. Substance Key/Substance Definitions

Substance Key

This table crosswalks a specific substance, listed by trade name or synonym, to the PCS value that would be used to represent that substance in either the Administration or New Technology section. The ICD-10-PCS value may be located in either the 6th-character Substance column or the 7th-character Qualifier column depending on the section/table to which it is classified. The most specific character is listed in the table.

Trade Name or Synonym	ICD-10-PCS Value	PCS Section
AIGISRx Antibacterial Envelope	Anti-Infective Envelope (A)	Administration (3)
Angiotensin II	Synthetic Human Angiotensin II	New technology (X)
Antimicrobial envelope	Anti-Infective Envelope (A)	Administration (3)
Axicabtagene Ciloeucel	Engineered Autologous Chimeric Antigen Receptor T-cell Immunotherapy (C)	New technology (X)
Bone morphogenetic protein 2 (BMP 2)	Recombinant Bone Morphogenetic Protein (B)	Administration (3)
CBMA (Concentrated Bone Marrow Aspirate)	Concentrated Bone Marrow Aspirate (Ø)	New technology (X)
Clolar	Clofarabine (P)	Administration (3)
Defitelio	Defibrotide Sodium Anticoagulant (9)	New technology (X)
DuraGraft® Endothelial Damage Inhibitor	Endothelial Damage Inhibitor (8)	New technology (X)
Factor Xa Inhibitor Reversal Agent, Andexanet Alfa	Andexanet Alfa, Factor Xa Inhibitor Reversal Agent (7)	New technology (X)
GIAPREZA™	Synthetic Human Angiotensin II	New technology (X)
Human angiotensin II, synthetic	Synthetic Human Angiotensin II	New technology (X)
Kcentra	4-Factor Prothrombin Complex Concentrate (B)	Administration (3)
KYMRIAH	Engineered Autologous Chimeric Antigen Receptor T-cell Immunotherapy	New technology (X)
Nesiritide	Human B-type Natriuretic Peptide (H)	Administration (3)
rhBMP-2	Recombinant Bone Morphogenetic Protein (B)	Administration (3)
Seprafilm	Adhesion Barrier (5)	Administration (3)
STELARA®	Other New Technology Therapeutic Substance (F)	New technology (X)
Tisagenlecleucel	Engineered Autologous Chimeric Antigen Receptor T-cell Immunotherapy	New technology (X)
Tissue Plasminogen Activator (tPA)(r- tPA)	Other Thrombolytic (7)	Administration (3)
Ustekinumab	Other New Technology Therapeutic Substance (F)	New technology (X)
Vistogard®	Uridine Triacetate (8)	New technology (X)
Voraxaze	Glucarpidase (Q)	Administration (3)
VYXEOS™	Cytarabine and Daunorubicin Liposome Antineoplastic (B)	New technology (X)
ZINPLAVA™	Bezlotoxumab Monoclonal Antibody (A)	New technology (X)
Zyvox	Oxazolidinones (8)	Administration (3)

Substance Definitions

This table crosswalks a PCS value, used in the Administration or New Technology section, to a specific substance. The specific substances are listed by trade name or synonym. The ICD-10-PCS value may be located in either the 6th-character Substance column or the 7th-character Qualifier column depending on the section/table to which it is classified.

ICD-10-PCS Value	Trade Name or Synonym	PCS Section
4-Factor Prothrombin Complex Concentrate (B)	**Includes:** Kcentra	Administration (3)
Adhesion Barrier (5)	**Includes:** Seprafilm	Administration (3)
Andexanet Alfa, Factor Xa Inhibitor Reversal Agent (7)	**Includes:** Factor Xa Inhibitor Reversal Agent, Andexanet Alfa	New technology (X)
Anti-Infective Envelope (A)	**Includes:** AIGISRx Antibacterial Envelope Antimicrobial envelope	Administration (3)
Bezlotoxumab Monoclonal Antibody (A)	**Includes:** ZINPLAVA™	New technology (X)
Clofarabine (P)	**Includes:** Clolar	Administration (3)
Concentrated Bone Marrow Aspirate (Ø)	**Includes:** CBMA (Concentrated Bone Marrow Aspirate)	New technology (X)
Cytarabine and Daunorubicin Liposome Antineoplastic (B)	**Includes:** VYXEOS™	New technology (X)
Defibrotide Sodium Anticoagulant (9)	**Includes:** Defitelio	New technology (X)
Endothelial Damage Inhibitor (8)	**Includes:** DuraGraft® Endothelial Damage Inhibitor	New technology (X)
Engineered Autologous Chimeric Antigen Receptor T-cell Immunotherapy (C)	**Includes:** Axicabtagene Ciloeucel KYMRIAH Tisagenlecleucel	New technology (X)
Glucarpidase (Q)	**Includes:** Voraxaze	Administration (3)
Human B-type Natriuretic Peptide (H)	**Includes:** Nesiritide	Administration (3)
Other New Technology Therapeutic Substance (F)	**Includes:** STELARA® Ustekinumab	New technology (X)
Other Thrombolytic (7)	**Includes:** Tissue Plasminogen Activator (tPA)(r-tPA)	Administration (3)
Oxazolidinones (8)	**Includes:** Zyvox	Administration (3)
Recombinant Bone Morphogenetic Protein (B)	**Includes:** Bone morphogenetic protein 2 (BMP 2) rhBMP-2	Administration (3)
Synthetic Human Angiotensin II	**Includes:** Angiotensin II GIAPREZA™ Human angiotensin II, synthetic	New technology (X)
Uridine Triacetate (8)	**Includes:** Vistogard®	New technology (X)

Appendix I. Character Meanings

Central Nervous System and Cranial Nerves 001–00X

Character Meanings

This Character Meaning table is provided as a guide to assist the user in the identification of character members that may be found in this section of code tables. It **SHOULD NOT** be used to build a PCS code.

Operation–Character 3		Body Part–Character 4		Approach–Character 5		Device–Character 6		Qualifier–Character 7	
1	Bypass	Ø	Brain	Ø	Open	Ø	Drainage Device	Ø	Nasopharynx
2	Change	1	Cerebral Meninges	3	Percutaneous	2	Monitoring Device	1	Mastoid Sinus
5	Destruction	2	Dura Mater	4	Percutaneous Endoscopic	3	Infusion Device	2	Atrium
7	Dilation	3	Epidural Space, Intracranial	X	External	4	Radioactive Element, Cesium-131 Collagen Implant	3	Blood Vessel
8	Division	4	Subdural Space, Intracranial			7	Autologous Tissue Substitute	4	Pleural Cavity
9	Drainage	5	Subarachnoid Space, Intracranial			J	Synthetic Substitute	5	Intestine
B	Excision	6	Cerebral Ventricle			K	Nonautologous Tissue Substitute	6	Peritoneal Cavity
C	Extirpation	7	Cerebral Hemisphere			M	Neurostimulator Lead	7	Urinary Tract
D	Extraction	8	Basal Ganglia			Y	Other Device	8	Bone Marrow
F	Fragmentation	9	Thalamus			Z	No Device	9	Fallopian Tube
H	Insertion	A	Hypothalamus					B	Cerebral Cisterns
J	Inspection	B	Pons					F	Olfactory Nerve
K	Map	C	Cerebellum					G	Optic Nerve
N	Release	D	Medulla Oblongata					H	Oculomotor Nerve
P	Removal	E	Cranial Nerve					J	Trochlear Nerve
Q	Repair	F	Olfactory Nerve					K	Trigeminal Nerve
R	Replacement	G	Optic Nerve					L	Abducens Nerve
S	Reposition	H	Oculomotor Nerve					M	Facial Nerve
T	Resection	J	Trochlear Nerve					N	Acoustic Nerve
U	Supplement	K	Trigeminal Nerve					P	Glossopharyngeal Nerve
W	Revision	L	Abducens Nerve					Q	Vagus Nerve
X	Transfer	M	Facial Nerve					R	Accessory Nerve
		N	Acoustic Nerve					S	Hypoglossal Nerve
		P	Glossopharyngeal Nerve					X	Diagnostic
		Q	Vagus Nerve					Z	No Qualifier
		R	Accessory Nerve						
		S	Hypoglossal Nerve						
		T	Spinal Meninges						
		U	Spinal Canal						
		V	Spinal Cord						
		W	Cervical Spinal Cord						
		X	Thoracic Spinal Cord						
		Y	Lumbar Spinal Cord						

Peripheral Nervous System Ø12–Ø1X

Character Meanings

This Character Meaning table is provided as a guide to assist the user in the identification of character members that may be found in this section of code tables. It **SHOULD NOT** be used to build a PCS code.

Operation–Character 3	Body Part–Character 4	Approach–Character 5	Device–Character 6	Qualifier–Character 7
2 Change	Ø Cervical Plexus	Ø Open	Ø Drainage Device	1 Cervical Nerve
5 Destruction	1 Cervical Nerve	3 Percutaneous	2 Monitoring Device	2 Phrenic Nerve
8 Division	2 Phrenic Nerve	4 Percutaneous Endoscopic	7 Autologous Tissue Substitute	4 Ulnar Nerve
9 Drainage	3 Brachial Plexus	X External	M Neurostimulator Lead	5 Median Nerve
B Excision	4 Ulnar Nerve		Y Other Device	6 Radial Nerve
C Extirpation	5 Median Nerve		Z No Device	8 Thoracic Nerve
D Extraction	6 Radial Nerve			B Lumbar Nerve
H Insertion	8 Thoracic Nerve			C Perineal Nerve
J Inspection	9 Lumbar Plexus			D Femoral Nerve
N Release	A Lumbosacral Plexus			F Sciatic Nerve
P Removal	B Lumbar Nerve			G Tibial Nerve
Q Repair	C Pudendal Nerve			H Peroneal Nerve
R Replacement	D Femoral Nerve			X Diagnostic
S Reposition	F Sciatic Nerve			Z No Qualifier
U Supplement	G Tibial Nerve			
W Revision	H Peroneal Nerve			
X Transfer	K Head and Neck Sympathetic Nerve			
	L Thoracic Sympathetic Nerve			
	M Abdominal Sympathetic Nerve			
	N Lumbar Sympathetic Nerve			
	P Sacral Sympathetic Nerve			
	Q Sacral Plexus			
	R Sacral Nerve			
	Y Peripheral Nerve			

Heart and Great Vessels 021–02Y

Character Meanings

This Character Meaning table is provided as a guide to assist the user in the identification of character members that may be found in this section of code tables. It **SHOULD NOT** be used to build a PCS code.

Operation–Character 3	Body Part–Character 4	Approach–Character 5	Device–Character 6	Qualifier–Character 7
1 Bypass	0 Coronary Artery, One Artery	0 Open	0 Monitoring Device, Pressure Sensor	0 Allogeneic
4 Creation	1 Coronary Artery, Two Arteries	3 Percutaneous	2 Monitoring Device	1 Syngeneic
5 Destruction	2 Coronary Artery, Three Arteries	4 Percutaneous Endoscopic	3 Infusion Device	2 Zooplastic OR Common Atrioventricular Valve
7 Dilation	3 Coronary Artery, Four or More Arteries	X External	4 Intraluminal Device, Drug-eluting	3 Coronary Artery
8 Division	4 Coronary Vein		5 Intraluminal Device, Drug-eluting, Two	4 Coronary Vein
B Excision	5 Atrial Septum		6 Intraluminal Device, Drug-eluting, Three	5 Coronary Circulation
C Extirpation	6 Atrium, Right		7 Intraluminal Device, Drug-eluting, Four or More OR Autologous Tissue Substitute	6 Bifurcation
F Fragmentation	7 Atrium, Left		8 Zooplastic Tissue	7 Atrium, Left
H Insertion	8 Conduction Mechanism		9 Autologous Venous Tissue	8 Internal Mammary, Right
J Inspection	9 Chordae Tendineae		A Autologous Arterial Tissue	9 Internal Mammary, Left
K Map	A Heart		C Extraluminal Device	A Innominate Artery
L Occlusion	B Heart, Right		D Intraluminal Device	B Subclavian
N Release	C Heart, Left		E Intraluminal Device, Two OR Intraluminal Device, Branched or Fenestrated, One or Two Arteries	C Thoracic Artery
P Removal	D Papillary Muscle		F Intraluminal Device, Three OR Intraluminal Device, Branched or Fenestrated, Three or More Arteries	D Carotid
Q Repair	F Aortic Valve		G Intraluminal Device, Four or More	E Atrioventricular Valve, Left
R Replacement	G Mitral Valve		J Synthetic Substitute OR Cardiac Lead, Pacemaker	F Abdominal Artery
S Reposition	H Pulmonary Valve		K Nonautologous Tissue Substitute OR Cardiac Lead, Defibrillator	G Atrioventricular Valve, Right OR Axillary Artery
T Resection	J Tricuspid Valve		M Cardiac Lead	H Transapical OR Brachial Artery
U Supplement	K Ventricle, Right		N Intracardiac Pacemaker	J Truncal Valve OR Temporary OR Intraoperative
V Restriction	L Ventricle, Left		Q Implantable Heart Assist System	K Left Atrial Appendage
W Revision	M Ventricular Septum		R Short-term External Heart Assist System	P Pulmonary Trunk

Continued on next page

Heart and Great Vessels Ø21–Ø2Y (Continued)

Operation–Character 3	Body Part–Character 4	Approach–Character 5	Device–Character 6	Qualifier–Character 7
Y Transplantation	N Pericardium		T Intraluminal Device, Radioactive	Q Pulmonary Artery, Right
	P Pulmonary Trunk		Y Other Device	R Pulmonary Artery, Left
	Q Pulmonary Artery, Right		Z No Device	S Pulmonary Vein, Right OR Biventricular
	R Pulmonary Artery, Left			T Pulmonary Vein, Left OR Ductus Arteriosus
	S Pulmonary Vein, Right			U Pulmonary Vein, Confluence
	T Pulmonary Vein, Left			V Lower Extremity Artery
	V Superior Vena Cava			W Aorta
	W Thoracic Aorta, Descending			X Diagnostic
	X Thoracic Aorta, Ascending/Arch			Z No Qualifier
	Y Great Vessel			

Upper Arteries Ø31–Ø3W

Character Meanings

This Character Meaning table is provided as a guide to assist the user in the identification of character members that may be found in this section of code tables. It **SHOULD NOT** be used to build a PCS code.

Operation–Character 3	Body Part–Character 4	Approach–Character 5	Device–Character 6	Qualifier–Character 7
1 Bypass	Ø Internal Mammary Artery, Right	Ø Open	Ø Drainage Device	Ø Upper Arm Artery, Right
5 Destruction	1 Internal Mammary Artery, Left	3 Percutaneous	2 Monitoring Device	1 Upper Arm Artery, Left OR Drug-coated Balloon
7 Dilation	2 Innominate Artery	4 Percutaneous Endoscopic	3 Infusion Device	2 Upper Arm Artery, Bilateral
9 Drainage	3 Subclavian Artery, Right	X External	4 Intraluminal Device, Drug-eluting	3 Lower Arm Artery, Right
B Excision	4 Subclavian Artery, Left		5 Intraluminal Device, Drug-eluting, Two	4 Lower Arm Artery, Left
C Extirpation	5 Axillary Artery, Right		6 Intraluminal Device, Drug-eluting, Three	5 Lower Arm Artery, Bilateral
H Insertion	6 Axillary Artery, Left		7 Intraluminal Device, Drug-eluting, Four or More OR Autologous Tissue Substitute	6 Upper Leg Artery, Right OR Bifurcation
J Inspection	7 Brachial Artery, Right		9 Autologous Venous Tissue	7 Upper Leg Artery, Left OR Stent Retriever
L Occlusion	8 Brachial Artery, Left		A Autologous Arterial Tissue	8 Upper Leg Artery, Bilateral
N Release	9 Ulnar Artery, Right		B Intraluminal Device, Bioactive	9 Lower Leg Artery, Right
P Removal	A Ulnar Artery, Left		C Extraluminal Device	B Lower Leg Artery, Left
Q Repair	B Radial Artery, Right		D Intraluminal Device	C Lower Leg Artery, Bilateral
R Replacement	C Radial Artery, Left		E Intraluminal Device, Two	D Upper Arm Vein
S Reposition	D Hand Artery, Right		F Intraluminal Device, Three	F Lower Arm Vein
U Supplement	F Hand Artery, Left		G Intraluminal Device, Four or More	G Intracranial Artery
V Restriction	G Intracranial Artery		J Synthetic Substitute	J Extracranial Artery, Right
W Revision	H Common Carotid Artery, Right		K Nonautologous Tissue Substitute	K Extracranial Artery, Left
	J Common Carotid Artery, Left		M Stimulator Lead	M Pulmonary Artery, Right
	K Internal Carotid Artery, Right		Z No Device	N Pulmonary Artery, Left
	L Internal Carotid Artery, Left			T Abdominal Artery
	M External Carotid Artery, Right			V Superior Vena Cava
	N External Carotid Artery, Left			X Diagnostic
	P Vertebral Artery, Right			Y Upper Artery
	Q Vertebral Artery, Left			Z No Qualifier
	R Face Artery			
	S Temporal Artery, Right			
	T Temporal Artery, Left			
	U Thyroid Artery, Right			
	V Thyroid Artery, Left			
	Y Upper Artery			

Lower Arteries Ø41–Ø4W

Character Meanings

This Character Meaning table is provided as a guide to assist the user in the identification of character members that may be found in this section of code tables. It **SHOULD NOT** be used to build a PCS code.

Operation–Character 3	Body Part–Character 4	Approach–Character 5	Device–Character 6	Qualifier–Character 7
1 Bypass	Ø Abdominal Aorta	Ø Open	Ø Drainage Device	Ø Abdominal Aorta
5 Destruction	1 Celiac Artery	3 Percutaneous	1 Radioactive Element	1 Celiac Artery OR Drug-coated Balloon
7 Dilation	2 Gastric Artery	4 Percutaneous Endoscopic	2 Monitoring Device	2 Mesenteric Artery
9 Drainage	3 Hepatic Artery	X External	3 Infusion Device	3 Renal Artery, Right
B Excision	4 Splenic Artery		4 Intraluminal Device, Drug-eluting	4 Renal Artery, Left
C Extirpation	5 Superior Mesenteric Artery		5 Intraluminal Device, Drug-eluting, Two	5 Renal Artery, Bilateral
H Insertion	6 Colic Artery, Right		6 Intraluminal Device, Drug-eluting, Three	6 Common Iliac Artery, Right OR Bifurcation
J Inspection	7 Colic Artery, Left		7 Intraluminal Device, Drug-eluting, Four or More OR Autologous Tissue Substitute	7 Common Iliac Artery, Left
L Occlusion	8 Colic Artery, Middle		9 Autologous Venous Tissue	8 Common Iliac Arteries, Bilateral
N Release	9 Renal Artery, Right		A Autologous Arterial Tissue	9 Internal Iliac Artery, Right
P Removal	A Renal Artery, Left		C Extraluminal Device	B Internal Iliac Artery, Left
Q Repair	B Inferior Mesenteric Artery		D Intraluminal Device	C Internal Iliac Arteries, Bilateral
R Replacement	C Common Iliac Artery, Right		E Intraluminal Device, Two OR Intraluminal Device, Branched or Fenestrated, One or Two Arteries	D External Iliac Artery, Right
S Reposition	D Common Iliac Artery, Left		F Intraluminal Device, Three OR Intraluminal Device, Branched or Fenestrated, Three or More Arteries	F External Iliac Artery, Left
U Supplement	E Internal Iliac Artery, Right		G Intraluminal Device, Four or More	G External Iliac Arteries, Bilateral
V Restriction	F Internal Iliac Artery, Left		J Synthetic Substitute	H Femoral Artery, Right
W Revision	H External Iliac Artery, Right		K Nonautologous Tissue Substitute	J Femoral Artery, Left OR Temporary
	J External Iliac Artery, Left		Y Other Device	K Femoral Arteries, Bilateral
	K Femoral Artery, Right		Z No Device	L Popliteal Artery
	L Femoral Artery, Left			M Peroneal Artery
	M Popliteal Artery, Right			N Posterior Tibial Artery
	N Popliteal Artery, Left			P Foot Artery
	P Anterior Tibial Artery, Right			Q Lower Extremity Artery
	Q Anterior Tibial Artery, Left			R Lower Artery

Continued on next page

Lower Arteries Ø41–Ø4W (Continued)

Operation–Character 3	Body Part–Character 4	Approach–Character 5	Device–Character 6	Qualifier–Character 7
	R Posterior Tibial Artery, Right			**S** Lower Extremity Vein
	S Posterior Tibial Artery, Left			**T** Uterine Artery, Right
	T Peroneal Artery, Right			**U** Uterine Artery, Left
	U Peroneal Artery, Left			**X** Diagnostic
	V Foot Artery, Right			**Z** No Qualifier
	W Foot Artery, Left			
	Y Lower Artery			

Upper Veins Ø51–Ø5W

Character Meanings

This Character Meaning table is provided as a guide to assist the user in the identification of character members that may be found in this section of code tables. It **SHOULD NOT** be used to build a PCS code.

Operation–Character 3		Body Part–Character 4		Approach–Character 5		Device–Character 6		Qualifier–Character 7	
1	Bypass	Ø	Azygos Vein	Ø	Open	Ø	Drainage Device	1	Drug-coated Balloon
5	Destruction	1	Hemiazygos Vein	3	Percutaneous	2	Monitoring Device	X	Diagnostic
7	Dilation	3	Innominate Vein, Right	4	Percutaneous Endoscopic	3	Infusion Device	Y	Upper Vein
9	Drainage	4	Innominate Vein, Left	X	External	7	Autologous Tissue Substitute	Z	No Qualifier
B	Excision	5	Subclavian Vein, Right			9	Autologous Venous Tissue		
C	Extirpation	6	Subclavian Vein, Left			A	Autologous Arterial Tissue		
D	Extraction	7	Axillary Vein, Right			C	Extraluminal Device		
H	Insertion	8	Axillary Vein, Left			D	Intraluminal Device		
J	Inspection	9	Brachial Vein, Right			J	Synthetic Substitute		
L	Occlusion	A	Brachial Vein, Left			K	Nonautologous Tissue Substitute		
N	Release	B	Basilic Vein, Right			M	Neurostimulator Lead		
P	Removal	C	Basilic Vein, Left			Y	Other Device		
Q	Repair	D	Cephalic Vein, Right			Z	No Device		
R	Replacement	F	Cephalic Vein, Left						
S	Reposition	G	Hand Vein, Right						
U	Supplement	H	Hand Vein, Left						
V	Restriction	L	Intracranial Vein						
W	Revision	M	Internal Jugular Vein, Right						
		N	Internal Jugular Vein, Left						
		P	External Jugular Vein, Right						
		Q	External Jugular Vein, Left						
		R	Vertebral Vein, Right						
		S	Vertebral Vein, Left						
		T	Face Vein, Right						
		V	Face Vein, Left						
		Y	Upper Vein						

Lower Veins Ø61–Ø6W

Character Meanings

This Character Meaning table is provided as a guide to assist the user in the identification of character members that may be found in this section of code tables. It **SHOULD NOT** be used to build a PCS code.

Operation–Character 3	Body Part–Character 4	Approach–Character 5	Device–Character 6	Qualifier–Character 7
1 Bypass	Ø Inferior Vena Cava	Ø Open	Ø Drainage Device	4 Hepatic Vein
5 Destruction	1 Splenic Vein	3 Percutaneous	2 Monitoring Device	5 Superior Mesenteric Vein
7 Dilation	2 Gastric Vein	4 Percutaneous Endoscopic	3 Infusion Device	6 Inferior Mesenteric Vein
9 Drainage	3 Esophageal Vein	7 Via Natural or Artificial Opening	7 Autologous Tissue Substitute	9 Renal Vein, Right
B Excision	4 Hepatic Vein	8 Via Natural or Artificial Opening Endoscopic	9 Autologous Venous Tissue	B Renal Vein, Left
C Extirpation	5 Superior Mesenteric Vein	X External	A Autologous Arterial Tissue	C Hemorrhoidal Plexus
D Extraction	6 Inferior Mesenteric Vein		C Extraluminal Device	P Pulmonary Trunk
H Insertion	7 Colic Vein		D Intraluminal Device	Q Pulmonary Artery, Right
J Inspection	8 Portal Vein		J Synthetic Substitute	R Pulmonary Artery, Left
L Occlusion	9 Renal Vein, Right		K Nonautologous Tissue Substitute	T Via Umbilical Vein
N Release	B Renal Vein, Left		Y Other Device	X Diagnostic
P Removal	C Common Iliac Vein, Right		Z No Device	Y Lower Vein
Q Repair	D Common Iliac Vein, Left			Z No Qualifier
R Replacement	F External Iliac Vein, Right			
S Reposition	G External Iliac Vein, Left			
U Supplement	H Hypogastric Vein, Right			
V Restriction	J Hypogastric Vein, Left			
W Revision	M Femoral Vein, Right			
	N Femoral Vein, Left			
	P Saphenous Vein, Right			
	Q Saphenous Vein, Left			
	T Foot Vein, Right			
	V Foot Vein, Left			
	Y Lower Vein			

Lymphatic and Hemic Systems Ø72–Ø7Y

Character Meanings

This Character Meaning table is provided as a guide to assist the user in the identification of character members that may be found in this section of code tables. It **SHOULD NOT** be used to build a PCS code.

Operation–Character 3		Body Part–Character 4		Approach–Character 5		Device–Character 6		Qualifier–Character 7	
2	Change	Ø	Lymphatic, Head	Ø	Open	Ø	Drainage Device	Ø	Allogeneic
5	Destruction	1	Lymphatic, Right Neck	3	Percutaneous	3	Infusion Device	1	Syngeneic
9	Drainage	2	Lymphatic, Left Neck	4	Percutaneous Endoscopic	7	Autologous Tissue Substitute	2	Zooplastic
B	Excision	3	Lymphatic, Right Upper Extremity	8	Via Natural or Artificial Opening Endoscopic	C	Extraluminal Device	X	Diagnostic
C	Extirpation	4	Lymphatic, Left Upper Extremity	X	External	D	Intraluminal Device	Z	No Qualifier
D	Extraction	5	Lymphatic, Right Axillary			J	Synthetic Substitute		
H	Insertion	6	Lymphatic, Left Axillary			K	Nonautologous Tissue Substitute		
J	Inspection	7	Lymphatic, Thorax			Y	Other Device		
L	Occlusion	8	Lymphatic, Internal Mammary, Right			Z	No Device		
N	Release	9	Lymphatic, Internal Mammary, Left						
P	Removal	B	Lymphatic, Mesenteric						
Q	Repair	C	Lymphatic, Pelvis						
S	Reposition	D	Lymphatic, Aortic						
T	Resection	F	Lymphatic, Right Lower Extremity						
U	Supplement	G	Lymphatic, Left Lower Extremity						
V	Restriction	H	Lymphatic, Right Inguinal						
W	Revision	J	Lymphatic, Left Inguinal						
Y	Transplantation	K	Thoracic Duct						
		L	Cisterna Chyli						
		M	Thymus						
		N	Lymphatic						
		P	Spleen						
		Q	Bone Marrow, Sternum						
		R	Bone Marrow, Iliac						
		S	Bone Marrow, Vertebral						
		T	Bone Marrow						

Eye Ø8Ø–Ø8X

Character Meanings

This Character Meaning table is provided as a guide to assist the user in the identification of character members that may be found in this section of code tables. It **SHOULD NOT** be used to build a PCS code.

Operation–Character 3	Body Part–Character 4	Approach–Character 5	Device–Character 6	Qualifier–Character 7
Ø Alteration	Ø Eye, Right	Ø Open	Ø Drainage Device OR Synthetic Substitute, Intraocular Telescope	3 Nasal Cavity
1 Bypass	1 Eye, Left	3 Percutaneous	1 Radioactive Element	4 Sclera
2 Change	2 Anterior Chamber, Right	7 Via Natural or Artificial Opening	3 Infusion Device	X Diagnostic
5 Destruction	3 Anterior Chamber, Left	8 Via Natural or Artificial Opening Endoscopic	5 Epiretinal Visual Prosthesis	Z No Qualifier
7 Dilation	4 Vitreous, Right	X External	7 Autologous Tissue Substitute	
9 Drainage	5 Vitreous, Left		C Extraluminal Device	
B Excision	6 Sclera, Right		D Intraluminal Device	
C Extirpation	7 Sclera, Left		J Synthetic Substitute	
D Extraction	8 Cornea, Right		K Nonautologous Tissue Substitute	
F Fragmentation	9 Cornea, Left		Y Other Device	
H Insertion	A Choroid, Right		Z No Device	
J Inspection	B Choroid, Left			
L Occlusion	C Iris, Right			
M Reattachment	D Iris, Left			
N Release	E Retina, Right			
P Removal	F Retina, Left			
Q Repair	G Retinal Vessel, Right			
R Replacement	H Retinal Vessel, Left			
S Reposition	J Lens, Right			
T Resection	K Lens, Left			
U Supplement	L Extraocular Muscle, Right			
V Restriction	M Extraocular Muscle, Left			
W Revision	N Upper Eyelid, Right			
X Transfer	P Upper Eyelid, Left			
	Q Lower Eyelid, Right			
	R Lower Eyelid, Left			
	S Conjunctiva, Right			
	T Conjunctiva, Left			
	V Lacrimal Gland, Right			
	W Lacrimal Gland, Left			
	X Lacrimal Duct, Right			
	Y Lacrimal Duct, Left			

Ear, Nose, Sinus Ø9Ø–Ø9W

Character Meanings

This Character Meaning table is provided as a guide to assist the user in the identification of character members that may be found in this section of code tables. It **SHOULD NOT** be used to build a PCS code.

Operation–Character 3		Body Part–Character 4		Approach–Character 5		Device–Character 6		Qualifier–Character 7	
Ø	Alteration	Ø	External Ear, Right	Ø	Open	Ø	Drainage Device	Ø	Endolymphatic
1	Bypass	1	External Ear, Left	3	Percutaneous	4	Hearing Device, Bone Conduction	X	Diagnostic
2	Change	2	External Ear, Bilateral	4	Percutaneous Endoscopic	5	Hearing Device, Single Channel Cochlear Prosthesis	Z	No Qualifier
3	Control	3	External Auditory Canal, Right	7	Via Natural or Artificial Opening	6	Hearing Device, Multiple Channel Cochlear Prosthesis		
5	Destruction	4	External Auditory Canal, Left	8	Via Natural or Artificial Opening Endoscopic	7	Autologous Tissue Substitute		
7	Dilation	5	Middle Ear, Right	X	External	B	Intraluminal Device, Airway		
8	Division	6	Middle Ear, Left			D	Intraluminal Device		
9	Drainage	7	Tympanic Membrane, Right			J	Synthetic Substitute		
B	Excision	8	Tympanic Membrane, Left			K	Nonautologous Tissue Substitute		
C	Extirpation	9	Auditory Ossicle, Right			S	Hearing Device		
D	Extraction	A	Auditory Ossicle, Left			Y	Other Device		
H	Insertion	B	Mastoid Sinus, Right			Z	No Device		
J	Inspection	C	Mastoid Sinus, Left						
M	Reattachment	D	Inner Ear, Right						
N	Release	E	Inner Ear, Left						
P	Removal	F	Eustachian Tube, Right						
Q	Repair	G	Eustachian Tube, Left						
R	Replacement	H	Ear, Right						
S	Reposition	J	Ear, Left						
T	Resection	K	Nasal Mucosa and Soft Tissue						
U	Supplement	L	Nasal Turbinate						
W	Revision	M	Nasal Septum						
		N	Nasopharynx						
		P	Accessory Sinus						
		Q	Maxillary Sinus, Right						
		R	Maxillary Sinus, Left						
		S	Frontal Sinus, Right						
		T	Frontal Sinus, Left						
		U	Ethmoid Sinus, Right						
		V	Ethmoid Sinus, Left						
		W	Sphenoid Sinus, Right						
		X	Sphenoid Sinus, Left						
		Y	Sinus						

Respiratory System ØB1–ØBY

Character Meanings

This Character Meaning table is provided as a guide to assist the user in the identification of character members that may be found in this section of code tables. It **SHOULD NOT** be used to build a PCS code.

Operation–Character 3	Body Part–Character 4	Approach–Character 5	Device–Character 6	Qualifier–Character 7
1 Bypass	Ø Tracheobronchial Tree	Ø Open	Ø Drainage Device	Ø Allogeneic
2 Change	1 Trachea	3 Percutaneous	1 Radioactive Element	1 Syngeneic
5 Destruction	2 Carina	4 Percutaneous Endoscopic	2 Monitoring Device	2 Zooplastic
7 Dilation	3 Main Bronchus, Right	7 Via Natural or Artificial Opening	3 Infusion Device	4 Cutaneous
9 Drainage	4 Upper Lobe Bronchus, Right	8 Via Natural or Artificial Opening Endoscopic	7 Autologous Tissue Substitute	6 Esophagus
B Excision	5 Middle Lobe Bronchus, Right	X External	C Extraluminal Device	X Diagnostic
C Extirpation	6 Lower Lobe Bronchus, Right		D Intraluminal Device	Z No Qualifier
D Extraction	7 Main Bronchus, Left		E Intraluminal Device, Endotracheal Airway	
F Fragmentation	8 Upper Lobe Bronchus, Left		F Tracheostomy Device	
H Insertion	9 Lingula Bronchus		G Intraluminal Device, Endobronchial Valve	
J Inspection	B Lower Lobe Bronchus, Left		J Synthetic Substitute	
L Occlusion	C Upper Lung Lobe, Right		K Nonautologous Tissue Substitute	
M Reattachment	D Middle Lung Lobe, Right		M Diaphragmatic Pacemaker Lead	
N Release	F Lower Lung Lobe, Right		Y Other Device	
P Removal	G Upper Lung Lobe, Left		Z No Device	
Q Repair	H Lung Lingula			
R Replacement	J Lower Lung Lobe, Left			
S Reposition	K Lung, Right			
T Resection	L Lung, Left			
U Supplement	M Lungs, Bilateral			
V Restriction	N Pleura, Right			
W Revision	P Pleura, Left			
Y Transplantation	Q Pleura			
	T Diaphragm			

Mouth and Throat 0C0–0CX

Character Meanings

This Character Meaning table is provided as a guide to assist the user in the identification of character members that may be found in this section of code tables. It **SHOULD NOT** be used to build a PCS code.

Operation–Character 3		Body Part–Character 4		Approach–Character 5		Device–Character 6		Qualifier–Character 7	
0	Alteration	0	Upper Lip	0	Open	0	Drainage Device	0	Single
2	Change	1	Lower Lip	3	Percutaneous	1	Radioactive Element	1	Multiple
5	Destruction	2	Hard Palate	4	Percutaneous Endoscopic	5	External Fixation Device	2	All
7	Dilation	3	Soft Palate	7	Via Natural or Artificial Opening	7	Autologous Tissue Substitute	X	Diagnostic
9	Drainage	4	Buccal Mucosa	8	Via Natural or Artificial Opening Endoscopic	B	Intraluminal Device, Airway	Z	No Qualifier
B	Excision	5	Upper Gingiva	X	External	C	Extraluminal Device		
C	Extirpation	6	Lower Gingiva			D	Intraluminal Device		
D	Extraction	7	Tongue			J	Synthetic Substitute		
F	Fragmentation	8	Parotid Gland, Right			K	Nonautologous Tissue Substitute		
H	Insertion	9	Parotid Gland, Left			Y	Other Device		
J	Inspection	A	Salivary Gland			Z	No Device		
L	Occlusion	B	Parotid Duct, Right						
M	Reattachment	C	Parotid Duct, Left						
N	Release	D	Sublingual Gland, Right						
P	Removal	F	Sublingual Gland, Left						
Q	Repair	G	Submaxillary Gland, Right						
R	Replacement	H	Submaxillary Gland, Left						
S	Reposition	J	Minor Salivary Gland						
T	Resection	M	Pharynx						
U	Supplement	N	Uvula						
V	Restriction	P	Tonsils						
W	Revision	Q	Adenoids						
X	Transfer	R	Epiglottis						
		S	Larynx						
		T	Vocal Cord, Right						
		V	Vocal Cord, Left						
		W	Upper Tooth						
		X	Lower Tooth						
		Y	Mouth and Throat						

Gastrointestinal System ØD1–ØDY

Character Meanings

This Character Meaning table is provided as a guide to assist the user in the identification of character members that may be found in this section of code tables. It **SHOULD NOT** be used to build a PCS code.

Operation–Character 3		Body Part–Character 4		Approach–Character 5		Device–Character 6		Qualifier–Character 7	
1	Bypass	Ø	Upper Intestinal Tract	Ø	Open	Ø	Drainage Device	Ø	Allogeneic
2	Change	1	Esophagus, Upper	3	Percutaneous	1	Radioactive Element	1	Syngeneic
5	Destruction	2	Esophagus, Middle	4	Percutaneous Endoscopic	2	Monitoring Device	2	Zooplastic
7	Dilation	3	Esophagus, Lower	7	Via Natural or Artificial Opening	3	Infusion Device	3	Vertical
8	Division	4	Esophagogastric Junction	8	Via Natural or Artificial Opening Endoscopic	7	Autologous Tissue Substitute	4	Cutaneous
9	Drainage	5	Esophagus	F	Via Natural or Artificial Opening with Percutaneous Endoscopic Assistance	B	Intraluminal Device, Airway	5	Esophagus
B	Excision	6	Stomach	X	External	C	Extraluminal Device	6	Stomach
C	Extirpation	7	Stomach, Pylorus			D	Intraluminal Device	9	Duodenum
D	Extraction	8	Small Intestine			J	Synthetic Substitute	A	Jejunum
F	Fragmentation	9	Duodenum			K	Nonautologous Tissue Substitute	B	Ileum
H	Insertion	A	Jejunum			L	Artificial Sphincter	H	Cecum
J	Inspection	B	Ileum			M	Stimulator Lead	K	Ascending Colon
L	Occlusion	C	Ileocecal Valve			U	Feeding Device	L	Transverse Colon
M	Reattachment	D	Lower Intestinal Tract			Y	Other Device	M	Descending Colon
N	Release	E	Large Intestine			Z	No Device	N	Sigmoid Colon
P	Removal	F	Large Intestine, Right					P	Rectum
Q	Repair	G	Large Intestine, Left					Q	Anus
R	Replacement	H	Cecum					X	Diagnostic
S	Reposition	J	Appendix					Z	No Qualifier
T	Resection	K	Ascending Colon						
U	Supplement	L	Transverse Colon						
V	Restriction	M	Descending Colon						
W	Revision	N	Sigmoid Colon						
X	Transfer	P	Rectum						
Y	Transplantation	Q	Anus						
		R	Anal Sphincter						
		U	Omentum						
		V	Mesentery						
		W	Peritoneum						

Hepatobiliary System and Pancreas ØF1–ØFY

Character Meanings

This Character Meaning table is provided as a guide to assist the user in the identification of character members that may be found in this section of code tables. It **SHOULD NOT** be used to build a PCS code.

Operation–Character 3	Body Part–Character 4	Approach–Character 5	Device–Character 6	Qualifier–Character 7
1 Bypass	Ø Liver	Ø Open	Ø Drainage Device	Ø Allogeneic
2 Change	1 Liver, Right Lobe	3 Percutaneous	1 Radioactive Element	1 Syngeneic
5 Destruction	2 Liver, Left Lobe	4 Percutaneous Endoscopic	2 Monitoring Device	2 Zooplastic
7 Dilation	4 Gallbladder	7 Via Natural or Artificial Opening	3 Infusion Device	3 Duodenum
8 Division	5 Hepatic Duct, Right	8 Via Natural or Artificial Opening Endoscopic	7 Autologous Tissue Substitute	4 Stomach
9 Drainage	6 Hepatic Duct, Left	X External	C Extraluminal Device	5 Hepatic Duct, Right
B Excision	7 Hepatic Duct, Common		D Intraluminal Device	6 Hepatic Duct, Left
C Extirpation	8 Cystic Duct		J Synthetic Substitute	7 Hepatic Duct, Caudate
D Extraction	9 Common Bile Duct		K Nonautologous Tissue Substitute	8 Cystic Duct
F Fragmentation	B Hepatobiliary Duct		Y Other Device	9 Common Bile Duct
H Insertion	C Ampulla of Vater		Z No Device	B Small Intestine
J Inspection	D Pancreatic Duct			C Large Intestine
L Occlusion	F Pancreatic Duct, Accessory			F Irreversible Electroporation
M Reattachment	G Pancreas			X Diagnostic
N Release				Z No Qualifier
P Removal				
Q Repair				
R Replacement				
S Reposition				
T Resection				
U Supplement				
V Restriction				
W Revision				
Y Transplantation				

Endocrine System 0G2–0GW

Character Meanings

This Character Meaning table is provided as a guide to assist the user in the identification of character members that may be found in this section of code tables. It **SHOULD NOT** be used to build a PCS code.

Operation–Character 3	Body Part–Character 4	Approach–Character 5	Device–Character 6	Qualifier–Character 7
2 Change	0 Pituitary Gland	0 Open	0 Drainage Device	X Diagnostic
5 Destruction	1 Pineal Body	3 Percutaneous	2 Monitoring Device	Z No Qualifier
8 Division	2 Adrenal Gland, Left	4 Percutaneous Endoscopic	3 Infusion Device	
9 Drainage	3 Adrenal Gland, Right	X External	Y Other Device	
B Excision	4 Adrenal Glands, Bilateral		Z No Device	
C Extirpation	5 Adrenal Gland			
H Insertion	6 Carotid Body, Left			
J Inspection	7 Carotid Body, Right			
M Reattachment	8 Carotid Bodies, Bilateral			
N Release	9 Para-aortic Body			
P Removal	B Coccygeal Glomus			
Q Repair	C Glomus Jugulare			
S Reposition	D Aortic Body			
T Resection	F Paraganglion Extremity			
W Revision	G Thyroid Gland Lobe, Left			
	H Thyroid Gland Lobe, Right			
	J Thyroid Gland Isthmus			
	K Thyroid Gland			
	L Superior Parathyroid Gland, Right			
	M Superior Parathyroid Gland, Left			
	N Inferior Parathyroid Gland, Right			
	P Inferior Parathyroid Gland, Left			
	Q Parathyroid Glands, Multiple			
	R Parathyroid Gland			
	S Endocrine Gland			

Skin and Breast ØHØ–ØHX

Character Meanings

This Character Meaning table is provided as a guide to assist the user in the identification of character members that may be found in this section of code tables. It **SHOULD NOT** be used to build a PCS code.

Operation–Character 3		Body Part–Character 4		Approach–Character 5		Device–Character 6		Qualifier–Character 7	
Ø	Alteration	Ø	Skin, Scalp	Ø	Open	Ø	Drainage Device	3	Full Thickness
2	Change	1	Skin, Face	3	Percutaneous	1	Radioactive Element	4	Partial Thickness
5	Destruction	2	Skin, Right Ear	7	Via Natural or Artificial Opening	7	Autologous Tissue Substitute	5	Latissimus Dorsi Myocutaneous Flap
8	Division	3	Skin, Left Ear	8	Via Natural or Artificial Opening Endoscopic	J	Synthetic Substitute	6	Transverse Rectus Abdominis Myocutaneous Flap
9	Drainage	4	Skin, Neck	X	External	K	Nonautologous Tissue Substitute	7	Deep Inferior Epigastric Artery Perforator Flap
B	Excision	5	Skin, Chest			N	Tissue Expander	8	Superficial Inferior Epigastric Artery Flap
C	Extirpation	6	Skin, Back			Y	Other Device	9	Gluteal Artery Perforator Flap
D	Extraction	7	Skin, Abdomen			Z	No Device	D	Multiple
H	Insertion	8	Skin, Buttock					X	Diagnostic
J	Inspection	9	Skin, Perineum					Z	No Qualifier
M	Reattachment	A	Skin, Inguinal						
N	Release	B	Skin, Right Upper Arm						
P	Removal	C	Skin, Left Upper Arm						
Q	Repair	D	Skin, Right Lower Arm						
R	Replacement	E	Skin, Left Lower Arm						
S	Reposition	F	Skin, Right Hand						
T	Resection	G	Skin, Left Hand						
U	Supplement	H	Skin, Right Upper Leg						
W	Revision	J	Skin, Left Upper Leg						
X	Transfer	K	Skin, Right Lower Leg						
		L	Skin, Left Lower Leg						
		M	Skin, Right Foot						
		N	Skin, Left Foot						
		P	Skin						
		Q	Finger Nail						
		R	Toe Nail						
		S	Hair						
		T	Breast, Right						
		U	Breast, Left						
		V	Breast, Bilateral						
		W	Nipple, Right						
		X	Nipple, Left						
		Y	Supernumerary Breast						

Subcutaneous Tissue and Fascia ØJØ–ØJX

Character Meanings

This Character Meaning table is provided as a guide to assist the user in the identification of character members that may be found in this section of code tables. It **SHOULD NOT** be used to build a PCS code.

Operation–Character 3		Body Part–Character 4		Approach–Character 5		Device–Character 6		Qualifier–Character 7	
Ø	Alteration	Ø	Subcutaneous Tissue and Fascia, Scalp	Ø	Open	Ø	Drainage Device OR Monitoring Device, Hemodynamic	B	Skin and Subcutaneous Tissue
2	Change	1	Subcutaneous Tissue and Fascia, Face	3	Percutaneous	1	Radioactive Element	C	Skin, Subcutaneous Tissue and Fascia
5	Destruction	4	Subcutaneous Tissue and Fascia, Right Neck	X	External	2	Monitoring Device	X	Diagnostic
8	Division	5	Subcutaneous Tissue and Fascia, Left Neck			3	Infusion Device	Z	No Qualifier
9	Drainage	6	Subcutaneous Tissue and Fascia, Chest			4	Pacemaker, Single Chamber		
B	Excision	7	Subcutaneous Tissue and Fascia, Back			5	Pacemaker, Single Chamber Rate Responsive		
C	Extirpation	8	Subcutaneous Tissue and Fascia, Abdomen			6	Pacemaker, Dual Chamber		
D	Extraction	9	Subcutaneous Tissue and Fascia, Buttock			7	Autologous Tissue Substitute OR Cardiac Resynchronization Pacemaker Pulse Generator		
H	Insertion	B	Subcutaneous Tissue and Fascia, Perineum			8	Defibrillator Generator		
J	Inspection	C	Subcutaneous Tissue and Fascia, Pelvic Region			9	Cardiac Resynchronization Defibrillator Pulse Generator		
N	Release	D	Subcutaneous Tissue and Fascia, Right Upper Arm			A	Contractility Modulation Device		
P	Removal	F	Subcutaneous Tissue and Fascia, Left Upper Arm			B	Stimulator Generator, Single Array		
Q	Repair	G	Subcutaneous Tissue and Fascia, Right Lower Arm			C	Stimulator Generator, Single Array Rechargeable		
R	Replacement	H	Subcutaneous Tissue and Fascia, Left Lower Arm			D	Stimulator Generator, Multiple Array		
U	Supplement	J	Subcutaneous Tissue and Fascia, Right Hand			E	Stimulator Generator, Multiple Array Rechargeable		
W	Revision	K	Subcutaneous Tissue and Fascia, Left Hand			H	Contraceptive Device		
X	Transfer	L	Subcutaneous Tissue and Fascia, Right Upper Leg			J	Synthetic Substitute		
		M	Subcutaneous Tissue and Fascia, Left Upper Leg			K	Nonautologous Tissue Substitute		
		N	Subcutaneous Tissue and Fascia, Right Lower Leg			M	Stimulator Generator		
		P	Subcutaneous Tissue and Fascia, Left Lower Leg			N	Tissue Expander		
		Q	Subcutaneous Tissue and Fascia, Right Foot			P	Cardiac Rhythm Related Device		
		R	Subcutaneous Tissue and Fascia, Left Foot			V	Infusion Device, Pump		
		S	Subcutaneous Tissue and Fascia, Head and Neck			W	Vascular Access Device, Totally Implantable		
		T	Subcutaneous Tissue and Fascia, Trunk			X	Vascular Access Device, Tunneled		
		V	Subcutaneous Tissue and Fascia, Upper Extremity			Y	Other Device		
		W	Subcutaneous Tissue and Fascia, Lower Extremity			Z	No Device		

Muscles ØK2–ØKX

Character Meanings

This Character Meaning table is provided as a guide to assist the user in the identification of character members that may be found in this section of code tables. It **SHOULD NOT** be used to build a PCS code.

Operation–Character 3	Body Part–Character 4	Approach–Character 5	Device–Character 6	Qualifier–Character 7
2 Change	Ø Head Muscle	Ø Open	Ø Drainage Device	Ø Skin
5 Destruction	1 Facial Muscle	3 Percutaneous	7 Autologous Tissue Substitute	1 Subcutaneous Tissue
8 Division	2 Neck Muscle, Right	4 Percutaneous Endoscopic	J Synthetic Substitute	2 Skin and Subcutaneous Tissue
9 Drainage	3 Neck Muscle, Left	X External	K Nonautologous Tissue Substitute	5 Latissimus Dorsi Myocutaneous Flap
B Excision	4 Tongue, Palate, Pharynx Muscle		M Stimulator Lead	6 Transverse Rectus Abdominis Myocutaneous Flap
C Extirpation	5 Shoulder Muscle, Right		Y Other Device	7 Deep Inferior Epigastric Artery Perforator Flap
D Extraction	6 Shoulder Muscle, Left		Z No Device	8 Superficial Inferior Epigastric Artery Flap
H Insertion	7 Upper Arm Muscle, Right			9 Gluteal Artery Perforator Flap
J Inspection	8 Upper Arm Muscle, Left			X Diagnostic
M Reattachment	9 Lower Arm and Wrist Muscle, Right			Z No Qualifier
N Release	B Lower Arm and Wrist Muscle, Left			
P Removal	C Hand Muscle, Right			
Q Repair	D Hand Muscle, Left			
R Replacement	F Trunk Muscle, Right			
S Reposition	G Trunk Muscle, Left			
T Resection	H Thorax Muscle, Right			
U Supplement	J Thorax Muscle, Left			
W Revision	K Abdomen Muscle, Right			
X Transfer	L Abdomen Muscle, Left			
	M Perineum Muscle			
	N Hip Muscle, Right			
	P Hip Muscle, Left			
	Q Upper Leg Muscle, Right			
	R Upper Leg Muscle, Left			
	S Lower Leg Muscle, Right			
	T Lower Leg Muscle, Left			
	V Foot Muscle, Right			
	W Foot Muscle, Left			
	X Upper Muscle			
	Y Lower Muscle			

Tendons 0L2–0LX

Character Meanings

This Character Meaning table is provided as a guide to assist the user in the identification of character members that may be found in this section of code tables. It **SHOULD NOT** be used to build a PCS code.

Operation–Character 3	Body Part–Character 4	Approach–Character 5	Device–Character 6	Qualifier–Character 7
2 Change	0 Head and Neck Tendon	0 Open	0 Drainage Device	X Diagnostic
5 Destruction	1 Shoulder Tendon, Right	3 Percutaneous	7 Autologous Tissue Substitute	Z No Qualifier
8 Division	2 Shoulder Tendon, Left	4 Percutaneous Endoscopic	J Synthetic Substitute	
9 Drainage	3 Upper Arm Tendon, Right	X External	K Nonautologous Tissue Substitute	
B Excision	4 Upper Arm Tendon, Left		Y Other Device	
C Extirpation	5 Lower Arm and Wrist Tendon, Right		Z No Device	
D Extraction	6 Lower Arm and Wrist Tendon, Left			
H Insertion	7 Hand Tendon, Right			
J Inspection	8 Hand Tendon, Left			
M Reattachment	9 Trunk Tendon, Right			
N Release	B Trunk Tendon, Left			
P Removal	C Thorax Tendon, Right			
Q Repair	D Thorax Tendon, Left			
R Replacement	F Abdomen Tendon, Right			
S Reposition	G Abdomen Tendon, Left			
T Resection	H Perineum Tendon			
U Supplement	J Hip Tendon, Right			
W Revision	K Hip Tendon, Left			
X Transfer	L Upper Leg Tendon, Right			
	M Upper Leg Tendon, Left			
	N Lower Leg Tendon, Right			
	P Lower Leg Tendon, Left			
	Q Knee Tendon, Right			
	R Knee Tendon, Left			
	S Ankle Tendon, Right			
	T Ankle Tendon, Left			
	V Foot Tendon, Right			
	W Foot Tendon, Left			
	X Upper Tendon			
	Y Lower Tendon			

Bursae and Ligaments ØM2–ØMX

Character Meanings

This Character Meaning table is provided as a guide to assist the user in the identification of character members that may be found in this section of code tables. It **SHOULD NOT** be used to build a PCS code.

Operation–Character 3		Body Part–Character 4		Approach–Character 5		Device–Character 6		Qualifier–Character 7	
2	Change	Ø	Head and Neck Bursa and Ligament	Ø	Open	Ø	Drainage Device	X	Diagnostic
5	Destruction	1	Shoulder Bursa and Ligament, Right	3	Percutaneous	7	Autologous Tissue Substitute	Z	No Qualifier
8	Division	2	Shoulder Bursa and Ligament, Left	4	Percutaneous Endoscopic	J	Synthetic Substitute		
9	Drainage	3	Elbow Bursa and Ligament, Right	X	External	K	Nonautologous Tissue Substitute		
B	Excision	4	Elbow Bursa and Ligament, Left			Y	Other Device		
C	Extirpation	5	Wrist Bursa and Ligament, Right			Z	No Device		
D	Extraction	6	Wrist Bursa and Ligament, Left						
H	Insertion	7	Hand Bursa and Ligament, Right						
J	Inspection	8	Hand Bursa and Ligament, Left						
M	Reattachment	9	Upper Extremity Bursa and Ligament, Right						
N	Release	B	Upper Extremity Bursa and Ligament, Left						
P	Removal	C	Upper Spine Bursa and Ligament						
Q	Repair	D	Lower Spine Bursa and Ligament						
R	Replacement	F	Sternum Bursa and Ligament						
S	Reposition	G	Rib(s) Bursa and Ligament						
T	Resection	H	Abdomen Bursa and Ligament, Right						
U	Supplement	J	Abdomen Bursa and Ligament, Left						
W	Revision	K	Perineum Bursa and Ligament						
X	Transfer	L	Hip Bursa and Ligament, Right						
		M	Hip Bursa and Ligament, Left						
		N	Knee Bursa and Ligament, Right						
		P	Knee Bursa and Ligament, Left						
		Q	Ankle Bursa and Ligament, Right						
		R	Ankle Bursa and Ligament, Left						
		S	Foot Bursa and Ligament, Right						
		T	Foot Bursa and Ligament, Left						
		V	Lower Extremity Bursa and Ligament, Right						
		W	Lower Extremity Bursa and Ligament, Left						
		X	Upper Bursa and Ligament						
		Y	Lower Bursa and Ligament						

Head and Facial Bones ØN2–ØNW

Character Meanings

This Character Meaning table is provided as a guide to assist the user in the identification of character members that may be found in this section of code tables. It **SHOULD NOT** be used to build a PCS code.

Operation–Character 3		Body Part–Character 4		Approach–Character 5		Device–Character 6		Qualifier–Character 7	
2	Change	Ø	Skull	Ø	Open	Ø	Drainage Device	X	Diagnostic
5	Destruction	1	Frontal Bone	3	Percutaneous	4	Internal Fixation Device	Z	No Qualifier
8	Division	3	Parietal Bone, Right	4	Percutaneous Endoscopic	5	External Fixation Device		
9	Drainage	4	Parietal Bone, Left	X	External	7	Autologous Tissue Substitute		
B	Excision	5	Temporal Bone, Right			J	Synthetic Substitute		
C	Extirpation	6	Temporal Bone, Left			K	Nonautologous Tissue Substitute		
D	Extraction	7	Occipital Bone			M	Bone Growth Stimulator		
H	Insertion	B	Nasal Bone			N	Neurostimulator Generator		
J	Inspection	C	Sphenoid Bone			S	Hearing Device		
N	Release	F	Ethmoid Bone, Right			Y	Other Device		
P	Removal	G	Ethmoid Bone, Left			Z	No Device		
Q	Repair	H	Lacrimal Bone, Right						
R	Replacement	J	Lacrimal Bone, Left						
S	Reposition	K	Palatine Bone, Right						
T	Resection	L	Palatine Bone, Left						
U	Supplement	M	Zygomatic Bone, Right						
W	Revision	N	Zygomatic Bone, Left						
		P	Orbit, Right						
		Q	Orbit, Left						
		R	Maxilla						
		T	Mandible, Right						
		V	Mandible, Left						
		W	Facial Bone						
		X	Hyoid Bone						

Upper Bones ØP2–ØPW

Character Meanings

This Character Meaning table is provided as a guide to assist the user in the identification of character members that may be found in this section of code tables. It **SHOULD NOT** be used to build a PCS code.

Operation–Character 3	Body Part–Character 4	Approach–Character 5	Device–Character 6	Qualifier–Character 7
2 Change	Ø Sternum	Ø Open	Ø Drainage Device OR Internal Fixation Device, Rigid Plate	X Diagnostic
5 Destruction	1 Ribs, 1 to 2	3 Percutaneous	4 Internal Fixation Device	Z No Qualifier
8 Division	2 Ribs, 3 or more	4 Percutaneous Endoscopic	5 External Fixation Device	
9 Drainage	3 Cervical Vertebra	X External	6 Internal Fixation Device, Intramedullary	
B Excision	4 Thoracic Vertebra		7 Autologous Tissue Substitute	
C Extirpation	5 Scapula, Right		8 External Fixation Device, Limb Lengthening	
D Extraction	6 Scapula, Left		B External Fixation Device, Monoplanar	
H Insertion	7 Glenoid Cavity, Right		C External Fixation Device, Ring	
J Inspection	8 Glenoid Cavity, Left		D External Fixation Device, Hybrid	
N Release	9 Clavicle, Right		J Synthetic Substitute	
P Removal	B Clavicle, Left		K Nonautologous Tissue Substitute	
Q Repair	C Humeral Head, Right		M Bone Growth Stimulator	
R Replacement	D Humeral Head, Left		Y Other Device	
S Reposition	F Humeral Shaft, Right		Z No Device	
T Resection	G Humeral Shaft, Left			
U Supplement	H Radius, Right			
W Revision	J Radius, Left			
	K Ulna, Right			
	L Ulna, Left			
	M Carpal, Right			
	N Carpal, Left			
	P Metacarpal, Right			
	Q Metacarpal, Left			
	R Thumb Phalanx, Right			
	S Thumb Phalanx, Left			
	T Finger Phalanx, Right			
	V Finger Phalanx, Left			
	Y Upper Bone			

Lower Bones ØQ2–ØQW

Character Meanings

This Character Meaning table is provided as a guide to assist the user in the identification of character members that may be found in this section of code tables. It **SHOULD NOT** be used to build a PCS code.

Operation–Character 3	Body Part–Character 4	Approach–Character 5	Device–Character 6	Qualifier–Character 7
2 Change	Ø Lumbar Vertebra	Ø Open	Ø Drainage Device	2 Sesamoid Bone(s) 1st Toe
5 Destruction	1 Sacrum	3 Percutaneous	4 Internal Fixation Device	X Diagnostic
8 Division	2 Pelvic Bone, Right	4 Percutaneous Endoscopic	5 External Fixation Device	Z No Qualifier
9 Drainage	3 Pelvic Bone, Left	X External	6 Internal Fixation Device, Intramedullary	
B Excision	4 Acetabulum, Right		7 Autologous Tissue Substitute	
C Extirpation	5 Acetabulum, Left		8 External Fixation Device, Limb Lengthening	
D Extraction	6 Upper Femur, Right		B External Fixation Device, Monoplanar	
H Insertion	7 Upper Femur, Left		C External Fixation Device, Ring	
J Inspection	8 Femoral Shaft, Right		D External Fixation Device, Hybrid	
N Release	9 Femoral Shaft, Left		J Synthetic Substitute	
P Removal	B Lower Femur, Right		K Nonautologous Tissue Substitute	
Q Repair	C Lower Femur, Left		M Bone Growth Stimulator	
R Replacement	D Patella, Right		Y Other Device	
S Reposition	F Patella, Left		Z No Device	
T Resection	G Tibia, Right			
U Supplement	H Tibia, Left			
W Revision	J Fibula, Right			
	K Fibula, Left			
	L Tarsal, Right			
	M Tarsal, Left			
	N Metatarsal, Right			
	P Metatarsal, Left			
	Q Toe Phalanx, Right			
	R Toe Phalanx, Left			
	S Coccyx			
	Y Lower Bone			

Upper Joints ØR2–ØRW

Character Meanings

This Character Meaning table is provided as a guide to assist the user in the identification of character members that may be found in this section of code tables. It **SHOULD NOT** be used to build a PCS code.

Operation–Character 3	Body Part–Character 4	Approach–Character 5	Device–Character 6	Qualifier–Character 7
2 Change	Ø Occipital-cervical Joint	Ø Open	Ø Drainage Device OR Synthetic Substitute, Reverse Ball and Socket	Ø Anterior Approach, Anterior Column
5 Destruction	1 Cervical Vertebral Joint	3 Percutaneous	3 Infusion Device	1 Posterior Approach, Posterior Column
9 Drainage	2 Cervical Vertebral Joint, 2 or more	4 Percutaneous Endoscopic	4 Internal Fixation Device	6 Humeral Surface
B Excision	3 Cervical Vertebral Disc	X External	5 External Fixation Device	7 Glenoid Surface
C Extirpation	4 Cervicothoracic Vertebral Joint		7 Autologous Tissue Substitute	J Posterior Approach, Anterior Column
G Fusion	5 Cervicothoracic Vertebral Disc		8 Spacer	X Diagnostic
H Insertion	6 Thoracic Vertebral Joint		A Interbody Fusion Device	Z No Qualifier
J Inspection	7 Thoracic Vertebral Joint, 2 to 7		B Spinal Stabilization Device, Interspinous Process	
N Release	8 Thoracic Vertebral Joint, 8 or more		C Spinal Stabilization Device, Pedicle-Based	
P Removal	9 Thoracic Vertebral Disc		D Spinal Stabilization Device, Facet Replacement	
Q Repair	A Thoracolumbar Vertebral Joint		J Synthetic Substitute	
R Replacement	B Thoracolumbar Vertebral Disc		K Nonautologous Tissue Substitute	
S Reposition	C Temporomandibular Joint, Right		Y Other Device	
T Resection	D Temporomandibular Joint, Left		Z No Device	
U Supplement	E Sternoclavicular Joint, Right			
W Revision	F Sternoclavicular Joint, Left			
	G Acromioclavicular Joint, Right			
	H Acromioclavicular Joint, Left			
	J Shoulder Joint, Right			
	K Shoulder Joint, Left			
	L Elbow Joint, Right			
	M Elbow Joint, Left			
	N Wrist Joint, Right			
	P Wrist Joint, Left			
	Q Carpal Joint, Right			
	R Carpal Joint, Left			
	S Carpometacarpal Joint, Right			
	T Carpometacarpal Joint, Left			
	U Metacarpophalangeal Joint, Right			
	V Metacarpophalangeal Joint, Left			
	W Finger Phalangeal Joint, Right			
	X Finger Phalangeal Joint, Left			
	Y Upper Joint			

Lower Joints ØS2–ØSW

Character Meanings

This Character Meaning table is provided as a guide to assist the user in the identification of character members that may be found in this section of code tables. It **SHOULD NOT** be used to build a PCS code.

Operation–Character 3	Body Part–Character 4	Approach–Character 5	Device–Character 6	Qualifier–Character 7
2 Change	Ø Lumbar Vertebral Joint	Ø Open	Ø Drainage Device OR Synthetic Substitute, Polyethylene	Ø Anterior Approach, Anterior Column
5 Destruction	1 Lumbar Vertebral Joint, 2 or more	3 Percutaneous	1 Synthetic Substitute, Metal	1 Posterior Approach, Posterior Column
9 Drainage	2 Lumbar Vertebral Disc	4 Percutaneous Endoscopic	2 Synthetic Substitute, Metal on Polyethylene	9 Cemented
B Excision	3 Lumbosacral Joint	X External	3 Infusion Device OR Synthetic Substitute, Ceramic	A Uncemented
C Extirpation	4 Lumbosacral Disc		4 Internal Fixation Device OR Synthetic Substitute, Ceramic on Polyethylene	C Patellar Surface
G Fusion	5 Sacrococcygeal Joint		5 External Fixation Device	J Posterior Approach, Anterior Column
H Insertion	6 Coccygeal Joint		6 Synthetic Substitute, Oxidized Zirconium on Polyethylene	X Diagnostic
J Inspection	7 Sacroiliac Joint, Right		7 Autologous Tissue Substitute	Z No Qualifier
N Release	8 Sacroiliac Joint, Left		8 Spacer	
P Removal	9 Hip Joint, Right		9 Liner	
Q Repair	A Hip Joint, Acetabular Surface, Right		A Interbody Fusion Device	
R Replacement	B Hip Joint, Left		B Resurfacing Device OR Spinal Stabilization Device, Interspinous Process	
S Reposition	C Knee Joint, Right		C Spinal Stabilization Device, Pedicle-Based	
T Resection	D Knee Joint, Left		D Spinal Stabilization Device, Facet Replacement	
U Supplement	E Hip Joint, Acetabular Surface, Left		E Articulating Spacer	
W Revision	F Ankle Joint, Right		J Synthetic Substitute	
	G Ankle Joint, Left		K Nonautologous Tissue Substitute	
	H Tarsal Joint, Right		L Synthetic Substitute, Unicondylar Medial	
	J Tarsal Joint, Left		M Synthetic Substitute, Unicondylar Lateral	
	K Tarsometatarsal Joint, Right		N Synthetic Substitute, Patello Femoral	
	L Tarsometatarsal Joint, Left		Y Other Device	
	M Metatarsal-Phalangeal Joint, Right		Z No Device	
	N Metatarsal-Phalangeal Joint, Left			
	P Toe Phalangeal Joint, Right			
	Q Toe Phalangeal Joint, Left			

Continued on next page

Lower Joints ØS2–ØSW (Continued)

Operation–Character 3	Body Part–Character 4		Approach–Character 5	Device–Character 6	Qualifier–Character 7
	R	Hip Joint, Femoral Surface, Right			
	S	Hip Joint, Femoral Surface, Left			
	T	Knee Joint, Femoral Surface, Right			
	U	Knee Joint, Femoral Surface, Left			
	V	Knee Joint, Tibial Surface, Right			
	W	Knee Joint, Tibial Surface, Left			
	Y	Lower Joint			

Urinary System ØT1–ØTY

Character Meanings

This Character Meaning table is provided as a guide to assist the user in the identification of character members that may be found in this section of code tables. It **SHOULD NOT** be used to build a PCS code.

Operation–Character 3	Body Part–Character 4	Approach–Character 5	Device–Character 6	Qualifier–Character 7
1 Bypass	Ø Kidney, Right	Ø Open	Ø Drainage Device	Ø Allogeneic
2 Change	1 Kidney, Left	3 Percutaneous	2 Monitoring Device	1 Syngeneic
5 Destruction	2 Kidneys, Bilateral	4 Percutaneous Endoscopic	3 Infusion Device	2 Zooplastic
7 Dilation	3 Kidney Pelvis, Right	7 Via Natural or Artificial Opening	7 Autologous Tissue Substitute	3 Kidney Pelvis, Right
8 Division	4 Kidney Pelvis, Left	8 Via Natural or Artificial Opening Endoscopic	C Extraluminal Device	4 Kidney Pelvis, Left
9 Drainage	5 Kidney	X External	D Intraluminal Device	6 Ureter, Right
B Excision	6 Ureter, Right		J Synthetic Substitute	7 Ureter, Left
C Extirpation	7 Ureter, Left		K Nonautologous Tissue Substitute	8 Colon
D Extraction	8 Ureters, Bilateral		L Artificial Sphincter	9 Colocutaneous
F Fragmentation	9 Ureter		M Stimulator Lead	A Ileum
H Insertion	B Bladder		Y Other Device	B Bladder
J Inspection	C Bladder Neck		Z No Device	C Ileocutaneous
L Occlusion	D Urethra			D Cutaneous
M Reattachment				X Diagnostic
N Release				Z No Qualifier
P Removal				
Q Repair				
R Replacement				
S Reposition				
T Resection				
U Supplement				
V Restriction				
W Revision				
Y Transplantation				

Female Reproductive System ØU1–ØUY

Character Meanings

This Character Meaning table is provided as a guide to assist the user in the identification of character members that may be found in this section of code tables. It **SHOULD NOT** be used to build a PCS code.

Operation–Character 3		Body Part–Character 4		Approach–Character 5		Device–Character 6		Qualifier–Character 7	
1	Bypass	Ø	Ovary, Right	Ø	Open	Ø	Drainage Device	Ø	Allogeneic
2	Change	1	Ovary, Left	3	Percutaneous	1	Radioactive Element	1	Syngeneic
5	Destruction	2	Ovaries, Bilateral	4	Percutaneous Endoscopic	3	Infusion Device	2	Zooplastic
7	Dilation	3	Ovary	7	Via Natural or Artificial Opening	7	Autologous Tissue Substitute	5	Fallopian Tube, Right
8	Division	4	Uterine Supporting Structure	8	Via Natural or Artificial Opening Endoscopic	C	Extraluminal Device	6	Fallopian Tube, Left
9	Drainage	5	Fallopian Tube, Right	F	Via Natural or Artificial Opening With Percutaneous Endoscopic Assistance	D	Intraluminal Device	9	Uterus
B	Excision	6	Fallopian Tube, Left	X	External	G	Intraluminal Device, Pessary	L	Supracervical
C	Extirpation	7	Fallopian Tubes, Bilateral			H	Contraceptive Device	X	Diagnostic
D	Extraction	8	Fallopian Tube			J	Synthetic Substitute	Z	No Qualifier
F	Fragmentation	9	Uterus			K	Nonautologous Tissue Substitute		
H	Insertion	B	Endometrium			Y	Other Device		
J	Inspection	C	Cervix			Z	No Device		
L	Occlusion	D	Uterus and Cervix						
M	Reattachment	F	Cul-de-sac						
N	Release	G	Vagina						
P	Removal	H	Vagina and Cul-de-sac						
Q	Repair	J	Clitoris						
S	Reposition	K	Hymen						
T	Resection	L	Vestibular Gland						
U	Supplement	M	Vulva						
V	Restriction	N	Ova						
W	Revision								
Y	Transplantation								

Male Reproductive System ØV1–ØVW

Character Meaning

This Character Meaning table is provided as a guide to assist the user in the identification of character members that may be found in this section of code tables. It **SHOULD NOT** be used to build a PCS code.

Operation–Character 3	Body Part–Character 4	Approach–Character 5	Device–Character 6	Qualifier–Character 7
1 Bypass	Ø Prostate	Ø Open	Ø Drainage Device	D Urethra
2 Change	1 Seminal Vesicle, Right	3 Percutaneous	1 Radioactive Element	J Epididymis, Right
5 Destruction	2 Seminal Vesicle, Left	4 Percutaneous Endoscopic	3 Infusion Device	K Epididymis, Left
7 Dilation	3 Seminal Vesicles, Bilateral	7 Via Natural or Artificial Opening	7 Autologous Tissue Substitute	N Vas Deferens, Right
9 Drainage	4 Prostate and Seminal Vesicles	8 Via Natural or Artificial Opening Endoscopic	C Extraluminal Device	P Vas Deferens, Left
B Excision	5 Scrotum	X External	D Intraluminal Device	S Penis
C Extirpation	6 Tunica Vaginalis, Right		J Synthetic Substitute	X Diagnostic
H Insertion	7 Tunica Vaginalis, Left		K Nonautologous Tissue Substitute	Z No Qualifier
J Inspection	8 Scrotum and Tunica Vaginalis		Y Other Device	
L Occlusion	9 Testis, Right		Z No Device	
M Reattachment	B Testis, Left			
N Release	C Testes, Bilateral			
P Removal	D Testis			
Q Repair	F Spermatic Cord, Right			
R Replacement	G Spermatic Cord, Left			
S Reposition	H Spermatic Cords, Bilateral			
T Resection	J Epididymis, Right			
U Supplement	K Epididymis, Left			
W Revision	L Epididymis, Bilateral			
X Transfer	M Epididymis and Spermatic Cord			
	N Vas Deferens, Right			
	P Vas Deferens, Left			
	Q Vas Deferens, Bilateral			
	R Vas Deferens			
	S Penis			
	T Prepuce			

Anatomical Regions, General ØWØ–ØWY

Character Meanings

This Character Meaning table is provided as a guide to assist the user in the identification of character members that may be found in this section of code tables. It **SHOULD NOT** be used to build a PCS code.

Operation–Character 3	Body Region–Character 4	Approach–Character 5	Device–Character 6	Qualifier–Character 7
Ø Alteration	Ø Head	Ø Open	Ø Drainage Device	Ø Vagina OR Allogeneic
1 Bypass	1 Cranial Cavity	3 Percutaneous	1 Radioactive Element	1 Penis OR Syngeneic
2 Change	2 Face	4 Percutaneous Endoscopic	3 Infusion Device	2 Stoma
3 Control	3 Oral Cavity and Throat	7 Via Natural or Artificial Opening	7 Autologous Tissue Substitute	4 Cutaneous
4 Creation	4 Upper Jaw	8 Via Natural or Artificial Opening Endoscopic	J Synthetic Substitute	9 Pleural Cavity, Right
8 Division	5 Lower Jaw	X External	K Nonautologous Tissue Substitute	B Pleural Cavity, Left
9 Drainage	6 Neck		Y Other Device	G Peritoneal Cavity
B Excision	8 Chest Wall		Z No Device	J Pelvic Cavity
C Extirpation	9 Pleural Cavity, Right			W Upper Vein
F Fragmentation	B Pleural Cavity, Left			X Diagnostic
H Insertion	C Mediastinum			Y Lower Vein
J Inspection	D Pericardial Cavity			Z No Qualifier
M Reattachment	F Abdominal Wall			
P Removal	G Peritoneal Cavity			
Q Repair	H Retroperitoneum			
U Supplement	J Pelvic Cavity			
W Revision	K Upper Back			
Y Transplantation	L Lower Back			
	M Perineum, Male			
	N Perineum, Female			
	P Gastrointestinal Tract			
	Q Respiratory Tract			
	R Genitourinary Tract			

Anatomical Regions, Upper Extremities ØXØ–ØXY

Character Meanings

This Character Meaning table is provided as a guide to assist the user in the identification of character members that may be found in this section of code tables. It **SHOULD NOT** be used to build a PCS code.

Operation–Character 3	Body Part–Character 4	Approach–Character 5	Device–Character 6	Qualifier–Character 7
Ø Alteration	Ø Forequarter, Right	Ø Open	Ø Drainage Device	Ø Complete OR Allogeneic
2 Change	1 Forequarter, Left	3 Percutaneous	1 Radioactive Element	1 High OR Syngeneic
3 Control	2 Shoulder Region, Right	4 Percutaneous Endoscopic	3 Infusion Device	2 Mid
6 Detachment	3 Shoulder Region, Left	X External	7 Autologous Tissue Substitute	3 Low
9 Drainage	4 Axilla, Right		J Synthetic Substitute	4 Complete 1st Ray
B Excision	5 Axilla, Left		K Nonautologous Tissue Substitute	5 Complete 2nd Ray
H Insertion	6 Upper Extremity, Right		Y Other Device	6 Complete 3rd Ray
J Inspection	7 Upper Extremity, Left		Z No Device	7 Complete 4th Ray
M Reattachment	8 Upper Arm, Right			8 Complete 5th Ray
P Removal	9 Upper Arm, Left			9 Partial 1st Ray
Q Repair	B Elbow Region, Right			B Partial 2nd Ray
R Replacement	C Elbow Region, Left			C Partial 3rd Ray
U Supplement	D Lower Arm, Right			D Partial 4th Ray
W Revision	F Lower Arm, Left			F Partial 5th Ray
X Transfer	G Wrist Region, Right			L Thumb, Right
Y Transplantation	H Wrist Region, Left			M Thumb, Left
	J Hand, Right			N Toe, Right
	K Hand, Left			P Toe, Left
	L Thumb, Right			X Diagnostic
	M Thumb, Left			Z No Qualifier
	N Index Finger, Right			
	P Index Finger, Left			
	Q Middle Finger, Right			
	R Middle Finger, Left			
	S Ring Finger, Right			
	T Ring Finger, Left			
	V Little Finger, Right			
	W Little Finger, Left			

Anatomical Regions, Lower Extremities ØYØ–ØYW

Character Meanings

This Character Meaning table is provided as a guide to assist the user in the identification of character members that may be found in this section of code tables. It **SHOULD NOT** be used to build a PCS code.

Operation–Character 3		Body Part–Character 4		Approach–Character 5		Device–Character 6		Qualifier–Character 7	
Ø	Alteration	Ø	Buttock, Right	Ø	Open	Ø	Drainage Device	Ø	Complete
2	Change	1	Buttock, Left	3	Percutaneous	1	Radioactive Element	1	High
3	Control	2	Hindquarter, Right	4	Percutaneous Endoscopic	3	Infusion Device	2	Mid
6	Detachment	3	Hindquarter, Left	X	External	7	Autologous Tissue Substitute	3	Low
9	Drainage	4	Hindquarter, Bilateral			J	Synthetic Substitute	4	Complete 1st Ray
B	Excision	5	Inguinal Region, Right			K	Nonautologous Tissue Substitute	5	Complete 2nd Ray
H	Insertion	6	Inguinal Region, Left			Y	Other Device	6	Complete 3rd Ray
J	Inspection	7	Femoral Region, Right			Z	No Device	7	Complete 4th Ray
M	Reattachment	8	Femoral Region, Left					8	Complete 5th Ray
P	Removal	9	Lower Extremity, Right					9	Partial 1st Ray
Q	Repair	A	Inguinal Region, Bilateral					B	Partial 2nd Ray
U	Supplement	B	Lower Extremity, Left					C	Partial 3rd Ray
W	Revision	C	Upper Leg, Right					D	Partial 4th Ray
		D	Upper Leg, Left					F	Partial 5th Ray
		E	Femoral Region, Bilateral					X	Diagnostic
		F	Knee Region, Right					Z	No Qualifier
		G	Knee Region, Left						
		H	Lower Leg, Right						
		J	Lower Leg, Left						
		K	Ankle Region, Right						
		L	Ankle Region, Left						
		M	Foot, Right						
		N	Foot, Left						
		P	1st Toe, Right						
		Q	1st Toe, Left						
		R	2nd Toe, Right						
		S	2nd Toe, Left						
		T	3rd Toe, Right						
		U	3rd Toe, Left						
		V	4th Toe, Right						
		W	4th Toe, Left						
		X	5th Toe, Right						
		Y	5th Toe, Left						

Obstetrics 1Ø2–1ØY

Character Meanings

This Character Meaning table is provided as a guide to assist the user in the identification of character members that may be found in this section of code tables. It **SHOULD NOT** be used to build a PCS code.

Ø: Pregnancy

Operation–Character 3		Body Part–Character 4		Approach–Character 5		Device–Character 6		Qualifier–Character 7	
2	Change	Ø	Products of Conception	Ø	Open	3	Monitoring Electrode	Ø	High
9	Drainage	1	Products of Conception, Retained	3	Percutaneous	Y	Other Device	1	Low
A	Abortion	2	Products of Conception, Ectopic	4	Percutaneous Endoscopic	Z	No Device	2	Extraperitoneal
D	Extraction			7	Via Natural or Artificial Opening			3	Low Forceps
E	Delivery			8	Via Natural or Artificial Opening Endoscopic			4	Mid Forceps
H	Insertion			X	External			5	High Forceps
J	Inspection							6	Vacuum
P	Removal							7	Internal Version
Q	Repair							8	Other
S	Reposition							9	Fetal Blood OR Manual
T	Resection							A	Fetal Cerebrospinal Fluid
Y	Transplantation							B	Fetal Fluid, Other
								C	Amniotic Fluid, Therapeutic
								D	Fluid, Other
								E	Nervous System
								F	Cardiovascular System
								G	Lymphatics & Hemic
								H	Eye
								J	Ear, Nose & Sinus
								K	Respiratory System
								L	Mouth & Throat
								M	Gastrointestinal System
								N	Hepatobiliary & Pancreas
								P	Endocrine System
								Q	Skin
								R	Musculoskeletal System
								S	Urinary System
								T	Female Reproductive System
								U	Amniotic Fluid, Diagnostic
								V	Male Reproductive System
								W	Laminaria
								X	Abortifacient
								Y	Other Body System
								Z	No Qualifier

Placement 2WØ–2Y5

Character Meanings

This Character Meaning table is provided as a guide to assist the user in the identification of character members that may be found in this section of code tables. It **SHOULD NOT** be used to build a PCS code.

W: Anatomical Regions

Operation–Character 3	Body Region–Character 4	Approach–Character 5	Device–Character 6	Qualifier–Character 7
Ø Change	Ø Head	X External	Ø Traction Apparatus	Z No Qualifier
1 Compression	1 Face		1 Splint	
2 Dressing	2 Neck		2 Cast	
3 Immobilization	3 Abdominal Wall		3 Brace	
4 Packing	4 Chest Wall		4 Bandage	
5 Removal	5 Back		5 Packing Material	
6 Traction	6 Inguinal Region, Right		6 Pressure Dressing	
	7 Inguinal Region, Left		7 Intermittent Pressure Device	
	8 Upper Extremity, Right		9 Wire	
	9 Upper Extremity, Left		Y Other Device	
	A Upper Arm, Right		Z No Device	
	B Upper Arm, Left			
	C Lower Arm, Right			
	D Lower Arm, Left			
	E Hand, Right			
	F Hand, Left			
	G Thumb, Right			
	H Thumb, Left			
	J Finger, Right			
	K Finger, Left			
	L Lower Extremity, Right			
	M Lower Extremity, Left			
	N Upper Leg, Right			
	P Upper Leg, Left			
	Q Lower Leg, Right			
	R Lower Leg, Left			
	S Foot, Right			
	T Foot, Left			
	U Toe, Right			
	V Toe, Left			

Y: Anatomical Orifices

Operation–Character 3	Body Orifice–Character 4	Approach–Character 5	Device–Character 6	Qualifier–Character 7
Ø Change	Ø Mouth and Pharynx	X External	5 Packing Material	Z No Qualifier
4 Packing	1 Nasal			
5 Removal	2 Ear			
	3 Anorectal			
	4 Female Genital Tract			
	5 Urethra			

Administration 3Ø2–3E1

Character Meanings

This Character Meaning table is provided as a guide to assist the user in the identification of character members that may be found in this section of code tables. It **SHOULD NOT** be used to build a PCS code.

Ø: Circulatory

Operation–Character 3	Body System/Region – Character 4	Approach–Character 5	Substance–Character 6	Qualifier–Character 7
2 Transfusion	3 Peripheral Vein	Ø Open	A Stem Cells, Embryonic	Ø Autologous
	4 Central Vein	3 Percutaneous	B 4-Factor Prothrombin Complex Concentrate	1 Nonautologous
	5 Peripheral Artery	7 Via Natural or Artificial Opening	G Bone Marrow	2 Allogeneic, Related
	6 Central Artery		H Whole Blood	3 Allogeneic, Unrelated
	7 Products of Conception, Circulatory		J Serum Albumin	4 Allogeneic, Unspecified
	8 Vein		K Frozen Plasma	Z No Qualifier
			L Fresh Plasma	
			M Plasma Cryoprecipitate	
			N Red Blood Cells	
			P Frozen Red Cells	
			Q White Cells	
			R Platelets	
			S Globulin	
			T Fibrinogen	
			V Antihemophilic Factors	
			W Factor IX	
			X Stem Cells, Cord Blood	
			Y Stem Cells, Hematopoietic	

C: Indwelling Device

Operation–Character 3	Body System/Region – Character 4	Approach–Character 5	Substance–Character 6	Qualifier–Character 7
1 Irrigation	Z None	X External	8 Irrigating Substance	Z No Qualifier

Continued on next page

Administration 3Ø2–3E1 (Continued)

E: Physiological Systems and Anatomical Regions

Operation–Character 3	Body System/Region–Character 4	Approach–Character 5	Substance–Character 6	Qualifier–Character 7
Ø Introduction	Ø Skin and Mucous Membranes	Ø Open	Ø Antineoplastic	Ø Autologous OR Influenza Vaccine
1 Irrigation	1 Subcutaneous Tissue	3 Percutaneous	1 Thrombolytic	1 Nonautologous
	2 Muscle	4 Percutaneous Endoscopic	2 Anti-infective	2 High-dose Interleukin-2
	3 Peripheral Vein	7 Via Natural or Artificial Opening	3 Anti-inflammatory	3 Low-dose Interleukin-2
	4 Central Vein	8 Via Natural or Artificial Opening Endoscopic	4 Serum, Toxoid and Vaccine	4 Liquid Brachytherapy Radioisotope
	5 Peripheral Artery	X External	5 Adhesion Barrier	5 Other Antineoplastic
	6 Central Artery		6 Nutritional Substance	6 Recombinant Human-activated Protein C
	7 Coronary Artery		7 Electrolytic and Water Balance Substance	7 Other Thrombolytic
	8 Heart		8 Irrigating Substance	8 Oxazolidinones
	9 Nose		9 Dialysate	9 Other Anti-infective
	A Bone Marrow		A Stem Cells, Embryonic	A Anti-infective Envelope
	B Ear		B Anesthetic Agent	B Recombinant Bone Morphogenetic Protein
	C Eye		E Stem Cells, Somatic	C Other Substance
	D Mouth and Pharynx		F Intracirculatory Anesthetic	D Nitric Oxide
	E Products of Conception		G Other Therapeutic Substance	F Other Gas
	F Respiratory Tract		H Radioactive Substance	G Insulin
	G Upper GI		K Other Diagnostic Substance	H Human B-type Natriuretic Peptide
	H Lower GI		L Sperm	J Other Hormone
	J Biliary and Pancreatic Tract		M Pigment	K Immunostimulator
	K Genitourinary Tract		N Analgesics, Hypnotics, Sedatives	L Immunosuppressive
	L Pleural Cavity		P Platelet Inhibitor	M Monoclonal Antibody
	M Peritoneal Cavity		Q Fertilized Ovum	N Blood Brain Barrier Disruption
	N Male Reproductive		R Antiarrhythmic	P Clofarabine
	P Female Reproductive		S Gas	Q Glucarpidase
	Q Cranial Cavity and Brain		T Destructive Agent	X Diagnostic
	R Spinal Canal		U Pancreatic Islet Cells	Z No Qualifier
	S Epidural Space		V Hormone	
	T Peripheral Nerves and Plexi		W Immunotherapeutic	
	U Joints		X Vasopressor	
	V Bones			
	W Lymphatics			
	X Cranial Nerves			
	Y Pericardial Cavity			

Measurement and Monitoring 4A0–4B0

Character Meanings

This Character Meaning table is provided as a guide to assist the user in the identification of character members that may be found in this section of code tables. It **SHOULD NOT** be used to build a PCS code.

A: Physiological Systems

Operation–Character 3	Body System–Character 4	Approach–Character 5	Function/Device–Character 6	Qualifier–Character 7
0　Measurement	0　Central Nervous	0　Open	0　Acuity	0　Central
1　Monitoring	1　Peripheral Nervous	3　Percutaneous	1　Capacity	1　Peripheral
	2　Cardiac	4　Percutaneous Endoscopic	2　Conductivity	2　Portal
	3　Arterial	7　Via Natural or Artificial Opening	3　Contractility	3　Pulmonary
	4　Venous	8　Via Natural or Artificial Opening Endoscopic	4　Electrical Activity	4　Stress
	5　Circulatory	X　External	5　Flow	5　Ambulatory
	6　Lymphatic		6　Metabolism	6　Right Heart
	7　Visual		7　Mobility	7　Left Heart
	8　Olfactory		8　Motility	8　Bilateral
	9　Respiratory		9　Output	9　Sensory
	B　Gastrointestinal		B　Pressure	A　Guidance
	C　Biliary		C　Rate	B　Motor
	D　Urinary		D　Resistance	C　Coronary
	F　Musculoskeletal		F　Rhythm	D　Intracranial
	G　Skin and Breast		G　Secretion	F　Other Thoracic
	H　Products of Conception, Cardiac		H　Sound	G　Intraoperative
	J　Products of Conception, Nervous		J　Pulse	H　Indocyanine Green Dye
	Z　None		K　Temperature	Z　No Qualifier
			L　Volume	
			M　Total Activity	
			N　Sampling and Pressure	
			P　Action Currents	
			Q　Sleep	
			R　Saturation	
			S　Vascular Perfusion	

B: Physiological Devices

Operation–Character 3	Body System–Character 4	Approach–Character 5	Function/Device–Character 6	Qualifier–Character 7
0　Measurement	0　Central Nervous	X　External	S　Pacemaker	Z　No Qualifier
	1　Peripheral Nervous		T　Defibrillator	
	2　Cardiac		V　Stimulator	
	9　Respiratory			
	F　Musculoskeletal			

Extracorporeal or Systemic Assistance and Performance 5AØ–5A2

Character Meanings

This Character Meaning table is provided as a guide to assist the user in the identification of character members that may be found in this section of code tables. It **SHOULD NOT** be used to build a PCS code.

A: Physiological Systems

Operation–Character 3	Body System–Character 4	Duration–Character 5	Function–Character 6	Qualifier–Character 7
Ø Assistance	2 Cardiac	Ø Single	Ø Filtration	Ø Balloon Pump
1 Performance	5 Circulatory	1 Intermittent	1 Output	1 Hyperbaric
2 Restoration	9 Respiratory	2 Continuous	2 Oxygenation	2 Manual
	C Biliary	3 Less than 24 Consecutive Hours	3 Pacing	3 Membrane
	D Urinary	4 24-96 Consecutive Hours	4 Rhythm	4 Nonmechanical
		5 Greater than 96 Consecutive Hours	5 Ventilation	5 Pulsatile Compression
		6 Multiple		6 Other Pump
		7 Intermittent, Less than 6 Hours per Day		7 Continuous Positive Airway Pressure
		8 Prolonged Intermittent, 6-18 hours per Day		8 Intermittent Positive Airway Pressure
		9 Continuous, Greater than 18 hours per Day		9 Continuous Negative Airway Pressure
				B Intermittent Negative Airway Pressure
				C Supersaturated
				D Impeller Pump
				F Membrane, Central
				G Membrane, Peripheral Veno-arterial
				H Membrane, Peripheral Veno-venous
				Z No Qualifier

Extracorporeal or Systemic Therapies 6AØ–6AB

Character Meanings

This Character Meaning table is provided as a guide to assist the user in the identification of character members that may be found in this section of code tables. It **SHOULD NOT** be used to build a PCS code.

A: Physiological Systems

Operation–Character 3	Body System–Character 4	Duration–Character 5	Qualifier–Character 6	Qualifier–Character 7
Ø Atmospheric Control	Ø Skin	Ø Single	B Donor Organ	Ø Erythrocytes
1 Decompression	1 Urinary	1 Multiple	Z No Qualifier	1 Leukocytes
2 Electromagnetic Therapy	2 Central Nervous			2 Platelets
3 Hyperthermia	3 Musculoskeletal			3 Plasma
4 Hypothermia	5 Circulatory			4 Head and Neck Vessels
5 Pheresis	B Respiratory System			5 Heart
6 Phototherapy	F Hepatobiliary System and Pancreas			6 Peripheral Vessels
7 Ultrasound Therapy	T Urinary System			7 Other Vessels
8 Ultraviolet Light Therapy	Z None			T Stem Cells, Cord Blood
9 Shock Wave Therapy				V Stem Cells, Hematopoietic
B Perfusion				Z No Qualifier

Osteopathic 7WØ

Character Meanings

This Character Meaning table is provided as a guide to assist the user in the identification of character members that may be found in this section of code tables. It **SHOULD NOT** be used to build a PCS code.

W: Anatomical Regions

Operation–Character 3	Body Region–Character 4	Approach–Character 5	Method–Character 6	Qualifier–Character 7
Ø Treatment	Ø Head	X External	Ø Articulatory-Raising	Z None
	1 Cervical		1 Fascial Release	
	2 Thoracic		2 General Mobilization	
	3 Lumbar		3 High Velocity-Low Amplitude	
	4 Sacrum		4 Indirect	
	5 Pelvis		5 Low Velocity-High Amplitude	
	6 Lower Extremities		6 Lymphatic Pump	
	7 Upper Extremities		7 Muscle Energy-Isometric	
	8 Rib Cage		8 Muscle Energy-Isotonic	
	9 Abdomen		9 Other Method	

Other Procedures 8CØ–8EØ

Character Meanings

This Character Meaning table is provided as a guide to assist the user in the identification of character members that may be found in this section of code tables. It **SHOULD NOT** be used to build a PCS code.

C: Indwelling Devices

Operation–Character 3	Body Region–Character 4	Approach–Character 5	Method–Character 6	Qualifier–Character 7
Ø Other procedures	1 Nervous System	X External	6 Collection	J Cerebrospinal Fluid
	2 Circulatory System			K Blood
				L Other Fluid

E: Physiological Systems and Anatomical Regions

Operation–Character 3	Body Region–Character 4	Approach–Character 5	Method–Character 6	Qualifier–Character 7
Ø Other Procedures	1 Nervous System	Ø Open	Ø Acupuncture	Ø Anesthesia
	2 Circulatory System	3 Percutaneous	1 Therapeutic Massage	1 In Vitro Fertilization
	9 Head and Neck Region	4 Percutaneous Endoscopic	6 Collection	2 Breast Milk
	H Integumentary System and Breast	7 Via Natural or Artificial Opening	B Computer Assisted Procedure	3 Sperm
	K Musculoskeletal System	8 Via Natural or Artificial Opening Endoscopic	C Robotic Assisted Procedure	4 Yoga Therapy
	U Female Reproductive System	X External	D Near Infrared Spectroscopy	5 Meditation
	V Male Reproductive System		Y Other Method	6 Isolation
	W Trunk Region			7 Examination
	X Upper Extremity			8 Suture Removal
	Y Lower Extremity			9 Piercing
	Z None			C Prostate
				D Rectum
				F With Fluoroscopy
				G With Computerized Tomography
				H With Magnetic Resonance Imaging
				Z No Qualifier

Chiropractic 9WB

Character Meanings

This Character Meaning table is provided as a guide to assist the user in the identification of character members that may be found in this section of code tables. It **SHOULD NOT** be used to build a PCS code.

W: Anatomical Regions

Operation–Character 3	Body Region–Character 4	Approach–Character 5	Method–Character 6	Qualifier–Character 7
B Manipulation	Ø Head	X External	B Non-Manual	Z None
	1 Cervical		C Indirect Visceral	
	2 Thoracic		D Extra-Articular	
	3 Lumbar		F Direct Visceral	
	4 Sacrum		G Long Lever Specific Contact	
	5 Pelvis		H Short Lever Specific Contact	
	6 Lower Extremities		J Long and Short Lever Specific Contact	
	7 Upper Extremities		K Mechanically Assisted	
	8 Rib Cage		L Other Method	
	9 Abdomen			

Index